WILEY SERIES IN NEUROBIOLOGY

R. Glenn Northcutt, Editor

NEURAL CONTROL OF
RHYTHMIC MOVEMENTS
IN VERTEBRATES

NEURAL CONTROL OF RHYTHMIC MOVEMENTS IN VERTEBRATES

Edited by

Avis H. Cohen

Section of Neurobiology and Behavior
Cornell University
Ithaca, New York

Serge Rossignol

Department of Physiology
University of Montreal
Montreal, Quebec, Canada

Sten Grillner

Nobel Institute for Neurophysiology
Karolinska Institute
Stockholm, Sweden

WILEY

A Wiley-Interscience Publication
JOHN WILEY & SONS
New York · Chichester · Brisbane · Toronto · Singapore

Library of Congress Cataloging in Publication Data:

Neural control of rhythmic movements in vertebrates.

    (Wiley series in neurobiology)
    "A Wiley-Interscience publication"
    Includes index.
    1. Vertebrates—Locomotion. 2. Nervous system—
Vertebrates. 3. Animal mechanics. I. Cohen, Avis H.
II. Rossignol, Serge, 1942– . III. Grillner,
Sten, 1941– . IV. Title: Rhythmic movements in
vertebrates. V. Series.

QP310.R45N48 1988   596'.01852   87-21573
ISBN 0-471-81968-9

Printed in the United States of America

10 9 8 7 6 5 4 3 2 1

CONTRIBUTORS

Lennart Brodin
Nobel Institute for
   Neurophysiology
Karolinska Institute
Stockholm, Sweden

James T. Buchanan
Nobel Institute for
   Neurophysiology
Karolinska Institute
Stockholm, Sweden

Avis H. Cohen
Section of Neurobiology
   and Behavior
Cornell University
Ithaca, New York

Trevor Drew
Center for Research in the
   Neurological Sciences
University of Montreal
Montreal, Quebec, Canada

Howard H. Ellenberger
Department of Kinesiology
University of California,
   Los Angeles
Los Angeles, California

Sumio Enomoto
Center for Research in the
   Neurological Sciences

University of Montreal
Montreal, Quebec, Canada

Jack L. Feldman
Department of Kinesiology
University of California,
   Los Angeles
Los Angeles, California

Israel M. Gelfand
Moscow State University and
   Institute of Problems of
   Information Transmission
Academy of Sciences of the USSR
Moscow, Soviet Union

Peter A. Getting
Department of Physiology
   and Biophysics
University of Iowa
Iowa City, Iowa

Sten Grillner
Nobel Institute for
   Neurophysiology
Karolinska Institute
Stockholm, Sweden

Ronald M. Harris-Warrick
Section of Neurobiology
   and Behavior
Cornell University
Ithaca, New York

Philip J. Holmes
Department of Theoretical
   and Applied Mechanics
Cornell University
Ithaca, New York

Nancy Kopell
Department of Mathematics
Boston University
Boston, Massachusetts

James P. Lund
Center for Research in the
   Neurological Sciences
University of Montreal
Montreal, Quebec, Canada

Donald R. McCrimmon
Department of Physiology
Northwestern University
Chicago, Illinois

Brian Mulloney
Department of Zoology
University of California
Davis, California

Grisja N. Orlovsky
Moscow State University and
   Institute of Problems of
   Information Transmission
Academy of Sciences of the USSR
Moscow, Soviet Union

Aftab E. Patla
Department of Kinesiology
University of Waterloo
Waterloo, Ontario, Canada

Donald H. Perkel
Psychobiology Department

University of California
Irvine, California

Richard H. Rand
Department of Theoretical
   and Applied Mechanics
Cornell University
Ithaca, New York

Serge Rossignol
Center for Research in the
   Neurological Sciences
University of Montreal
Montreal, Quebec, Canada

Mark L. Shik
Moscow State University and
   Institute of Problems of
   Information Transmission
Academy of Sciences of the USSR
Moscow, Soviet Union

Jeffrey C. Smith
Department of Kinesiology
University of California,
   Los Angeles
Los Angeles, California

Dexter F. Speck
Department of Physiology
   and Biophysics
University of Kentucky
Lexington, Kentucky

Peter Wallén
Nobel Institute for
   Neurophysiology
Karlinska Institute
Stockholm, Sweden

SERIES PREFACE

Neuroscience is a rapidly expanding interdisciplinary field that is yielding significant insights into the organization and function of nervous systems. An outgrowth of several more traditional disciplines—Animal Behavior, Comparative Biology, Cybernetics, Neuroanatomy, Neurochemistry, Neurophysiology, and Physiological Psychology—Neuroscience arose because of many reasons, but central to the focus of Neuroscience is the growing realization that no single approach or discipline can fully explain how nervous systems are organized; how they come into being ontogenetically, as well as phylogenetically; how a specific nervous system works and what operational principles are applicable to most, if not all, nervous systems.

From subcellular organelles and processes to entire networks mediating behavior, the complexity and diversity exhibited by nervous systems is staggering. The goal of Neuroscience is to understand how these complex and diverse systems work as devices for information processing, control, and communication. Unlike artificial devices that are man-made and thus specifically designed to solve limited, well-defined sets of problems, nervous systems are the result of a historical process called evolution. Thus their analysis is further confounded by the fact that they have arisen opportunistically and without optimal design. Understanding how they have arisen, how they have adapted to solve problems that are virtually unlimited, is a challenge that can not be met by a single discipline. Although individual neuroscientists will continue to focus on specific questions related to a particular facet of neural organization or a single species, achievement of the goals of Neuroscience demands an eclectic approach that is rapidly becoming its hallmark.

The Wiley Series in Neurobiology reflects this eclecticism, and the Series will present work ranging from subcellular to behavioral topics, from specialized monographs to contributions spanning several disciplines. As a forum in which nervous systems are viewed and analyzed from widely different perspectives, it is hoped that these offerings will not only provide information to researchers in all disciplines of Neuroscience, but will also provide further stimulation for an eclectic approach to the evolution, organization, and function of nervous systems.

R. GLENN NORTHCUTT

Ann Arbor, Michigan

PREFACE

The neural origin of different motor acts has been the interest of neuroscientists since the last century. During the 1960s, rapid progress took place with the development of invertebrate "simple" preparations by Wilson, Wiersma, Kennedy, and others. In parallel, experimentally amenable vertebrate preparations permitting the study of ongoing behavior were developed by von Euler, Sears, Lund, Orlovsky, and Shik. As time has gone by, it has become clear that different rhythmic motor patterns are coordinated by an interaction between a detailed neuronal network, often referred to as a central pattern generator (CPG), residing within the central nervous system and peripheral signals arising as a consequence of the movements themselves. This organization appears rather general, although the specific solutions differ somewhat according to the species and the motor acts. Beginning in the 1960s with studies of the specific motor patterns and the description of the general organizational features underlying the motor acts, we have now also reached a level of knowledge in the vertebrate sphere such that we can ask meaningful questions about the cellular bases of behavior, which until recently have been exclusive to the invertebrate field.

The work of many of the authors of this volume has shaped the field. In their chapters they draw upon a range of organisms, movements, and perspectives. In the relatively simple nervous systems of invertebrates, considerable progress has been made in determining the functional constituents of CPGs. The chapters by Getting and Harris-Warrick relate the insights gained from the wealth of material obtained from the invertebrate studies. Getting outlines the structural elements of CPGs and their functional roles, while Harris-Warrick describes how neuromodulators function to regulate and restructure the circuits. Their chapters are intended to highlight some of the principles that are useful to better understand vertebrate systems treated in the subsequent chapters.

In hopes of moving the field forward, the authors highlight critical issues and speculate regarding the significance of what is known. For example, Gelfand, Orlovsky, and Shik compare the control of locomotion and scratch; Rossignol, Lund, and Drew compare sensory afferents and their control of locomotion, respiration, and mastication. Cohen compares locomotion across vertebrates in order to gain insights into the organization and evolution of the locomotor pattern generator. Grillner, Buchanan, Wallén, and Brodin compare undulatory movements of several species with a more in-depth treatment of the lamprey pattern generator for swimming. Feldman, McCrimmon, Smith, and Speck examine what is known or suspected regarding the mechanisms underlying generation of respiration and the same is done by Lund and Enomoto for mastication.

The final four chapters offer a unique view of theoretical and modeling techniques that will be of use in a range of fields. In the chapter by Kopell as well as the one by Rand, Cohen, and Holmes, the organization of CPGs has been likened to that of chains of mutually coupled nonlinear oscillators. However, such structures do not lend themselves easily to manipulation or intuition. With this in mind the chapters present coupled oscillator theory in a form largely accessible to the mathematically untrained reader. The work is relatively new and represents an attempt to use techniques and concepts developed by mathematicians in an area of motor control particularly suited for such cross-fertilization. The chapter by Mulloney and Perkel reviews and evaluates the role of synthetic models, which have been the more traditional method for conceptualizing the structure of neural circuits. Such models have been in general use for some time, especially in the literature dealing with invertebrate CPGs. Finally, Patla presents an analytic approach to the study of motor output to help extract some basic features out of seemingly more complex data.

The book is largely intended for neuroscientists, but not necessarily those studying motor control. Our hope is that many of the questions raised in the various chapters will soon be answered and give rise to a new generation of insights and directions.

Avis H. Cohen
Serge Rossignol
Sten Grillner

CONTENTS

Chapter One

NEURAL CONTROL OF LOCOMOTION IN LOWER VERTEBRATES

From Behavior to Ionic Mechanisms

STEN GRILLNER
JAMES T. BUCHANAN
PETER WALLÉN
LENNART BRODIN

Nobel Institute for Neurophysiology
Karolinska Institute
Stockholm, Sweden

When a fish swims, its nervous system activates muscle fibers which in turn produce active movements that interact with the surrounding water. In this chapter we will focus on how the nervous system generates the undulatory movements which are transmitted from head to tail and which provide the propulsive thrust. We will proceed from a description of the actual movement and muscle activity to the underlying nervous mechanisms.

1

1   MOVEMENT AND MUSCLE ACTIVITY

1.1   Lateral Body Undulations

The amphioxus and cyclostomes lack paired fins and locomote by means of an undulatory wave of increasing amplitude which is transmitted along the body from head to tail. In principle, a similar type of propagation occurs in most fish (Figure 1), such as the eel and the cod, and also in amphibian larvae (Kahn et al., 1982). Fish with paired fins use these for postural stability and steering control but also to maneuver and propel the body at a slow speed, but for ordinary steady or rapid swimming most species depend on body propulsion (cf Gray, 1933a,b, 1968).

Fish, such as the the lamprey, eel, and trout, have been investigated during swimming in a swimmill and their bodily movements have been filmed while simultaneously recording muscle activity with intramuscular electrodes in several segments along the body. In general, a laterally directed wave travels with an increasing amplitude from rostral to caudal. As the wave travels caudally, it pushes the body forward through the water. If the speed of the wave is 1.0 m per second, the fish usually moves forward through the water at a speed of 0.7–0.8 m per second (cf Lighthill, 1969). This relation applies to most velocities except the lowermost at which the amplitude of the wave decreases (Grillner and Kashin, 1976; cf Bainbridge, 1958, 1961; Williams, 1986). The wave is created by rhythmic alternating contractions occurring in all segments at the same frequency. However, each caudal segment is delayed somewhat in relation to its rostral neighbor (Figure 2). Between adjacent segments the delay is a fixed proportion of the cycle duration (usually 1%), and over the entire body the lag will consequently be between 50–100% of the cycle duration depending on the number of segments. This constant phase lag will create the travelling wave. The phase lag between the rostral and the caudal part will remain almost identical regardless of the speed of swimming. The rate of

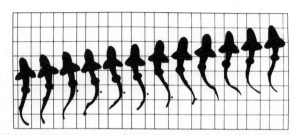

FIGURE 1. Silhouettes of a swimming dogfish, drawn from photographs taken at 100 ms intervals, illustrate the rostral-to-caudal propagation of the lateral body bends. The dots indicate the peak of one bend as it propagates caudally during forward swimming. (From Gray, 1968.)

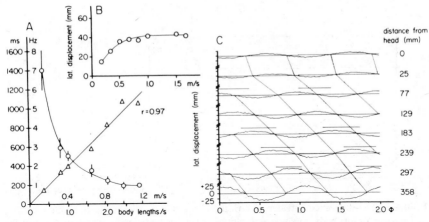

FIGURE 2. Phase lags and lateral displacement during swimming. (A) This graph illustrates the relation between forward velocity of a swimming eel versus cycle duration (circles) and, inversely, cycle frequency (triangles). Cycle frequency increases with increasing swim velocity. (B) The relation between swim velocity and lateral displacement of the tail fin of a trout (280 mm long). (C) The lateral displacement of the body of a swimming eel at eight different body levels (distance from head indicated at right). The plot shows that lateral displacement of the body wave increases as it propagates caudally. The caudal propagation of the wave is emphasized by the dotted lines connecting the zero displacement points. The periods of EMG activity are indicated below levels 2, 4, 5, and 6. (From Grillner and Kashin, 1976.)

alternation varies from very low values as 0.2 Hz to values as high as 25 Hz when a trout makes a run (Grillner and Kashin, 1976). The rate of alternation is proportional to the speed of swimming (Figure 2) except for the lowermost velocities (Bainbridge, 1961).

The mechanical wave travelling down the body clearly results from the wave of muscle contractions, but it is modified by the interaction with the surrounding water through the resistance to the lateral movements and the fact that the longitudinal wave pushes the animal forward. In fact the mechanical wave often has a different and somewhat longer phase lag than the electromyographical wave (Figure 3; Grillner, Rossignol and Wallén in Grillner and Kashin, 1976).

The muscle fibers have a longitudinal orientation and extend from the myoseptum of the rostral border of the segment to the caudal myoseptum. The myotome of each segment has a complex conical shape divided into an upper epaxial and lower hypaxial part in relation to the vertebrae, which most readers will have noticed when eating cooked fish. The muscle fibers in adjacent parts of two myotomes have approximately the same orientation, if the muscle fibers are followed from one vertebra, and then from one myotome to another, they form an arc extending over approximately 15 segments between "insertions" in the vertebral column. This is presumably a biomechanical advantage (cf Grillner and Kashin, 1976).

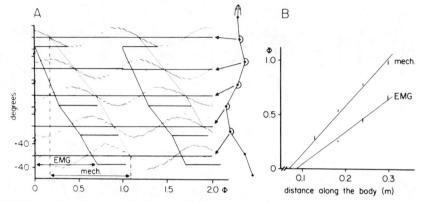

FIGURE 3. The difference between electrical and mechanical phase lags during swimming. (A) This graph plots body angle of a swimming eel at five body levels during two cycles. The periods of EMG activity are indicated by the bars below each line and their onsets are connected by solid lines. The onsets of the corresponding bending phases are connected by dotted lines. As indicated at the bottom of the graph, the mechanical lag is greater than the EMG lag. (B) This graph plots the mechanical and EMG phase lags at five different body levels (mean ± S.E., n = 10). (From Grillner and Kashin, 1976.)

Most fish have a lateral portion of red muscle fibers, like mackerels and herrings, which are slowly contracting and lack propagated action potentials (cf Bone, 1975). The larger part of the myotome is composed of white and intermediate muscle fibers which contract relatively fast and have propagated action potentials. During slow swimming mainly the red lateral portion is active, but as the speed of swimming increases the powerful white fibers are recruited (Figure 4; Hudson, 1973; Grillner, 1974; Grillner and Kashin, 1976). The duration of the locomotor burst in any given segment varies with the speed of swimming, but it remains a constant proportion of the cycle duration (20–40%; Grillner, 1974; Wallén & Williams, 1984). The myotomes of the primitive cyclostomes are also composed of longitudinal muscle fibers extending between the myosepta but they are arranged in a somewhat different way from that of teleosts and elasmobranchs. Modules with an inner part of longitudinal white muscle fibers and a surrounding outer part of red fibers extend from the notochord to the skin. Each myotome is composed of a number of such modules packed from dorsal to ventral. Separate motoneurons supply slow and fast muscle fibers (Rovainen, 1979). The amphioxus has yet another type of myotome with segmental flattened muscle fibers like lamellae (Flood, 1968). The muscle fiber membrane tapers into a fine axon-like process which projects to the spinal cord. The arrangement is unusual in that the motoneurons synapse on these muscle fiber processes at the surface of the spinal cord, corresponding to the ventral root exit.

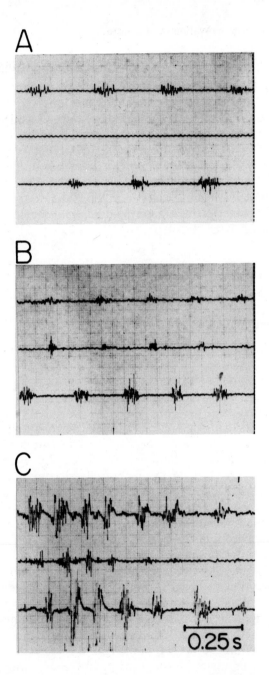

FIGURE 4. EMG activity of red and white muscles of a trout during forward swimming at three different velocities: (A) = 0.4, (B) = 1.0, (C) = 1.3 m/s. Bipolar copper wire electrodes, insulated except for the tip, were inserted into the red lateral muscles (top records) in the middle of the white epaxial muscles at the same level (middle records), and in the red muscles of the contralateral side (bottom records). There was no activity in the white muscles at the slowest speed, but activity appeared in B at a swim frequency of about 4 Hz. (From Grillner and Kashin, 1976.)

1.2   Propulsion by Rostrocaudal Waves Propagated Along Fins

Some fish, like the sea horse, transmit rapid waves along their extended dorsal fins, but no detailed physiologic studies of their locomotion have been performed. The ray and the skate have very extended pectoral fins along which a caudally directed wave is propagated through alternating contractions of the dorsal and the ventral parts of the fin muscles. During forward swimming the two fins act in synergy, but under certain conditions, as during turning, the fins may be uncoupled. The amplitude of the caudally transmitted wave increases from the rostral to the middle portion and there is a constant phase lag between adjacent myotomes (Droge and Leonard, 1983a; Leonard, 1986).

2   NEURAL CONTROL OF LOCOMOTION: SUPRASPINAL MECHANISMS

2.1   Locomotor Areas in the Brainstem

To survive, an animal must be able to move in a fashion which is well adapted to the demands of the environment. It is well known that mammals can perform well-adapted movements even after a decortication (cf Grillner, 1985). For example, decorticate mammals can locomote in search of food and can eat or drink. This type of well-adapted behavior seems to depend on the basal ganglia and the ventral pallidum and their projections to the mesencephalon near the cuneiform nucleus and/or the adjacent pedunculopontine nucleus (Garcia-Rill, 1986; Garcia-Rill and Skinner, 1986). Stimulation in this area can elicit well-controlled locomotion (Shik and Orlovsky, 1976; Gelfand et al., Chapt. 6). A transection through the caudal diencephalon leaves us with a preparation which can be made to walk by brainstem stimulation, but the movements are now stereotyped and not adapted to the environment. Without brainstem stimulation such a preparation essentially displays decerebrate rigidity.

In fish very little is known about the role of the basal ganglia in the control of locomotion except that mesencephalic fish have been reported to display inactivity similar to decerebrate rigidity (cf Grillner, 1981) but well-coordinated swimming can be elicited by sensory stimuli in a variety of species. Stimulation in the mesencephalon was first reported to elicit locomotion by Kashin et al. (1974) in the teleost carp.

In the lamprey brainstem-spinal cord in vitro preparation, tonic stimulation (e.g., 20 Hz) of a circumscribed area located in parallel with the midline throughout the rhombencephalon and part of the mesencephalon (Figure 5) can elicit the swimming motor pattern (McClellan and Grillner, 1984). A similar rhombencephalic area within the reticular formation can elicit steady, well-coordinated swimming in the dogfish. If the animal is rendered motionless by curare, the same type of motor pattern can be re-

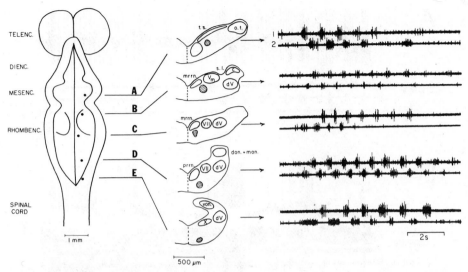

FIGURE 5. Lamprey brain stem regions from which swimming activity could be elicited with extracellular electrical stimulation. Systematic stimulation (1 ms pulses at 20 Hz) of the brain stem revealed a low-threshold (1.5–3.0 μA), circumscribed region extending from the mesencephalon to the caudal rhombencephalon which could induce fictive swimming. The effective sites were marked by current lesioning and are indicated by the dots in the whole brain drawing and by the shaded region of the transverse sections. Abbreviations: c, cerebellum; don., dorsal octavolateralis nucleus; dV, descending sensory tract of V; mon., medial octavolateralis nucleus; mrrn., mesencephalic rhombencephalon reticular nucleus; o.t., optic tectum; prrn., posterior rhombencephalon reticular nucleus; s.l., sulcus limitans; t.s., torus semicircularis; von., ventral octavolateralis nucleus; Vm, motor nucleus of V; VII, sensory nucleus of VII; X, vagus motor nucleus. (From McClellan and Grillner, 1984.)

corded in the ventral roots (Grillner and Wallén, 1984), which shows that movement-related feedback is not required to elicit the basic pattern of coordination. However, a stimulation in the mesencephalon in the dogfish gave rise to a combination of locomotion along with steering control "commands." For instance, a stimulation in the left mesencephalon gave rise to a turning response to the left as indicated by a bending of the body towards that side combined with appropriate adjustments of the pectoral and pelvic fins. Stimulation in the midline in mesencephalon gave rise to swimming movements in the upward (dorsal stimulation) or the downward (ventral stimulation) direction. It appeared that these steering control signals were superimposed or added to the propulsive locomotor synergy.

2.2   Activity of Brainstem Neurons During Fictive Locomotion

Reticulospinal neurones from the mesencephalic, superior, middle, and posterior reticular nucleus of the rhombencephalon (cf Nieuwenhuys,

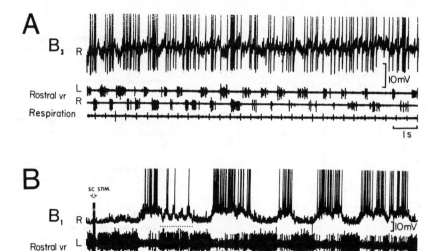

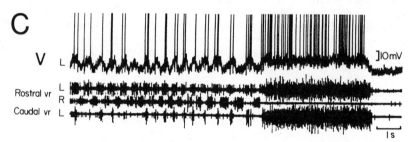

FIGURE 6. The activity of reticulospinal neurons (bulbar Müller cells and V-cells) during fictive swimming and other motor activity. (A) The cell B_3 shows a depolarization and modulation of firing frequency in phase with the ipsilateral rostral (gill region) ventral root (vr) activity (L, left; R, right). The respiratory activity was recorded in the 10th cranial nerve. (B) A short train of stimuli applied to the cut caudal end of the spinal cord (SC stim.) could induce a long lasting period of activity both in the B_1 cell and the rostral and caudal (between segments 10–20) ventral roots. The cell depolarized and spiked in phase with the ipsilateral ventral root activity, and slightly hyperpolarized during contralateral ventral root activity. (C) During fictive swimming and during tonic activity in the ipsilateral ventral roots, this V-cell had a pattern of activity similar to that of B cells. Note time and voltage calibration (intracellular trace) in each set of recordings. (From Kasicki and Grillner, 1986.)

1972; Rovainen, 1979) are phasically modulated during fictive locomotion in the lamprey brainstem-spinal cord preparation (Kasicki and Grillner, 1986). The activity is in phase with the efferent motor activity on the ipsilateral side of the rostral spinal cord (Figure 6). These neurons include the large mesencephalic, isthmic, and bulbar reticulospinal Müller cells and the caudally located V-cells. The large Mauthner cells with their crossed axons are modulated in phase with the contralateral ventral root activity. When the fictive locomotor activity is powerful, the reticulospinal neurons are often spiking, whereas at low level locomotor activity the phasic oscillations are usually subthreshold. Many of these reticulospinal neurons monosynaptically excite both motoneurons and excitatory and inhibitory premotor interneurons in the spinal cord (Rovainen, 1974b; Buchanan, 1982; Buchanan and Grillner, 1987 and unpubl.). Consequently, their activity will affect the excitability of the spinal cord during locomotion.

In mammals, the locomotor related oscillations in bulbospinal neurons disappear or decrease markedly after removal of the cerebellum. The lamprey has a very small cerebellum (Heier, 1948). If it is removed, the reticulospinal oscillations continue unchanged.

2.3 Modulation of Fictive Swimming by Single Reticulospinal Neurons

The large reticulospinal Müller cells are known to have powerful monosynaptic connections to ipsilateral motoneurons and to inhibitory and excitatory premotor interneurons in the spinal cord (Rovainen, 1974b; Buchanan, 1982; Buchanan and Grillner, 1987). Stimulation of some of the Müller cells (M_3, B_1, B_2) in the lamprey brainstem-spinal cord preparation can modify the rate of ongoing fictive swimming induced by the application of excitatory amino acids (Buchanan and Cohen, 1982). Sometimes it can also initiate swimlike movements (Rovainen, 1983). To what extent the bulbar Müller cells take part in the normal initiation and maintenance of continuous locomotion is unknown. It would seem likely that other reticulospinal neurons are important for providing a continuous drive signal. The fast-conducting large Müller cells may be particularly important in the context of steering control and perhaps in the control of the rapid modifications of the rate of swimming (Grillner, 1981; Buchanan and Cohen 1982; Grillner and Wallén, 1984) necessary in escape or attack.

3 NEURAL CONTROL OF LOCOMOTION: SPINAL MECHANISMS

3.1 Locomotion after a Spinal Transection

What happens to the locomotor movements if the spinal cord is transected? In a few species such as the teleost eel and the elasmobranch dogfish, the part of the body caudal to the transection exhibits slow, spontaneous, well-coordinated movements which will move the animal forward (Steiner, 1886; Bethe, 1899; Gray and Sand, 1936; Grillner, 1974). These movements and the pattern of muscle activity resemble those of the intact fish (Figure 7). If sensory stimuli (e.g., to the tailfin mechanoreceptors) are applied, the cycle duration shortens markedly with a maintained

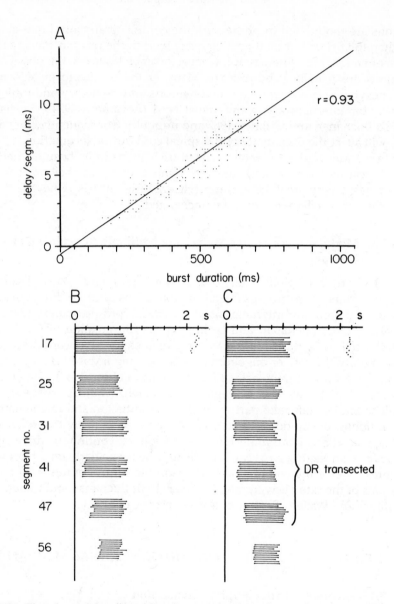

FIGURE 7. Phase lag and the effect of dorsal root transection in the swimming spinal dogfish. (A) The graph shows the time lag of EMG onsets between two electrodes in the red lateral muscle separated by 25 segments (normalized to delay/segment) versus burst duration (equivalent to period length). (B) Periods of EMG activity in a swimming spinal dogfish are shown for 10 cycles at 6 different body levels (segment number indicated at left). (C) The dorsal roots of segments 30 to 50 were bilaterally transected. (From Grillner and Kashin, 1976.)

intersegmental coordination and the speed of swimming increases (Grillner, 1974).

Most species do not display swimming activity after a spinal transection, but when the tailfin is touched or subjected to moderate pressure most species display a short bout of locomotor activity consisting of a few cycles or sometimes a longer period of activity. This applies to tadpoles, various teleost fish, and cyclostomes. In the spinal lamprey, which is not spontaneously active, continuous swimming is induced if it is placed in a water current as in a "swimmill" (Wallén and Williams, 1984). This activity is well-coordinated, showing burst activity and phase lags similar to that of the intact lamprey. How other species react in a water current after a spinal transection has not been studied, but it is conceivable that some of the other nonactive species would also swim continuously.

In most experimental situations, spinal swimming preparations have been held fixed in relation to the experimental chamber (cf Grillner, 1974; Poon, 1980; Ayers et al., 1983). The hydrodynamic situation is then very different from that of ordinary swimming. The fixed animal will produce an undulatory wave which will exert a caudal pressure on the water as the wave propagates backwards. In the normal case, this pressure will move the animal forwards with a speed being around 70–80% of the backward velocity of the wave (cf Lighthill, 1969). Thus the resistance to the caudal propagation of the wave is much greater when the animal is fixed and the forward velocity is zero. On the other hand, the resistance to the lateral undulation is greater in running water (swimmill) than in stationary water (fixed preparation). These hydrodynamic factors are obviously of paramount importance. Everything else being equal, the locomotor movement produced under the two conditions must be different. Under stationary conditions, the lateral undulations must become larger, and the resistance for the rostro-caudal wave will be greater. Unfortunately, this distinction was overlooked by Ayers et al. (1983), who compared the movements of intact swimming lamprey with those of fixed spinal preparations without realizing the fundamental difference between the two situations.

Some spinal animals can be induced to perform actual swimming movements by pharmacologic means. The spinal lamprey in which the entire spinal cord has been exposed generates undulatory movements when an excitatory amino acid is administered to the bath (Poon, 1980). The spinal stingray (see above) performs dorsal to ventral swimming movements propagated along its enlarged pectoral fins when L-dopa is applied in a similar way (Williams et al., 1981). In the latter case the duration of the bursts in each cycle is somewhat prolonged. In the tadpole, excitatory amino acids can also elicit swimming movements (Dale and Roberts, 1984, 1985).

Thus, in a number of species locomotor movements can be elicited by the spinal cord after a complete transection of the connections to the brainstem. Accordingly, the spinal cord contains a neural network of sufficient complexity to generate an undulatory wave transmitted along the body. In some species the excitability level of these circuits is high and they generate spontaneous swimming, whereas in others they need additional excitation from the brainstem, sensory fibers, or by pharmacologic agents to come into operation.

3.2   Evidence for a Central Pattern Generator

Research conducted in the last decade has shown that the isolated spinal cord, deprived of all movement-related sensory information, can produce a motor pattern. This pattern clearly resembles that of locomotion with alternating burst activity in each segment and an intersegmental coordination with a constant phase lag (Grillner et al., 1976; Cohen and Wallén, 1980). Such a demonstration constitutes proof that the spinal cord contains a central pattern generator (CPG) for locomotion. The lamprey spinal cord *in vitro* can produce a motor pattern with a similar phase lag, burst, and cycle duration as the spinal and intact lamprey swimming in a swimmill (Figure 8; Wallén and Williams, 1984). In principle, the same results have been obtained in the spinal dogfish (Grillner et al., 1976), the decerebrate stingray (Droge and Leonard, 1983b; Leonard, 1986) and the frog embryo (Roberts et al., 1981, 1986). In the latter cases, the movements were suppressed by curarizing the spinal animals. By contrast, the *Bufo* tadpole is reported to change the intersegmental coordination upon immobilization so that all segments become active in a synchronized fashion (Stehouwer and Farel, 1980). The motor patterns recorded under these deprived conditions tend to exhibit a lower rate than normal and the motor pattern may vary more. However, despite these limitations it should be noted that the range of activity can overlap entirely with that of intact animals (cf Brodin et al., 1985).

For a long period of time, Gray (1950) and his colleagues (Gray and Sand, 1936; Lissman, 1946a,b; Roberts, 1969) claimed that locomotor movements depended entirely on sensory signals, whereas von Holst (1935, 1954) advocated the opposite view, namely, that central mechanisms were all that mattered. These claims were largely based on experiments in which a dorsal root transection had been performed. The observations were usually made by visual inspection rather than actual recordings. Even if they were not generally accepted, von Holst's findings were correct. In retrospect, it can be said that his reasoning was based on partially inconclusive experiments. The recent demonstration of intraspinal mechanoreceptors in lamprey (Grillner et al., 1981a, 1982a, 1984) invalidates all conclusions drawn from deafferentation experiments in which animals have executed movements of the spine—and thus the spinal cord—even if all dorsal roots have been transected.

The isolated spinal cord can produce a coordinated pattern if left intact in its entirety. Moreover, the pattern-generating capacity is distributed

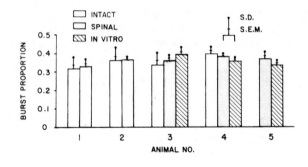

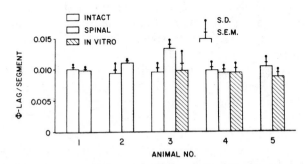

FIGURE 8. Comparison of locomotor burst duration and intersegmental phase lag between the intact lamprey and the spinal and in vitro preparations. The electromyographic activity of intact lampreys was recorded in different segments along the body while swimming freely (five preparations). The motor burst in each swim cycle constitutes a constant proportion of the cycle and the lag between the onset of the motor burst in adjacent segments constitutes a constant fraction (around 1 percent) of the swim cycle duration (that is phase lag/segment) regardless of the actual cycle duration. The spinal cords of the same animals were subsequently transected and their swimming activity was recorded from the same electrodes. Later, the spinal cords of the same animals were dissected free, fictive swimming was induced by an activation of NMDA receptors, and the efferent activity was recorded from different ventral roots by suction electrodes. In these five animals, the burst duration and phase lag remained very similar in the three different types of preparation. The swim frequency for the in vitro preparation ranged between 0.05 and 7 Hz and that for the intact animal from 0.5 to more than 7 Hz. (Modified from Wallén and Williams 1984.)

along the cord so that if the cord is transected into several pieces, each piece can be made to generate coordinated activity, even when only a few segments are left intact (Grillner, 1974; Cohen and Wallén, 1980; Grillner et al., 1982b). The excitability along the spinal cord appears to vary monotonically along the cord, but the degree and the sign of the gradient varies unsystematically across spinal cord pieces (Cohen, 1986).

A spinal cord divided longitudinally has the potential to produce coordinated burst activity in the tadpole (Roberts et al., 1986). In the lamprey the results are less clearcut. After isolation, the right and left spinal cord halves display tonic activity. However, if low doses of strychnine are added, reproducible rapid locomotorlike bursts occur (Grillner et al., 1986), that are similar to the bilaterally synchronous bursts observed by Cohen and Harris-Warrick (1984). The unilateral burst patterns observed in dogfish, ray, and lamprey have also been interpreted to suggest that there are bilateral pattern generators (Leonard, 1986; Grillner and Wallén, 1982; Grillner et al., 1986).

3.3 Action of Movement-Related Sensory Feedback on the Locomotor Pattern Generator

Although the interneuronal network can operate without sensory information, movement-related sensory information is of crucial importance. In both lamprey and dogfish, the central spinal network (CPG) generating locomotion is strongly affected by sensory signals (Grillner and Wallén, 1977; 1982, Grillner et al., 1981a, Buchanan and Cohen, 1982). Figure 9 shows a curarized dogfish preparation in which fictive locomotor activity is recorded in the ventral roots. If the caudal part of the body is moved back and forth, simulating the actual swimming movements, the motor bursts are entrained from the first movement cycle. The movements may be faster or slower than the resting fictive swimming rate, albeit within a certain range of frequencies. The phase relations between the applied movement and the efferent motor bursts resemble those which occur during active swimming.

This experimental situation is favorable for investigating the sensory effects on the CPG, but under normal conditions the situation is reversed so that the ventral root activity will induce the movements instead. One significance of this sensory control system lies in the possibility to adapt the swimming movement to external perturbations, such as those that will occur when a fish swims in water currents or turbulence. In addition, it is likely that these sensory mechanisms are important to produce the ordinary locomotor synergy during conditions when the movement pattern changes rapidly as during turning or when the speed of swimming increases. In the latter case, the velocity of the caudally directed travelling wave increases markedly during the phase of acceleration, which in turn changes the conditions with regard to the resistance to movements in the lateral direction. Another extreme example is provided by the situation in which a fish swims through water and then attempts to burrow by swimming into the soft sand of a sandbank. The resistance of the forward movement suddenly becomes much greater but the lateral resistance becomes smaller. The changes seen in the movement pattern from locomotion to burrowing will be produced by the new hydromechanical situation (see also Section 3.1) as well as modification of the efferent motor pattern which result from the changed sensory input (Grillner and Wallén, 1984).

The neural mechanism utilized by sensory neurons to control the CPG is not established, but all data are compatible with a scheme as presented

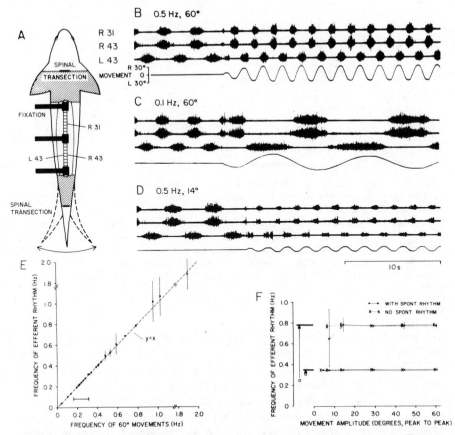

FIGURE 9. Entrainment of fictive swimming by imposed sinusoidal tail movements in a spinal dogfish. (A) Schematic drawing of the preparation indicating the three rigid fixation points on the vertebral column and the three ventral root recordings (L, left; R, right). The animal was paralyzed with curare. (B–D) Ventral root recordings showing spontaneous swimming activity which could be entrained by imposed tail movements (bottom traces). (E) The close correlation between frequency of the imposed movement and the entrained rhythm for a broad range of movement rates (fixed movement amplitude of 60° peak-to-peak). The horizontal bar indicates the frequency range of the spontaneous rhythm. Data points are means ± S.D., n = 10 (F) The effect of movement amplitude on entrainment. Two imposed frequencies (horizontal bars), 0.35 or 0.78 Hz, were given at various amplitudes when spontaneous swimming was present (dots) or not present (crosses). Data points are means ± S.D., n = 10. Mean burst frequency of the spontaneous rhythms (n = 10; S.D. = 0.01 Hz) in each of the two movement sessions is indicated by the open circles. Vertical arrows indicate the discrepancy between the spontaneous rhythm and the imposed movement. (From Grillner and Wallén, 1982.)

15

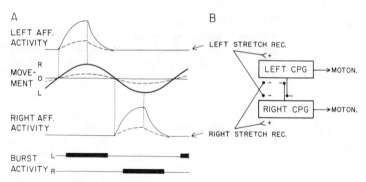

FIGURE 10. Proposed scheme to explain the entrainment of the central pattern generators (CPG) by imposed movements. (A) Schematically, the afferent (aff.) activity will start approximately when the movement passes the zero transition point and will reach a maximum at the extreme position (dotted lines). A lower movement amplitude will cause a reduced afferent discharge (dashed curves). The approximate timings of the entrained bursts are indicated below (L, left; R, right). (B) Proposed scheme of the central effects of the afferent signals. Stretch receptors activated when the left side is stretched are assumed to excite (+) the CPG in the left hemisegment and inhibit (−) the right CPG and vice versa (Grillner and Wallén, 1982).

in Figure 10. In principle, the afferent activity on one side would enhance the ipsilateral CPG activity and suppress the activity on the contralateral side. The lamprey spinal cord is supplied with intraspinal mechanoreceptors (Figure 11) which are used to sense the lateral undulation of the body and have an input to the spinal CPG (Grillner et al., 1981a, 1982a, 1984). However, peripheral receptors may also contribute (Buchanan and Cohen, 1982). Whether intraspinal receptors are of importance in fish is not yet established, but the results from dogfish support this possibility (Grillner and Wallén, 1982) and snakes appear to have similar types of intraspinal receptors (Schroeder and Richardson, 1985).

The movement-related feedback discussed here has a potent effect on the spinal network responsible for coordinating the locomotor movements. Generality of the mechanism underlying the control system is suggested by the striking similarities with the system controlling walking in mammals (Grillner, 1981, 1985).

3.4   Phase-Dependent Modulation of Sensory Signals

Sensory stimuli applied to the tailfin can elicit swimming or enhance already ongoing swimming. Short-lasting mechanical stimuli applied to the tailfin will enhance the ongoing phase of locomotion. Thus, for instance, if a stimulus occurs during myotomal activity on the left side, the movement to the left will become enhanced and vice versa (Figure 12). This gating of reflex effects is a direct or indirect consequence of the CPG activity (Grillner et al., 1977; Wallén, 1980). A response pattern of this type is behaviorally meaningful. It is important that a fish be able to adapt the response pattern to be appropriate to the ongoing phase of locomotion. In the case described here, mechanical stimuli will affect the tailfin during swimming so that the animal can respond to problems such as a piece of seaweed or, more seriously, a predator nibbling on the tailfin. Again, these effects in fish resemble the phase-dependent gating observed during walking in mammals (Forssberg et al., 1977).

4 SPINAL CIRCUITRY GENERATING LOCOMOTION

Most information regarding the neuronal circuitry of the CPG is from the adult lamprey CNS. We will, therefore, focus our description on this spe-

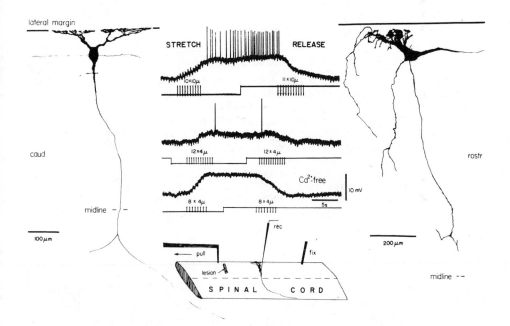

FIGURE 11. The edge cell as an intraspinal stretch receptor in the lamprey. Depolarizing responses to longitudinal stretch of the lateral margin of the spinal cord. The upper two sets of recordings are from the edge cell to the right (reconstruction after Lucifer yellow injection); the lower set is from the edge cell to the left. The upper traces show the intracellularly recorded depolarizations of the edge cells' membrane potentials induced by stretch of the cord. Stretches were applied and released in several 10 or 4 μm steps as indicated by the vertical lines. Note that the depolarization to stretch still occurred in Ca^{2+}-free solution (bottom set of traces), indicating that it is not mediated by chemical synaptic transmission. Lowermost drawing: The experimental arrangement for applying longitudinal stretches to the resting in situ length. The axon of cell A crossed the midline and had a descending branch, cell B had an ipsilaterally ascending axon. (Modified from Grillner, Williams, and Lagerbäck, 1984.)

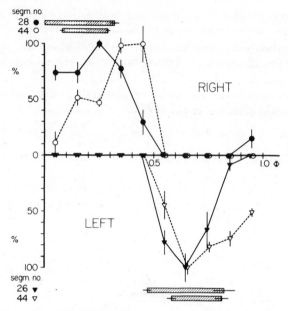

FIGURE 12. Phase dependence of EMG response amplitude to electrical stimulation of the tail fin during swimming in a spinal dogfish. Stimuli were given at different points in the swim cycle by varying the delay triggered from an EMG burst. The cycle is normalized with respect to the onset of EMG activity in the right segment no. 28. Response amplitude was measured from rectified and filtered EMG records and expressed as a percent of the maximum response (means ± S.E.). Circles indicate responses on the right side (R28, filled; R44, open), and triangles indicate the responses on the left side (L26, filled; L44, open). The horizontal bars indicate the mean duration (± S.D.) of EMG activity calculated from the normal swim cycle preceding each response cycle. Right side responses (upwards) occurred up to phase 0.5, when the pattern reversed to the left side (downwards). Note that large amplitude responses were not restricted to periods of EMG activity. (From Grillner, Rossignol, and Wallén, 1977.)

cies, although some pertinent information is available from other species. A particularly important preparation is the frog embryo (near hatching), which was developed by Alan Roberts and his associates. However, in the frog embryo the control system for locomotion is not yet fully developed (Roberts et al., 1981, 1986).

In the lamprey, activity in the spinal pattern generators for locomotion is initiated from the brainstem by long descending reticulospinal neurons (McClellan and Grillner, 1984; McClellan, 1984, 1986). The ability to produce rhythmic locomotor activity in one segment coordinated with the activity in adjacent segments is distributed throughout the spinal cord (see above).

4.1 Spinal Motoneurons Are Output Elements but Are Not Part of the Pattern-Generating Network

Vertebrate motoneurons are, in general, thought to serve only as output elements, and the following experiment in the lamprey has established that this is the case. All motoneurons of one segment were activated during fictive locomotion by continuous repetitive antidromic stimulation of the ventral roots (e.g., 20 Hz). If motoneurons were part of the pattern-generating circuitry, the resulting abnormal activity in one segment should have affected the pattern recorded in the adjacent rostral and caudal ventral roots (Wallén and Lansner, 1984). However, no effects were observed. We can, therefore, conclude that interneurons distributed throughout the spinal cord must be able to produce the output pattern and that motoneurons serve solely or primarily as output elements.

4.2 Pattern of Activity in Premotor Interneurons and Motoneurons During Fictive Locomotion

In each swimcycle, motoneurons supplying both slow and fast muscle fibers receive phasic excitation followed by phasic inhibition (Fig. 13;

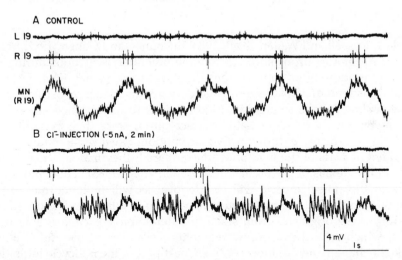

FIGURE 13. Chloride-dependent inhibition of lamprey motoneurons during fictive swimming. (A) Oscillations of membrane potential of a motoneuron (MN) and the ventral root activity from the right (R) and left (L) sides of segment 19 in a preparation of 38 segments during fictive swimming (induced with 0.3 mM D-glutamate). (B) Reversal of the repolarizing phase by intracellular injection of chloride ions from a 3M potassium chloride microelectrode using −5 nA of hyperpolarizing current for 2 minutes. The reversal reveals two phases: an excitatory phase coincident with the ipsilateral ventral root discharges and an inhibitory phase coincident with the contralateral ventral root discharges. (From Russell and Wallén, 1983.)

TABLE 1. Interaction Between some Spinal Premotor Interneurons and
Motoneurons[a]

Presynaptic	Postsynaptic				
		Inh.			Putative
	MN	CCin	LIN	EIN	Transmitters
EIN (ipsi)	+	+	+		EAA
Inh. CCIN (contra)	−	−	−		Glycine
LIN (ipsi)	(−)	−			
5-HT IN (bilat)	(+)	(+)	(+)		5-HT, TK
Ret. sp.	+	+	+	+	EAA
Ret. sp.	+	(+)	+		CCK
Ret. sp.					5-HT

[a]Data compiled from Brodin et al., 1986, 1987; Buchanan, 1982; Buchanan and Grillner, 1987; Ohta et al., 1987; Rovainen, 1974a,b; van Dongen et al., 1985a,b. Presynaptic neurons are indicated to the left; EIN, excitatory premotor interneurons; CCIN, the inhibitory crossed interneurons; LIN, lateral interneurons; 5-HT IN, local spinal midline interneurons; Ret. sp., different reticulospinal neurons including the large Müller cells. The type of postsynaptic receptors are indicated; EAA, excitatory amino acids; TK, tachykinins; CCK, cholecystokinins. Spinal sensory cells, relay interneurons, and crossed excitatory interneurons are not included. The different postsynaptic neurons are indicated in the different vertical columns.

Table 1; Russell and Wallén, 1980, 1983; Buchanan and Cohen, 1982; Kahn, 1982). All motoneurons show membrane potential oscillations during fictive locomotion. Slow motoneurons discharge more readily while fast motoneurons tend to display subthreshold membrane potential oscillations at least at slow rates of swimming. Motoneurons supplying the same part of the myotome receive essentially identical input since their cycle-to-cycle variations correspond during fictive locomotion. However, if motoneurons to different parts of the myotome are compared, they may differ considerably in the details of the oscillations (Wallén et al., 1985). Thus, motoneurons to the dorsal muscle will be identical as will motoneurons to the ventral muscle, but the two groups may be quite different. The phasic excitatory drive originates from small ipsilateral spinal excitatory interneurons, which extend over a few segments (Dale, 1986; Dale and Grillner, 1986; Buchanan and Grillner, 1987). At least part of the midcycle inhibition of the motoneurons originates from crossed interneurons which have a main long descending axon. These are inhibitory CC interneurons (Buchanan, 1982; Buchanan and Cohen, 1982). Local inhibitory interneurons may also take part in the inhibition of motoneurons (Grillner et al., 1986).

The inhibitory premotor interneurons (CCINs) are initially excited at the same time as the ipsilateral motoneurons or even before (Fig. 14), but subsequently the inhibitory CCINs become inhibited while the motoneurons are still excited (Buchanan and Cohen, 1982, Kahn, 1982). This inhibition originates, at least partially, from ipsilateral inhibitory neurons with

a long descending axon. They are called lateral interneurons (LINs, Rovainen, 1974a) and are active in phase with the ipsilateral motoneurons. The
inhibitory CCINs thus have a phase-advanced excitation which leads to an
inhibition of contralateral motoneurons, CCINs, and LINs. Inhibitory
CCINs can be subdivided into two categories dependent on their reticulospinal input (Buchanan, 1982).

4.3 Neurons that Utilize NMDA and Kainate Receptors Are Critical for the Generation of Locomotion

Primary sensory neurons, reticulospinal neurons, and premotor interneurons in the lamprey release a transmitter—probably glutamate and/or as-

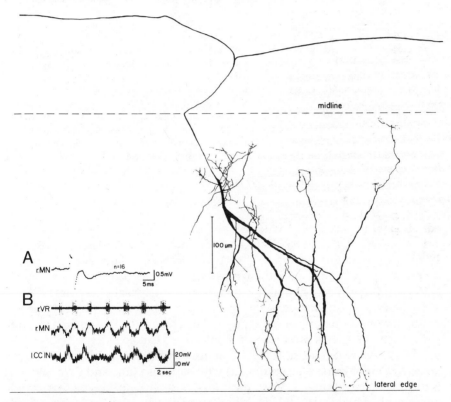

FIGURE 14. Drawing of an inhibitory CC interneuron injected intracellularly with Lucifer
yellow in the lamprey spinal cord. (A) The average of 16 intracellularly recorded inhibitory
postsynaptic potentials produced by the CC interneuron in a contralateral motoneuron (MN)
located in the same segment (0.9 mm rostrally). (B) Fictive swimming (0.15 mM D-glutamate)
was recorded as rhythmic ventral root (VR) activity. The CC interneuron exhibited a depolarizing phase during the repolarizing phase of its postsynaptic motoneuron. Thus, when this
CC interneuron fired action potentials during swimming, it would contribute to the inhibitory
phase of the motoneuron.

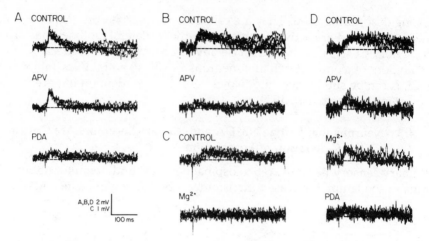

FIGURE 15. Three types of excitatory postsynaptic potentials (EPSPs) in lamprey motoneurons. Intracellular recordings of EPSPs were made in Mg^{2+}-free solution and in the presence of 5 μM strychnine. The EPSPs were evoked by extracellular stimulation of single axons. (A) A "fast" EPSP which was unaffected by 100 μM 2-amino-5-phosphonovalerate (APV), an N-methyl-D-aspartate (NMDA) receptor antagonist, but was reduced by 2 mM cis-2,3-piperidine dicarboxylate (PDA), an antagonist of both NMDA and kainate receptors. (B) A "slow" EPSP which was reduced by 100 μM APV. (C) Another "slow" EPSP reduced by 2 mM Mg^{2+}. (D) A "mixed" EPSP of which the slow, long-duration component was selectively reduced by 100 μM APV or 1 mM Mg^{2+} leaving an initial, fast component. Both slow and fast components were reduced by 2 mM PDA. Dashed lines indicate resting potential, and the arrows in A and B indicate spontaneous PSPs which were not seen during antagonist application (From Grillner, Wallén, Dale, Brodin, Buchanan, and Hill, 1987.)

partate—which activates excitatory amino acid receptors (Buchanan and Grillner, 1987; Dale, 1986; Dale and Grillner, 1986; Christenson et al., 1986). The excitatory amino acid receptors can be subdivided into three different types named after their most selective agonist. They are called NMDA (N-methyl-D-aspartate) kainate and quisqualate receptors (Watkins, 1981). The unitary excitatory postsynaptic potentials (EPSPs) of premotor interneurons are in a range between 0.3–1.9 mV (Buchanan and Grillner, 1987). EPSPs produced by single axons can be of three types (Figure 15), (1) with rapid-rise time (6.5 milliseconds) and rapid decay due to an activation of kainate receptors, (2) with slow-rise time and decay which is due to an activation of NMDA receptors, and (3) a mixed type with rapid onset and slow decay due to simultaneous activation of kainate and NMDA receptors (Dale and Grillner, 1986). The large reticulospinal Müller cells elicit EPSPs with an early electric component followed by a chemical component of up to 8–9 mV which is due to a mixed kainate/NMDA synapse (Christenson et al., 1986).

During locomotion all phasic excitation of the motoneurons appears to be due to an activation of kainate and NMDA receptors (Dale, 1986; Dale

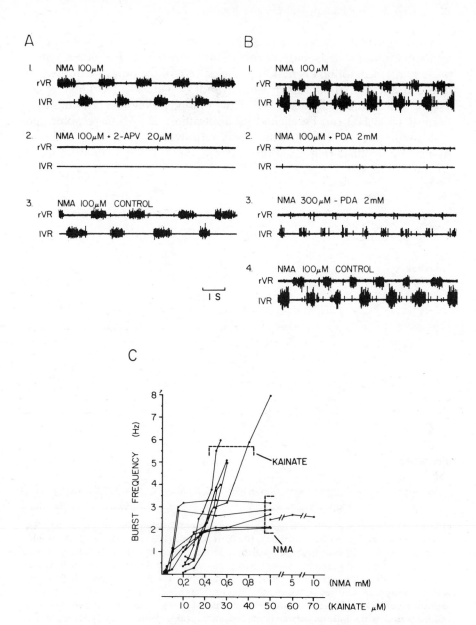

FIGURE 16. Induction of fictive swimming by N-methyl-D,L-aspartate (NMA) and kainate, and the sensitivity of NMA-induced swimming to excitatory amino acid antagonists in the lamprey spinal cord. (A) The blocking action of 20 μM 2-APV on fictive swimming induced by 100 μM NMA. (B) The blocking action of 2 mM PDA on fictive swimming induced by 100 μM NMA and the incomplete blocking action of 2 mM PDA when the NMA concentration was raised to 300 μM. (C) Swim burst frequency versus concentration of NMA and kainate in six lampreys. Concentration was increased every fifth minute. (From Brodin, Grillner, and Rovainen, 1985.)

and Grillner, 1986). A very unspecific excitation is caused by bath-applied excitatory amino acids but, nevertheless, it releases the motor output underlying locomotion even though the pattern of the output requires precise coordination (Poon 1980; Cohen and Wallén, 1980; Grillner et al., 1981b; Wallén and Williams, 1984). Slow to moderately fast rates of swimming (0.05–3 Hz) can be elicited by application of NMDA-receptor agonists (Grillner et al., 1981b), while faster rate swimming (1–8 Hz) is elicited by kainate agonists (Fig. 16, Brodin et al., 1985). If the swimming motor

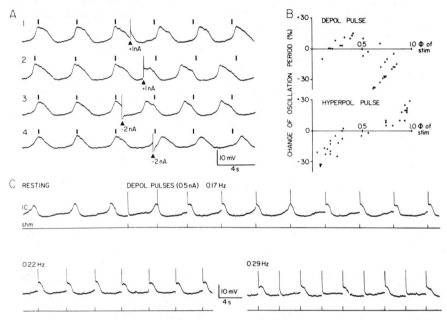

FIGURE 17. The effects of shortlasting de- and hyperpolarizing current pulses on TTX-resistant membrane potential oscillations. (A) Both positive (1,2) and negative (3,4) stimulus pulses (20 ms; arrows) can affect the oscillation period and cause rhythm resetting. Vertical bars indicate normal occurrence of oscillation peaks during undisturbed activity. (B) Phase-response curves for the stimulation effects exemplified in A. The phase of the oscillatory cycle at which a stimulus occurred (Phase of stim; abscissa) has been plotted versus its effect on the oscillation period (percentage increase (+) or decrease (−), as compared to the control value and measured as the interval between depolarization peaks; ordinate). Depolarizing pulses (upper graph) delivered early in the cycle in general caused prolongation of the oscillation period (cf. A:1), whereas the same type of stimulus occurring later gave period shortening (cf. A:2). Hyperpolarizing pulses gave opposite effects (lower graph; cf. A:3,4). (C) Entrainment of oscillatory activity by repetitive brief stimulus pulses. Depolarizing pulses (0.5 nA, 50 ms) were delivered at a rate slightly higher (0.17 Hz) than "rest" rate of oscillations resulting in 1:1 entrainment, which was maintained with the rate increased to 0.22 Hz. A further frequency increase gave incomplete entrainment (0.29 Hz; 1:2 correlation). (From Wallén and Grillner, 1985.)

NMDA induced TTX-resistant
oscillations

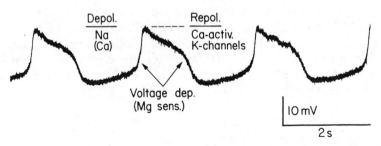

FIGURE 18. Schematic representation of some factors which contribute to NMDA receptor-evoked TTX-resistant membrane potential oscillations, based on ion substitution experiments. NMDA causes a gradual depolarization and the voltage-dependent properties of the NMDA-channels, which require the presence of magnesium, will suddenly swing the membrane potential to a depolarized level. The depolarizing current is carried mainly by Na⁺, and is partly counteracted by voltage-sensitive K⁺-channels. The voltage-dependent properties will eventually support the repolarization down to a hyperpolarized level. (From Grillner, Wallén, Dale, Brodin, Buchanan, and Hill, 1987.)

pattern is elicited by brainstem stimulation or by sensory stimuli, the entire swimming motor pattern can be blocked by antagonists of both NMDA and kainate receptors. On the other hand, NMDA receptor antagonists will only block the slow—but not the fast-swimming activity (Brodin and Grillner, 1985a,b). Thus, naturally evoked locomotion also utilizes the activation of NMDA and kainate receptors.

NMDA and kainic acid activate very different types of channels. Whereas a kainate receptor activates a fast conventional conductance increase, an activation of NMDA receptors gates voltage-dependent ionophores (MacDonald et al., 1982; Moore et al., 1986). At a resting membrane potential the NMDA-gated channels may be closed, but at a more depolarized level the ionophores will open. The voltage dependence is due to the presence of Mg^{2+} in the extracellular fluid (Nowak et al., 1984; Mayer et al., 1984; Mayer and Westbrook, 1985; cf Brodin and Grillner, 1986). Activation of NMDA receptors thus adds a new property to a cell. The NMDA receptor can switch the cell from a state in which the NMDA ionophores are closed to one in which they are open. Furthermore, they will contribute a depolarizing current due to a passage of Na⁺ and Ca^{2+} ions. In fact, such a cell can exhibit TTX-resistant, pacemakerlike oscillations by switching between these two stable states (Figure 17; Sigvardt and Grillner, 1981; Sigvardt et al., 1985; Grillner and Wallén, 1985b; Wallén and Grillner, 1985, 1987). The oscillations are due to the voltage-dependent property of the NMDA channels and to a gradual activation of Ca^{2+}-dependent K⁺ channels during the depolarized phase (Figure 18; Grillner and Wallén, 1985b; Wallén and Grillner, 1987). The latter is caused by the entry of Ca^{2+} through the NMDA channels (MacDermott et al., 1986). Although functionally isolated cells will exhibit such NMDA-induced oscillations, the activity of neurons will, under ordinary conditions, be coordinated by their synaptic interactions. This NMDA-induced property, however, gives the cells of the neuronal network different membrane properties from those encountered under resting conditions. This is a factor which must be incorporated into any model of how the network operates.

4.4   The Role of Glycine and the Nonrole of GABA in the Generation of "Fictive Swimming"

Glycine causes a hyperpolarization of spinal neurons which is blocked by strychnine (Homma and Rovainen, 1978). The unitary inhibitory postsynaptic potentials (IPSPs) produced by the crossed inhibitory CC interneurons in motoneurons are also blocked by strychnine and can thus be expected to be glycinergic (Buchanan, 1982). In fact, the entire inhibition of motoneurons during fictive locomotion is blocked by strychnine (Dale, 1986). The inhibitory CCINs of the two sides mutually inhibit each other and can thus be expected to contribute to the reciprocal alternation of the two sides of one segment. They may also play a role in intersegmental coordination (cf Buchanan, 1986).

A possible way to test whether glycinergic neurons are important in the locomotor network is to administer a low concentration of strychnine to produce a partial receptor blockade (Grillner and Wallén, 1980). When this is done, the rate of fictive locomotion increases markedly, demonstrating that the pattern-generating circuitry is directly affected. Moreover, at a critical dose of strychnine, the alternation between left and right side can be replaced by synchronous activity on the two sides (Cohen and Harris-Warrick, 1984). Thus, the alternation is dependent on glycinergic mechanisms, possibly mediated by the inhibitory CCINs.

Gamma-aminobutyric acid (GABA) is presumably also an inhibitory transmitter in the lamprey spinal cord since glutamic acid decarboxylase is present (Wald et al., 1981). Moreover, GABA-containing neurons have been demonstrated by immunohistochemical methods (Dale, Storm-Mathiesen and Grillner, unpubl.). An activation of GABA-receptors causes a hyperpolarization and a conductance increase for Cl^- ions (Homma and Rovainen, 1978). However, GABA interneurons do not seem to be of critical importance during fictive locomotion since an administration of GABA antagonists does not affect the motor pattern. On the other hand, interneurons in the pattern-generating circuitry have GABA receptors since the rate of fictive swimming is depressed if GABA is applied (Grillner and Wallén, 1980).

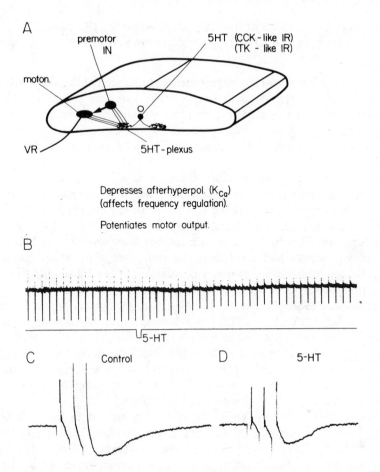

FIGURE 19. 5-HT causes a depression of the afterhyperpolarization (AHP) in lamprey motoneurons and premotor interneurons. (A) Schematic representation of the lamprey spinal cord. Midline 5-HT interneurons, which also contain CCK-like and tachykinin-like immunoreactivity (IR), distribute their dendrites in a ventromedial plexus into which both motoneurons and premotor interneurons send their dendrites. (B) A continuous recording of the membrane potential of a moteneuron during repeated intracellular stimulation at 0.3 Hz. At each stimulation the cell is stimulated three times with an interval of 20 ms (compare C,D). Note the accumulated afterhyperpolarization (AHP) following the action potentials and the marked reduction in amplitude of the AHP directly after an ejection of 5-HT onto the ventral surface of the spinal cord just outside the ventromedial plexus. The AHPs are shown with higher time resolution before (C) and after (D) ejection of 5-HT. (From Grillner, Wallén, Dale, Brodin, Buchanan, and Hill, 1987.)

4.5   5-HT Depression of the Ca^{2+} Dependent K$^+$ Channels Underlying the After Hyperpolarization Affects the Frequency Regulation

5-hydroxytryptamine (5-HT) interneurons are located along the midline of the spinal cord (Harris-Warrick et al., 1985; van Dongen et al., 1985b). Their processes form varicosities in close proximity to the dendrites belonging to motoneurons, LINs, and CCINs (van Dongen et al., 1985a). In addition, there are two descending 5-HT projections from the brainstem (Brodin et al., 1986).

The frequency regulation of a neuron is to a large extent due to the afterhyperpolarization which follows the action potential (Gustafsson, 1974). In most spinal neurons the late phase of the afterhyperpolarization is due to an activation of Ca^{2+}-dependent potassium channels by the Ca^{2+} ions which enter during the action potential (for lamprey, see Hill et al., 1985). Any process which modulates the amplitude of the afterhyperpolarization will also affect the frequency regulation. When 5-HT is applied outside motoneurons, the afterhyperpolarization is markedly depressed (van Dongen et al., 1986; Wallén et al, 1986), through an action on the Ca^{2+} dependent K$^+$ channels (Fig. 19). As a consequence, the motoneurons will react to other excitatory inputs with a higher discharge rate, everything else being equal (Wallén et al., 1986). This mechanism for rate modulation is presumably used by the 5-HT neurons. It is yet another synaptic mechanism which has to be considered when trying to understand the operation of the neural network generating locomotion.

When 5-HT is applied during NMDA or D-glutamate induced fictive locomotion it potentiates each motor burst markedly (Grillner and Wilén, unpubl.; Harris-Warrick and Cohen, 1985), consistent with the 5-HT effects on the afterhyperpolarization. It also causes a prolongation of each burst and, thus, a slowing of the rate of swimming, rather than an increase in frequency, which might not have been expected at first (van Dongen et al., 1985a).

4.6   How the Segmental Rhythmic Activity May Come About: Rhythmogenesis and Initiation

The neurons contained within approximately 1.5–2 segments can generate alternating activity (Grillner et al., 1982b) and the isolated ipsilateral spinal cord (around 5 segments) can be made to produce rhythmic bursting (Grillner et al., 1986).

When inspecting the circuit discussed below in Figure 20, it appears intuitively likely that it could produce rhythmic alternating activity if the excitability is high in the different neurons (see below). There is one piece of information missing, and that is the origin of the segmental input to the EINs. They have an inhibitory input during fictive locomotion coinciding with the contralateral burst activity possibly originating from contralateral

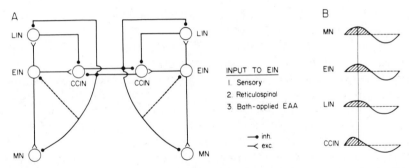

FIGURE 20. A proposed circuit to account for the origin of the swimming rhythm in the lamprey spinal cord. (A) The circuit is based upon demonstrated synaptic interactions among the illustrated cell classes. The key unit of the circuit for rhythmogenesis is the reciprocal inhibition between CC interneurons (CCIN) on opposite sides of the spinal cord and the inhibition of ipsilateral CC interneurons from lateral interneurons (LIN). The LIN inhibition limits the activity of the CCINs, thus allowing activity to begin on the contralateral side. The excitatory interneurons (EIN) provide rhythmic excitation of motoneurons and interneurons, and if they synapse upon other excitatory interneurons, they might also provide for sustaining excitatory drive to the circuit. Although inhibition of excitatory interneurons by CC interneurons has not been demonstrated (hence the dashed lines indicating the connection), excitatory interneurons do receive rhythmic inhibition during fictive swimming consistent with CC interneuron input. Excitatory interneurons receive direct excitation from reticulospinal cells, polysynaptic excitation from sensory afferents, and are excited by bath-applied excitatory amino acids (EAA). (B) Schematic representation of membrane potential oscillations of the cell types of the circuit during fictive swimming. The shaded regions above the dashed line indicates the approximate period of excitation; the region below is the approximate period of inhibition. The CC interneurons are about 15% of a cycle phase advanced in relation to the other cell types. See text for further details and references.

CCINs. Whether the EINs mutually facilitate each other to a limited degree or not is unknown.

Let us consider the circuit of Figure 20. If we assume that there is an inhibitory input to the excitatory interneurons (EINs) from crossed CC interneurons (CCINs), a simple circuit emerges in which the EINs and the CCINs of the two sides could interact in a reciprocal fashion. When the neurons of one side are active, the contralateral side will be inhibited by the inhibitory CCINs and vice versa. The inhibition from the lateral interneurons to the CCINs is presumably responsible for the early inhibition of the CCINs during fictive locomotion and thereby the phase advance of the spike activity of the CCINs. The short-lasting CCIN excitation due to the lateral IN activity may be very important. When the CCINs are inhibited the contralateral neurons will become disinhibited and, if their background excitation is sufficiently high, a contralateral burst will be initiated. If the contralateral EINs become activated, they would turn on the CCINs of that side, which, subsequently, would effectively shut off the bursts of the first side. The interaction between EINs, lateral interneurons (LINs), and CCINs could thus provide an intuitively satisfactory explanation for the rhythmogenesis.

In this model, the early inhibition of CCINs caused by LINs is important. The earlier the CCIN spike activity is inhibited, the earlier the contralateral side will turn on due to disinhibition. However, all the ideas discussed here must be corroborated by developing a model of the network. Such a model would have the appropriate properties of the different types of neurons under the appropriate type of synaptic drive. For instance, the duration and amplitude of the afterhyperpolarization (cf 5-HT effects), and the activation of synaptic voltage dependent ionophores (e.g., NMDA) are two out of many factors which will modify the properties of a given type of neuron (cf also Wallén et al., 1984). Even if the circuit of Figure 20 captures many important features of the "full" explanation, there are a number of facts which remain to be explained. First, the small ipsilateral inhibitory interneurons (Grillner et al., 1986 and unpubl.) may take part, and it is uncertain whether the entire midcycle inhibition of motoneurons can be ascribed to crossed inhibitory CCIN activity (Wallén, unpubl.). Second, the circuit above cannot satisfactorily explain the bursting observed in the isolated longitudinally hemisected spinal cord (cf. however above, Section 3.2) or the synchronous activity. Third, the large lateral interneurons are only present in the rostral two-thirds of the spinal cord (Rovainen, 1974a), but smaller neurons of the same functional type may exist in the caudal spinal cord (Tang and Selzer, 1979). Fourth, the role of the crossed excitatory CCINs (Buchanan, 1982) during fictive locomotion is unclear but they have been found to be active in phase and out of phase with the ipsilateral activity.

If the circuit of Figure 20 is a significant part of the oscillator circuit, then it is easy to understand that any process which would excite only the EINs (or all three types of neurons) of the two sides simultaneously could lead to a rhythmic alternating activity. Locomotion can be initiated from (1) long reticulospinal neurons (McClellan and Grillner, 1984), (2) sensory stimuli (McClellan and Grillner 1983), and (3) bath-applied excitatory amino acids (Poon, 1980; Cohen and Wallén, 1980; Grillner et al., 1981b; Brodin et al., 1985). We know, or it can be inferred, that all three types of stimuli will excite the EINs (Buchanan and Grillner, 1987; Christenson et al., 1986). Consequently, a fairly imprecise excitability increase could activate the network. The circuitry within the network could then result from the "self organizing" interactions among the different inhibitory interneurons.

The peripheral feedback (Grillner et al., 1984) which can entrain the locomotor activity (Grillner et al., 1981a; Grillner and Wallén, 1982) presumably exerts its effects on the interneuronal circuitry, but exactly at what level is not yet known. Activity in dorsal sensory cells can also modify the motor pattern (Buchanan and Cohen, 1982), and they have input to all cell types considered in Figure 20.

4.7   Intersegmental Coordination

Pieces of the spinal cord, whether short (5 segments) or long (50 segments), can maintain a phase lag of approximately 1% of the cycle duration between adjacent segments from rostral to caudal (Wallén and Williams, 1984). This means that the bursts of a caudal segment will start later and also terminate later. The time delay corresponding to the phase lag of 1% will vary 50 fold when going from very slow swimming at 0.2 Hz to very fast at 10 Hz (Table 2). The corresponding "conduction velocity" of the excitation from segment to segment would change from 0.04 m per second to 2.0 m per second. It is obvious that a phase lag of this type cannot be explained by axonal conduction delays since they are constant for any given type of axon (Table 2). The excitability of the different independent parts of the spinal cord does not vary in any systematic fashion if the spinal cord is split into several pieces (Cohen, 1986). However, in each part there can be a rostrocaudal lag (Grillner, 1974; Wallén and Williams, 1984). Let us further review what is known about the intersegmental projections of the three types of neurons or what can be predicted from available data.

1. **Excitatory interneurons (EINs)** project both to rostral and caudal segments, but the rostral projection is not longer than 2 or 3 segments and the caudal not longer than 7–8 segments (Dale, 1986; Dale and Grillner, 1986). Let us furthermore assume that they are of only one category and that they excite both motoneurons, LINs and CCINs, in all segments to which they project (Buchanan and Grillner, 1987). Whether the excitatory interneurons mutually excite each other or not is unknown.

2. The **lateral interneurons (LINs)** send long axons throughout the larger part of the spinal cord (Rovainen, 1974a) and they inhibit CC interneurons (Buchanan, 1982).

3. The **inhibitory CC interneurons (CCINs)** inhibit contralateral spinal motoneurons, CC interneurons, and lateral interneurons and possi-

TABLE 2.   Comparison of the Time Lags between Consecutive Segments at Different Velocities (rates) of Swimming in the Pysiological Range

Intersegmental Coordination	Axonal Conduction Velocity
Segmental phase lag 1%	LIN 2.0 m per s^{-1}
Intersegmental distance 2 mm	CCIN 1.4 m·s^{-1}
Segm. time lag at 10 Hz 1 ms (2.0 m·s^{-1})	EIN 0.6 m·s^{-1}
Segm. time lag at 5 Hz 2 ms (1.0 m·s^{-1})	Ret.sp (Mü) 3.5 m·s^{-1}
Segm. time lag at 1 Hz 10 ms (0.2 m·s^{-1})	Ret.sp (V) 2.0 m·s^{-1}
Segm. time lag at 0.2 Hz. 50 ms (0.04 m·s^{-1})	

The computation is based on a lamprey of a length of 0.2 m. For comparison the axonal conduction velocities of different propriospinal neurons are shown.

bly also the excitatory interneurons, mainly at the same level and in the caudal direction. The average length of the CC interneuron axon is unknown, but the orthodromic action potential has been recorded 30 segments caudal to the location of the soma. In most instances however, pieces of 10–20 segments have been used (Buchanan, 1982).

For the sake of a simplifying discussion, let us assume that there is one circuit of the type shown in Figure 20 in each segment and, furthermore, that tonic excitation from an extrinsic source will affect all excitatory interneurons in all segments to approximately the same degree. Moreover, let us assume as in Figure 20 that the CCINs inhibit the EINs. The more caudally located EINs will then be subject to inhibition from a larger number of CCINs than the rostral segments. This will lead to a deeper inhibition of the caudal than the rostral segments. It might, therefore, possibly take longer for the EINs of the more caudal segments to recover and initiate spike activity and a ventral root burst. In that case, a segmental lag would result from differences in the degree of inhibition along the spinal cord. Moreover, the more caudally located CCINs will also be subject to a more pronounced inhibition from contralateral CCINs. This also might lead to a later recovery of the CCINs and, consequently, they will become active and inhibit the contralateral side at a somewhat later point than the corresponding inhibition will occur in more rostral segments. This condition might lead to a later termination of the burst activity in the more caudal segments. The arrangements of the inhibitory interneurons will, in each separate piece of the spinal cord, result in a rostrocaudal excitability gradient.

Furthermore, Rovainen (1985, 1986), on indirect grounds, has suggested that there are crossed ascending EINs, and thus they would increase the excitability in rostral segments and promote a rostrocaudal excitability gradient. Whether the rostrocaudal gradient (referred to here) and the general synaptic organization is sufficient to explain the rostrocaudal phase lag can only be tested by modelling based on the identified circuitry and known properties of the neurons (cf Kopell, Chapt. 10; Mulloney, Chapt. 11; Rand et al., Chapt. 9).

5   CONCLUDING REMARKS

In this review we have discussed how fish swim and how the nervous system controls the swimming behavior. We have been mainly concerned with the propulsive synergy and have only dealt to a very limited degree with the more sophisticated steering control and adaptive aspects of the locomotor control. A number of reticulospinal neurons are active during fictive locomotion and they will presumably enhance the excitability of a number of spinal neurons. A spinal network based on identified interneurons and their known connections is discussed and it appears likely that it could be an essential component in the spinal pattern-generating circuitry. The different types of neurons and their transmitters and synaptic effects are considered in some detail, emphasizing the novel synaptic effects exerted by, for instance, NMDA receptors and 5-HT. Although the spinal central network is essential, it appears equally important to emphasize that a potent sensory control can adapt and modify any ongoing swim cycle to the current environmental demands in any particular moment. The cellular bases of locomotor behavior in a lower vertebrate are beginning to be unravelled, but there is a long way to go before we have reached the level already achieved in some invertebrate systems (like Tritonia; Getting, 1986; Getting, Chapt. 4) or the lobster stomatogastric system (Selverston and Moulins, 1985; cf Getting, Chapt. 4). With regard to our understanding of complex behavior in higher vertebrates, it is very encouraging that the general organization of the locomotor system in the lamprey resembles that of the frog embryo and also that of mammals (see Grillner, 1985; Grillner and Wallén, 1985a; Stein 1978, 1983). Thus, we may hope that studies of the lamprey CNS may contribute to the understanding of the cellular bases of mammalian motor behavior, which appears so inaccessible due to the vast number of neurons (cf also Cohen, Chapt. 5).

REFERENCES

Ayers, J., G. A. Carpenter, S. Currie, and J. Kinch (1983). Which behaviour does the lamprey central motor program mediate. *Science*, **221**:1312–1314.

Bainbridge, R. (1958). The speed of swimming of fish as related to size and to the frequency and amplitude of tail beat. *J. Exp. Biol.*, **35**:109–133.

Bainbridge, R. (1961). Problems of fish locomotion. *Zool. Soc. (Lond.) Symposia*, **5**:13–32.

Bethe, A. (1899). Die Locomotion des Haifisches (Scyllium) und ihre Beziehungen zu den einzelnen Gehirntheilen und zum Labyrinth. *Pflugers Arch. Ges. Physiol.*, **765**:470–493.

Bone, Q. (1975). Muscular and energetic aspects of fish swimming. In *Swimming and Flying in Nature*, Vol. 2. T. Y. Wu, C. J. Brokaw, and C. Brennen, eds. Plenum Press, New York, pp. 493–528.

Brodin, L., J. T. Buchanan, T. Hökfelt, S. Grillner, and A. A. J. Verhofstad (1986). A spinal projection of 5-hydroxytryptamine neurons in the lamprey brain stem: evidence from combined retrograde tracing and immunohistochemistry. *Neuroscience*, **67**:53–57.

Brodin, L., J. T. Buchanan, T. Hökfelt, S. Grillner, F. Rehfeld, P. Frey, A. A. J. Verhofstad, G. J. Dockray, and H. Walsh (1987). Immunohistochemical studies of cholecystokinin (CCK)-like peptides and their relation to 5-HT, CGRP and bombesin immunoreactivities in the brainstem and spinal cord of lampreys. *J. Comp. Neurol.*, in press.

Brodin, L. and S. Grillner (1985a). The role of putative excitatory amino acid neurotransmitters in the initiation of locomotion in the lamprey spinal cord. I. The effects of excitatory amino acid antagonists. *Brain Res.*, **360**:139–148.

Brodin, L. and S. Grillner (1985b). The role of putative excitatory amino acid neurotransmitters in the initiation of locomotion in the lamprey spinal cord. II. The effects of amino acid uptake inhibitors. *Brain Res.*, **360**:149–158.

Brodin, L. and S. Grillner (1986). Effects of magnesium on fictive locomotion induced by activation of N-Methyl-D-aspartate (NMDA) receptors in the lamprey spinal cord in vitro. *Brain Res.*, **380**:244–252.

Brodin, L., S. Grillner, and C. M. Rovainen (1985). NMDA, kainate and quisqualate receptors and the generation of fictive locomotion in the lamprey spinal cord. *Brain Res.*, **325**:302–306.

Buchanan, J. T. (1982). Identification of interneurons with contralateral caudal axons in the lamprey spinal cord: synaptic interactions and morphology. *J. Neurophysiol.*, **47**:961–975.

Buchanan, J. T. (1986). Premotor interneurones in the lamprey spinal cord: morphology, synaptic interactions, and activities during fictive swimming. In *Neurobiology of Vertebrate Locomotion*, S. Grillner, P. S. G. Stein, D. G. Stuart, H. Forssberg, and R. M. Herman, eds. Macmillan, London, pp. 321–334.

Buchanan, J. T. and A. H. Cohen (1982). Activities of identified interneurons, motoneurons, and muscle fibers during fictive swimming in the lamprey and effects of reticulospinal and dorsal cell stimulation. *J. Neurophysiol.*, **47**:948–960.

Buchanan, J. and S. Grillner (1987). Newly identified "Glutamate interneurons" and their role in locomotion in the lamprey spinal cord. *Science*, **236**:312–314.

Christenson, J., L. Brodin, J. Buchanan, N. Dale, and S. Grillner (1986). Sensory afferent and descending fiber mediated excitation of lamprey spinal neurons; effects of excitatory amino acid antagonists. *Neurosci. Lett.*, Suppl. 26, S161.

Cohen, A. H. (1986). The intersegmental coordinating system of the lamprey; experimental and theoretical studies. In *Neurobiology of Vertebrate Locomotion*, S. Grillner, P. S. G. Stein, D. G. Stuart, H. Forssberg, and R. M. Herman, eds. Macmillan, London, pp. 371–382.

Cohen, A. H. and R. M. Harris-Warrick (1984). Strychnine eliminates alternating motor output during fictive locomotion in the lamprey. *Brain Res.*, **293**:164–167.

Cohen, A. H. and P. Wallén (1980). The neuronal correlate of locomotion in fish. "Fictive swimming" induced in an in vitro preparation of the lamprey spinal cord. *Exp. Brain Res.*, **41**:11–18.

Dale, N. (1986). Excitatory synaptic drive for swimming mediated by amino acid receptors in the lamprey. *J. Neurosci.*, **6**:2662–2675.

Dale, N. and S. Grillner (1986). Dual component synaptic potentials in the lamprey mediated by excitatory amino acid receptors. *J. Neurosci.*, **6**:2653–2661.

Dale, N. and A. Roberts (1984). Excitatory amino acid receptors in *Xenopus* embryo spinal cord and their role in the activation of swimming. *J. Physiol.*, **348**:527–543.

Dale, N. and A. Roberts (1985). Dual-component amino acid-mediated synaptic potentials: Excitatory drive for swimming in *Xenopus* embryos. *J. Physiol.*, **363**:35–59.

Droge, M. H. and R. B. Leonard (1983a). The swimming pattern in intact and decerebrated sting rays. *J. Neurophysiol.*, **50**:162–177.

Droge, M. H. and R. B. Leonard (1983b). Swimming rhythm in decerebrated, paralyzed sting rays: normal and abnormal coupling. *J. Neurophysiol.*, **50**:178–191.

Flood, P. R. (1968). Structure of the segmental trunk muscle in *Amphioxus. Zeitschr. für Zehforsch.*, **84**:389–416.

Forssberg, H., S. Grillner, and S. Rossignol (1977). Phasic gain control of reflexes from the dorsum of the paw during spinal locomotion. *Brain Res.*, **132**:121–139.

Garcia-Rill, E. (1986). The basal ganglia and the locomotor regions. *Brain Res. Rev.*, **11**:47–64.

Garcia-Rill, E. and R. D. Skinner (1986). The basal ganglia and the mesencephalic locomotor region. In *Neurobiology of Vertebrate Locomotion*, S. Grillner, P. S. G. Stein, D. G. Stuart, H. Forssberg, and R. M. Herman, eds. Macmillan, London, pp. 77–104.

Getting, P. A. (1986). Understanding central pattern generators: insights gained from the study of invertebrate systems. In *Neurobiology of Vertebrate Locomotion*, S. Grillner, P. S. G. Stein, H. Forssberg, D. G. Stuart, and R. M. Herman, eds. Macmillan, London, pp. 231–244.

Gray, J. (1950). The role of peripheral sense organs during locomotion in the vertebrates. *Symp. Soc. Exp. Biol.*, **4**:112–126.

Gray, J. (1968). *Animal Locomotion*. Weidenfeld and Nicolson, London.

Gray, J. (1933a). Studies in animal locomotion. I. The movement of fish with special reference to the eel. *J. Exp. Biol.*, **10**:88–103.

Gray, J. (1933b). Studies in animal locomotion. II. The relationship between waves of muscular contraction and the propulsive mechanism of the eel. *J. Exp. Biol.*, **10**:386–400.

Gray, J. and A. Sand (1936). The locomotory rhythm of the dogfish (*Scyllium canicula*). *J. Exp. Biol.*, **13**:200–209.

Grillner, S. (1974). On the generation of locomotion in the spinal dogfish. *Exp. Brain Res.*, **20**:459–470.

Grillner, S. (1981). Control of locomotion in bipeds, tetrapods and fish. In *Handbook of Physiology, Sect. 1. The Nervous System Vol. II. Motor Control.* V. B. Brooks, ed. Waverly Press, Maryland, pp. 1179–1236.

Grillner, S. (1985). Neurobiological bases of rhythmic motor acts in vertebrates. *Science*, **228**:143–149.

Grillner, S., L. Brodin, K. Sigvardt, and N. Dale (1986). On the spinal network generating locomotion in lamprey: Transmitters, membrane properties and circuitry. In *Neurobiology of Vertebrate Locomotion*. S. Grillner, P. S. G. Stein, D. G. Stuart, H. Forssberg, and R. M. Herman, eds. Macmillan, London, pp. 335–352.

Grillner, S. and S. Kashin (1976). On the generation and performance of swimming in fish. In *Neural Control of Locomotion, Vol. 18*. R. M. Herman, S. Grillner, P. S. G. Stein, and D. G. Stuart, eds. Plenum Press, New York, pp. 181–202.

Grillner, S., A. McClellan, and C. Perret (1981a). Entrainment of the spinal pattern generators for swimming by mechanosensitive elements in the lamprey spinal cord in vitro. *Brain Res.*, **217**:380–386.

Grillner, S., A. McClellan, and K. Sigvardt (1982a). Mechanosensitive neurons in the spinal cord of the lamprey. *Brain Res.*, **235**: 169–173.

Grillner, S., A. McClellan, K. Sigvardt, P. Wallén, and M. Wilén (1981b). Activation of NMDA-receptors elicits "fictive locomotion" in lamprey spinal cord in vitro. *Acta Physiol. Scand.*, **113**:549–551.

Grillner, S., A. McClellan, K. Sigvardt, P. Wallén, and T. Williams (1982b). On the neural generation of "fictive locomotion" in a lower vertebrate nervous system, in vitro. In *Brain Stem Control of Spinal Mechanisms*, B. Sjölund and A. Björklund, eds. Fernström Foundation Series No. 1, Elsevier, New York, pp. 273–295.

Grillner, S., C. Perret, and P. Zangger (1976). Central generation of locomotion in the spinal dogfish. *Brain Res.*, **109**:255–269.

Grillner, S., S. Rossignol, and P. Wallén (1977). The adaptation of a reflex response to the ongoing phase of locomotion in fish. *Exp. Brain Res.*, **30**:1–11.

Grillner, S. and P. Wallén (1977). Is there a peripheral control of the central pattern generators for swimming in dogfish? *Brain Res.*, **127**:291–295.

Grillner, S. and P. Wallén (1980). Does the central pattern generation for locomotion in lamprey depend on glycine inhibition? *Acta Physiol. Scand.*, **110**:103–105.

Grillner, S. and P. Wallén (1982). On peripheral control mechanisms acting on the central pattern generators for swimming in the dogfish. *J. Exp. Biol.*, **98**:1–22.

Grillner, S. and P. Wallén (1984). How does the lamprey central nervous system make the lamprey swim? *J. Exp. Biol.*, **112**:337–357.

Grillner, S. and P. Wallén (1985a). Central pattern generators for locomotion, with special reference to vertebrates. *Ann. Rev. Neurosci.*, **8**: 233–261.

Grillner, S. and P. Wallén (1985b). The ionic mechanisms underlying NMDA receptor induced, TTX resistant membrane potential oscillations in lamprey neurons active during locomotion. *Neurosci. Lett.*, **60**:289–294.

Grillner, S., P. Wallén, N. Dale, L. Brodin, J. Buchanan, and R. Hill (1987). Transmitters, membrane properties and network circuitry in the control of locomotion in lamprey. *Trends Neurosci.* **10**:34–41.

Grillner, S., T. Williams, and P. Å. Lagerbäck (1984). The edge cell, a possible intraspinal mechanoreceptor. *Science*, **223**:500–503.

Gustafsson, B. (1974). Afterhyperpolarization and the control of repetitive firing in spinal neurons of the cat. *Acta Physiol., Scand. Suppl.* 416.

Harris-Warrick, R. M. and A. H. Cohen (1985). Serotonin modulates the central pattern generator for locomotion in the isolated lamprey spinal cord. *J. Exp. Biol.*, **116**:27–46.

Harris-Warrick, R. M., J. C. McPhee, and J. A. Filler (1985). Distribution of serotonergic neurons and processes in the lamprey spinal cord. *Neuroscience*, **14**:1127–1140.

Heier, P. (1948). Fundamental principles in the structure of the brain. A study of the brain of *Petromyzon fluviatilis*. *Acta Anat. Suppl.*, **8**:1–213.

Hill, R. H., P. Århem, and S. Grillner (1985). Ionic mechanisms of three types of functionally different neurons in the lamprey spinal cord. *Brain Res.*, **358**:40–52.

Holst, E. von. (1935). Erregungsbildung und Erregungsleitung im Fischrucken-mark. *Pflugers Arch. Ges. Physiol.*, **235**:345–359.

Holst, E. von. (1954). Relations between the central nervous system and the peripheral organs. *Brit. J. Anim. Behav.*, **2**:89–94.

Homma, S. and C. M. Rovainen (1978). Conductance increases produced by glycine and γ-aminobutyric acid in lamprey interneurons. *J. Physiol.*, **279**:231–252.

Hudson, K. C. L. (1973). On the function of the white muscles in teleosts at intermediate swimming speeds. *J. Exp. Biol.*, **58**:509–522.

Kahn, J. A. (1982). Patterns of synaptic inhibition in motoneurones and interneurones during fictive swimming in the lamprey as revealed by Cl⁻-injections. *J. Comp. Physiol.*, **147**:189–194.

Kahn, J. A., A. Roberts, and S. Kashin (1982). The neuromuscular basis of swimming movements in embryos of the amphibian *Xenopus laevis*. *J. Exp. Biol.*, **99**:175–184.

Kashin, S., A. G. Feldman, and G. N. Orlovsky (1974). Locomotion of fish evoked by electrical stimulation of the brain. *Brain Res.*, **82**:41–47.

Kasicki, S. and S. Grillner (1986). Müller cells and other reticulospinal neurons are phasically active during fictive locomotion in the isolated nervous system of the lamprey. *Neurosci. Lett.*, **69**:239–243.

Leonard, R. B. (1986). Locomotion in rays and tadpole. In *Neurobiology of Vertebrate Locomotion*. S. Grillner, P. S. G. Stein, D. G. Stuart, H. Forssberg, and R. M. Herman, eds. Macmillan, London, pp. 157–172.

Lighthill, M. J. (1969). Hydrodynamics of aquatic animal propulsion. *Ann. Rev. Fluid Mech.*, **1**:413–446.

Lissman, H. W. (1946a). The neurological basis of the locomotory rhythm in the spinal dogfish (*Scyllium canicula, Acanthias vulgaris*). I. Reflex behaviour. *J. Exp. Biol.*, **23**:143–161.

Lissman, H. W. (1946b). The neurological basis of the locomotory rhythm in the spinal dogfish (*Scyllium canicula, Acanthias vulgaris*). II. The effect of deafferentation. *J. Exp. Biol.*, **23**:162–176.

MacDermott, A. B., M. L. Mayer, G. L. Westbrook, S. J. Smith, and J. L. Barker (1986). NMDA receptor activation increases cytoplasmic calcium concentration in cultured spinal cord neurons. *Nature*, **321**:519–522.

MacDonald, J. F., A. V. Porietis, and J. M. Wojtowicz (1982). L-aspartic acid induces a region of negative slope conductance in the current-voltage relationship of cultured spinal cord neurons. *Brain Res.*, **237**:248–253.

Mayer, M. L. and G. L. Westbrook (1985). The action of N-methyl-D-aspartic acid on mouse spinal neurons in culture. *J. Physiol.*, **361**:65–90.

Mayer, M. L., G. L. Westbrook, and P. B. Guthrie (1984). Voltage-dependent block by Mg^{2+} of NMDA responses in spinal cord neurons. *Nature*, **309**:261–263.

McClellan, A. D. (1984). Descending control and sensory gating of fictive swimming and turning responses elicited in an in vitro preparation of the lamprey brainstem spinal cord. *Brain Res.*, **302**:151–162.

McClellan, A. D. (1986). Command system for initiating locomotion in fish and amphibians: parallels to initiation systems in mammals. In *Neurobiology of Verte-*

brate Locomotion. S. Grillner, P. S. G. Stein, D. G. Stuart, H. Forssberg, and R. M. Herman, eds. Macmillan, London, pp. 3–20.

McClellan, A. D. and S. Grillner (1983). Initiation and sensory gating of "fictive" swimming and withdrawal responses in an in vitro preparation of the lamprey spinal cord. *Brain Res.*, **269**:237–250.

McClellan, A. D. and S. Grillner (1984). Activation of "fictive swimming" by electrical microstimulation of brainstem locomotor regions in an in vitro preparation of the lamprey central nervous system. *Brain Res.*, **300**:357–361.

Moore, L. E., R. H. Hill, and S. Grillner (1986). Voltage clamp analysis of NMDA induced oscillating spinal neurons. *Acta Physiol. Scand.*, **128**:20A.

Nieuwenhuys, R. (1972). Topological analysis of the brainstem of the lamprey, *Lampetra fluviatilis. J. Comp. Neurol.*, **145**:165–178.

Nowak, L., P. Bregestovski, P. Ascher, A. Herbet, and A. Prochiantz (1984). Magnesium gates glutamate-activated channels in mouse central neurones. *Nature,* **307**:462–465.

Ohta, Y., L. Brodin, J. T. Buchanan, T. Hökfelt, and S. Grillner (1987). Morphology and activity of transmitter-identified reticulospinal neurons in the lamprey. *Abstr. 2nd World Congress of Neuroscience. Neuroscience, S643.*

Poon, M. L. T. (1980). Induction of swimming in lamprey by L-DOPA and amino acids. *J. Comp.Physiol.*, **136:** 337–344.

Roberts, A., J. A. Kahn, S. R. Soffe, and J. D. W. Clarke (1981). Neural control of swimming in a vertebrate. *Science*, **213**:1032–1034.

Roberts, A., S. R. Soffe, and N. Dale (1986). Spinal interneurons and swimming in frog embryos. In *Neurobiology of Vertebrate Locomotion,* S. Grillner, P. S. G. Stein, D. G. Stuart, H. Forssberg, and R. M. Herman, eds. Macmillan, London, pp. 279–306.

Roberts, B. L. (1969). Spontaneous rhythms in the motoneurons of spinal dogfish (*Scyliorhinus canicula*). *J. Mar. Biol. Assoc. U. K.*, **49**:33–49.

Rovainen, C. M. (1974a). Synaptic interactions of identified nerve cells in the spinal cord of the sea lamprey. *J. Comp. Neurol.*, **154**:189–206.

Rovainen, C. M. (1974b). Synaptic interactions of reticulospinal neurons and nerve cells in the spinal cord of the sea lamprey. *J. Comp. Neurol.*, **154**:207–224.

Rovainen, C. M. (1979). Neurobiology of lampreys. *Physiol. Rev.*, **59**:1007–1077.

Rovainen, C. M. (1983). Neurophysiology. In *The Biology of Lampreys Vol. 3*, M. W. Hardisty and I. C. Potter, eds. Academic Press, New York, pp. 1–136.

Rovainen, C. M. (1985). Effects of groups of propriospinal interneurons on fictive swimming in the isolated spinal cord of the lamprey. *J. Neurophysiol.*, **54**:959–977.

Rovainen, C. M. (1986). The contribution of multisegmental interneurons to the longitudinal coordination of fictive swimming in the lamprey. In *Neurobiology of Vertebrate Locomotion.* S. Grillner, P. S. G. Stein, D. G. Stuart, H. Forssberg, and R. M. Herman, eds. Macmillan, London, pp. 353–370.

Russell, D. F. and P. Wallén (1980). On the pattern generator for fictive swimming in the lamprey, *Ichthyomyzon unicuspis. Acta Physiol. Scand.*, **108**:9A.

Russell, D. F. and P. Wallén (1983). On the control of myotomal motoneurons during "fictive swimming" in the lamprey spinal cord in vitro. *Acta Physiol. Scand.*, **117**:161–170.

Schroeder, D. M. and S. C. Richardson (1985). Is the intimate relationship between ligaments and marginal specialized cells in the snake spinal cord indicative of a CNS mechanoreceptor? *Brain Res.*, **328**:145–149.

Selverston, A. I. and M. Moulins (1985). Oscillatory neural networks. *Ann. Rev. Physiol.*, **47**:29–48.

Shik, M. L. and G. N. Orlovsky (1976). Neurophysiology of locomotor automatism. *Physiol. Rev.*, **56**:465–501.

Sigvardt, K. A., and S. Grillner (1981). Spinal neuronal activity during fictive locomotion in the lamprey. *Soc. Neurosci.*, **7**:362.

Sigvardt, K. A., S. Grillner, P. Wallén, and P. A. M. van Dongen (1985). Activation of NMDA receptors elicits fictive locomotion and bistable membrane properties in the lamprey spinal cord. *Brain Res.*, **336**:390–395.

Stehouwer, D. J. and P. B. Farel (1980). Central and peripheral controls of swimming in anuran larvae. *Brain Res.*, **195**:323–335.

Stein, P. S. G. (1978). Motor systems, with special reference to the control of locomotion. *Ann. Rev. Neurosci.*, **1**:61–81.

Stein, P. S. G. (1983). The vertebrate scratch reflex. *Symp. Soc. Exp. Biol.*, **37**:383–403.

Steiner, I. (1886). Über das Centralnervensystem der grünen Eidechse, nebst weiteren Untersuchungen über das des Haifisches. *Sitzungsberichten der K. Preuss. Akad. Wissensch.*, **32**:539–543.

Tang, D. and M. E. Selzer (1979). Projections of lamprey spinal neurons determined by the retrograde axon transport of horseradish peroxidase. *J. Comp. Neurol.*, **188**:629–645.

Van Dongen, P. A. M., S. Grillner, and T. Hökfelt (1986). 5-Hydroxytryptamine (serotonin) causes a reduction in the afterhyperpolarization following the action potential in lamprey motoneurons and premotor interneurons. *Brain Res.*, **366**:320–325.

Van Dongen, P. A. M., T. Hökfelt, S. Grillner, A. A. J. Verhofstad, and A. W. M. Steinbusch (1985a). Possible target neurons of 5-HT fibres in the lamprey spinal cord: immunohistochemistry combined with intracellular staining with Lucifer yellow. *J. Comp. Neurol.*, **234**:523–535.

Van Dongen, P. A. M., T. Hökfelt, S. Grillner, A. A. J. Verhofstad, H. W. M. Steinbusch, A. C. Cuello, and L. Terenius (1985b). Immunohistochemical demonstration of some putative neurotransmitters in the lamprey spinal cord and spinal ganglia: 5-hydroxytryptamine-, tachykinin-, and neuropeptide-Y-immunoreactive neurons and fibers. *J. Comp. Neurol.*, **234**:501–522.

Wald, U., M. E. Selzer, and N. R. Krieger (1981). Glutamic acid decarboxylase in sea lamprey (*Petromyzon marinus*): characterization, localization and developmental changes. *J. Neurochem.*, **36**: 363–368.

Wallén, P. (1980). On the mechanisms of a phase dependent reflex occurring during locomotion in dogfish. *Exp. Brain Res.*, **39**:193–202.

Wallén, P., J. Buchanan, S. Grillner, and T. Hökfelt (1986). 5-HT modifies frequency regulation and inherent membrane potential oscillations in lamprey neurons. *Abstr. 1st International Congress of Neuroethology,* Tokyo, Japan.

Wallén, P., P. Grafe, and S. Grillner (1984). Phasic variations of extracellular potassium during fictive swimming in the lamprey spinal cord in vitro. *Acta Physiol. Scand.,* **120,**457–463.

Wallén, P. and S. Grillner (1985). The effects of current passage on NMDA induced, TTX resistant membrane potential oscillations in lamprey neurons active during locomotion. *Neurosci. Lett.,* **56:**87–93.

Wallén, P. and S. Grillner (1987). N-methyl-D-aspartate receptor-induced, inherent oscillatory activity in neurons active during fictive locomotion in the lamprey. *J. Neurosci.,* in press.

Wallén, P., S. Grillner, J. L. Feldman, and S. Bergelt (1985). Dorsal and ventral myotome motoneurons and their input during fictive locomotion in lamprey. *J. Neurosci.,* **5:**654–661.

Wallén, P. and A. Lansner (1984). Do the motoneurons constitute a part of the spinal network generating the swimming rhythm in the lamprey? *J. Exp. Biol.,* **113:**493–497.

Wallén, P. and T. L. Williams (1984). Fictive locomotion in the lamprey spinal cord in vitro compared with swimming in the intact and spinal animal. *J. Physiol.,* **347:**225–239.

Watkins, J. C. (1981). Pharmacology of excitatory amino acid transmitters. In *Amino Acid Neurotransmitters,* F. V. DeFeudis and P. Mandel, eds. Raven Press, New York, pp. 205–212.

Williams, B. J., M. H. Droge, K. Hester, and R. B. Leonard (1981). Induction of swimming in the high spinal stingray by L-DOPA. *Brain Res.,* **220:**208–213.

Williams T. L. (1986). Mechanical neural patterns underlying swimming by lateral undulations: Review of studies on fish, amphibia and lamprey. In *Neurobiology of Vertebrate Locomotion,* S. Grillner, P. S. G. Stein, D. Stuart, H. Forssberg, and R. Herman, eds. Macmillan, London, pp. 141–156.

Chapter Two

THE GENERATION OF MASTICATION BY THE MAMMALIAN CENTRAL NERVOUS SYSTEM

JAMES P. LUND
SUMIO ENOMOTO

Center for Research in Neurological Sciences
Department of Stomatology, Faculty of Dental Medicine
University of Montreal
Montreal, Quebec, Canada

1 INTRODUCTION

Like locomotion and respiration, the system controlling mastication is based on a central pattern generator. It is an intermittent rhythmical act like locomotion, but the need to synchronously control bilateral structures (mandible, lips, and tongue), in a cycle in which the pattern of muscular activity is different in the two major phases, makes the system somewhat similar to respiration. The musculoskeletal system of the jaws is so related to diet, and, thus, to an animal's ecological niche, that it is a major determinant of phylogeny, and each phylum has developed characteristic forms of mastication.

In order to efficiently accomplish the gathering and preparation of different classes of food, the mammalian dentition has differentiated and evolved along several lines. The anterior teeth have become specialized for food procurement, while the posterior teeth have developed features useful for food preparation that are dependent on diet. In turn, the shape of the teeth governs, in part, the form of the masticatory movements: for instance, the long interlocking canine teeth of adult male monkeys limit the lateral movements of the mandible. Another determining factor is the shape of the two temporomandibular joints. When the socket is flat and loose, the mandibular condyles are free to swing and slide, as they do in most herbivores. On the other hand, deep, tight cylindrical sockets, that are typical of the cat and other carnivores, force the mandible to swing about a fulcrum passing through the two joints.

The general plan of the mammalian masticatory musculature is directly derived from a more primitive reptilian model that was primarily used for the procurement of food (Turnbull, 1970). It is based upon three distinct groups of jaw closing muscles—the temporalis group, the masseter group, and the pterygoid group—and one jaw opening group—the digastric—as shown in Figure 1. The major adaptive types of masticatory systems have been classified by Turnbull (1970), in a way which differs only slightly from other workers (eg., Schumacher, 1980).

2 THE CLASSIFICATION OF MASTICATORY SYSTEMS

1. *Generalized Group* The jaws, teeth, and muscles of this group, which includes marsupials, primitive eutherian mammals, primates, and man, have diverged least from the reptilian model. The teeth are numerous and relatively unspecialized; the temporalis is the dominant muscle, and movement of the jaw is restricted laterally. We have descriptions of the movements of mastication of one primitive member of this group, the opossum (Hiiemae, 1976), as well as the macaque monkey (Luschei and Goodwin, 1974), and man (Ahlgren, 1976; Moller, 1966; Hannam et al., 1977).

2. *Specialized Group I, carnivore-shear or scissors type.* The anterior teeth of this group are specialized for the seizing of prey, while the premolars and molars slide past one another to shear meat into pieces that are often swallowed with little processing. The temporomandibular joints act as simple hinges, around which the dominant temporalis and powerful masseters swing the mandible closed. Much of our knowledge of the control of jaw movement comes form one member of this group, the domestic cat. Gorniak and Gans (1980) and Thexton et al. (1980) have analyzed the masticatory movements in detail.

3. *Specialized Group II, ungulate-grinding or mill type.* The anterior teeth of this group have become specialized for the cropping of forage, which is then transported by the tongue to the crested or lophed posterior teeth. These have evolved so that fibrous plant foods can be efficiently broken down by three types of masticatory strokes: the vertical, the side-to-side

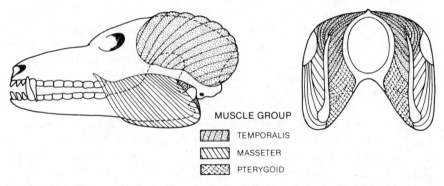

FIGURE 1. A diagram of lateral and cross-sectional views of the basic plan of the masticatory apparatus, redrawn from Turnbull (1970). The three major jaw closing muscle groups are shown.

milling movement characteristic of this group, and a less-developed movement using an anterior-posterior slide. The temporalis muscles are small, while the masseter gorup is highly developed and specialized for lateral grinding. De Vree and Gans (1976) have carried out an EMG study of one member of the group, the pigmy goat.

4. *Specialized Group III, rodent-gnawing or anterior shift type.* This group, which includes rodents and lagomorphs (rabbits and hares), has a jaw that operates in two different positions. Most of the anterior teeth are lost, and the incisors that remain are chisel-shaped. Behind these is a distinctive gap (diastema). When the jaw is protruded for gnawing, the posterior teeth are disengaged; when it is retruded for milling on the posterior teeth, the incisors are taken out of function. So that this can occur, the joint is modified to allow the long anterior-posterior slide. Some species grind on the molar teeth using a combination of vertical and lateral movements; others use horizontal and anterior-posterior strokes. The temporalis muscles are the smallest of all groups, while the masseter muscles have evolved into complex, many-layered structures. The mastication of the rat (Weijs and Datuma, 1975), hamster (Gorniac, 1977), guinea pig (Byrd, 1981), and the rabbit (Weijs and Dantuma, 1981), have been described in detail.

3   A DESCRIPTION OF MASTICATION

With the exception of the first few strokes following ingestion, and those that precede swallowing, the pattern of mastication of individual animals and species has been considered to be stereotyped (Luschei and Goodwin, 1974; Luschei and Goldberg, 1981; Weijs and Dantuma, 1981). However, just as the pattern of locomotion depends on the terrain, there are differences in the form of the cycle that are related to the texture and size of the food particles (Luschei and Goodwin, 1974; Thexton et al., 1980). It is presumably because of this that the form of the cycle gradually changes from the time that the food is ingested until it is swallowed. However, if we create conditions comparable to walking on a treadmill by using a substance that does not change in size or texture, such as chewing gum, then the movements can be very regular (A. G. Hannam, personal communication).

Animals of the Generalized Group and Specialized Group II (Crompton and Hiiemae, 1970; Hiiamae and Kay, 1973; Luschei and Goodwin, 1974; Herring and Scapino, 1973; Ahlgren, 1976) use two forms of mastication. The first, called "chopping" by Ahlgren (1966) and "puncture-crushing" by Hiiemae and Crompton (1971), is used at the start of feeding to bite off large pieces of food with the cheek teeth and to reduce them in size. These movements are followed by a sequence of cycles of more regular form that are called "chewing" (Hiiemae, 1978). If the food is already in lumps that can be picked up with the incisors, these are tossed back to the cheek teeth with a movement of the head. The food is then chewed between the molar and premolar teeth until it is ready for swallowing. Food is shifted from one side of the mouth to the other by movements of the head and tongue. Almost all animals chew on one side at a time (called the working side), but shift the bolus from one side to another every few strokes. Unlike primitive man, most modern humans have a preferred working side, and rarely chew on the other, the balancing side. In contrast, some species such as rats can chew on both sides at once (Hiiemae and Ardran, 1968, Weijs and Dantuma, 1975).

3.1 The Chewing Cycle

Despite the fact that many descriptions of the movements of mastication have been published for a number of species (Hiiemae, 1976, 1978), no universal nomenclature for the phases of the cycle has been accepted. Luschei and Goldberg (1981) suggested that we use the terminology that Hiiemae proposed (1976, 1978), because it has the advantages of simplicity and applicability to all species that have been studied. Hiiemae defined the start of the masticatory cycle as the point of maximum jaw opening, and divided it into three phases, which are: the closing stroke, the power stroke, and the opening stroke. However, another manner of dividing the chewing cycle is needed to describe alterations in the structure of the cycle, such as those that occur when the food is changed (e.g., Thexton, et al., 1980). To fill this need, Hiiemae (1976, 1978) divided the cycle into fast closing (FC), slow closing (SC), slow opening (SO) and fast opening (FO) phases. Although this is a useful nomenclature, we believe that it can be improved. First of all, the SO phase defined by Hiiemae is sometimes made up of two parts, as she indicates in some of her figures (Hiiemae 1978, Fig. 3). When the cycle is long, the initial opening is followed by a

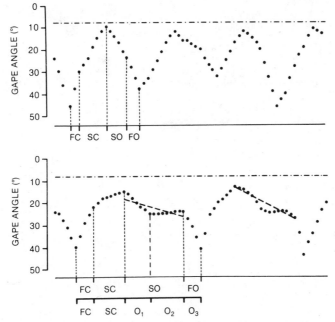

FIGURE 2. This data has been redrawn from Thexton et al. (1970). It shows the gape angle of the mandible of an awake cat chewing cooked liver measured from cineradiographs. The two series of cycles were recorded at different times during a single sequence of movements. Thexton et al. divided the cycles into four phases (FC, SC, SO, FO), and calculated a mean velocity during SO (broken line). We suggest that there are three opening phases, as shown below.

phase in which the mandible is almost stationary. This is illustrated in the lower part of Figure 2 that uses data taken from Thexton et al. (1980), and in an example of mastication in the lightly anesthetised rabbit (Fig. 3A and 3B). Since, at least in the rabbit (Fig. 3B), the instantaneous velocity in the "slow opening" phase can be higher than in "fast opening", these terms are not universally applicable. Instead, we suggest a system of nomenclature analogous to the one used for locomotion to divide the period of extension. Thus, the initial phase of opening becomes O_1, the second, O_2, and the late phase, O_3 (Fig. 2). We suggest the term "transition phase" for the O_2 component because, when there are long pauses in a sequence of chewing cycles, these always occur at this phase of the cycle. Then, the new masticatory cycle starts with a digastric burst at the end of the transition phase and ends with the following one.

A comparison of the parameters of movement gives more support to the idea that the masticatory cycle begins and ends in O_2 and not at the point of maximum opening. Thexton et al. (1980) have shown that the velocity of opening, maximum gape and the velocity of closure co-vary in the cat.

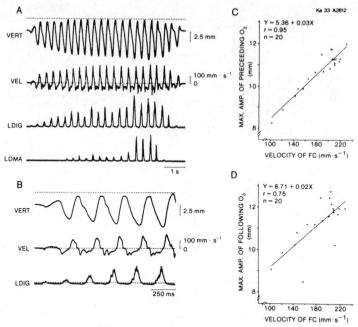

FIGURE 3. Data reanalyzed from study of Olsson et al. (1986). The records come from a lightly anesthetized rabbit chewing on a rubber tube. The full sequence of vertical movements is shown in A, together with the velocity and integrated activity of the digastric and deep masseter muscles of the left side. The first five cycles have been expanded in B. In C and D, we have graphed the maximum velocity recorded in FC against the maximum amplitude of the preceeding and following $O3$.

This is also true in the monkey (Lund and Lamarre, 1974) and in the rabbit, where we can show in addition, that the maximum velocity of FC is more closely related to the preceding O_3 than to the one that follows (Figure 3C).

3.2 Muscle Activity

Jaw opening in the rabbit is begun by the balancing-side lateral pterygoid, followed by the digastrics and geniohyoid muscles (Weijs and Dantuma, 1981), although when the movements are very slow, the initial fall of the jaw in O_1 is probably passive, since no muscles are active at this time. The form and action of the lateral pterygoid is very dependent on the species. In the cat, it is a single muscle that is only active during closure (Gorniak and Gans, 1980). The lateral pterygoid of man and monkeys has two well-defined bellies, and it is only the inferior that initiates opening (Grant, 1973; McNamara, 1973). The superior belly is active in closure, when it appears to retard posterior displacement of the mandibular condyle (Luschei and Goodwin, 1974).

Closure of the mandible in the cat starts with a simultaneous contraction of both zygomaticotemporal muscles (the deepest layer of the masseter complex) and the other major closing muscles are recruited early in FC. There is a slight horizontal swing of the mandible in this phase towards the working side that is brought about by asymmetrical activity in some of the pairs of closing muscles. The deep temporalis on the working side and the medial pterygoid on the balancing side are more active than their contralateral homologues (Gorniak and Gans, 1980). Similarly, the wide lateral swing to the working side that characterizes chewing in species like the rabbit is caused by bilateral asymmetry in muscle activity. Furthermore, Weijs and Dantuma (1981) showed that there appears to be independent control of the recruitment of the compartments of the multipinnate masseter. The superficial layer of the balancing side is first active, and this is followed by the recruitment of deeper and deeper layers. The layers of the working-side masseter are recruited in the opposite sequence. Although no data exists, it is probable that the compartments of the medial pterygoid muscle are similarly controlled.

Thexton et al. (1980) saw on their cineradiographs that FC appeared to end when the teeth came in contact with the food bolus, and it is presumably the resistance of the food to compression that reduces the velocity of closure in the SC phase. The contraction of the closer muscles builds in the first half of SC (Gorniak and Gans, 1980: Weijs and Dantuma, 1981). Records of periodontal receptor firing in rabbits confirm that pressure begins to be applied to the teeth at the transition from FC to SC, and that it increases in the first half of SC (Appenteng et al., 1982). When mastication is produced by electrical stimulation of the cerebral cortex with the mouth empty, FC continues until the upper and lower teeth contact (Lund et al., 1984).

3.3   Variations in Movement Pattern

The number of cycles needed by cats to prepare the food bolus for swallowing and, to a lesser extent, cycle duration, increase with the size and toughness of the pieces of food consumed (Thexton et al., 1980). These authors showed that the duration of the parts of the cycle that they define as SO (O_1 and O_2) is more closely related to cycle duration than is that of the other phases (Thexton et al., 1980). It seems from their data (Fig. 2) and from our data on rabbits (Fig. 3B) that O_1 changes immediately into O_3 when the cycle time is short. O_2 only appears when the cycle duration is long and, in the natural situation, it may be present to allow more time for food manipulation.

After analysing the mandibular movements that an awake rabbit makes when eating chow, we have found that the cycles at the start, middle, and end of the sequence have different characteristics. Figure 4 shows that the initial movements of the sequence (perhaps corresponding to "puncture-

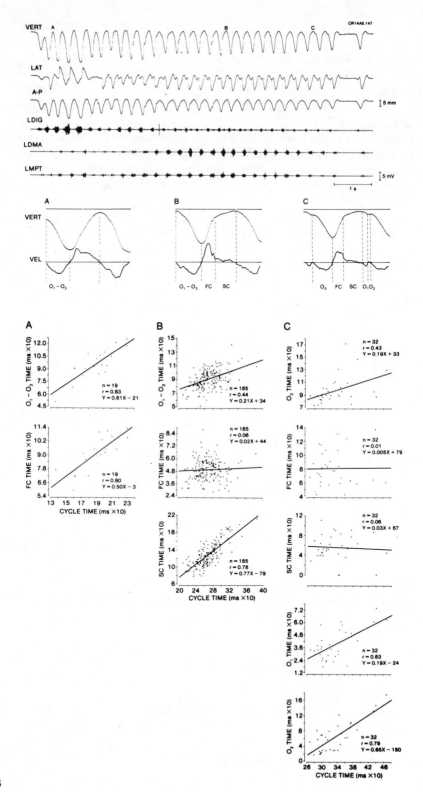

48

crushing" in other animals) are simple in form. They are made up of a single opening phase O_1–O_3 and a fast closing phase (FC), and the duration of both of these varies with cycle duration. As the food is broken up, the SC phase develops, and its length becomes the major determinant of cycle duration in the middle of the sequence. Finally, the opening phase breaks down into its three components late in the sequence, and it is the transition phase, O_2, that lengthens most when the cycle duration increases.

4   THE CONTROL OF MASTICATION

Mastication is one of the types of rhythmical movements that are made by the coordinated action of masticatory, facial, lingual, neck, and supra- and infra-hyoid muscles. It can be distinguished on sight from respiration, lapping, sucking, and swallowing, but there have been no attempts to define the common elements in these patterns. Several writers have speculated that, as the teeth erupt, the masticatory pattern generator may develop from circuits that pattern sucking or lapping (e.g., Dellow, 1969, 1976).

The facial, tongue, and jaw muscles are coupled differently in the three patterns (for instance, the orbicularis oris relaxes during jaw opening in mastication, but contracts during sucking). Clearly, the power stroke of the jaw is in the opening direction during sucking and in the closing direction during mastication. Furthermore, even if it is entirely separate, the masticatory central pattern generator (CPG) must be linked to the swallowing and respiratory centers because the two rhythms become entrained.

The role of sensory inputs in the control of mastication is discussed in the chapter by Rossignol et al. in this book. The rest of this chapter will summarize what is known about the many areas of the brain that have been implicated in the control of mastication. Under normal conditions, they probably act in concert. However, this last point is difficult to verify with classic anatomical and physiological methods. One study that does support the concept was published by Goldberg et al. (1980). The authors stimulated the masticatory area of the motor cortex (see below) at low frequency for 45 min. after an injection of [^{14}C]- or [^{3}H]deoxyglucose. Auto-

---

FIGURE 4. Jaw movements and EMG activity were recorded from an awake rabbit during mastication (top). Note the change in the pattern of movement as the series progresses. The sections labeled A, B, and C have been expanded (bottom), and the phases of the cycle have been identified. The graphs show the relationships between phase and cycle duration for the three types of cycles. (Schwartz, Enomoto and Lund, unpublished data.)

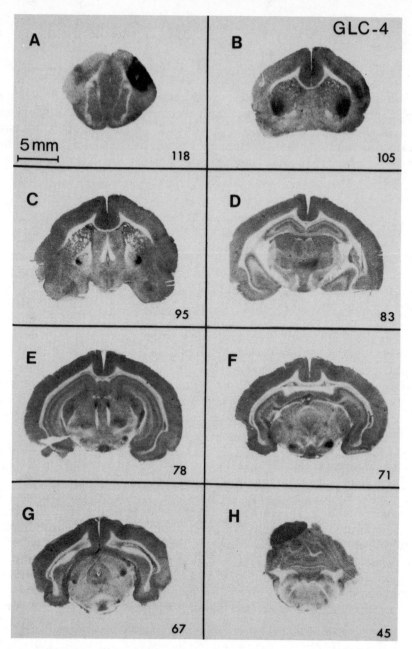

FIGURE 5. Photographs of eight levels of the brain of a guinea pig in which the motor cortex was stimulated after injecting [³H] deoxyglucose. A shows the increased levels of metabolic activity (black) surrounding the stimulation site on the left, and in the contralateral cortex. The striatum (B), globus pallidus (C), pars reticulata of the substantia nigra (E and F), and the lateral part of the deep layer of the superior colliculus (G) were labeled on both sides, while the thalamus was labeled ipsilaterally (D). No cell groups in the brain stem showed an increase in deoxyglucose uptake apart from the trigeminal nuclei (e.g., H). (Data from Goldberg et al., 1980.)

radiographs of serial sections of the whole brain were developed. Areas of high metabolic activity take up large amounts of deoxyglucose and these show up as dark areas on the film. The area surrounding the stimulating electrode and a contralateral mirror focus increased their metabolism, as did parts of a number of subcortical structures. These included the striatum, globus pallidus, the pars reticulata of the substantia nigra, subthalamic nucleus, red nucleus, the deep layers of the superior colliculus and a pretectal nucleus (Fig. 5). The labeling was bilateral. In addition, a ventral region of the thalamus was labeled ipsilaterally.

There is other evidence linking these areas to the control of orofacial movements. First, the labeled area of the putamen corresponds to that which receives an input from the anterolateral orofacial region of the cortex in the rat (Webster, 1961). There is somatotopic orofacial representation in the putamen and pallidum of cats and monkeys (Lidsky et al., 1978; Schneider and Lidsky, 1981; Liles, 1979; Neafsey et al., 1978; Crutcher and Delong, 1984a) and neurons in the putamen, pallidum, and substantia nigra, pars reticulata discharge during ingestive movements (Lidsky et al., 1975; Soltysik et al., 1975; Delong et al., 1983; Mora et al., 1977; Nishino et al., 1985; Schultz, 1986), but no attempts were made by the authors to relate neural activity to the pattern of movement. Mastication has been produced by stimulation of the striatum of the rabbit (Lund and Dellow, 1971), but without contrary evidence, it is safest to assume that the effects were due to the excitation of corticobulbar fibers of passage. The dorsomedial segment of the red nucleus that was labeled with deoxyglucose may be the site of origin of trigeminorubral fibers (Edwards, 1972), while the tectal layer may be the site of termination of nigrotectal projection described by Graybiel (1978) in the cat.

In addition to the regions that increase metabolism when the cortex is stimulated, there are several limbic areas that must activate the CPG, because repetitive stimulation of the lateral amygdaloid nucleus (Kawamura and Tsukamoto, 1960; Nakamura and Kubo, 1978), lateral hypothalamus, anterior commissure (Lund and Dellow, 1973), and lateral habenular nucleus (Lund, unpublished observations) causes mastication.

Presumably through its actions on the striatum, apomorphine causes rhythmical jaw movements in guinea pigs that are different from those that arise spontaneously under ketamine anesthesia (Lambert et al., 1986). It is interesting that these are stopped by lesions of the superior colliculus, whereas cortically evoked mastication continues (Chandler and Goldberg, 1984).

4.1 The Brain Stem

Nevertheless, just as in respiration, only the brain stem is essential for mastication. Bazett and Penfield (1922) were the first to show this conclusively. They decerebrated cats above the pons and kept them alive for up to three weeks. These animals not only swallowed, but chewed food if it was inserted into the back of the mouth. Other people have shown that the basic movements of the jaw, and the accompanying coordinated action of the tongue and lips of decerebrate animals, occur in response to sensory inputs, and to the electrical stimulation of the corticobulbar tracts or sites in the mesencephalic reticular formation close to the locomotor region (Miller, 1920; Bremer, 1923; Lund and Dellow, 1971; Dellow and Lund, 1971; Sumi, 1971; Nozaki et al., 1986b).

Like the other movements discussed in this book, the basic rhythm can be generated without sensory feedback (Sumi, 1970; Dellow and Lund, 1971; Lund and Dellow, 1973; Nakamura et al., 1976). The fictive movements that have been studied were most commonly produced by electrical stimulation of the CNS, although the patterns of activity that arise upon stimulating the mouth, or spontaneously during ketamine anaesthesia, have been studied (Lund and Dellow, 1973; Goldberg and Tal, 1978; Chandler and Goldberg, 1982).

There are many similarities between the movements and the fictive motor pattern. When mastication is evoked by repetitive stimulation of the corticobulbar pathways, there is a gradual increase in mylohyoid nerve activity (supplying the mylohyoid and digastric muscles) that terminates in the first burst of the sequence. Tonic activity in the masseteric nerve is inhibited concurrently: thereafter, activity alternates in the two nerves, and this is not changed by paralysis (Dellow and Lund, 1971; Lund, 1976). Similarly, there are two groups of rhythmically active tongue motoneurons in the hypoglossal nucleus, one that fires during jaw opening, the other during jaw closing, and no changes occur in the pattern when the rabbits are paralysed (Sumi, 1970). Dellow and Lund (1971) proved that the basic masticatory pattern was centrally generated by eliminating all other hypotheses. They isolated the brain stem by severing the spinal cord, brachial and cervical nerves to remove all afferent inputs from unblocked intrafusal muscle fibers, vascular or respiratory mechanoreceptors. In addition, they showed that the timing was not provided by rhythmical changes in vascular or respiratory pressure waves in the brain stem. Finally, they proved that the constant frequency of trigeminal and hypoglossal motoneuron bursts was not due to regularity in the input by stimulating the corticobulbar tracts with trains of shocks of random frequency.

Nevertheless, the masticatory cycle time depends on input parameters. As the mean stimulus frequency is raised from threshold, the frequency of movement, and of trigeminal motoneuron bursts, rises rapidly to reach a maximum of 4–5 Hz in the rabbit (Dellow and Lund, 1971) and close to 2 Hz in the cat (Nakamura et al., 1976). Raising the stimulus voltage causes a small increase in this maximum output frequency (Dellow and Lund, 1971). Although this is not changed by paralysis, (Dellow and Lund, 1971), it can be increased by tonic stretch of the jaw closing muscles, which also raises the amplitude of the masseteric nerve bursts (Nakamura et al., 1976).

Mastication can also be produced by inflating a small balloon between the tongue and hard palate of the rabbit (Lund and Dellow, 1971), and the rhythmical activity evoked in the hypoglossal nerve by this stimulus, or by tonic pressure applied to the anterior hard palate, persist after paralysis (Lund and Dellow, 1973; Juch et al., 1985). Subthreshold central and peripheral stimuli sum to produce movements or fictive rhythmical activity (Lund and Dellow, 1973).

4.2 Motoneurons

The slow membrane potential fluctuations that produce the rhythmical activity of trigeminal motoneurons have been studied during fictive mastication in the cat and guinea pig. First of all, these studies show that the slow potentials in digastric and masseteric motoneurons are not mirror images. The digastric motoneurons of the cat fire bursts 150–300 ms long, that contain up to 30 spikes at frequencies of 30–250 Hz (Kubo et al., 1981). In both species, the action potentials are superimposed on rhythmical depolarizing waves that fall to resting levels in the jaw closing phase of the cycle (Nakamura and Kubo, 1978; Nakamura et al., 1978; Kubo et al., 1981; Goldberg et al., 1982; Figure 6A). Hypoglossal motoneurons behave similarly (Sahara et al., 1983). In contrast, the dominant feature of the records from masseter motoneurons are the large hyperpolarizing potentials that

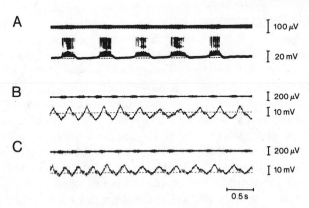

FIGURE 6. Rhythmical digastric nerve activity (upper traces) and intracellular potentials induced in digastric (A) and masseter motoneurons (B,C), by repetitive stimulation of the cortical masticatory area of the paralysed cat. B and C were recorded from the same neuron before (B) and after an intravenous injection of strychnine nitrate. The broken line represents the resting membrane potential preceding stimulation. (Data modified from (A) Kubo et al. (1981) and Enomoto et al. (1987) Neurosci. Res. 4:396–412.

occur during the jaw opening phase. They are probably axosomatic IPSPs because they are easily reversed by intracellular Cl^- injections (Nakamura and Kubo, 1978; Chandler and Goldberg, 1982). The rhythmical IPSPs alternate with depolarizing potentials that are usually too small to cause firing (Fig. 6B). Nevertheless, when the masseteric motoneurons do discharge, they fire as many as 10 action potentials/cycle, at frequencies of up to 60 Hz (Nakamura and Kubo, 1978; Kubo et al., 1981), and, when sensory feedback is added, they seem to be capable of discharging at higher rates (Goldberg and Tal, 1978).

Neither the suprahyoid nor tongue muscles contain significant numbers of muscle spindles (for refs., see Rossignol et al., this book), so the lack of rhythmical inhibition of digastric and hypoglossal motoneurons supports Sears (1964) hypothesis, developed for respiration, that the inhibition serves to inhibit the stretch reflex (Nakamura et al., 1980; Goldberg and Chandler, 1981). Because they are not hyperpolarized, digastric motoneurons are able to participate in the protective jaw opening reflex response to the stimulation of high threshold afferents during jaw closing (Lund et al., 1981; Lund and Olsson, 1983; Rossignol et al., this book).

When mastication is caused by stimulation of the lowest threshold sites in the guinea pig cortex, the digastric depolarizing potential contains EPSP subunits that follow each cortical shock at a latency of about 8 ms. The concurrent hyperpolarizing wave in the jaw closing motoneurons also contains stimulus-linked IPSP subunits, and both of the subunits wax and wane cyclically (Goldberg et al., 1982; Chandler and Goldberg, 1982). On the basis of these data, Chandler and Goldberg (1982) have suggested that masticatory pattern generation is fundamentally different from that of locomotion and respiration. In their model, they postulate that cortical stimulation activates the CPG and short-latency pathways at the same time. This is undoubtedly true. However, the second proposition, that the CPG only modulates the interneurons on the corticobulbar pathway, and has no other means of controlling the motoneurons, does not seem to be tenable for the following reasons. First, if one stimulates the part of the cortical masticatory area that overlaps the jaw motor area, then the EMG pattern is dominated by stimulus-linked activity; however, this component fades when the site of stimulation is shifted to the posterolateral part of the masticatory cortex, showing that the CPG must have other ports of access to the motoneurons (Lund et al., 1984). Second, Enomoto et al. (1986) have found that some rhythmical hyperpolarization of masseteric motoneurons persists after short-latency cortical and trigeminal nerve IPSPs have been blocked by the glycine antagonist, strychnine (Fig. 6C). The residual rhythmical component was sensitive to tetanus toxin.

Both Enomoto et al. (1986), and Chandler et al., (1985b), showed that the production of the basic rhythm of mastication is not dependent on glycine, although both glycine and serotonin may play a role in controlling EMG burst duration and amplitude (Chandler et al., 1985a and b).

4.3   Premotor Neurons

The areas of origin of the corticobulbar pathways, and sites at which they terminate in the trigeminal and reticular nuclei, have been described recently (Landgren and Olsson 1980; Travers and Norgren, 1983; Yasui et al., 1985). It is enough to mention that axons from sensory and motor cortex terminate in the Vth main sensory nucleus, supra- and intertrigeminal areas, and all subdividions of the spinal trigeminal nucleus and adjacent reticular formation (Kawana and Kusama, 1968; Kuypers, 1958a and b; Wold and Brodal, 1973; Mizuno et al., 1968; Dunn and Tolbert, 1982; Tashiro et al., 1983; Travers and Norgren, 1983; Yasui et al., 1985). Additionally, some areas of the medial pontomedullary reticular formation receive fibers from the masticatory area of the cat's orbital cortex (Yasui et al., 1985). Neurons in all these areas respond at short latency to cortical and peripheral nerve stimulation (Darian-Smith and Yokota, 1966; Limanskii and Gura, 1969; Porter, 1967; Nozaki et al., 1983; Sessle et al., 1981; Landgren and Olsson, 1983; Olsson et al., 1986). Although many of these cortical inputs may control sensory transmission rather than mastication (Sessle et al., 1981; Kim et al., 1986), all the nuclei receiving them project to the Vth, VIIth, and XIIth motor nuclei (Holstege and Kuypers, 1977; Holstege et al., 1977; Mizuno et al., 1983, Landgren et al., 1984; Nozaki et al., 1983; Sahara et al., 1983).

Trigeminal interneurons have never been carefully classified, but it seems that some components that are prominent in the spinal cord are missing in the brain stem. For instance, there is no evidence that trigeminal, facial, or hypoglossal motoneurons have recurrent collaterals (Cajal, 1911; Lorente de No, 1933), and they do not show signs of recurrent or reciprocal inhibiton (Kidokoro et al., 1968; Porter, 1965). Consequently, Renshaw cells, 1A inhibitory interneurons, or their equivalents are unlikely to exist in these motor nuclei. Interneurons in the supratrigeminal nucleus, which probably cause inhibition of masseteric motoneurons during the jaw opening reflex (Kidokoro et al., 1968b; Goldberg and Nakamura, 1968; Nakamura et al., 1973, 1978), are not active during fictive mastication (Kubo et al., 1981). Similarly, neurons in the intertrigeminal area, main sensory trigeminal nucleus, nucleus oralis, and medullary dorsal horn, do not fire rhythmically during mastication unless their receptive fields are stimulated, despite the fact that their responses to peripheral or cortical inputs are modulated by the CPG (Olsson et al., 1986; Kim et al., 1986). Therefore, it seems unlikely that corticobulbar interneurons, or those interneurons on the reflex pathways, are essential to rhythm generation.

4.4   The Site of Pattern Generation

Recording unit activity in awake cats (Nakamura et al., 1980, 1982) and lesioning or isolating small areas of the brain stem of guinea pigs (Nozaki

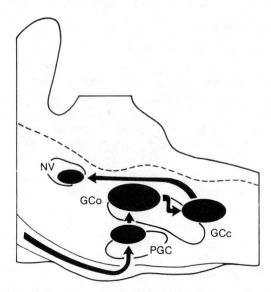

FIGURE 7. Schematic diagram showing the input from the pyramidal tract to the cell groups of the medulla that elaborate the masticatory rhythm. Redrawn from Nakamura (1985). PGC, n. reticularis paragigantocellularis; GCo, n. gigantocellularis, pars oralis; GCc, n. gigantocellularis, pars caudalis.

et al., 1986a and b), has helped to identify those parts of the brain stem that seem to be essential for pattern generation. The structures required for the induction of rhythmical activity in trigeminal motoneurons by pyramidal tract stimulation seem to be the medial bulbar reticular formation and the parts of the pons containing the trigeminal nuclei. Figure 7 summarizes the connections proposed by Nakamura (1986), on the basis of these experiments. When mastication is induced by stimulation of the cerebral cortex, the pyramidal tract is the only input of importance to the brain stem, because unilateral section of this pathway abolishes the action of the ipsilateral cortex. The corticobulbar input activates neurons in the most dorsal part of N. reticularis paragigantocellularis and the overlying region (dPGC), and is strongest in the contralateral side. Injections of HRP into dPCG confirmed the predominance of the contralateral projection (Nozaki et al., 1986b). Repetitive stimulation of dPGC can cause rhythmical motoneuronal firing, and it must be an essential link to the rhythm generating elements, because a lesion of one dPGC blocks the effects of contralateral, but not ipsilateral, cortical stimulation. The neurons of the dPGC appear to induce rhythmical activity in the oral part of N. reticularis gigantocellularis (GCo), which, in turn, entrains neurons in the region dorsolateral to the caudal parts of the same nucleus (dGCc). Finally digastric motoneurons can be monosynaptically excited from dGCc.

Just as in locomotion (Arshavsky et al., 1977; Drew et al., 1986), the output of the CPG is transmitted to the cerebellum by a group of neurons in the lateral reticular nucleus (Marini and Sogiu, 1985), but these seem to be located much further caudally than neurons that are driven by the spinal cord rhythm generators (Drew et al., 1986).

5 THE ROLE OF THE SENSORIMOTOR CORTEX

Ferrier (1886) was the first to show that mastication was represented in the cerebral cortex when he found that repetitive electrical stimulation of the cerebral hemispheres of several species of animal could evoke complex, coordinated rhythmical movements of the jaws.

When defined by electrical stimulation, the masticatory area of humans, monkeys, and cats is separate from the jaw, face, and tongue representations in area 4. It is found at the lateral end of area 6 in man and monkeys and probably extends into area 44 (Beevor and Horsley, 1894; Vogt and Vogt, 1919; Magnus et al., 1952; Foerster, 1931; Lund and Lamarre, 1974); in the cat, it is located at the rostral end of the orbital gyrus (Magoun et al., 1933; Morimoto and Kawamura, 1973; Ward and Clark, 1935; Nakamura et al., 1980), where area 6a meets areas 3b and 43 (Landgren and Olsson, 1980).

Neurons in these areas receive inputs from the oral cavity and other parts of the upper alimentary tract (Lund and Sessle, 1974; Lund and Lamarre, 1974; Landgren, 1957; Landgren and Olsson, 1980). These regions do not project directly to trigeminal, facial, or hypoglossal motoneurons (Walberg, 1957; Kuypers, 1958a et b; Mizuno et al., 1968; Wold and Brodal, 1973) but, nevertheless, macroelectrode stimulation with single pulses or brief trains produces short latency responses in the motoneurons that, at first sight, are the same as those produced by similar stimulation of area 4: excitation of the jaw-opening motoneurons and inhibition of the jaw-closing motoneurons (Hoffman and Luschei, 1980; refs.).

In the monkey, a very discrete representation of the other two groups of muscles directly involved in manipulating the food bolus (the facial and lingual muscles) is revealed by microstimulation of area 4 (Kubota, 1976; McGuinness et al., 1980). However, microstimulation of the adjacent precentral jaw area in awake or sedated monkeys usually produces bilateral effects in several masticatory muscles, the most common of which is inhibition of the closing muscles at latencies as short as 7 ms and activation of the digastric muscles. On rare occasions, one or more jaw-closing muscles are excited (Clark and Luschei, 1974; Hoffman and Luschei, 1980; McGuinness et al., 1980). It seems surprising that this technique yields so little evidence that the jaw muscles are represented as a mosaic, as are other groups of muscles that appear to need a similar degree of voluntary control (Asanuma and Rosen, 1972). To explain this, Hoffman and Luschei (1980) hypothesize that there may be a detailed representation of the jaw closing muscles in area 4, but that this is superimposed upon a widespread and powerful inhibitory system. Presumably, electrical stimulation excites both, and inhibition usually wins. Certainly, the firing pattern of many neurons in area 4 is consistent with the idea that they exert fine control over the jaw-closing muscles (see later). More detail on these effects and those that can be obtained by stimulation of the sensory cortex can be found in reviews by Luschei and Goldberg, (1981), Dubner et al. (1978), and Landgren and Olson (1980).

In species in which the cortex is less differentiated, such as the guinea pig and rabbit, the masticatory area overlaps the jaw area of the traditional motor map (Godlberg et al., 1982; Lund et al., 1984). Repetitive electrical stimulation of the center of the area of superimposition causes short latency (4–7 ms) twitch contractions of both digastric muscles at a threshold that is less than that of mastication, and there appears to be some sites from which the contralateral lateral pterygoid can be concurrently excited (Lambert et al., 1985). Increasing the stimulus intensity gives a pattern of muscular activity that is a combination of rhythmic bursts and short latency effects that follow each stimulus pulse (Chandler & Goldberg, 1982; Lund et al., 1984; Nozaki et al., 1986).

5.1   Rhythmical Movements Produced by Stimulation of the Masticatory Area

Masticatory movements begin with inhibition of postural activity in the closer muscles (Lund et al., 1977; Beaulieu, 1978; Fig. 8). This is also the case when twitch contractions of limb muscles are produced by stimulation of the motor cortex (Gahery and Nieoullon, 1978) and is reminiscent of the postural adjustments that precede voluntary or reflex movements (Massion, 1984). The stimulus threshold for inhibition of closer muscle EMG activity is considerably lower than the threshold for rhythmical movements (Lund et al., 1977). As the stimulus intensity is increased above the threshold for inhibition, the digastric muscles become tonically active: when it is raised again, the digastric activity begins to alternate with bursts in the closer muscles. The sequence ends with the mandible falling to its approximate resting position during O_2.

Ferrier described the movements made by the rabbit, guinea pig, and rat as a "frequently repeated chumping and munching action of the jaws," and many people writing after him have confirmed that the movements evoked in several species, including man, look like natural chewing (see Luschei and Goldberg, 1981 and Lund et al., 1984, for details). In the cat, another pattern of rhythmical movements that look like lapping is given by stimulation of sites just ventral to those giving mastication (Magoun, Ranson, and Fisher, 1933; Morimoto and Kawamura, 1973), and rhythmic

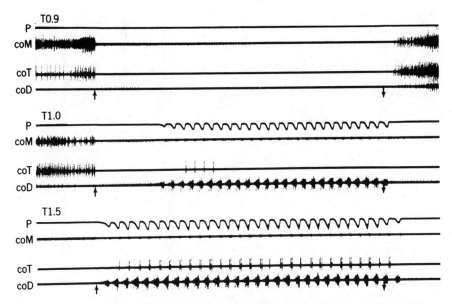

FIGURE 8. Recording of vertical jaw position (P), left masseter (coM), temporalis (coT), and digastric muscles (coD) made while repetitively stimulating the right masticatory area through an electrode implanted in the cortex of an anesthetized rabbit. Ten-second train of shocks, 1 ms in duration at a frequency of 45 Hz, were delivered between the arrows at intensities below (TO.9), above (T1.5) and at the threshold (T1.0) of mastication. (Data rephotographed from Beaulieu, 1978.)

licking and retching have been evoked from other foci (Hess, Akert, and McDonald, 1952). Even within the category of movements that are called mastication, there are slight variations in form that are related to the site of stimulation of the orbital cortex (Morimoto and Kawamura, 1973). This finding confirmed early work on the rabbit (Rethi, 1893; Bremer, 1923).

Bremer (1923) found that there is a cortical representation of the three basic patterns of mastication used by a rabbit: gnawing, vertical mastication, and the ruminatory or milling type of chewing. He obtained the first type by stimulating the most anterior region of the masticatory area of awake animals. The middle part of the area yielded vertical mastication, while the final type of movement was represented posteriorly. These findings were recently extended by Lund et al. (1984), who stimulated the cortex of anesthetized rabbits while recording jaw movement and EMG activity. They also reported that the form of the movements depends on the location of the stimulating electrode, as is shown in Figure 9. They were not able to evoke true gnawing in this preparation and speculated that it may be suppressed by anesthesia. The movements that were produced by threshold stimulation of the most anterior sites were almost entirely the result of rhythmical contractions of the jaw-opening muscles,

KANIN-49

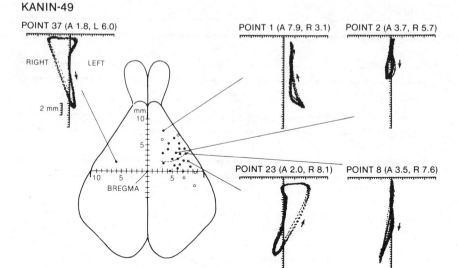

FIGURE 9. Drawing of the cerebral cortex of a rabbit showing all stimulus sites on the right from which mastication could be evoked by repetitive stimulation (filled circles). The dashed line divides the anterior vertical masticatory area from the posterior zone. The envelopes of movement, as seen from in front of the animal, are shown at the right. On the left is an example of movements produced by stimulation of the left cortex. (Figure from Lund et al., 1984.)

although increasing the stimulus intensity caused some increase in closer EMG amplitude. In contrast, the stimulation of posterior sites gave movements in which the mandible swung to the contralateral side during FC and returned to the midline in SC with the molar teeth in contact. During this phase, the sound of grinding teeth was often heard. If a site close to the junction between the two areas was stimulated, the movement changed from vertical mastication to the ruminatory type as the stimulus intensity was increased. This was apparently due to stimulus spread, because the movements evoked from sites rostral or caudal to the border remained true to type when the stimulus voltage was increased, although the frequency and amplitude rose to maxima that were site-dependent. The maximum frequency of vertical masticatory movements (>5 Hz) was greater than that of the grinding movements (<4.5 Hz). The dependency of the frequency of mastication on the intensity and/or frequency of stimulation had already been shown (Kawamura and Tsukamoto, 1960; Sumi, 1969; Dellow and Lund, 1971; Nakamura et al., 1976).

Thus, unlike the midbrain locomotor region, where the change from walking to trotting to galloping depends on stimulus intensity (Shik et al., 1966), there is a *kinesiotopic* representation of the masticatory patterns in the sensorimotor cortex.

5.2   The Effects of Lesions of the Sensorimotor Cortex

The early studies of lesioned and decorticate animals summarized by Bremer (1923) led to very general conclusions because nothing could be measured. Luschei and Goodwin (1975) tried to improve on this by training monkeys in a reaction time biting task before placing lesions in the face area and in the masticatory area. Unilateral lesions caused little impairment, but after bilateral lesions of the face area, the reaction time was prolonged and force control lost or severely compromised. Although these deficits could be reduced by retraining, voluntary control was never completely restored. In contrast, these monkeys could eat immediately after surgery (Larson et al., 1980; Luschei and Goldberg, 1981), but the masticatory movements were smaller than normal in vertical and lateral amplitude, even after many weeks. They tipped their heads back to swallow, as do rabbits without the sensorimotor cortex, perhaps because they have trouble forming a food bolus (Bremer, 1923).

The descriptions of symptoms caused by large bilateral lesions of the masticatory area are confusing. Two series of experiments have been published by Luschei and collaborators (Goodwin and Luschei, 1975; Larson et al., 1981) and comments were made on the results of the first study in the review by Luschei and Goldberg 1981). In the first study, the monkeys had few problems with the voluntary biting task, and we were originally left with the impression that the masticatory area is of little importance in motor control (Goodwin and Luschei, 1975). When the results were discussed again by Luschei and Goldberg (1981), they stated that these monkeys did not eat for several days after surgery and had to be fed with an intragastric tube. Later, the monkeys began to eat softened biscuits and eventually were able to eat normally. The two monkeys described by Larson et al. (1981) seemed to do much better after lesions of the masticatory area. However, nine days after a unilateral lesion in their monkey M, the rate of chewing on the ipsilateral side was lower than normal due to a lengthening of the opening phase by 100–200 ms. Only transient difficulties were reported to have occurred after the lesion on the other side, but the envelope of movement, recorded when chewing on the right 93 days afterwards, looks extremely irregular (Larson et al., 1981; Figure 2).

5.3   The Activity of Neurons of the Face Area During Mastication and Biting

Kubota and Niki (1971) were the first to record from cortical neurons in the jaw and face areas of awake monkeys during mastication. Half the units were related to jaw opening and half to closing, and the increase in firing frequency preceded EMG activity in the muscle. When the load on the muscles was increased, the periods of neural and muscular activity were lengthened, so that, although the firing frequency did not increase, the number of spikes/cycle went up. Perhaps the most interesting finding of

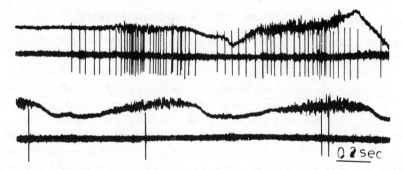

FIGURE 10. Recording of a pyramidal tract neuron from the face area of an awake monkey (lower trace) and the EMG of a digastric muscle (upper trace). This neuron fired strongly during the opening phase of the first two cycles of mastication, but rarely by the eighth and ninth cycles. (Reproduced with permission from Kubota and Niki, 1971.)

this study was that the activity of many neurons was high at the start of a sequence of movements, but fell rapidly as the series progressed (Fig. 10). This was confirmed by Hoffman and Luschei (1980) in their study of voluntary biting. They recorded neurons within a cortical area from which jaw muscle activity could be modified by microstimulation. They were able to confirm an earlier report that neurons here change their activity prior to a conditioned bite (Luschei, Garthwaite, and Armstrong, 1971) and to add the finding that some units increase their firing rate with the biting force. Furthermore, when sinusoidal movements were applied to the bar on the lower teeth, the firing frequency of most neurons was modulated in a way that suggested that they received inputs from muscle spindles or perhaps periodontal pressoreceptors, as do neurons in the corresponding area of the cat (Lund and Sessle, 1974; Landgren and Olsson, 1980). Despite all this evidence of their participation in the control of biting, the patterns of activity of 60% of the task-related neurons, and all of another small group of neurons that discharged during licking, were unrelated to mastication. Even when a neuron did fire in rhythmic bursts during chewing, the relationship between firing frequency and EMG amplitude was reported to be much less consistent than during voluntary biting (Hoffman and Luschei, 1980).

If we take them at their face value, the experiments described above lead to the conclusion that this region of cortex participates in the control of voluntary biting, the manipulation of the food bolus after it is put in the mouth, and in the first movements of mastication (perhaps of the puncture-crush type), but that it contributes little once rhythmical chewing is established. However, just as in locomotion, the motor cortex may have to intervene during mastication if something unforseen happens (finding a bone in the food or an obstacle on the path), or if the food or terrain is unusual (eating toffee or walking on a ladder). Situations analogous to these are being investigated for locomotion (Armstrong, 1987, Drew, personal communication) and need to be for mastication.

5.4   Single Unit Recording in the Masticatory Area

The only relevant study was published by Lund and Lamarre (1974), who recorded in the area while monkeys voluntarily opened their mouths and stuck out their tongues, rhythmically slapped their lips, and chewed. Stimulation of the center of the region caused rhythmical mastication with well-coordinated movements of the lips and tongue, and 75% of the neurons in

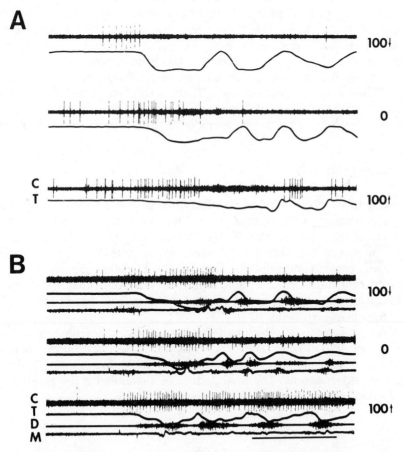

FIGURE 11. The behavior of two neurons in the masticatory area of the cerebral cortex of an awake monkey. The microelectrode record (C) and vertical jaw movement (T) are shown, with the addition of digastric and masseter EMGs in B. Both neurons began to fire before the start of the first voluntary jaw opening movement to receive a liquid reward. They discharged strongly during this movement, but were rarely active during the opening phase of the subsequent rhythmical movements unless these were opposed by a load (100 g). (Modified from Lund and Lamarre, 1974.)

this central area had patterns of activity that were related to the movements. A number, classified as weakly phasic jaw-opening neurons, had properties like the majority of face area neurons; they discharged strongly during voluntary movements, but were weakly related to the rhythmical movements, unless loads were applied to aid or oppose opening (Fig. 11). Another group were more strongly phase-related and, for some of these, firing frequency was correlated to the velocity and displacement of the jaw during opening. Many of them seemed to have an input from the muscle spindles in the closing muscles. The removal of this large population of neurons controlling opening could explain why this phase slows after the cortex was lesioned by Larson et al. (1980). In contrast with the face area, where the majority of phasically related neurons fired during jaw closure (Hoffman and Luschei, 1980), very few neurons in the masticatory area fired preferentially during the early FC phase, although a number were active in SC and appeared to receive inputs from periodontal pressoreceptors. Others that seemed to fire most strongly during movements of the tongue had lingual receptive fields. These results suggested that the masticatory area has a role in initiating movement and in controlling the rhythmical movements using tactile, periodontal, and proprioceptive feedback.

6   CONCLUSIONS

The way in which rhythmical mastication is generated and controlled has much in common with respiration and locomotion. The basic features of the pattern are produced in the brain stem. Inputs from higher centers and from the mouth probably drive neurons in the dorsal part of the nucleus reticularis paragigantocellularis. These connect to other groups of reticular neurons that transform the tonic input into a rhythm, that is then transmitted to several cranial motor nuclei. The details of these processes are only now being worked out.

A repertory of masticatory patterns is spacially represented in the cerebral cortex and in other subcortical structures. Cortical output neurons connect with the pattern generator, directly with motoneurons and with reflex arc interneurons. The final pattern of movement is the result of the interaction of these signals and peripheral feedback.

REFERENCES

Ahlgren, J. (1976). Masticatory movements in man. In *Mastication*, D. J. Anderson adn B. Matthews, eds. John Wright and Sons, Bristol, pp. 119–130.

Appenteng, K., J. P. Lund, and J. J. Seguin (1982). Intraroral mechanoreceptor activity during jaw movement in the anesthetized rabbit. *J. Neurophysiol.*, **48**:27–37.

Armstrong, D. M. (1986).Supraspinal contributions to the initiation and control of locomotion in the cat. *Prog. Neurobiol.*, **26**:273–361.

Armstrong, D. M. (1987). The motor cortex and locomotion in the cat. In *Neurobiology of Vertebrate Locomotion*, S. Grillner, H. Forssberg, P. S. G. Stein, and D. Stewart, eds. Macmillan, London.

Arshavsky, Y. I., I. M. Gelfand, G. N. Orlovsky, and G. A. Pavlova (1978). Messages conveyed by spinocerebellar pathways during scratching in the cat. I. Activity of neurons of the lateral reticular nucleus. *Brain Res.*, **151**:479–491.

Asanuma, H. and I. Rosén (1972). Topographical organization of cortical efferent zones projecting to distal forelimb muscles in the monkey. *Exp. Brain Res.*, **14**:243–256.

Bazett, H. C. and W. G. Penfield (1922). A study of the Sherrington decerebrate animal in the chronic as well as acute condition. *Brain*, **45**:185–265.

Beaulieu, M. (1978). *Etude de la Mastication Rythmique Induite par Stimulation Corticale*. Thesis, Université de Montréal.

Beevor, C. E. and V. Horsley (1894). A further minute analysis by electrical stimulation of the so-called motor region (facial area) of the cortex cerebri in the monkey *(Macacus sinicus)*. *Phil. Trans. Roy. Soc. B.*, **185**:39–81.

Bremer, F. (1923). Physiologie nerveuse de la mastication chez le chat et le lapin. Réflexes de mastication. Réponses masticatrices corticales et centre cortical du gout. *Arch. Int. Physiol.*, **21**:308–352.

Byrd, K. E. (1981). Mandibular movement and muscle activity during mastication in the guinea pig *(Cavia porcellus)*. *J. Morphol.*, **170**:147–169.

Cajal, S. R. Y. (1911). *Histologie du Système Nerveux de l'Homme et des Vertebrés*. Azoulay, L. trans. Maloine, Paris.

Chandler, S. H. and L. J. Goldberg (1984). Differentiation of the neural pathways mediating cortically induced and dopaminergic activation of the central pattern generator (CPG) for rhythmical jaw movements in the anesthetized guinea pig. *Brain Res.*, **323**:297–301.

Chandler, S. H. and L. J. Goldberg (1982). Intracellular analysis of synaptic mechanisms controlling spontaneous and cortically induced rhythmical jaw movements in the guinea pig. *J. Neurophysiol.*, **48**: 126–138.

Chandler, S. H., L. J. Goldberg, and B. Alba (1985). Effects of a serotonin agonist and antagonist on cortically induced rhythmical jaw movements in the anesthetized guinea pig. *Brain Res.* **344**:201–206.

Chandler, S. H., S. A. Nielsen, and L. J. Goldberg (1985). The effects of a glycine antagonist (strychnine) on cortically induced rhythmical jaw movements in the anesthetized guinea pig. *Brain Res.* **325**:181–186.

Clark, R. W. and E. S. Luschei (1974). Short latency jaw movement produced by low intensity intracortical microstimulation of the precentral face area in monkeys. *Brain Res.*, **70**:144–147.

Crompton, A. W. and K. M. Hiiemae (1970). Molar occlusion and mandibular movements during occlusion in the American opossum, *Didelphis marsupialis. J. Linn. Soc. (Zool.)*, **49**:21–47.

Crutcher, M. D. and M. R. Delong (1984). Single cell studies of primate putamen. I. Functional organization. *Exp. Brain Res.*, **53**:233–243.

Darian-Smith, I. and T. Yokota (1966). Corticofugal effects on different neuron types within the cat's brain stem activated by tactile stimulation of the face. *J. Neurophysiol.*, **29**:185–206.

De Vree, F. and C. Gans (1976). Mastication in pygmy goats *"Capra hircus"*. *Ann. Soc. Roy. Zool. Belg.*, **105**:255–306.

Delong, M. R., M. D. Crutcher, and A. P. Georgopoulos (1983). Relations between movement and single cell discharge in the substantia nigra of the behaving monkey. *J. Neurosc.*, **3**:1599–1606.

Dellow, P. G. (1969). Control mechanisms of mastication. *Ann. Aust. Coll. Dent. Surg.*, **2**:81–95.

Dellow, P. G. (1976). The general physiological background of chewing and swallowing. In *Mastication and Swallowing*. B. J. Sessle and A. G. Hannam, eds., Univ. Toronto Press., Toronto. pp. 6–9.

Dellow, P. G. and J. P. Lund (1971). Evidence for central timing of rhythmical mastication. *J. Physiol.*, **215**:1–13.

Drew, T., R. Dubuc, and S. Rossignol (1986). Discharge patterns of reticulospinal and other reticular neurons in chronic, unrestrained cats walking on a treadmill. *J. Neurophysiol.*, **55**:375–401.

Dubner, R., B. J. Sessle, and A. T. Storey (1978). *The Neural Basis of Oral and Facial Function.* Plenum Press, New York, pp. 160–165.

Dunn, R. C. and D. L. Tolbert (1982). The corticotrigeminal projection in the cat. A study of the organization of cortical projections to the spinal trigeminal nucleus. *Brain Res.*, **240**:13–25.

Edwards, S. B. (1972) The ascending and descending projections of the red nucleus in the cat: an experimental study using an autoradiographic tracing method. *Brain Res.*, **48**:45–63.

Ferrier, D. (1886). *The Function of the Brain,* 2nd ed. Smith & Elder, London.

Foerster, O. The cerebral cortex in man. *Lancet*, **221**:309–312.

Gahery, Y. and A. Nieoullon (1978). Postural and kinetic coordination following cortical stimuli which induce flexion movements in the cats limbs. *Brain Res.*, **149**:25–37.

Goldberg, L. J. and S. H. Chandler (1981). Evidence for patten generator control of the effect of spindle offerent input during rhythmical jaw movements. *Can. J. Physiol. Pharmacol.*, **59**:707–712.

Goldberg, L. J., S. H. Chandler, and M. Tal (1982). Relationship between jaw movements and trigeminal motoneuron membrane-potential fluctuations during cortically induced rhythmical jaw movements in the guinea pig. *J. Neurophysiol.*, **48**: 110–125.

Goldberg, L. J., J. Courville, J. P. Lund, and J. S. Kauer (1980). Increased uptake of ^{3}H and ^{14}C labeled deoxyglucose in localized regions of the brain during stimulation of the motor cortex. *Can. J. Physiol. Pharmacol.*, **58**:1086–1091.

Goldberg, L. J. and Y. Nakamura (1968). Lingually induced inhibition of masseteric motoneurons. *Experimentia*, **24**:371–373.

Goldberg, L. J. and M. Tal (1978). Intracellular recording in trigeminal motoneurons of the anesthetized guinea pig during rhythmic jaw movements. *Exp. Neurol.*, **58**:102–110.

Goodwin, G. M. and E. S. Luschei (1975). Discharge of spindle afferents form jaw-closing muscles during chewing in alert monkeys. *J. Neurophysiol.*, **38**:560–571.

Gorniak, G. C. (1977). Feeding in golden hamsters. *Mesocricetus auratus. J. Morphol.*, **154**:427–458.

Gorniak G. C. and C. Gans (1980). Quantitative assay of electromhograms during mastication in domestic cats *(Felis catus). J. Morphol.*, **163**:253–281.

Grant, P. G. (1973). Lateral pterygoid: two muscles? *Amer. J. Anat.*, **138**:1–10.

Graybiel, A. M. (1978). Organization of the nigrotectal connection: an experimental tracer study in the cat. *Brain Res.*, **143**:339–348.

Hannam, A. G., R. E. Decou, J. D. Scott, and W. W. Wood (1977). The relationship between dental occlusion, muscle activity, and associated jaw movement in man. *Arch Oral Biol.*, **22**:25–32.

Herring, S. W. and R. P. Scapino (1973). Physiology of feeding in miniature pigs. *J. Morphol.*, **141**:427–460.

Hess, W. R., K. C. Akert, and D. A. McDonald (1952). Functions of the orbital gyri of cats. *Brain*, **75**:244–258.

Hiiemae, K. M. (1976). Masticatory movements in primitive mammals. In *Mastication*, D. J. Anderson and B. Matthews, eds. Wright, Bristol, pp. 105–118.

Hiiemae, K. M. (1978). Mammalian mastication: a review of the activity of the jaw muscles and the movements they produce in chewing. In *Development, Function and Evolution of Teeth*, P. M. Butler and K. A. Joysey, eds. Academic Press, London, pp. 359–398.

Hiiemae, K. M. and G. M. Ardran (1968). A cineradiographic study of feeding in *Rattus norvegicus. J. Zool.*, **154**:139–154.

Hiiemae, K. M. and A. W. Crompton (1971). A cinefluorographic study of feeding in the American opossum, *Didelphis marsupialis*. In *Dental morphology and evolution*, Dahlberg, A. A. ed., Univ. Chicago Press, Chicago, pp. 299–334.

Hiiemae, K. M. and R. F. Kay (1983). Evolutionary trends in the dynamics of primate mastication. In: *Symp. IVth Int. Congr. Primat. Vol. 3. Craniofacial Biology of Primates*. Zingeser, M. R. ed., Karger, Basle, pp. 28–64.

Hoffman, D. S. and E. S. Luschei (1980). Responses of monkey precentral cortical cells during a controlled jaw bite task. *J. Neurophysiol.*, **44**:333–348.

Holstege, G. and H. G. J. M. Kuypers (1977). Propriobulbar fibre connections to the trigeminal, facial and hypoglossal motor nuclei. 1. An anterograde degeneration study. *Brain*, **100**:239–264.

Holstege, G., H. G. J. M. Kuypers, and J. J. Dekker (1977). The organization of the bulbar fibre connections to the trigeminal, facial, and hypoglossal motor nuclei. II. An autoradiographic tracing study in the cat. *Brain*, **100**:265–286.

Jüch, P. J. W., J. D. Van Willigen, M. L. Broekhuijsen, and C. M. Ballintijn (1985). Peripheral influences on the central pattern-rhythm generator for tongue movements in the rat. *Arch. Oral Biol.*, **30**:415–421.

Kawamura, Y. and S. Tsukamoto (1960). Analysis of jaw movements from the cortical jaw motor area and amygdala. *Jpn. J. Physiol.*, **10**:471–488.

Kawana, E. and T. Kusama (1968). Projections form the anterior part of the coronal gyrus to the thalamus, the spinal trigeminal complex and the nucleus of the solitary tract in cats. *Proc. Jpn. Acad.*, **44**:176–181.

Kidokoro, Y., K. Kubota, S. Shuto, and R. Sumino (1968a). Reflex organization of cat masticatory muscles. *J. Neurophysiol.*, **31**:695–708.

Kidokoro, Y., K. Kubota, S. Shuto, and R. Sumino (1968b). Possible interneurons responsible for reflex inhibition of motoneurons of jaw-closing muscles from the inferior dental nerve. *J. Neurophysiol.* **31**:709–716.

Kim, J. S., M. C. Bushnell, G. H. Duncan, and J. P. Lund (1986). The modulation of sensory transmission through the medullary dorsal horn during cortically driven mastication. *Can. J. Physiol. Pharmacol.*, **64**:999–1005.

Kubo, Y., S. Enomoto, and Y. Nakamura (1981). Synaptic basis of orbital cortically induced rhythmical masticatory activity of trigeminal motoneurons in immobilized cats. *Brain Res.*, **230**:97–110.

Kubota, K. (1976). Motoneuron mechanisms: suprasegmental controls. In *Mastication and Swallowing*. B. J. Sessle and A. G. Hannam, eds. Univ. of Toronto Press, Toronto, pp. 60–75.

Kubota, K. and H. Niki (1971). Precentral cortical unit activity and jaw movement in chronic monkeys. In *Oral-facial Sensory and Motor Mechanisms*. R. Dubner and Y. Kawamura, eds. Appleton-Century-Crofts, New York, pp. 365–379.

Kuypers, H. G. J. M. (1958a). Some projections from the peri-central cortex to the pons and lower brain stem in monkey and chimpanzee. *J. Comp. Neurol.*, **110**: 221–255.

Kuypers, H. G. J. M. (1958b). An anatomic analysis of cortico-bulbar connexions to the pons and lower brain stem in the cat. *J. Anat.*, **92**:198–218.

Lambert, R. W., L. J. Goldberg, and S. H. Chandler (1985). The relationship between cortically induced mandibular movements and lateral pterygoid and digastric muscle EMG activity in the anesthetized guinea pig. *Brain Res.*, **329**:7–17.

Lambert, R. W., L. J. Goldberg, and S. H. Chandler (1986). Comparison of mandibular movement trajectories and associated patterns of oral muscle electromyographic activity during spontaneous and apomorphine-induced rhythmic jaw movements in the guinea pig. *J. Neurophysiol.*, **55**:301–319.

Landgren, S. (1957). Convergence of tactile, thermal, and gustatory impulses on single cortical cells. *Acta Physiol. Scand.*, **40**:210–221.

Landgren, S., and K. A. Olsson (1980). Low threshold afferent projections from the oral cavity and the face to the cerebral cortex of the cat. *Exp. Brain Res.*, **39**:133–147.

Landgren, S. and K. A. Olsson (1983). Cortical and trigeminal convergence in the intertrigeminal nucleus. *Soc. Neurosci. Abs.*, **9**:1–4.

Landgren, S., K. A. Olsson, and K. G. Westberg (1984). Bulbar neurons with axonal projections to the trigeminal motor nucleus. *Neurosci. Lett. Suppl.*, **18**:S60.

Larson, C. R., K. E. Byrd, C. R. Garthwaite, and E. S. Luschei (1980). Alterations in the pattern of mastication after ablations of the lateral precentral cortex in rhesus macaques. *Exp. Neurol.*, **70**:638–651.

Larson, C. R., A. Smith, and E. S. Luschei (1981). Discharge characteristics and stretch sensitivity of jaw muscle afferents in the monkey during controlled isometric bites. *J. Neurophysiol.*, **46**:130–142.

Lidsky, T. I., N. A. Buchwald, C. D. Hull, and M. S. Levine (1975). Pallidal and entopeduncular single unit activity in cats during drinking. *Electroencephal. Clin. Neurophysiol.*, **39**:79–84.

Lidsky, T. I., J. H. Robinson, F. J. Denaro, and P. M. Weinhold (1978). Trigeminal influences on entopeduncular units. *Brain Res.*, **141**:227–234.

Liles, S. L. (1979). Topographic organization of neurons related to arm movement in the putamen. In *Advances in Neurology*, vol. 23, T. N. Chase, N. S. Wexler, and A. Barbeau, eds., Raven Press, New York, pp. 155–162.

Limanskii, Y. P. and E. V. Gura (1969). Corticofugal influences on neurons of the main trigeminal sensory nucleus. *Neirofiziol.*, **1**:47–53.

Lorente De Nó, R. (1933). Vestibulo-ocular reflex arc. *Arch. Neurol. Psychiat.*, **30**:245–291.

Lund, J. P. (1976). Evidence for a central neural pattern generator regulating the chewing cycle. In: *Mastication*, D. J. Anderson and B. Matthews, eds., Wright, Bristol, pp. 204–212.

Lund, J. P. and P. G. Dellow (1971). The influence of interactive stimuli on rhythmical masticatory movements in rabbit. *Arch Oral Biol.*, **16**:215–223.

Lund, J. P. and P. G. Dellow (1973). Rhythmical masticatory activity of hypoglossal motoneurons responding to an oral stimulus. *Exp. Neurol.*, **40**:243–246.

Lund, J. P. and Y. Lamarre (1974). Activity of neurons in the lower precentral cortex during voluntary and rhythmical jaw movements in the monkey. *Exp. Brain Res.*, **19**:282–299.

Lund, J. P., T. Murakami, and M. Beaulieu (1977). An electromyographic investigation of rhythmical jaw movements evoked by repetitive electrical stimulation of the sensorimotor cortex of the rabbit. *Proc. Int. U. Physiol. Sci.*, **13**:458.

Lund, J. P. and K. A. Olsson (1983). The importance of reflexes and their control during jaw movement. *Trends Neurosci.*, **6**:458–463.

Lund, J. P., S. Rossignol, and T. Murakami (1981). Interactions between the jaw-opening reflex and mastication. *Can. J. Physiol. Pharmacol.*, **59**:683–690.

Lund, J. P., K. Sasamoto, T. Murakami, and K. A. Olsson (1984). Analysis of rhythmical jaw movements produced by electrical stimulation of motor-sensory cortex of rabbits. *J. Neurophysiol.*, **52**:1014–1029.

Lund, J. P. and B. J. Sessle (1974). Oral-facial and jaw muscle afferent projections to neurons in cat frontal cortex. *Exp. Neurol.* **45**:314–331.

Luschei, E. S., C. R. Garthwaite, and M. E. Armstrong (1971). Relationship of firing patterns of units in face area of monkey precentral cortex to conditioned jaw movements. *J. Neurophysiol.*, **34**:552–561.

Luschei, E. S. and L. J. Goldberg (1981). Neural mechanisms of mandibular control: mastication and voluntary biting. In *Handbook of Physiology, Section 1: Motor Control, Vol II*, V. B. Brooks, ed., American Physiological Society, Washington, pp. 1237–1274.

Luschei, E. S. and G. M. Goodwin (1974). Patterns of mandibular movement and jaw muscle activity during mastication in the monkey. *J. Neurophysiol.*, **37**:954–966.

Luschei, E. S. and G. M. Goodwin (1975). Role of monkey precentral cortex in control of voluntary jaw movements. *J. Neurophysiol.*, **38**:146–157.

Magnus, O., W. Penfield, and H. Jasper. Mastication and consciousness in epileptic seizures. *Acta Psychiat. Neurol. Scand.* **27**:91–114.

Magoun, H. W., S. W. Ranson, and C. Fisher (1933). Corticofugal pathways for mastication, lapping, and other motor functions in the cat. *Arch. Neurol. Psychiat.*, **30**:292–308.

Marini, G. and M. L. Sotgiu (1985). Single unit activity in lateral reticular nucleus during cortically evoked masticatory movements in rabbits. *Brain Res.*, **337**:287–292.

Massion, J. (1984). Postural changes accompanying voluntary movements. Normal and pathological aspects. *Human Neurobiol.*, **2**:261–267.

McGuinness, E., D. Sivertsen, and J. M. Allman (1980). Organization of the face-representation macaque motor cortex. *J. Comp. Neurol.*, **193**:591–608.

McNamara, J. A. (1973). The independent functions of the two heads of the lateral pterygoid muscle. *Amer. J. Anat.*, **138**:197–206.

Miller, F. R. (1920). The cortical paths for mastication and deglutition. *J. Physiol.*, **53**:473–478.

Mizuno, N., E. K. Sauerland, and C. D. Clemente (1968). Projections from the orbital gyrus in the cat. I. To brain stem structures. *J. Comp. Neurol.* **133**:463–476.

Mizuno, N., Y. Yasui, S. Nomura, K. Itoh, A. Konishi, M. Takada, and M. Kudo (1983). A light and electron microscopic study of premotor neurons for the trigeminal motor nucleus. *J. Comp. Neural.*, **215**:290–298.

Møller, E. (1966). The chewing apparatus: an electromyograph study of the action of the muscles of mastication and its correlation to facial morphology. *Acta Physiol. Scand.* **69**: (Suppl) 280.

Mora, F., G. J. Mogenson, and E. T. Rolls (1977). Activity of neurons in the region of the substantia nigra during feeding in the monkey. *Brain Res.*, **133**:267–276.

Morimoto, T. and Y. Kawamura (1973). Properties of tongue and jaw movements elicited by stimulation of the orbital agyrus of the cat. *Arch. Oral. Biol.*, **18**:361–372.

Nakamura, Y. (1985). Localization and functional organization of masticatory rhythm generator in the lwoer brain stem reticular formation. *Neurosci. Lett.*, *(suppl.)* **20**:S3–S4.

Nakamura, Y., L. J. Goldberg, N. Mizuno, and C. D. Clemente (1978). Effects of hypoglossal afferent stimulation on masseteric motoneurons in cats. *Exp. Neurol.*, **61**:1–14.

Nakamura, Y. and Y. Kubo (1978). Masticatory rhythm in intracellular potential of trigeminal motoneurons induced by stimulation of orbital cortex and amygdala in cats. *Brain Res.*, **148**:504–509.

Nakamura, Y., Y. Kubo, S. Nozaki, and M. Takatori (1976). Cortically induced masticatory rhythm and its modification by tonic peripheral inputs in immobilized cats. *Bull. Tokyo Med. Dent. Univ.*, **23**:101–107.

Nakamura, Y., S. Mori, and H. Nagashima (1973). Origin and central pathways of crossed inhibitory effects of afferents form the masseteric muscle on the masseteric motoneuron of the cat. *Brain Res.*, **57**:29–42.

Nakamura, Y., M. Takatori, Y. Kubo, S. Nozaki, and S. Enomoto (1980). Possible roles of lower brain stem reticular formation in jaw position and jaw movement,

In *Jaw Position and Jaw Movement*. K. Kubota, Y. Nakamura and G.-H. Schumacher, eds. VEB Verlag Volk und Gesundheit, Berlin, pp. 309–321.

Neafsey, E. J., C. D. Hull, and N. A. Buchwald (1978). Preparation for movement in the cat. II. Unit activity in the basal ganglia and thalamus. *Electroencephal. Clin. Neurophysiol.*, **44**:714–723.

Nishino, H., T. Ono, M. Fukuda, and K. Sasaki (1985). Monkey substantia nigra (pars reticular) neuron discharges during operant feeding. *Brain Res.*, **334**:190–193.

Nozaki, R., S. Enomoto, and Y. Nakamura (1983). Identification and input-output properties of bulbar reticular neurons involved in the cerebral cortical control of trigeminal motoneurons in cats. *Exp. Brain Res.*, **49**:363–372.

Nozaki, S., A. Iriki, and Y. Nakamura (1986). Role of corticobulbar projection neurons in cortically induced rhythmical masticatory jaw-opening movement in the guinea pig. *J. Neurophysiol.*, **55**:826–845.

Nozaki, S., A. Iriki, and Y. Nakamura (1986). Localization of central rhythm generator involved in cortically induced rhythmical masticatory jaw-opening movement in the guinea pig. *J. Neurophysiol.*, **55**:806–825.

Olsson, K. Å., K. Sasamoto, and J. P. Lund (1986). Modulation of transmission in rostral trigeminal sensory nuclei during chewing. *J. Neurophysiol.*, **55**:56–75.

Porter, R. (1965). Synaptic potentials in hypoglossal motoneurons. *J. Physiol.*, **180**:209–244.

Porter, R. (1967). Cortical actions on hypoglossal motoneurons in cats: a proposed role for a common internuncial cell. *J. Physiol.*, **193**:295–308.

Rethi, L. (1893). Das Rindenfeld, die subcorticalen Bahnen und das Coordinationscentrum und Schluckens. *Sitzungsb. Akad. Wissensch. Mathnaturw. Cl.*, **102**:359–377.

Sahara, Y., M. Katoh, and Y. Nakamura (1983). Nature of cortically induced rhythmical masticatory activity of hypoglossal motoneurons in cats. *J. Physiol. Soc. Japan*, **45**:428.

Schneider, J. S. and T. I. Lidsky (1981). Processing of somatosensory information in striatum of behaving cats. *J. Neurophysiol.* **45**:841–851.

Schultz, W. (1986). Activity of pars reticula neurons of monkey substantia nigra in relation to motor, sensory, and complex events. *J. Neurophysiol.*, **55**:660–677.

Schumacher, G.-H. (1980). Comparative functional anatomy of jaw muscles. In *Jaw Position and Jaw Movement*. K. Kubota, Y. Nakamura, and G.-H. Schumacher, eds. VEB Verlag volk und gesundheit, Berlin, pp. 76–93.

Sears, T. A. (1964). Investigations on respiratory motoneurons of the thoracic spinal cord. *Prog. Brain Res.* **12**:259–273.

Sessle, B. J., J. W. Hu, R. Dubner, and G. E. Lucier (1981). Functional properties of neurons in cat trigeminal subnucleus caudalis (medullary dorsal horn). II. Modulation of responses to noxious and nonnoxious stimuli by periaqueductal gray, nucleus raphe magnus, cerebral cortex, and afferent influences, and effect of naloxone. *J. Neurophysiol.*, **45**:193–207.

Shik, M. L., F. V. Severin, and G. M. Orlovsky (1966). Control of walking and running by means of electrical stimulation of the mid-brain. *Biophysics*, **11**:757–765.

Soltysik, S., C. D.Huyll, N. A. Buchwald, and T. Fekete (1975). Single unit activity in basal ganglia of monkeys during performance of a delayed response task. *Electroencephal. Clin. Neurophysiol.*, **39**:65–78.

Sumi, T. (1969). Some properties of cortically-evoked swallowing and chewing in rabbits. *Brain Res.*, **15**:107–120.

Sumi, T. (1970). Activity in single hypoglossal fibers during cortically induced swallowing and chewing in rabbits. *Pflugers Arch.*, **314**:329–346.

Sumi, T. (1971). Modification of cortically evoked rhythmic chewing and swallowing from midbrain and pons. *Jpn. J. Physiol.*, **21**:489–506.

Tashiro, T., T. Matsuyama, and S. Higo (1983). Distribution of cells of origin of the corticotrigeminal projections to the nucleus caudalis of the spinal trigeminal complex in the cat. A horseradish peroxidase (HRP) study. *Exp. Neurol.*, **80**:178–185.

Thexton, A. J., K. M. Hiiemae, and A. W. Crompton (1980). Food consistency and bite size as regulators of jaw movement during feeding in the cat. *J. Neurophysiol.*, **44**:456–474.

Travers, J. B., and R. Norgren (1983). Afferent projections to the oral motor nuclei in the rat. *J. Comp. Neurol.*, **220**: 280–298.

Turnbull, W. E. (1970). Mammalian masticatory apparatus. *Fieldiana: Geology*, **18**:153–356.

Vogt, C. and O. Vogt (1919). Ergebnisse unserer Hirnforschung. *J. Psychol. Neurol.*, **25**:277–462.

Walberg, F. (1957). Do the motor nuclei of the cranial nerves receive corticofugal fibers? An experimental study int he cat. *Brain*, **80**:597–605.

Ward, J. and S. L. Clark (1935). Specific responses elicitable from subdivisions of the motor cortex of the ceerebrum of the cat. *J. Comp. Neurol.* **63**:49–64.

Webster, K. E. Cortico-striate interrelations in the albino rat. *J. Anat.*, **95**:532–544.

Weijs, W. A. and R. Dantuma (1975). Electromyography and mechanics of mastication in the albino rat. *J. Morphol.*, **146**:1–34.

Weijs, W. A. and R. Datuma (1981). Functional anatomy of the masticatory apparatus in the rabbit *(Oryctolagus cuniculus)*. *Neth. J. Zool.*, **31**:99–147.

Wold, J. E. and A. Brodal. The projection of cortical sensorimotor regions onto the trigeminal neurons in the cat. An experimental anatomical study. *Neurobiol.*, **3**:353–375.

Yasui, Y., K. Itoh, A. Mitani, M. Takada, and N. Mizuno (1985). Cerebral cortical projections to the reticular regions around the trigeminal motor nucleus in the cat. *J. Comp. Neurol.* **241**:348–356.

Chapter Three

GENERATION OF RESPIRATORY PATTERN IN MAMMALS

JACK L. FELDMAN*
JEFFREY C. SMITH*
DONALD R. McCRIMMON
HOWARD H. ELLENBERGER*
DEXTER F. SPECK†

Department of Physiology
Northwestern University
Chicago, Illinois

> . . . it is true that my tactic is to make sweeping categorical statements. Whether or not this is a fault . . . is debatable. My own feeling is that it leads more quickly to the solution of scientific problems than a cautious sitting on the fence.‡

1 INTRODUCTION

The control of movements and regulation of homeostatic mechanisms represent the major actions of the mammalian brain. While significant progress has been made in elucidating cellular and synaptic properties, projections and neurotransmitters of individual nerve cells and systems, there exists a large gap in our understanding of how these properties are

*Present address: Systems Neurobiology Laboratory, Department of Kinesiology, University of California, Los Angeles, Los Angeles, California.
†Present address: Department of Physiology and Biophysics, University of Kentucky, Lexington, Kentucky.
‡E. Mayr, *The Growth of Biological Thought*, Harvard University Press, Cambridge Mass., 1982, p. 9.

integrated to produce complex behaviors. The impulse activity of a single motoneuron does not produce a meaningful movement; rather complex spatiotemporal discharge patterns of many groups of motoneurons is required; these are driven by a large number of interneurons. Thus, in order to unravel the mechanisms underlying the production of movements, the collective interactions of many neurons must be understood. Likewise, knowledge of the manner in which the activity of large collections of neurons is orchestrated is necessary to understand homeostatic regulation.

Homeostasis requires the coordinated movement of skeletal musculature for breathing; a central neural circuit is required to generate and control the rhythmic movements. Thus, the neural control system for respiration represents an ideal system for the study of intrinsic mechanisms underlying both the central generation of preprogrammed movement as well as other integrative actions of the mammalian nervous system. The question we wish to address is: *How does the central nervous system (CNS) integrate the activity of individual neurons and populations of neurons to produce appropriate respiratory movements?* We present limited background material and focus on hypotheses and speculation concerning this question; the reader is referred to several recent reviews for detailed background (Cohen, 1979; von Euler, 1983; Feldman, 1986).

What must the CNS do in the control of breathing? *First*, the CNS must produce a rhythm that underlies the periodic cycle of expansion and contraction of the respiratory pump. *Second*, this rhythm must be translated into a precisely coordinated pattern of discharge of the various populations of motoneurons innervating respiratory muscles. *Third*, the CNS must adapt and adjust this pattern so that the appropriate ventilation of the lung is maintained for blood gas and acid-base homeostasis. *Fourth*, the CNS must integrate respiratory movements with other body movements—speech (Bunn and Mead, 1971), postural changes, locomotion (Bramble and Carrier, 1983), chewing (Luschei and Goldberg, 1982), and swallowing (Miller, 1982)—preferably at minimal energy expenditure (Milic-Emili and Petit, 1960). The adaptation, adjustment and integration of respiratory movements is based on information derived from mechanoreceptors; the regulation of blood gases and pH requires peripheral and central chemoreception.

2   GLOBAL DESCRIPTION OF THE RESPIRATORY PATTERN

A large number of motoneuronal pools, extending from sites in the brain stem to lumbar regions of the spinal cord, are engaged for the act of breathing under various conditions. The respiratory motor apparatus controlled by these motoneurons consists of: (1) the diaphragm (the major inspiratory muscle in mammals) and musculature of the thorax and abdomen which are innervated by spinal motoneurons and collectively constitute the respiratory pump; (2) the laryngeal and pharyngeal muscles, innervated by cranial motoneurons, which control the upper airway and modulate respiratory airflow resistance; and (3) tracheal and bronchial smooth muscle, whose tone is modulated by vagal motoneurons, which also modulate airflow resistance.

A precise spatiotemporal pattern of respiratory motoneuronal activity (Fig. 1) determines the integrated muscle forces acting on the respiratory

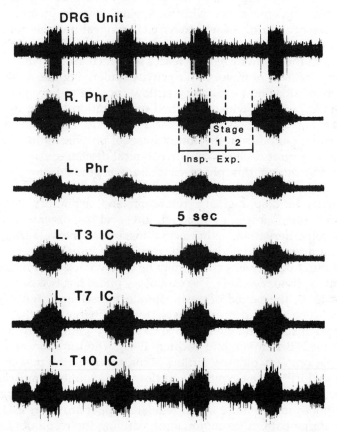

FIGURE 1. A precise spatiotemporal pattern of periodic motoneuronal activity is necessary for ventilation. Recordings are shown from several nerves innervating respiratory muscles that alter the configuration of the thorax and were obtained from an anesthetized, paralyzed, mechanically ventilated cat. The left and right phrenic nerves (L. Phr and R. Phr.) innervate the diaphragm and the (left) intercostal nerves (e.g., T3 IC, T7 IC,T10 IC) innervate the intercostal, parasternal, and paravertebral muscles. The neuromechanical coupling is as in all mammalian skeletal muscles; the coupling between the coordinated muscle contraction and the actual movement of the lung is complex. Inspiration is the period from the abrupt onset of phrenic motoneuronal activity to its abrupt decline. Expiration consists of two stages: Stage 1, during which there is *post-inspiratory* discharge of phrenic motoneurons and Stage 2. Modified from Feldman, 1986. DRG: dorsal respiratory group, a concentration of inspiratory modulated neurons in the ventrolateral nucleus of the solitary tract in the medulla.

pump and controlling airflow resistance. During eupnea (resting normal breathing) in awake humans and other mammals there is phasic inspiratory activity of the diaphragm and parasternal intercostal muscles. As breathing efforts increase, such as during hypercapnea (increased arterial Pco_2) or hypoxia (decreased arterial Po_2), phasic inspiratory activity appears in the external intercostal muscles, and activity in the diaphragm and parasternal intercostal muscles increases. Expiratory muscles of the thorax and abdomen are usually not phasically active during quiet breathing, but they become active with increasing drive to breathe, reaching maximal activity during heavy exercise. Laryngeal motoneurons are frequently active during both inspiratory and expiratory phases of the breathing cycle and their activity also increases with increased drive.

The basic pattern of motor nerve activity underlying the alternating periods of inspiratory and expiratory airflow consists of two phases, inspiration and expiration, with the period of expiration having two distinct subphases (Fig. 1). The inspiratory phase of activity (neural inspiration) is defined as the period from the abrupt onset of phrenic motoneuronal discharge to its abrupt decline. The stereotypical discharge pattern of spinal motoneurons during this phase consists of a gradual augmenting discharge that terminates abruptly. The abrupt decline in phrenic nerve activity results in diaphragmatic relaxation and expiratory airflow. The relaxation is often slowed by residual, low-level *post-inspiratory* discharge in the phrenic nerve (and other active inspiratory nerves) lasting up to several hundred milliseconds, which retards the initial expiratory airflow. The next burst of phrenic activity may be delayed a second or more from the end of expiratory airflow. The expiratory phase has two distinct neural phases: *stage 1*, the period of post-inspiratory discharge, and *stage 2*, the period between the end of post-inspiratory discharge and the beginning of the next inspiration, when active expiratory efforts may be present (Richter, 1982; Ballantyne and Richter, 1984). The duration of expiration and the pattern of expiratory airflow is controlled by the post-inspiratory discharge which brakes expiratory airflow, the expiratory muscle activity which promotes expiratory airflow, and the laryngeal, pharyngeal, and airway smooth muscle tone which regulates upper airway resistance. The basic discharge pattern for motoneurons driving the respiratory pump as depicted in Figure 1 is present over a wide range of respiratory requirements.

The discharge patterns of laryngeal and pharyngeal motoneurons controlling airway resistance is somewhat different from the pattern of activity of motoneurons driving the respiratory pump. The inspiratory pattern of discharge of laryngeal and pharyngeal motoneurons (Fig. 5) has an abrupt onset and precedes the appearance of phrenic motoneuronal activity by up to several hundred milliseconds. Activity then remains at a plateau level or declines throughout the rest of inspiration, terminating no later than the end of the phrenic burst. This laryngeal abductor motoneuronal discharge pattern insures reduced airway resistance during inspiration.

3   RHYTHM GENERATION

3.1   Site

In mammals, respiratory rhythm of a normal character persists following decerebration and decerebellation. Subsequent transection at the spino-medullary junction permanently abolishes respiratory rhythmic discharge of the phrenic and intercostal nerves but does not markedly affect the respiratory activity of cranial nerves (Hukuhara, 1976; St. John, Bartlett, Knuth, and Hwang, 1981). In vitro preparations support these observations. In fact, Adrian and Buytendijk (1931) presented the first evidence of central pattern generation in vertebrates using an in vitro model of respiratory rhythmogenesis. With cotton wick electrodes, they recorded a regular periodic pattern of field potentials from the isolated goldfish brainstem. The temporal pattern of these potentials resembled the respiratory rhythm in the intact animals (see Fig. 4 in Adrian and Buytendijk, 1931). Recently, recording from the isolated, in vitro brain stem-spinal cord of neonatal rats, Suzue (1984) observed rhythmic discharges in the spinal ventral roots containing phrenic motoneuronal axons. Using this preparation, we have also observed such rhythmic respiratory motor discharges in cranial and spinal ventral roots (Fig. 2; Smith and Feldman, 1985, 1986, 1987a,b). Transection at the spinomedullary junction of this preparation abolishes rhythmic respiratory discharge on the spinal nerves without markedly affecting the rhythmic discharge on cranial nerves. Thus, the brainstem is the site for respiratory rhythmogenesis.*

Within the brainstem of the deeply anesthetized or decerebrate cat, neurons with respiratory modulated spiking patterns are concentrated in, but not restricted to, several clusters, referred to as the dorsal (DRG), ventral (VRG), and pontine (PRG) respiratory groups (See Fig. 4 in Feldman, 1986). The DRG corresponds to the ventrolateral nucleus of the solitary tract; the VRG roughly corresponds to the nucleus ambiguus-retroambigualis and extends from the rostral cervical spinal cord through the medulla to the retrofacial nucleus (the most rostral portion is referred to as the Bötzinger Complex). The PRG corresponds to the region of the medial parabrachial, lateral parabrachial and Kölliker-Fuse nuclei in the rostral dorsolateral pons (Feldman, 1986).

---

*Some authors have claimed a spinal source for respiratory rhythmicity. These results are equivocal, since all reports of apparently normal respiratory movements in spinalized animals could be accounted for by: (1) peripheral feedback (non-paralyzed animals), due to either the reflex effects of respiratory related contractions of muscles innervated by cranial nerves, e.g. sternocleidomastoid, or segmental afferents activated by non-respiratory phrenic or intercostal motoneuronal activity, and (2) driving of phrenic nerve activity by spinal locomotor activity (paralyzed animals). In the absence of descending respiratory drive, locomotor activity could drive phrenic nerve activity in a manner resembling normal breathing (Viala and Freton, 1983). There is evidence that locomotion entrains respiration in intact animals (Bramble and Carrier, 1983; Eldridge and Millhorn, 1984).

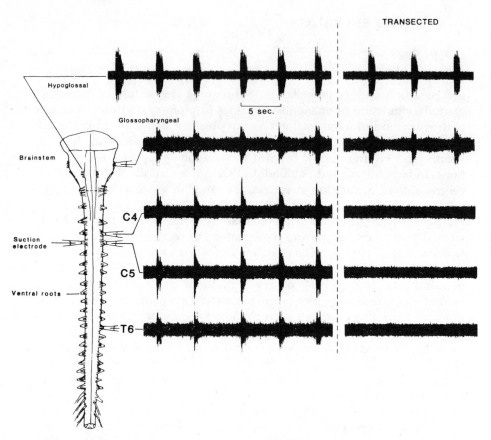

FIGURE 2. The mammalian central nervous system is capable, in the absence of afferent input, of generating the rhythmic activity that underlies breathing movements. Such rhythms can even be obtained in an *in vitro* neonatal rat spinal cord-brainstem preparation (Smith and Feldman, 1985, 1987a,b; see also Suzue, 1984). At left is a drawing of the neonatal spinal cord with suction electrode recordings from various roots shown at the right. Transection of the neuraxis at the spinomedullary junction abolishes spinal motoneuronal activity related to respiration whereas cranial motoneuronal activity remains unaffected.

The DRG and VRG have been hypothesized for many years to contain the circuitry responsible for respiratory rhythm generation (e.g., Cherniack and von Euler, 1980; Mitchell and Berger, 1981; Wyman, 1977). Yet, after more than a decade of searching, *no* evidence has been presented that provides strong support for this hypothesis. In fact, there is considerable evidence that the DRG and VRG (DRG-VRG) are not necessary for the generation of respiratory rhythm:

1. The majority of neurons in the DRG-VRG project down the spinal cord, providing the rhythmic respiratory drive to phrenic, intercostal and abdominal motoneurons (see Fig. 1 for an example of DRG neuronal ac-

tivity). We tested the involvement of these bulbospinal neurons in the generation of respiratory rhythm by observing the effects on phrenic motoneuronal discharge of synchronous activation of their axons, produced by stimulating the descending tracts in the upper cervical spinal cord (Feldman, McCrimmon, and Speck, 1984). We presumed that if these bulbospinal neurons generated rhythm, or sent collaterals directly to regions generating rhythm (see Fig. 1 in Feldman, McCrimmon, and Speck, 1984), their synchronous activation should phase-shift or reset the rhythm. These perturbations did not affect the timing of respiratory motor nerve activity, which strongly suggests a limited role, if any, for these neurons in generating the rhythm.

2. Perhaps a subset of brain stem neurons located in the DRG-VRG are important in generating respiratory rhythm. Several authors have postulated a class of DRG-VRG inspiratory neurons that actively inhibit other DRG-VRG inspiratory neurons ("off-switch" neurons) and are responsible for the termination of inspiratory discharge (Bradley, von Euler, Martilla, and Roos, 1973; Feldman, 1976; Feldman and Cowan, 1976; Feldman, Cohen, and Wolotsky, 1976b). We tested this possibility by analyzing the cross-correlations of impulse activity of pairs of DRG-VRG neurons recorded simultaneously (Feldman, Sommer, and Cohen, 1980; Feldman and Speck, 1983). An analysis of over 400 pairs of neurons in this study, as well as in other studies, has not revealed such a class of neurons. In fact, the predominant mechanism for the impulse discharge synchronization of DRG-VRG inspiratory neurons is likely shared inputs, perhaps from a source outside the DRG-VRG.

3. The observations discussed in 1 and 2 of course do not exclude all possible mechanisms for rhythm generation in the DRG-VRG. Other possibilities are limited by the observation that extensive electrolytic lesions carefully confined to the DRG and/or VRG do not significantly affect the periodicity of phrenic motoneuronal activity.* These lesions markedly reduce the amplitude of phrenic nerve activity, in proportion to the amount

*Perturbations made using focal cooling or kainic acid lesions in the region of the DRG can produce marked changes in respiratory period (Berger and Cooney, 1982; Koepchen et al, 1974, 1985; Morin-Surin et al, 1985). These different results may be due to the different nature of the pertubations. However, it is also possible that the alterations in timing seen were due to perturbations affecting regions outside the limited confines of the DRG into the medial region of the solitary nucleus or ventral and lateral into the reticular formation. Koepchen, for example, reports (1985) that the maximal effect on phrenic nerve discharge due to cooling occurs when the probe is centered 500-750 μm *lateral* to the vlNTS, the anatomical correlate of the DRG. This region of the reticular formation would be affected even if the cooling probe were centered in the DRG. Kainic acid lesions, although they *may* spare axons in the region of injection, can be transported (by diffusion or local circulation) considerable distances from the injection site. Thus, Berger and Cooney (1982) placed their kainate containing electrode in the DRG and nonetheless reported significant destruction of the hypoglossal nucleus, which is >750 μm from their injection site. Although neurons in the hypoglossal nucleus, *per se*, are unlikely to alter rhythm, it suggests that more subtle and therefore undetected destruction in other regions may produce such effects.

of DRG-VRG tissue destroyed; this effect is likely due to destruction of premotor neurons. Although alternative interpretations are possible (see discussion in Speck and Feldman, 1982), these results indicate that the DRG and/or VRG are not exclusive sites, if at all, for generating rhythm.

Where, then, might the respiratory rhythm be generated in the brain? Regions identified as projecting to the DRG-VRG are logical candidates. These include:

a. *Pontine respiratory group.* Reciprocal connections between the DRG-VRG and the PRG have been identified. The possible role of the PRG in generation of respiratory rhythm is discussed below (see: Section 3.5; Bertrand and Hugelin, 1971; Feldman, 1976).

b. *Paragigantocellularis lateralis (PGCL) and "retrotrapezoid" (RTN) nuclei.* We have observed a marked projection to the VRG from two distinct adjacent groups of cells near the ventral medullary surface in cat (Ellenberger, Smith, McCrimmon, and Feldman, 1985; Andrezik, Chan-Palay, and Palay 1981). One of the cell groups lies ventral to the medial division of the facial nucleus within approximately 500 μm of the medullary surface, extending rostrally with the facial nucleus to about the level of the caudal end of the nucleus of the trapezoid body. Since much of this group lies immediately caudal to the trapezoid nucleus and occupies a position relative to the facial nucleus and medullary surface similar to the caudal pole of the trapezoid nucleus, we refer to this group as the *retro*trapezoid nucleus (RTN). Cell bodies of the rostral PGCL neurons projecting to the VRG-DRG are located slightly medial and dorsal to retrotrapezoid cells, medial to the facial nucleus, and are also concentrated more caudally in the brain stem ventral and medial to the retrofacial nucleus.

Cell groups near the ventral medullary surface are of particular interest, since superficial perturbations of this region, such as cooling (Cherniack, von Euler, Homma, and Kao, 1979), superfusion of solutions of differing pH (Ahmed and Loeschcke, 1982), topical procaine, GABA (Yamada, Norman, Hamosh, and Gillis, 1982), and electrical stimulation (Trouth, Loeschke, and Berndt, 1973), produce marked alterations in the respiratory pattern. These responses have been hypothesized to be due to perturbation of the putative intracranial (central) chemoreceptors, i.e., structures monitoring brain pH (or related variables), thought to lie near the ventral surface. von Euler et al. (1985) observed that focal cooling in the caudal paragigantocellular nuclear region can profoundly affect breathing pattern. We have found that electrical stimulation in these regions can markedly affect breathing pattern (Connelly, Ellenberger and Feldman; Smith and Feldman, unpublished observations). More detailed studies will be necessary to determine if these nuclei are involved in rhythmogenesis and/or intracranial chemoreception.

c. *Regions ventral and lateral to the DRG proper.* Cooling (Koepchen, Lazar, and Borchert, 1985), focal lesions (Morin-Surin, Denavit-Saubie, Champagnat, and Boudinot, 1985), or picomole amounts of excitatory amino acids (McCrimmon, Feldman, and Speck, 1985, 1986) ventral and lateral to the DRG produce profound alterations in respiratory timing. Neurons discharging with a respiratory periodicity have not been reported to be concentrated in these regions in deeply anesthetized cats (see, however, King, 1980; King and Knox, 1984); nevertheless, the proximity to DRG neurons would allow for non-spiking rhythm generating cells to drive respiration.

d. *Suprapontine sites.* Sites rostral to the brain stem may be important in rhythmogenesis (Bassal and Bianchi, 1982; Gauthier, Monteau, and Dussardier, 1983; Harper, Frysinger, Trelease, and Marks, 1984). Although breathing pattern maintains an essentially normal character in decerebrates, this does not exclude a contribution from suprapontine sites when the neuraxis is intact.

3.2   Mechanisms

A central problem in understanding respiratory pattern generation is the determination of the mechanisms underlying rhythmogenesis. Neural rhythms may be explicable in terms of the membrane properties in special groups of cells, i.e., pacemaker cells (see below) or may only emerge as a dynamic property of a complex neural network. Without a precise description of the location of the respiratory oscillator, it is impossible to determine the detailed circuitry and neuronal properties that would permit the development and/or testing of comprehensive models of pattern generation. Yet, possible mechanisms are suggested by existing data on respiratory motor patterns and from hypotheses concerning rhythm generation in other systems, especially invertebrates; respiratory neurobiologists are not without speculations.

Neural circuits that generate rhythms as well as models that simulate oscillations are not hard to come by. The problem we face in understanding the mechanisms underlying respiratory rhythmogenesis is the lack of information necessary to test *detailed* models. Conceptual models may be useful, however, in providing a framework in which to interpret data and for designing further experiments. Such models for rhythmogenesis fall into at least 3 categories (Fig. 3):

1. Timing and detailed spatiotemporal pattern are generated together (e.g., Bradley, von Euler, Martilla, and Roos 1973; Feldman and Cowan, 1975; Fig. 3A). This model is not meant to include the trivial case of separate generation of timing and pattern simply lumped into one compartment.
2. Timing and basic discharge ramp are generated together, e.g., a sinewave generator, and serve as input to a network that produces the detailed spatiotemporal pattern (Fig. 3B). Thus, in this model, the timer provides input to the burst pattern generator that affects its

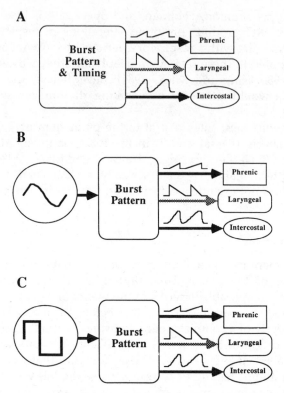

FIGURE 3. Three distinct ways periodic respiratory pattern could be generated. See text for details.

global output but does not determine the detailed discharge pattern among the various motoneuron pools.

3. Timing and burst generation are distinct functions (e.g., Feldman, 1981). A gate turns on and off the circuitry that produces the detailed spatiotemporal burst pattern of the different motoneuron pools (Fig. 3C). The timer provides no specific input to the burst pattern generator that affects the magnitude and pattern of its output.

We argue below that 2 or 3 represents the most likely organization for the circuitry underlying respiratory pattern generation.

3.3   Compartmentalization of Function

One important consideration is the apparent compartmentalization of function in the production of a rhythmic respiratory pattern (Fig. 4). Thus, the motor side of the system, including the motoneurons *and* bulbospinal premotor neurons play no (or a limited) role in the generation of respiratory rhythm. These neurons receive rhythmic input, which they integrate with other central and peripheral inputs in producing the command sent to the respiratory muscles; their function can be classified as *sensorimotor integration*. Rhythm generation arises from neurons presynaptic to the premotor neurons, at locales yet unknown.

Since a significant component of the central pattern generator is concerned with sensorimotor integration and is separate from the rhythm generator, *per se*, we propose that these functions are distinct (Fig. 4; Feldman, 1981, 1986; Feldman and Smith, 1986). This would suggest models like Figures 3B or 3C. An extension of this hypothesis is that the mechanisms controlling the evolution of a burst of motoneuronal discharge are independent of those mechanisms that determine burst duration, e.g., Figure 3C.

The functional separation of the mechanisms controlling the timing of an individual phase from those generating the burst pattern within a phase is evident in the response to several different experimental perturbations.

1. *Pulmonary stretch receptor activation.* Our experimental paradigm has been to use a respiratory cycle-triggered pump (lung inflations by the pump are triggered by phrenic nerve activity) in anesthetized or decerebrate paralyzed cats. We typically compare the respiratory motor nerve (or neuronal) activity during control cycles when the lungs are inflated during the period of phrenic motoneuronal discharge (neural inspiration) with test cycles when the inflation protocol is altered. A test cycle may have

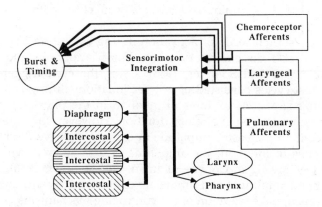

FIGURE 4. Considerable evidence suggests that different neuronal networks are concerned with generation of the rhythm underlying respiration (e.g. a neural sine-wave generator or a series of temporal gates) and with the sensorimotor integration that effects the final pattern of motoneuronal activity (central burst pattern generation with afferent influences). See Figure 3B,C. Afferents can directly affect timing or the motoneuronal burst pattern (see Figure 5).

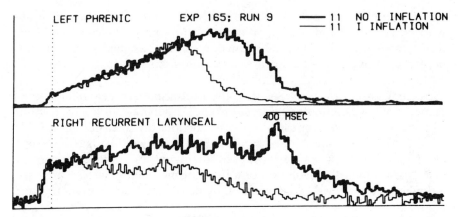

FIGURE 5. Cycle triggered histograms of phrenic and recurrent laryngeal nerve activity demonstrating the profound and discrete influences of pulmonary stretch receptor activity on phase timing and burst pattern (Feldman & Speck, 1983).

lung inflation withheld or shifted to the period of phrenic motoneuronal silence (neural expiration). Withholding lung inflation, for example, results in prolonged inspiratory nerve discharge, but has little or no effect on phrenic motoneuronal discharge at equivalent times when comparing test and control cycles (Fig. 5; Feldman, Cohen, and Wolotsky, 1976a; Cohen and Feldman, 1979, 1984; Feldman and Speck, 1983). Thus, the timing is altered with no necessary change in the evolution of the phrenic nerve burst. Yet, there is a change in the amplitude of recurrent laryngeal nerve discharge. This indicates that pulmonary stretch receptor afferents can affect global phase timing and selectively affect the pattern of different motoneuron pools.

Pulmonary stretch receptor activation during expiration also produces differential effects on expiratory nerve burst amplitude and duration (Cohen, Feldman, and Sommer, 1986). Using the cycle-triggered pump paradigm, test cycles consisted of ~ 1 sec inflations during *mid-expiration* in anesthetized cats. At all rates of inflation in the physiological range, lung inflation prolonged expiratory duration. However, low rates of inflation produced an increased amplitude in expiratory nerve discharge; yet, at higher rates of inflation, the amplitude of expiratory nerve discharge decreased (see Fig. 12 in Cohen, Feldman, and Sommer, 1986). Since the effects on burst amplitude and timing are distinctly different, these results suggest a functional separation of the controlling mechanisms.

2. *Chemoreceptor activation.* The addition of CO_2 to the inspired gas mixture activates chemoreceptors and increases the rate of augmentation of the burst of inspiratory motoneuronal discharge but inspiratory duration remains relatively unaltered. A simple explanation is that CO_2 mostly affects mechanisms controlling the burst evolution but leaves relatively unaffected those mechanisms generating timing (Feldman, 1981).

3. *Microinjection.* We have recently discovered that extremely small injections (0.2–2 nanoliters; 0.2–20 picomoles) of excitatory amino acids into discrete regions of the VRG can have profound dose-dependent effects on phrenic nerve discharge (McCrimmon, Feldman, and Speck, 1986). At many sites, there is only a change in the amplitude of the integrated phrenic nerve discharge, with no associated change in burst duration or overall timing of the bursting. At other sites there was either no effect or a change in both burst amplitude and timing.

4. *Brain stem lesions.* Lesions in the DRG-VRG that reduce the amplitude of phrenic nerve activity do not affect the timing of the burst (Speck and Feldman, 1982).

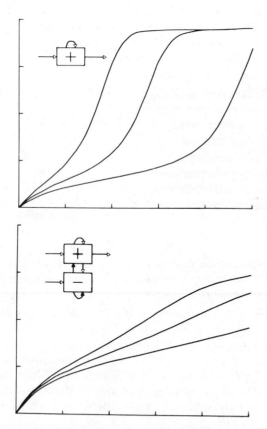

FIGURE 6. The generation of the stereotypic augmenting motoneuronal burst pattern may be due to recurrent interactions within a neuronal circuit. These graphs represent the firing pattern of model neuronal populations with 3 levels of tonic input. Ordinate: Population activity; abscissa: Time in units of population time constants. Top: Recurrent excitation will result in an augmenting burst. In the absence of nonlinear or accommodative synaptic or membrane properties, recurrent excitation leads rapidly to maximal firing. Bottom: The addition of recurrent inhibition to this network results in a quasi-linear augmenting burst, similar to that seen in many respiratory neurons (Feldman and Cowan, 1976).

Thus, it is reasonable to separately consider the mechanisms for: (1) generation of the discharge pattern during inspiration and expiration; and, (2) generation of the signals controlling the duration of inspiration and expiration (Fig. 6; Feldman, 1986).

3.3.1 Generation of the Discharge Pattern During Inspiration and Expiration

1. *Recurrent excitation.* A diffusely interconnected network of tonically driven or spontaneously active population of mutually excitatory neurons would develop steadily increasing activity following release from inhibition (Fig. 6; Feldman and Cowan, 1976). If such a network consisted of neurons lacking accommodative properties, then there would be an exponential rather than a linear rate of increasing discharge (Fig. 6, top). An exponential pattern of discharge is seen in convulsant states (e.g., following administration of strychnine) and during gasping but not during eupnea. Addition of recurrent inhibition to the network tends to linearize the developing pattern of discharge. A recurrent network of excitation and inhibition has the additional feature of exhibiting a step-ramp pattern of activity (Fig. 6, bottom), which is commonly seen in respiratory motor nerve activity and premotor and motoneuronal membrane potentials. There is no direct evidence of recurrent excitation among brainstem bulbospinal neurons or of recurrent inhibition between *identified* DRG-VRG neurons.

2. *Network inhibition.* Inhibitory interactions among neurons would also be expected to play a role in shaping the burst pattern (recurrent inhibition) and in reciprocal inhibition (Feldman and Grillner, 1983).

3. *Pacemaker-like activity.* See Section 3.4.

4. *Plateau and slow postsynaptic potentials.* When primed, cells in the lobster stomatogastric ganglion respond to a short depolarizing pulse with a long plateau depolarization and associated spiking; plateau potentials may terminate spontaneously or in response to a short hyperpolarizing pulse (Russell and Hartline, 1982). Such plateaus might be important in generating bursts in vertebrate neurons. If plateau potentials are important, only brief input pulses would be necessary to turn the bursts on and off.

Synaptic potentials with time courses of seconds have been observed (Jan and Kuffler, 1979; Harris-Warrick, Chapter 8). Thus, at synapses releasing transmitters that produce slow, potent postsynaptic potentials, a brief input may be sufficient to trigger the generation of a burst lasting seconds.

5. *Postinhibitory rebound.* Many neurons exhibit a rebound depolarization and associated impulse activity following a sudden release from hyperpolarization due to IPSPs or injected current. Such a mechanism has been postulated to underlie the early peak, slow decrementing discharge of neurons which fire during stage 1 of expiration, such as early expiratory

(Feldman and Cohen, 1978) or post-inspiratory neurons (Richter, 1982) or abrupt inspiratory burst onset. Following an abrupt decrease in IPSPs at the end of inspiration, these neurons depolarize rapidly in early expiration and produce a burst of impulses. Consistent with this hypothesis, early expiratory neurons exhibit an increased burst discharge when the peak amplitude of the preceding inspiratory burst is increased, presumably along with the associated reciprocal inhibition of expiratory neurons (Feldman and Cohen, 1978).

6. *Extracellular K^+ accumulation.* Accumulation of extracellular K^+ depolarizes neurons. Thus, tightly clustered neurons or dendrites might show gradually augmenting patterns of activity in response to tonic inputs, since as K^+ accumulated extracellularly, impulse discharge rates would increase. Potassium activity, a_{K^+}, in the region of DRG-VRG inspiratory neurons fluctuates in phase with the respiratory cycle (Richter, Camerer, and Sonnhof, 1978). These changes are probably pre-synaptic in origin since: (1) a_{K^+} increases precede local neuronal spiking, and (2) antidromic activation of DRG-VRG neurons does not markedly alter a_{K^+}.

If K^+ accumulation is important, then a restriction could be placed on prolonged neuronal discharges, since presynaptic release of neurotransmitter would be attenuated due to depolarization of axon terminals and postsynaptic discharge should be limited by depolarization block. However, synaptic activity increases throughout the entire inspiratory cycle (Ballantyne and Richter, 1984). Moreover, in mechanically ventilated animals, respiratory neurons can fire for periods > 1 hour, e.g., during apneusis (prolonged and continuous—plateau—inspiratory activity) or during electrical stimulation, with no obvious accommodation.

3.3.2 Generation of the Signals Controlling the Duration of Inspiration and Expiration

Considerable interest has focused on the neural basis for the transition from inspiration to expiration and *vice versa*. The following mechanisms have been proposed as contributing neural events:

1. *Pacemaker-like Activity.*   See Section "Inhibition and Pacemaker Neurons."

2. *Fatigue or Accommodation.*   One of the first modern models of neural rhythmogenesis of a two phase movement was Brown's half-center model (1914). Reciprocal inhibition between the centers generating each phase would ensure that only one phase would be active at any time. Each phase generator would have a bimodal distribution of states: active in the absence of inhibition or silent in the presence of inhibition. The activity of each phase would be limited by the inherent fatiguability of its constituent neurons; thus, alterations between the two phases would develop as the substrate for one phase fa-

tigued, removing the inhibition from the other. Such an arrangement is unlikely for respiration, since, under the appropriate conditions, a single phase can last for minutes or longer, with no evidence of fatigue.

3. *Postsynaptic Inhibition.*   Impulse activity of a neuron may be terminated by a barrage of IPSPs. Many models of respiratory rhythmogenesis have proposed that a population of neurons, often called *off-switch* neurons, produce a burst of IPSPs that terminates inspiration. Neurons with the predicted spike discharge pattern are found in the DRG; however, they do not appear to be inhibitory (Feldman and Speck, 1983; Cohen and Feldman, 1984). Such a population, if it did exist elsewhere, would be an important component of the respiratory oscillator.

4. *Disfacilitation.*   The removal of excitatory inputs to inspiratory (or expiratory) premotor or motor neurons would result in phase termination. This could result from presynaptic inhibition, late arriving impulses that cause shunting of EPSPs, or simply the removal of impulses causing inspiratory drive EPSPs. This begs the question, however, of the ultimate source of these inputs.

3.4   Inhibition and Pacemaker Neurons

Inhibition is undoubtedly important in respiratory pattern generation. Recurrent inhibition (see above) may be important in shaping burst pattern. Reciprocal inhibition may function to assure silence in inspiratory neurons during expiration and *vice versa*. Inhibition has been hypothesized to produce phase termination. We have exploited a novel in vitro mammalian brain stem-spinal cord preparation (Smith and Feldman, 1985, 1987b; Suzue, 1984) to test the role of Cl^--dependent synaptic inhibition in pattern generation (Feldman and Smith, 1986; Smith and Feldman, 1986, 1987a). We selectively changed the medium bathing the brain stem from a mock brain extracellular fluid (ECF) to a Cl^--free ECF, or to ECF containing Cl^- channel blockers/antagonists to the inhibitory neurotransmitters γ-aminobutyric acid (GABA) or glycine (Gly). None of the antagonists, nor Cl^--free fluid disrupted the rhythm of spontaneous respiratory motor bursts recorded on cranial nerves IX, X, and XII and spinal cervical nerves C4, and C5 and thoracic ventral roots. However, blocking synaptic inhibition increased burst durations and amplitudes. These results suggest that Cl^--dependent inhibition is not essential for the generation of respiratory rhythm in this preparation, but contributes to the shaping of the motor burst pattern.

Although our results pertain to Cl^--dependent inhibition, we hypothesize that inhibitory interactions are not necessary for generation of respiratory rhythm; termination of phase bursting by disfacilitation is sufficient for rhythmogenesis in vitro. The role of inhibition in controlling burst duration may be to assure burst termination in intact animals where sensory inputs might lead to spurious phase reactivation. If this latter hypothesis were correct, neural pacemaker activity could underlie the periodicity of mammalian respiration. Neural pacemakers can give rise to the gradually augmenting pattern of discharge characteristic of respiratory motoneurons (Feldman and Cleland, 1982). Since neurons in the DRG-VRG do not appear to have pacemaker-like properties except under special circumstances that may or may not be physiologically relevant (Dekin, Richerson, and Getting, 1985), other, as yet undetermined, sites may contain the hypothetical pacemakers.

3.5 State-Dependence of the Mechanisms Generating Respiratory Pattern

Respiration is the only rhythmic movement of skeletal muscles that is continuous throughout life in mammals. It is the only purposeful movement active in all sleep-wake states. This does not mean, however, that the same neural elements generate the pattern in all states. In fact, since the respiratory pattern changes in basic character in the different sleep-wake states, it is possible that different pattern generators produce respiratory movements in each state. Parsimony, however, would argue for some degree of overlap. There is evidence that the PRG, in the region of the Kölliker-Fuse and parabrachial nuclei in the dorsolateral rostral pons, may have a state-dependent role in the generation of the respiratory pattern (Feldman, 1986).

In anesthetized or decerebrate preparations where phasic pulmonary stretch receptor activity is controlled by a cycle triggered pump, respiratory-modulated PRG neuronal activity is readily observed only during respiratory cycles when inflation of the lung is withheld (Feldman, Cohen, and Wolotsky, 1976a,b). During cycles with inflation, there is little or no respiratory modulated PRG neuronal activity (Fig. 7A). Following lesions in the PRG, apneusis (prolonged—several seconds to hours—inspiratory periods) will develop, but only in the *absence* of lung inflation (Fig. 7D). Nanoliter injections of excitatory amino acids into the Kölliker-Fuse nucleus during expiration will produce, almost immediately, an inspiratory motoneuronal burst and an associated resetting of the rhythm (McCrimmon, Feldman, Speck, Ellenberger, and Smith, 1986). Thus, either phasic pulmonary stretch-receptor input or an intact PRG are required for respiratory motor pattern to be stereotypic (Fig. 7A–C); with neither, a significant abnormality develops (Fig. 7D). We assert that this represents direct evidence of a state-dependent change in the circuitry involved in generation of respiratory pattern. Under more natural conditions, the degree of respiratory modulation of PRG neurons varies with the sleep-wake cycle (Lydic and Orem, 1979; Sieck and Harper, 1980). This may represent normally occurring state-dependent changes in the circuitry controlling respiration and may underlie the profound changes in control of breathing seen in different sleep-wake states.

INTACT - With Lung Inflation

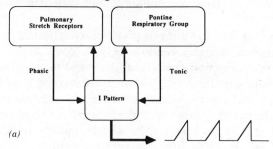

(a)

INTACT - Without Lung Inflation

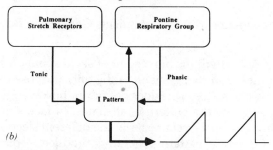

(b)

PRG LESIONS - With Lung Inflation

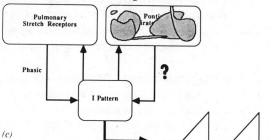

(c)

PRG LESIONS - Without Lung Inflation

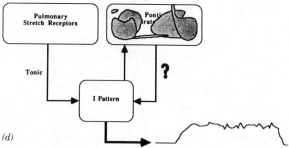

(d)

FIGURE 7. Either or both phasic pulmonary stretch receptor activity or PRG neuronal activity are necessary to generate a normal respiratory pattern in the decerebrate or anesthetized cat. *Intact* means that basic brainstem and spinal cord circuits for breathing are not lesioned. Panels A–D show the effects of alterations in stretch receptor or PRG activity on motor outflow. Hatched areas of PRG indicate presence of lesions. See text for details.

4   SENSORIMOTOR INTEGRATION: RESPIRATORY PREMOTOR NEURONS AS A DISPLACED MOTOR SYSTEM

The central respiratory drive command to spinal motoneurons is transmitted from the brain stem to the spinal cord via bulbospinal neurons. Considerable evidence suggests that a significant component of this projection is monosynaptic:

1. Cross-correlation histograms of the discharge of phrenic and/or intercostal nerves relative to the time of occurrence of impulses in bulbospinal neurons often show a short-latency, rapidly rising peak. This peak can be interpreted as an indicator of a monosynaptic projection, although alternative interpretations are possible. It has been argued that these peaks may indicate: a. A disynaptic projection, mediated by spinal interneurons, such as in descending control of limb motoneurons. Yet, anatomical studies demonstrate a dominant projection of bulbospinal neurons directly to the respiratory motoneuron pools (see below). b. A spurious correlation due to a correlated discharge of a non-bulbospinal neuron with a bulbospinal neuron that makes the true connection (Kirkwood & Sears, 1985). Yet, we observed pairs of brain stem neurons that had a strongly correlated timing of impulse discharges, but only one neuron showed a correlation to phrenic nerve discharge (Feldman and Speck, 1983).

2. Anterograde labeling of the projections of bulbospinal VRG neurons shows a marked projection often restricted to the regions of phrenic and intercostal motoneurons (Feldman, Loewy, and Speck, 1985; Ellenberger, McKenna, and Feldman, 1985). Some injection sites do show, in addition, a projection to (likely) propriospinal interneurons (Aoki, 1981) in the upper cervical spinal cord. These presumed propriospinal interneurons appear to project directly to intercostal, but only indirectly to phrenic, motoneurons (Lipski and Duffin, 1985). These results suggest both monosynaptic and multisynaptic descending bulbospinal projections, with the phrenic motoneurons seemingly receiving a strong monosynaptic input.

The apparent monosynaptic descending control of the diaphragm *appears* in distinct contrast to the current picture of control of limb musculature, where descending control of motoneurons is largely mediated by segmental interneurons. Yet, we would argue that the basic organization of command, premotor, and motor neurons is similar in limb muscle and diaphragm and suggest a common paradigm for sensorimotor integration (Fig. 8). We arrive at this opinion by consideration of the signals provided by afferents activated by movement. In limb muscle control, a descending command, relayed through segmental interneurons, alters the firing rate

DESCENDING MOTOR CONTROL
(OVERSIMPLIFIED)

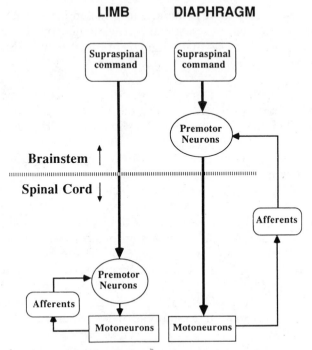

FIGURE 8. The basic organization of command, premotor, and motor neurons may be similar in the systems controlling limb or diaphragm (for ventilation) and suggest a common paradigm for sensorimotor integration. See text for details.

of the appropriate motoneurons, resulting in a coordinated movement. This movement activates afferents in the limb, which enter the nervous system in segments proximal to the location of the premotor interneurons that receive the descending command. Thus, some premotor interneurons can integrate descending command with afferent signals to provide immediate adjustment in the command to the motoneurons.

In diaphragm control, the rhythmic command, which is of supraspinal origin, is relayed to the motoneurons by premotor neurons whose somas are located (quite distant) in the brain stem. The resultant movement activates afferents. Since it is movement of the *lung* that results in ventilation, it should not be surprising that the brain is very interested in the status of the lung (lung volume, rate of expansion-contraction, etc.). Signals containing such information, arising from receptors in the lung, enter the brain via *cranial nerves* and synapse in the region of the solitary tract nuclei, which includes the DRG. In fact, some afferents synapse on bulbospinal inspiratory premotor neurons (Averill, Cameron, and Berger, 1984). Thus, some respiratory premotor neurons integrate afferent signals with respiratory drive to allow for immediate changes in the command to phrenic (and intercostal) motoneurons. In principle, therefore, both the diaphragm and limb control systems share an arrangement of descending command, premotor neuron, motoneuron, and movement-activated afferent organization. The difference is in the physical distance between the cell somas of premotor and motor neurons; the associated differences in conduction velocity are insignificant (typically, descending respiratory impulses take 2–6 ms to reach phrenic motoneurons).

The anatomical differences and functional similarities between respiratory and limb motor control might be explained by considering the evolution of the respiratory system. In fish the pattern generator and motoneurons controlling respiratory movements of the branchial musculature of the gills is located in the brain stem. This anatomy is similar to limb motor control circuitry in mammals, where premotor and motoneurons are often quite proximate. With further evolutionary development from fish to mammals, the innervation of the branchiomeric or homologous* muscles for respiratory control was maintained. Evolution added the lung and associated musculature of the diaphragm, thorax, and abdomen. For the control of these respiratory muscles, the brain used the already existing substrate for rhythmogenesis and premotor control in the brain stem, and directly targeted the cervical and thoracic motoneuron pools with long descending axons. Thus, in comparison with the spinal mechanisms for limb motor control, the control system for the mammalian respiratory pump may be considered a *displaced motor system.*

The displacement of the respiratory premotor network distant from the motoneurons in concentrated clusters in the brain stem presents a distinct advantage for studying the premotor or motoneuronal systems. For example, we were able to examine the effects of synchronous antidromic activation of a large fraction of the bulbospinal premotor neurons on respiratory pattern (Feldman, McCrimmon, and Speck, 1984). The unique anatomy may offer other opportunities for testing hypotheses of premotorneuronal organization difficult or impossible to implement in systems controlling, for example, limb, jaw or eye muscles.

5 UNIQUE PROPERTIES OF THE CENTRAL RESPIRATORY NETWORK

Uninterrupted breathing is required for life; inefficient breathing compromises life. An important feature of the respiratory system in mammals

---

*Muscles subserving a respiratory function in mammals (e.g., pharyngeal and laryngeal muscles) are derived from the mesoderm of the branchial arches and are innervated by cranial motoneurons (special visceral efferents, Brodal, 1981, p450).

must therefore be reliability, fatigue resistance and efficiency. Such design optimization would include gas exchange, muscle and pump mechanics, and neural control; we wish to comment on the latter.

The robustness of the respiratory system has led many to suggest that the neural control system may be highly redundant and widely distributed. This would certainly make it resistant to local insults. Under more global challenges such as anoxia or severe hypoglycemia (e.g., insulin shock), the central generation of respiratory pattern is also resistant to failure as the last consequential neural function to fail. Two properties aside from redundancy or distribution may contribute to this relative resistance to failure: (1) local regulation of blood flow in the brain may maximize brain stem circulation during such conditions; and, (2) respiratory neurons may be inherently or, because of special local environment, more tolerant of extreme conditions than other neurons. We hypothesize that the neurons controlling respiration have distinct properties underlying the system's resilience when compared to other neurons.

It is notable that the use of deoxyglucose uptake as a marker of neuronal activity (Sokoloff, 1977) has not explicitly labeled DRG or VRG neurons (Grippi, Rossiter, Davies, Pack, and Fishman, 1985; Kostreva, 1983; Kostreva, Zuperku, and Feldman, unpublished observations), even though these neurons are obviously active. This failure to label (which could have non-metabolic causes) may indicate special metabolic properties of respiratory neurons. The whole brain, on the average, does not appear to have the metabolic machinery for gluconeogenesis or anerobic metabolism; yet, such mechanisms may be present in discrete parts of the brain concerned with respiration.

There is regular periodic release of neurotransmitters by respiratory premotor neurons and likely by neurons providing the respiratory drive to these premotor neurons. Under normal, but especially extreme conditions, any compromise of synaptic function would reduce ventilation. This would suggest that the neurotransmitters be efficiently used. For example, a transmitter that is inactivated by reuptake, as opposed to enzymatic degradation, would be more energy efficient; the excitatory and inhibitory amino acids are examples of the former. Recent evidence suggests a role for excitatory amino acids or related pepides as the neurotransmitters of respiratory bulbospinal premotor neurons (McCrimmon, Smith, Ellenberger, and Feldman, 1986; McCrimmon, Smith, and Feldman, 1986). We would also argue that the axonal terminals function as autonomously as possible relative to the cell somas. This would reduce the need for energetically expensive anterograde and retrograde transport systems. This is consistent with our observation that bulbospinal and intrinsic brain stem respiratory neurons do not appear to transport horseradish peroxidase (antero- and retrograde) (Kalia, Feldman, and Cohen, 1981; Ellenberger, Smith, McCrimmon, and Feldman, 1986) or tritiated amino acids (Feldman, Loewy, and Speck, 1985) as well as other neurons in the brain stem, e.g., red nucleus (Gibson, Hansma, Houk, and Robinson, 1983), i.e., for similar protocols, considerably less material appears to be transported by respiratory neurons.

All of this is highly speculative and based on anecdotal observations. Yet, we would call attention to such matters, as recognition of possible unique or extreme properties may provide a handle for understanding central respiratory function.

6 SUMMARY

In conclusion, understanding the central control and generation of respiratory movements may be both simpler (e.g., gating as a means of controlling phase duration) and more complex (e.g., coordination of discharge in diverse motoneuronal pools) than usually considered. Although neurobiological techniques will provide part of the necessary information, understanding the act of breathing may provide the remaining necessary perspective to unravel its secrets.

REFERENCES

Adrian, E. D. and F. J. J. Buytendijk (1931). Potential changes in the isolated brain stem of goldfish. *J. Physiol.*, **71**:121–135.

Ahmad, H. R. and H. H. Loeschcke (1982). Transient and steady state responses of pulmonary ventilation to the medullarly extracellular pH after approximately rectangular changes in alveolar PCO_2 *Pflüg. Arch.*, **395**:285–292.

Andrezik, J. A., V. Chan-Palay, and S. L. Palay (1981). The nucleus paragigantocellularis lateralis in the rat. Demonstration of afferents by retrograde transport of horseradish peroxidase. *Anat. Embryol.*, **161**:373–390.

Aoki, M., S. Mori, K. Kawahara, H. Watanabe, and N. Ebata (1980). Generation of spontaneous respiratory rhythm in high spinal cats. *Brain Res.*, **202**:51–63.

Averill, D. B., W. E. Cameron, and A. J. Berger (1984). Monosynaptic excitation of dorsal medullary respiratory neurons by slowly adapting pulmonary stretch receptors. *J. Neurophysiol.*, **52**:771–785.

Ballantyne. D. and D. W. Richter (1984). Post-synaptic inhibition of bulbar inspiratory neurones in the cat. *J. Physiol.* **348**:67–87.

Bassal, M. and A. L. Bianchi (1982). Inspiratory onset or termination induced by electrical stimulation of the brain. *Respir. Physiol.*, **50**:23–40.

Berger, A. J. and K. A. Cooney (1982). Ventilatory effects of kainic acid injection of the ventrolateral solitary nucleus. *J. Appl. Physiol.: Respirat. Environ. Exercise Physiol.*, **52**:131–140.

Bertrand, F. and A. Hugelin (1971). Respiratory synchronizing function of nucleus parabrachialis medialis: pneumotaxic mechanisms. *J. Neurophysiol.*, **34**:189–207.

Bianchi, A. L. (1971). Localisation et étude des neurones respiratoires bulbaires.

Mise en jeu antidromique par stimulation spinale ou vagale. *J. Physiol. (Paris)*, **63**:5–40.

Bianchi, A. L. and J. C. Barillot (1982). Respiratory neurons in the region of the retrofacial nucleus: pontile, medullary, spinal, and vagal projections. *Neurosci. Lett.*, **31**:277–282.

Bradley, G. W., C. von Euler, I. Marttila, and B. Roos (1973). A model of the central and reflex inhibition of inspiration in the cat. *Biol. Cybernetics*, **19**:105–116.

Bramble, D. M. and D. R. Carrier (1983). Running and breathing in mammals. *Science*, **219**:251–256.

Brodal, A. (1981). *Neurological Anatomy*, 3rd ed., Oxford University Press, London.

Brown, T. G. (1914). On the nature of the fundamental activity of the nervous centres: together with an analysis of the conditioning of rhythmic activity in progression, and a theory of the evolution of function in the nervous system. *J. Physiol.*, **48**:18–46.

Bunn, J. C. and J. Mead (1971). Control of ventilation during speech. *J. Appl. Physiol.*, **31**:870–872.

Cherniack, N. S., C. von Euler, I. Homma, and F. F. Kao (1979). Graded changes in central chemoreceptor input by local temperature changes on the ventral surface of medulla. *J. Physiol.*, **287**:191–211.

Cherniack, N. S. and C. von Euler (1980). Central neural and reflex control of breathing. In *Assessment of Pulmonary Performance*, (ed. A. P. Fishman), ed. McGraw-Hill, New York, pp. 69–75.

Cohen, M. I. (1979). Neurogenesis of respiratory rhythm in the mammal. *Physiol. Rev.*, **59**:1105–1173.

Cohen, M. I. and J. L. Feldman (1977). Models of respiratory phase switching. *Fed. Proc.*, **36**:2367–2374.

Cohen, M. I. and J. L. Feldman (1984). Discharge properties of dorsal medullary inspiratory neurons: relation to pulmonary afferent and phrenic efferent discharge. *J. Neurophysiol.*, **51**:753–776.

Cohen, M. I., J. L. Feldman, and D. Sommer (1985). Caudal medullary expiratory neurone and internal intercostal nerve discharge in the cats: Effects of lung inflation. *J. Physiol.*, **368**:147–178.

Dekin, M. S., P. A. Getting, and G. B. Richerson (1985). Thyrotropin-releasing hormone induces rhythmic bursting in neurons of the nucleus tractus solitarius. *Science*, **229**:67–69.

Eldridge, F. L., D. E. Millhorn, and T. Waldrop (1981). Exercise hypernea and locomotion: parallel activation from the hypothalamus. *Science*, **211**:844–846.

Ellenberger, H. H., J. C. Smith, D. R. McCrimmon, and J. L. Feldman (1985). A projection from a discretely localized cell group of the rostral medulla to the ventral respiratory group in the cat. *Soc. Neurosci. Abs.* **11**:1143.

Ellenberger, H. H., K. E. McKenna, and J. L. Feldman (1986). Efferent projections of the ventral respiratory group of the rat. *Fed. Proc.*, **45**:872.

Euler, C. von (1983). On the central pattern generator for the basic breathing rhythmicity. *J. Appl. Physiol.*, **55**:1647–1659.

Euler, C. von., K. Budzinska, T. Pantaleo, Y. Yamamoto, and F. F. Kao (1984). Some organizational features of the respiratory pattern generator and its output as revealed by focal cold block of different medullary structures. In *Neurogenesis of Central Respiratory Rhythm*, A. L. Bianchi, and M. Denavit-Saubie, eds. MTP Press, Hingham, MA, pp. 45–51.

Feldman, J. L. (1976). A network model for control of inspiratory cutoff by the pneumotaxic center with supportive experimental data in cats. *Biol. Cybernetics*, **21**:131–138.

Feldman, J. L. (1981). Interactions between medullary respiratory neurons. *Fed. Proc.*, **40**:2384–2388.

Feldman, J. L. (1986). Neurophysiology of Respiration in Mammals. In *Handbook of Physiology; Section 1: The Nervous System; Volume IV*, F. E. Bloom, ed. American Physiology Society, pp. 463–524.

Feldman, J. L. and C. L. Cleland (1982). Possible roles of pacemaker neurons in mammalian respiratory rhythmogenesis. In *Cellular Pacemakers*, Vol. II, D. O. Carpenter, ed. Wiley, New York, pp. 104–128.

Feldman, J. L. and M. I. Cohen (1978). Relation between expiratory duration and rostral medullary expiratory neuronal discharge. *Brain Res.*, **141**:172–178.

Feldman, J. L., M. I. Cohen, and P. Wolotsky (1976a). Powerful inhibition of pontine respiratory neurons by pulmonary afferents. *Brain Res.*, **104**:341–346.

Feldman, J. L., M. I. Cohen, and P. Wolotsky (1976b). Phasic pulmonary afferent activity drastically alters the respiratory modulation of neurons in the rostral pontine pneumotaxic center. In I.N.S.E.R.M. Colloquium: *Respiratory Centers and Afferent Systems*, B. Duron, ed. Edition INSERM, Paris, France, pp. 95–105.

Feldman, J. L. and J. D. Cowan (1975). Large scale activity in neural nets I: Theory with applications to motoneuron pool responses. *Biol. Cybernetics*, **17**:29–38.

Feldman, J. L. and J. D. Cowan (1975). Large scale activity in neural nets II: A model for the brainstem respiratory oscillator. *Biol. Cybernetics*, **17**:39–51.

Feldman, J. L. and H. Gautier (1976). The interaction of pulmonary afferents and pneumotaxic center in control of respiratory pattern in cats. *J. Neurophysiol.*, **39**:31–44.

Feldman, J. L. and S. Grillner (1983). Control of vertebrate respiration and locomotion. *The Physiologist*, **26**:310–316.

Feldman, J. L., A. D. Loewy, and D. F. Speck (1985). Projections from the ventral respiratory group to phrenic and intercostal motoneurons in cat: An autoradiographic study. *J. Neuroscience*, **8**:1993–2000.

Feldman, J. L., D. R. McCrimmon, and D. F. Speck (1984). Effect of synchronous activation of medullary respiratory premotor neurons on phrenic nerve discharge in cats. *J. Physiol.*, **347**:241–254.

Feldman, J. L., D. Sommer, and M. I. Cohen (1980). Short time scale correlations between discharges of medullary respiratory neurons. *J. Neurophysiol.* **43**:1284–1295.

Feldman, J. L. and J. C. Smith (1986). Separate generation of oscillation and motor burst pattern for mammalian respiration: *in vitro* studies. *Soc. Neurosci. Abs.*, **12**:791.

Feldman, J. L. and D. F. Speck (1983). Interactions among inspiratory neurons in the dorsal and ventral respiratory groups in cat medulla. *J. Neurophysiol.*, **49**:472–490.

Fedorko, L. and E. G. Merrill (1984). Axonal projections from rostral expiratory neurones of the Bötzinger complex to medulla and spinal cord in the cat. *J. Physiol.*, **350**:487–496.

Gauthier, P., R. Monteau, and M. Dussardier (1983). Inspiratory on-switch evoked by mesencephalic stimulation. *Exp. Brain. Res.*, **51**:261–270.

Gibson, A. R., D. I. Hansma, J. C. Houk, and F. R. Robinson (1984). A sensitive low artifact TMB procedure for the demonstration of WGA-HRP in the CNS. *Brain Res.*, **298**:235–241.

Grippi, M., C. Rossiter, R. Davies, A. Pack, and A. P. Fishman (1985). Metabolic mapping of vagal afferent activity in the cat medulla using the[14] C-2-deoxyglucose method. *Fed. Proc.*, **44**:1585.

Harper, R. M., R. C. Frysinger, R. B. Trelease, and J. D. Marks (1984). State-dependent alteration of respiratory timing by stimulation of the central nucleus of the amygdala. *Brain Res.*, **306**:1–8.

Hukuhara, T. Jr. (1976). Functional organization of brain stem respiratory neurons and its afferences. In *Respiratory Centres and Afferent Systems*, B. Duron, ed. INSERM, Paris, pp. 41–53.

Iscoe, S., J. L. Feldman, and M. I. Cohen (1979). Properties of inspiratory termination studied by superior laryngeal and vagal nerve stimulation. *Resp. Physiol.*, **36**:353–366.

Jan, Y. N., L. Y. Jan, and S. W. Kuffler (1979). A peptide as a possible transmitter in sympathetic ganglia of the frog. *Proc. Natl. Acad. Sci.*, **76**:1501–1505.

Kalia, M., J. L. Feldman, and M. I. Cohen (1979). Afferent projections to the inspiratory neuronal region of the ventrolateral nucleus of the tractus solitarius. *Brain Res.*, **171**:135–141.

King, G. W. (1980). Brain stem blood vessels and the organization of the lateral reticular formation in the medulla oblongata of the cat. *Brain Res.*, **191**:253–259.

King, G. W. and C. K. Knox (1984). Types and locations of respiratory-related neurones in lateral tegmental field of cat oblongata. *Brain Res.*, **295**:301–315.

Kirkwood, P. A., T. A. Sears, and J. G. Davies (1984). Cross-correlation analysis of the connections between bulbospinal neurones and respiratory motoneurones. In *Neurogenesis of Central Respiratory Rhythm*, A. L. Bianchi and M. Denavit-Saubie, eds. MTP Press, Hingham, MA, pp. 216–222.

Koepchen, H. P., H. Lazar, and J. Borchert (1974). On the role of the nucleus infrasolitarius in the determination of respiratory periodicity. *Proc. Intl. Union Physiol. Sci.*, **11**:81.

Koepchen, H. P., D. Klussendorf, H. Lazar, and T. Hukuhara (1984). Conclusions on respiratory rhythmogenesis drawn from lesion and cooling experiments predominantly in the region of ventrolateral nucleus of solitary tract. In *Neurogenesis of Central Respiratory Rhythm*, A. L. Bianchi and M. Denavit-Saubie, eds. MTP Press, Hingham, MA, pp. 77–81.

Kostreva, D. R. (1983). Functional mapping of cardiovascular reflexes and the heart using 2- [14C]Deoxyglucose. *The Physiologist*, **26**:333–350.

Lipski, J. and J. Duffin, (1986). An electrophysiological investigation of propriospinal inspiratory neurons in the upper cervical cord of cat. *Exp. Brain. Res.* **61**:625–637.

Lydic, R. and J. Orem (1979). Respiratory neurons of the pneumotaxis center during sleep and wakefulness. *Neurosci. Lett.*, **15**:187–192.

Luschei, E. S. and L. J. Goldberg (1982). Neural mechanisms of mandibular control: mastication and voluntary biting. In *Handbook of Physiology, Section 1: The Nervous System, Volume II*, V. Brooks, ed. Am Physiol. Soc., Bethesda, Md., pp. 1237–1274.

Luscher, H. R., P. Ruenzel, and E. Heneman (1983). Composite EPSPs in motoneurons of different sizes before and during PTP: Implications for transmission failure and its relief in Ia projections. *J. Neurophysiol.*, **49**:269–289.

McCrimmon, D. R., J. L. Feldman, and D. F. Speck (1987). Role of the dorsal respiratory group in the processing of afferent signals from vagal and superior laryngeal nerves. *Exp. Brain Res.* in press.

McCrimmon, D. R., J. L. Feldman, and D. F. Speck (1985). Respiratory motor discharge altered by picomole glutamate (GLU) injection into the ventral respiratory group (VRG) of cat. *Fed. Proc.*, **44**:428.

McCrimmon, D. R., J. L. Feldman, and D. F. Speck, (1986). Respiratory motoneuronal activity is altered by picomole injections of glutamate in the cat brainstem. *J. Neuroscience*, **6**:2384–2392.

McCrimmon, D. R., J. L. Feldman, D. F. Speck, H. H. Ellenberger, and J. C. Smith (1987). Functional heterogeneity of dorsal, ventral and pontine respiratory groups revealed by micropharmacological techniques. In *Neurobiology of the Control of Breathing, 10th Nobel Symposium*, C. von Euler and H. Lagercrantz, eds. Raven Press, New York, pp. 201–208.

McCrimmon, D. R., J. C. Smith, H. H. Ellenberger, and J. L. Feldman (1986). Possible excitatory amino acid mediation of inspiratory synaptic drive to spinal motoneurons in neonatal rat. *Soc. Neurosci. Abs.*, **12**:387.

McCrimmon, D. R., J. C. Smith, and J. L. Feldman (1986). Role of excitatory amino acids in transmitting respiratory drive to spinal motoneurons studied *in vitro*. *Fed. Prod.*, **45**:519.

Mendelson, M. (1971). Oscillator neurons in crustacean ganglia. *Science* **171**:1170–1173.

Milic-Emili, G. and J. M. Petit (1960). Mechanical efficiency of breathing. *J. Appl. Physiol.* **15**:359–362.

Miller, A. D., E. Ezure, and I. Suzuki (1985). Control of abdominal muscles by brain stem respiratory neurons in the cat. *J. Neurophysiol.*, **54**:155–167.

Miller, A. J. (1982). Deglutition. *Physiol. Rev.* **62**:129–184.

Mitchell, R. A. and A. J. Berger (1981). In *Lung Biology in Health and Disease: Regulation of Breathing*. Vol. 17. Pt. 1, Chapt. 8, pp. 541–620.

Morin-Surin, M. P., M. Denavit-Saubie, J. Champagnat, and E. Boudinot (1984). Differentiation of two respiratory areas in the cat medulla using kainic acid. *J. Resp. Physiol.*, **58**:323–334.

Richter, D. W., H. Camerer, and U. Sonnhof (1978). Changes in extracellular potassium during the spontaneous activity of medullary respiratory neurons. *Pflüg, Arch.*, **376**:139–149.

Richter, D. W. (1982). Generation and maintenance of the respiratory rhythm. *J. Expt. Biol.*, **100**:93–107.

Russell, D. F. and D. K. Hartline (1982). Slow active potentials and bursting motor patterns in pyloric network of the lobster, *Panulirus interruptus. J. Neurophysiol.*, **48**:914–937.

Saint-John, W. M., D. Bartlett, Jr., K. V. Knuth, and J. C. Hwang (1981). Brain stem genesis of automatic ventilatory patterns independent of spinal mechanisms. *J. Appl. Physiol. Respirat. Environ. Exercise Physiol.*, **51**:204–210.

Sieck, G. C. and R. M. Harper (1980). Pneumotaxic area neuronal discharge during sleep-waking states in the cat. *Exp. Neurol.*, **67**:79–102.

Smith, J. C. and J. L. Feldman (1985). Motor patterns for respiration and locomotion generated by an *in vitro* brainstem-spinal cord from neonatal rat. *Soc. Neurosci. Abs.*, **11**:24.

Smith, J. C. and J. L. Feldman (1986). Role of chloride-dependent synaptic inhibition in respiratory pattern generation. Studies in an *in vitro* mammalian brainstem-spinal cord preparation. *Fed. Proc.*, **45**:518.

Smith, J. C. and J. L. Feldman (1987a). Central respiratory pattern generation studied in an in vitro mammalian brainstem-spinal cord preparation. In: *Respiratory Muscles and Their Neuromotor Control*, G. C. Sieck, S. Gondevia and W. C. Cameron, eds. A. R. Liss, Inc., New York. pp. 27–36.

Smith, J. C. and J. L. Feldman. In vitro brainstem spinal cord preparations for study of motor systems for mammallian respiration and locomotion. *J. Neurosci. Methods. In press.*

Sokoloff, L. (1977). Relation between physiological function and energy metabolism in the central nervous system. *J. Neurochem.* **28**:897–916.

Speck, D. F. and J. L. Feldman (1982). Effects of microstimulation and microlesion in dorsal and ventral respiratory groups in medulla of cat on respiratory outflow. *J. Neuroscience*, **2**:744–757.

Suzue, T. (1984). Respiratory rhythm generation in the *in vitro* brain stem-spinal cord preparation of the neonatal rat. *J. Physiol.*, **354**:173–183.

Trouth, C. O., H. H. Loeschcke, and J. Berndt (1973). A superficial substrate on the ventral surface of the medulla oblongata influencing respiration. *Pflüg. Arch.*, **339**:135–152.

Viala, D. and E. Freton (1983). Evidence for respiratory and locomotor pattern generators in the rabbit cervico-thoracic cord and for their interactions. *Exp. Brain Res.*, **49**:247–256.

Wyman, R. J. (1977). Neural generation of the breathing rhythm. *Ann. Rev. Physiol.* **39**:417–448.

Yamada, K. A., W. P. Norman, P. Hamosh, and R. A. Gillis (1982). Medullary ventral surface GABA receptors affect respiratory and cardiovascular function. *Brain Res.*, **248**:71–78.

Chapter Four

COMPARATIVE ANALYSIS OF INVERTEBRATE CENTRAL PATTERN GENERATORS

PETER A. GETTING

Department of Physiology and Biophysics
University of Iowa
Iowa City, Iowa

1 INTRODUCTION

In the early 1960's, two observations were made which formed the basis for much of contemporary research on the organization of invertebrate motor systems. In 1964, Wiersma and Ikeda showed that stimulation of single neurons in the nerve cord of the crayfish could elicit coordinated behavioral acts. These cells were termed *command neurons*. Because the nature of the motor act elicited did not depend upon the pattern of stimulation. The command signals were regarded largely as "permissive." Their major role was viewed as signalling to the motor system when or when not to generate a particular motor pattern (Kennedy, 1973; Larimer, 1976; Kennedy and Davis, 1977). The generation of an appropriate sequence or pattern of motor output was religated to the motor network itself. In the case of rhythmic behaviors, the motor network is referred to as a *pattern generator*. At about the same time, Wilson (1961), showed that the isolated central nervous system of a locust could produce the motor pattern for flight in the absence of sensory feedback. This observation validated the concept that complex rhythmic behaviors could be generated by pattern generators contained within the central nervous system. A *central pattern generator* (CPG) is viewed as an assembly of neurons which, by virtue of their intrinsic properties and synaptic interactions, is capable of generating and controlling the spatial and temporal activity of motor neurons. The involvement of CPGs in numerous rhythmic behaviors has now been amply demonstrated (see Delcomyn, 1980 and Grillner, 1977 for review). With these concepts of a command system and a CPG serving as a focus, the thrust of research shifted towards determining how the command and pattern generation functions were implemented at the cellular, synaptic, and network levels.

2 THE HOPE

As a group, the invertebrates provided an alluring opportunity to pursue this quest. They display a diverse repertoire of rhythmic behaviors. But perhaps most attractive is the fact that their central nervous systems contain relatively few neurons, many of which are comparatively large and can be identified as individuals. The neurons can be penetrated either singly or in groups with microelectrodes, and their activity can be recorded and manipulated during the generation of motor activity. In addition, they could be morphologically characterized by dye injection. Because of these features, invertebrate preparations were coined "simple systems" (Fentress, 1975; Usherwood and Newth, 1975). These systems held the promise of allowing a thorough specification of the neurons and their synaptic interactions participating in a particular behavior. The hope was that, by analyzing the CPGs for different rhythmic systems, a relatively small number of mechanisms for pattern generation would emerge. If these mechanisms were conserved from animal to animal or behavior to behavior, then perhaps similar mechanisms would be involved in the generation of rhythmic motor responses in more complex systems such as those of the vertebrates. The purpose of this chapter is to describe some of the insights discovered about the organization of invertebrate central pattern generators and to offer a few general correlations which may assist in understanding and approaching more complex systems.

The first point is that the neuronal circuits controlling complex rhythmic behaviors in these invertebrate systems can be determined. The relevant neurons including sensory neurons, interneurons, and motor neurons can be located and analyzed. The role and firing pattern of these cells during generation of motor activity can be characterized. Their synaptic interactions can be mapped and measured. Even their intrinsic membrane properties can be uncovered (for review see Roberts and Roberts, 1983). This process, although still incomplete, has taken longer than many of us expected. In my own experience with *Tritonia*, it has taken over 10 years to describe, in relative detail, the neuronal mechanisms controlling the generation of the escape swimming motor program (Getting, 1983a). The reasons for taking so long are multiple. First, although the networks consist of a relatively small number of neurons, they can be very complex. For example, the CPG for *Tritonia* swimming contains at least twelve premotor interneurons. The pyloric system of the lobster stomatogastric ganglion contains fourteen neurons (Selverston et al., 1983). Likewise, the pattern generator controlling heartbeat in leech also consists of fourteen neurons (Calabrese and Peterson, 1983). The identity of these neurons was not usually obvious, and locating them required persistence as well as some luck.

Second, characterizing the synaptic connectivity between the CPG neurons is not trivial. This is usually done by pairwise intracellular recording. Given even the relatively small number of cells involved, mapping of the synaptic connectivity can be an arduous task. For example, there are 132 possible monosynaptic pathways between the 12 CPG neurons for swimming in *Tritonia*. Most of these possible pathways have been tested. Remarkably, 79 of the 132 possible connections are known to exist (Getting, 1981, 1983c) revealing the complexity of the network. Progress was further complicated by the presence of unexpected phenomena such as graded transmitter release from electrically coupled presynaptic neurons (Eisen and Marder, 1982) and multicomponent synaptic potentials (Getting, 1981). These problems required the invention and application of equally ingenious experimental approaches (e.g., cell "killing" techniques by photoinactivation (Miller and Selverston, 1979) and voltage clamp of neurons within an operating network (Lennard et al., 1980). The results of these mapping studies are usually represented as "ball-and-stick" circuit diagrams. Figure 1 shows the proposed diagrams and the sequence of firing for neurons within the CPG for swimming in *Tritonia* (A), the pyloric rhythm in lobster (B), and the control of heartbeat in leech (C). While the number of cell types involved in these CPGs is small, the pattern of synaptic connectivity is by no means simple.

Third, as our knowledge increased about how these networks function, it became apparent that the "ball-and-stick" diagrams were woefully inadequate. Although these diagrams show the identity of the cell types, their pattern of synaptic connectivity, and the sign of the interactions (excitatory or inhibitory), important information concerning the strength, time course, or mechanism of the synaptic action is not apparent. Nor do these diagrams include information about the intrinsic properties of each cell type. Intrinsic properties play a significant role in determining how a cell will respond to its synaptic input. Thus, CPGs turned out to be more complex than was anticipated.

Before any CPG had been described, several theoretical schemes had been proposed for the generation of cyclic patterned activity. It has become customary to divide these into two categories. First, patterned bursts could arise from the endogenous membrane properties of single neurons. In fact, "burster" neurons have been described in a number of invertebrates and

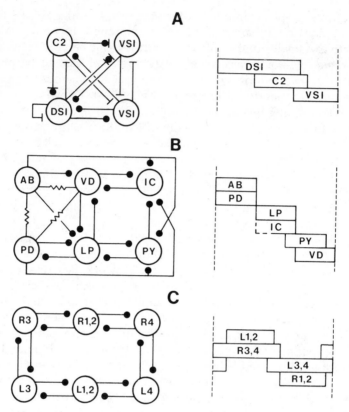

FIGURE 1. Neuronal networks forming the CPG for (A) swimming in *Tritonia* (Getting, 1983a), (B) pyloric rhythm in lobster (Selverston et al., 1983), and (C) heart beat control in leech (Calabrese and Peterson, 1983). In each panel, the synaptic connectivity is shown on the left. Excitatory connections are shown as T-bars, inhibitory connections as filled circles, and electrical synapses by the resistor symbol. Multi-action synapses are shown as mixed symbols. Nomenclature for cell types as per Getting (1983a) and Calabrese and Peterson (1983). On the right is a schematized summary of the temporal firing pattern within a single cycle.

produce recurrent bursts as a consequence of their time and voltage dependent ionic conductances (Alving, 1968; Berridge and Rapp, 1979; Meech, 1979). Alternatively, patterned bursts could emerge as a consequence of synaptic interactions within a network of otherwise mundane neurons. Network oscillators can be further divided into subgroups depending upon the nature and pattern of synaptic connectivity (Friesen and Stent, 1978; Kristan, 1980). It was hoped that this limited number of relatively simple schemes would provide a basis for explaining pattern generation in many diverse systems.

A number of CPGs have now been characterized to varying degrees and have been reviewed recently (Roberts and Roberts, 1983). In comparing these systems, one is struck by the diversity of networks and mechanisms. It appears that no two pattern generators are alike. Each seems to be a unique entity with its own set of peculiarities and properties. This point is illustrated by the diversity in synaptic connectivity within the three CPGs shown in Figure 1. Both the *Tritonia* swim system (A) and the lobster pyloric system (B) produce three-phase burst patterns within a single cycle as illustrated by the right-hand panel. These diagrams show the firing times of the corresponding neurons in the circuit diagrams. Yet, the neural circuits which produce these similar patterns are very different. The *Tritonia* circuit is characterized by a mix of both excitatory and inhibitory synapses. The pyloric network is dominated by inhibitory connections with only a few electrical synapses. These systems share similar output patterns, but these are generated by very different networks. In contrast, the lobster pyloric network (B) and the leech heart network (C) are both dominated by inhibitory connections with many reciprocal inhibitory pairs; yet, these two networks produce remarkably different temporal burst patterns. There appear to be multiple ways of generating similar patterns, and similar networks can produce diverse patterns. Unfortunately, it has not proven possible to parcel out the known CPGs into meaningful subsets. On theoretical grounds, this result should have been expected. Glass and Young (1979) have shown that four neurons, connected by either excitation or inhibition, could, in theory, generate cyclic patterns using any of 256 possible network structures. The initial expectation that only a small number of CPG types could explain a diverse repertoire of rhythmic behaviors was perhaps naive. Our error may not have been in expecting something to be conserved, but at the level at which this conservation occurred.

As will be discussed in detail later, the generation of patterned activity does not depend solely upon endogenous bursting properties or solely upon network interactions. Instead, the existence and form of the pattern seem to depend on a complex interaction between network, synaptic, and cellular properties. This understanding has led to an alternative view of what may be conserved from one system to the next. Pattern generating networks appear to share a common pool of "building block" mechanisms linked together in different combinations. Each combination could generate a different pattern thereby explaining the diversity of rhythmic behaviors. If this were true, CPG networks involved in diverse behaviors might appear different on the surface, but, in fact, be related by a common dependence on conserved mechanisms.

3   BUILDING BLOCKS OF A CPG

To gain some insight into what the building block mechanisms may be, it is helpful to consider, on theoretical grounds, what is necessary for a neuronal system to produce self-sustaining oscillations (not requiring phasic external input). Two features are easily recognizable. First, one action must inevitably be followed by its antagonistic action (sign reversal). Thus, excitation (or firing) of a neuron within a CPG must be followed by inhibition of the same neuron. Likewise, inhibition must lead to excitation (or firing). For example, excitation to initiate a burst must ultimately be followed by inhibition to terminate the burst. It is important to be clear on what is meant by excitation and inhibition. These terms apply to any process (cellular or synaptic) that increases or decreases, respectively, the likelihood of producing a spike (or membrane polarization in the case of nonspiking neurons). Inhibition could include (1) activation of an intrinsic membrane current that tends to hyperpolarize the cell, (2) synaptic inhibition, or (3) its functional equivalent, loss of excitation. The second major feature of an oscillatory system is that there must be a delay between the initial action and its antagonist (Friesen and Block, 1984). A delay is necessary so that one process (excitation or inhibition) can be expressed before the onset of its inevitable opposite action. In general, these delays are relatively long and close in duration to cycle period. With these ideas in mind, can we identify processes which give rise to excitation or inhibition, sign reversal from one to the other, and delays? These processes are likely to provide the "building blocks" for oscillatory CPGs.

It has proven convenient to divide the "building blocks" into three categories (Getting, 1983b; Selverston et al., 1983): those associated with properties intrinsic of single cells (cellular); those governing the action of single synapses (synaptic); and those describing the assembly of cells and synapses into circuits (network). In this section, I will describe some of the building block mechanisms currently thought to be involved in pattern generation. The following section illustrates how these building blocks can be assembled into functional pattern generator networks.

3.1 Cellular Properties

Central neurons contain more numerous and complex ionic currents than originally described by Hodgkin and Huxley (1952) for the squid axon. Different combinations of these currents can impart to cells radically divergent response characteristics (for review see Adams et al., 1980, Berridge and Rapp, 1979, Meech, 1979; Noble, 1983). For the purposes of this discussion, the underlying ionic currents are not so important as the nature of the response characteristics to which they give rise. Some important cellular properties which contribute to pattern generation are:

1. *Threshold.* This property determines the level of excitation needed for a neuron to start firing. Clearly, a cell with a high threshold (far from resting membrane potential) will require depolarization in order to fire. An auto-active cell which fires tonically without excitation can produce patterned activity simply by receiving phasic inhibition.

Both high threshold and auto-active neurons can be found within a single CPG network (Getting, 1983b). Recently, an interesting new twist has been added by the discovery of neurons in the lobster stomatogastric system which fire spikes only at membrane potentials between -60 mV and -30 mV (Robertson and Moulins, 1981, Robertson and Moulins, 1984). If these cells are depolarized beyond -30 mV, spiking ceases. Thus, these cells could produce two bursts for each cyclic depolarization; one as the depolarization increases towards -30 mV and a second as the membrane potential decreases from above -30mV.

2. *Spike-frequency Adaptation.*   This property is manifested as a decrease in spike frequency with time during sustained depolarization. Spike frequency adaptation is associated with the activation of slow outward potassium currents (Brown and Adams, 1979; Hume and Getting, 1982; Meech, 1978). Adaptation is a self-inhibitory process because it depends upon the recent firing history of the cell, and tends to decrease the responsiveness of the cell to further firing. Spike frequency adaptation can serve to shape burst structure (Hume and Getting, 1982b) and contribute to regulation of cycle period (Getting, 1983b).

3. *Postburst Hyperpolarization (PBH).*   Following a burst of spikes, many neurons become hyperpolarized for a period of time ranging from milliseconds to seconds (depending upon the strength and duration of the preceding burst). The postburst hyperpolarization appears to be a manifestation of a mechanism similar to that responsible for spike-frequency adaptation (Hume and Getting, 1982; Meech, 1974). Both characteristics are usually found together. Postburst hyperpolarization is also a self-inhibitory process producing an inhibition delayed until after a burst.

4. *Postinhibitory Rebound (PIR).*   This process is the inverse of PBH, and is expressed as a transient depolarization (excitation) following hyperpolarization (inhibition). If the depolarization exceeds threshold, the cell may fire a burst of spikes. PIR provides a mechanism to *delay* excitation until after inhibition. It has been implicated in the gastric mill system of lobsters (Mulloney and Selverston, 1974; Selverston and Mulloney, 1974) and the swimming systems of *Melibe* (Thompson, 1974) and *Clione* (Satterlie, 1985a). The ionic mechanism of PIR is largely unknown (but see Jones et al., 1983).

5. *Delayed Excitation (DE).*   Delayed excitation is manifested as a delay between the onset of a depolarizing stimulus and the first spike. The delay may range up to several seconds in molluscan neurons (Getting, 1983c) to several hundreds of milliseconds for mammalian cells (Dekin and Getting, 1984). These delays are too long to be attributed to the charging time of the membrane capacitance. The delay instead

results from the activation of a transient outward potassium current (Byrne et al., 1979; Byrne, 1980; Dekin and Getting, 1984; Getting, 1983c). This form of delayed excitation is different from the delayed firing caused by PIR. Delayed excitation is manifested *during* a depolarizing input while PIR produces delayed firing *after* an inhibitory input. Delayed excitation appears to play a role in phasing burst activity within the CPG for swimming in *Tritonia* (Getting, 1983c).

6. *Plateau Potentials.* Neurons displaying plateau potentials have two membrane potential states: A resting state and a depolarized state (Russell and Hartline, 1978). Transitions from the resting to the depolarized state can be induced (triggered) by short depolarizing inputs. This state can be maintained for considerable lengths of time (tens to hundreds of milliseconds) before it either spontaneously reverts to the resting state or is actively converted by a short hyperpolarizing stimulus. Plateau potentials provide a mechanism for translating transient input events into sustained responses. Neurons with this ability have been identified in the lobster stomatogastric system (Dickinson and Nagy, 1983; Russell and Hartline, 1978) and the swimming system of *Clione* (Archavsky et al. 1985 a,b).

7. *Endogenous and Conditional Bursters.* As a class, burster neurons are characterized by their ability to produce recurrent bursts. A true endogenous burster produces bursts in the absence of any synaptic actions from other neurons (Alving, 1968). A second subset of burster neurons, called conditional bursters, express bursting properties only upon synaptic or neurohumoral activation (Anderson and Baker, 1981; Levitan et al., 1979). These last two properties (6 and 7) are sometimes lumped together and called "bursting pacemaker properties" (BPP). These properties provide mechanisms intrinsic to the cell for self-excitation or self-inhibition.

3.2   Synaptic Properties

Neurons hardly, if ever, act individually, but are subject to a variety of influences impinging upon them from other cells. The nature and properties of these synaptic interactions play an important role in determining how a cell responds. The following list of synaptic properties is limited to those associated with the production of postsynaptic potentials. Neuromodulatory and neurohumoral actions are covered in another chapter.

1. *Sign, Strength, and Time Course of Action.* The most straightforward synaptic property is its sign. Synapses are either excitatory (increasing the probability of a spike) or inhibitory (decreasing the likelihood of a spike). In addition to the sign, synaptic actions may vary in strength and time course. Qualitatively, the difference between

"strong" and "weak" synaptic action can be easily appreciated but quantification has proven more difficult. Synaptic strength can be measured in a variety of ways. One measure is the size of the post-synaptic potential (PSP) or synaptic conductance. A second measure is the degree to which the activation of a synapse influences the activity or firing pattern of the postsynaptic cell. These two measures may not be covariant. For example, a small IPSP may have a profound inhibitory effect if its reversal potential is close to spike threshold and its conductance is large. Finally, the time course of synaptic action can vary from cell to cell and synapse to synapse. For example, the duration of the monosynaptic PSPs generated by different cells within the CPG network for *Tritonia* swimming differ by a factor of 30 (Getting, 1981). The time course of action is particularly important in determining summation properties which in turn regulate the duration of synaptic action relative to a cycle period. A "fast" synapse may act only during part of a cycle while "slow" synapses may exert their action over many cycles (Getting, 1981, 1983b). Finally, temporal properties (facilitation or depression) must also be considered.

2. *Nature of Synaptic Mechanism.* Synapses can be either chemical or electrical. Chemical PSPs can be produced by either a conductance increase or decrease. Likewise, electrical synapses can pass current in both directions or can be rectifying. All of these properties influence not only the character of each PSP but also how the PSPs from different sources will interact.

3. *Transmitter Release Properties.* Transmitter release is a continuous function of presynaptic membrane potential (Graubard, 1978). If the threshold for detectable release is high, then transmitter will be released only when the terminal is invaded by a spike. In this case, the information transmitted by the synapse depends only upon the temporal pattern of spikes in the presynaptic cell. If the threshold for transmitter release is low, then the presynaptic neuron can release transmitter in a graded manner. For this type of synapse, subthreshold potentials, as well as spikes, regulate the signal being transmitted (Graubard et al., 1983).

4. *Multicomponent Synaptic Potentials.* A synapse need not mediate only one action (either excitation or inhibition) but may produce multiple effects on a single postsynaptic neuron. For example, cerebral cell 2 (C2) within the *Tritonia* swim system forms monosynaptic connections with the dorsal swim interneurons (DSI) (Getting, 1981). The PSPs generated in the DSI have two temporally distinct components. The initial action is a depolarization, which excites the DSI, followed by a long-lasting hyperpolarization that inhibits the DSI. In effect, the sign of this synaptic connection changes from excitation to inhibition. Even more complex monosynaptic connections, having

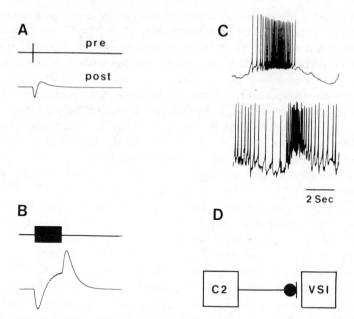

FIGURE 2. Integrative properties of a multi-action, inhibitoryexcitatory synapse. (A) Computer simulated, unitary I-EPSP produced by a single presynaptic spike. The parameters of the simulated unitary I-EPSP were chosen so as to match the relative time course and amplitude of the synaptic potential from C2 to VSI-A within the *Tritonia* swim CPG. (B) Compound PSP produced when the simulated synapse was activated by a presynaptic burst (10 Hz for 2 seconds) to mimic the activity of C2 during a swim. The compound PSP shows an initial inhibitory phase lasting approximately 1 second. Despite on-going activity in the presynaptic cell, the PSP becomes depolarizing. At the termination of the presynaptic burst, a large depolarization is observed producing delayed excitation. (C) Simultaneous intracellular recordings from C2 and a VSI-A during a single swim cycle. The VSI is inhibited during the C2 burst but is strongly excited by a large PSP following the C2 burst. Time scale in C also applies to A and B. (D) Circuit notation for the multiaction I-E synapse. From Getting, 1983b.

up to four components, are observed in the flexion motor neurons of *Tritonia* (Hume and Getting, 1982a). The mechanism for producing multiple actions appears to reside in the interaction of a single transmitter substance with multiple postsynaptic receptors (Kehoe, 1972). This type of synapse adds yet another set of important parameters including the temporal order of action as well as the relative amplitude and time course of each component. Multiaction synapses can lead to a number of interesting and unexpected integrative properties (Getting, 1983b). Figure 2 shows an example of a two-component inhibitory-excitatory synaptic potential which mediates inhibition *during* the presynaptic burst but excitation *following* the presynaptic burst. The excitation following the inhibition is not a form of post-inhibitory rebound which would be an intrinsic property of the postsynaptic cell, but rather reflects the difference in relaxation times for the two synaptic actions elicited by the neurotransmitter.

3.3 Network Properties

In addition to cellular and synaptic properties, certain patterns of connectivity have been recognized as important in pattern generation. These are shown diagrammatically in Figure 3.

1. *Mutual Excitation.* Figure 3A shows a ring of three mutually excitatory cells. Each neuron excites its neighbor and *vice versa*. The connections may be chemical, electrical, or both. One feature of mutually excitatory connections is to promote synchronous firing within the population and is commonly found between synergistic neurons (Getting, 1981; Hartline, 1979).

2. *Recurrent Cyclic Inhibition.* This network is characterized by a ring of neurons interconnected by inhibitory connections (Figure 3B). A recurrent cyclic inhibitory network can, in theory, produce as many different activity phases within a cycle as the number of cells within the ring (Friesen and Stent, 1978; Szekely, 1965). In addition, this network configuration could produce sustained, oscillation without the necessity to invoke additional cellular or synaptic properties. Although no motor program is known to be generated by this network, it has been implicated as a possible mechanism to coordinate the multiphasic limb movements in urodela (54) and the segmental un-

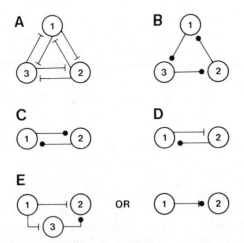

FIGURE 3. Network configurations. (A) Mutual excitation, (B) recurrent cyclic inhibition, (C) reciprocal inhibition, (D) feedback inhibition, and (E) parallel excitation-inhibition. Synaptic symbols as in Figure 1.

dulations of leech swimming (Friesen and Stent, 1977; but see Kristan and Weeks, 1983 for review of leech swimming).

3. *Reciprocal Inhibition.*   A network formed by two neurons (or groups) that inhibit each other is called reciprocal inhibition (Figure 3C), a simple form of recurrent cyclic inhibition. Although this network has been invoked as an oscillator, a reciprocal inhibitory network requires the addition of other properties either synaptic or cellular in order to display oscillation. One feature of a reciprocal inhibitory network is to promote asynchrony in firing and is commonly encountered between antagonistic neurons (Getting, 1983b, c; Miller and Selverston, 1982b; Mulloney and Selverston, 1974; Satterlie, 1985a; Selverston et al., 1976; Thompson, 1974).

4. *Feedback Inhibition.*   Figure 3D shows a simplified diagram of a negative feedback network. Cell 1 excites cell 2 which in turn inhibits cell 1. Under most circumstances, such a network would be stable and not produce oscillation. Increases in the activity of cell 1 inevitably lead to an increased inhibition of cell 1. If, however, cell 1 is made self-excitatory and cell 2 has a high threshold with strong inhibition of cell 1, this network could, in theory, produce a patterned output (Friesen and Stent, 1978).

5. *Parallel Excitation and Inhibition.*   In this network configuration, a single postsynaptic cell is both excited and inhibited by the same presynaptic cell. These two opposite actions may be mediated by separate pathways (Figure 3E, left) (Getting, 1983c; Getting and Dekin, 1985) or by a single multiaction synapse (Figure 3E, right) (Getting, 1983b). If the strength and time course of the two actions are equal, such a connectivity pattern makes little sense. If, however, the time course of one action is longer than the other, then this configuration can lead to a temporal reversal in the sign of synaptic action (delayed excitation or delayed inhibition—see Fig. 2 for an example). In addition, if the two actions are mediated by separate pathways and are subject to independent modulation, this configuration could produce either excitation or inhibition depending upon which pathway dominates (see Getting and Dekin, 1985).

This list of network configurations is necessarily incomplete, for there are many conceivable ways to interconnect two, three, or even four neurons, especially given the diversity of synaptic properties.

In looking through the list of cellular, synaptic, and network properties, one is struck by the fact that, with the exception of the burster neurons and the recurrent cyclic inhibition network, none of these properties in their own right is capable of producing self-sustaining oscillatory activity. In fact, many of these properties are commonly ascribed to neurons not associated with central pattern generators. There appears, therefore, to be little "special" about a CPG network at least in terms of its constituent mechanisms. The ability of a CPG to generate rhythmic, patterned activity must arise from (1) the specific "building block" mechanisms used; and (2) the manner in which they are assembled and interact. A major lesson we should learn from the study of invertebrate CPGs is that these systems do not function by a single mechanism but rather by the interaction ("cooperatively" as Selverston et al., put it, 1983) between many mechanisms.

4   ASSEMBLING A CPG

Having discussed some of the potential building block mechanisms, the next question to ask is how are these mechanisms assembled into functional networks. Let us look at a few examples of how the building blocks listed above could mediate the features of sign reversal and delay necessary for an oscillatory system. For example, there are numerous ways to accomplish a delay in excitation by combining the building blocks in different ways. One possibility is to combine synaptic inhibition with postinhibitory rebound (PIR). The synaptic property would provide an initial inhibition while PIR would cause excitation but delayed until after the inhibition. A second possibility would be a multiaction, inhibitory-excitatory synapse as illustrated in Figure 2. A third mechanism for delaying excitation would be to combine a small excitatory synaptic input with a high spike threshold in the postsynaptic cell. In this case, repetitive firing of the presynaptic cell would be required to depolarize the postsynaptic cell to threshold, thus producing a delay in the onset of firing. Finally, a fourth scheme for producing delayed excitation incorporates synaptic excitation with the activation of voltage- and time-dependent potassium currents within the postsynaptic cell (Getting, 1983c). One could construct similar lists for producing delayed inhibition. We have no a priori reason why one of these mechanisms should be used in preference to the others. In fact, all seem to be used.

Recently, it has been possible to characterize the CPG networks for several rhythmic behaviors in sufficient detail to identify many of the relevant building blocks and to uncover how these mechanisms contribute to pattern generation. An explanation of any CPG must account for two important aspects of the pattern: (a) the *existence* of a repeating pattern; and (b) the *form* of the activity within a cycle. This raises several questions. Why is the activity cyclic? What determines cycle period? What determines burst lengths and strengths? How are phase relationships established and maintained? These are not always independent considerations. To illustrate the interactive nature of the building block mechanisms in pattern generation, I have chosen two systems: The escape swimming system of the mollusc *Tritonia,* and the pyloric network of the lobster stomatogastric system. A detailed description of these systems has recently appeared (Roberts and Roberts, 1983).

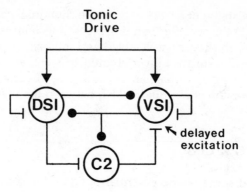

FIGURE 4. Simplified neuronal circuit for the swim CPG in *Tritonia*. Synaptic symbols as in Figure 1.

In response to noxious epithelial stimuli, *Tritonia* swim by making a series of alternating dorsal and ventral flexions (Getting, 1983a). The motor pattern for swimming is generated by at least three groups of premotor interneurons. Figure 1A shows the typical burst pattern of the interneurons during a swim cycle. A simplified circuit diagram of the synaptic connectivity is shown in Figure 4. The existence of a patterened output from this network depends upon synaptic interactions within the network. If any one of the three cell groups is removed, the remaining cells are incapable of pattern generation. Likewise, if each cell type is isolated from synaptic interactions, then the isolated cell is incapable of endogenous burst production. This system appears to be a true "network oscillator". But this is not to say that the cellular properties of each cell type do not play an important role in determining cycle period and the form of the pattern.

A cycle starts with a dorsal swim interneuron (DSI) burst. Cerebral cell 2 (C2) is silent because it has a high threshold and the ventral swim interneuron (VSI) is silent because it is inhibited by DSI. As DSI continues to fire, it excites C2 to threshold. Firing in C2 begins to depolarize one of the VSI. This VSI is, however, endowed with a transient potassium current which is turned on by depolarization. As the excitatory input from C2 depolarizes the VSI, the potassium current is activated, thus slowing the depolarization and delaying the onset of firing in VSI. Once VSI comes on, it inhibits both DSI and C2. When C2 goes off, VSI no longer receives additional excitatory input so the VSI burst terminates as the residual excitation decays. The basis for pattern generation in this system is reciprocal inhibition, paralleled by delayed excitation. Cycle period is determined by a combination of (1) the magnitude of the tonic drive, (2) the strength and time course of the synaptic interactions, (3) the high threshold level of C2, (4) the degree of spike frequency adaptation in each cell type, and (5) the magnitude of the delay between the initial depolarization of VSI and its inhibition of DSI (Getting, 1983b). Phase relationships particularly between DSI and VSI are maintained by reciprocal inhibition.

The swim network as shown in Figure 4 is not self-sustaining. Although excitation of DSI eventually leads to excitation of its antagonist VSI (through C2), there is no comparable, delayed excitatory pathway from VSI to DSI. At the termination of a VSI burst, the DSI are released from inhibition, but there is no phasic excitatory pathway from VSI to initiate a new cycle. If delayed excitation from VSI to DSI were present, then the network would become self-sustaining. As the network stands, continued oscillation requires tonic excitation of DSI to provide for the onset of the next cycle. In fact, *Tritonia* swim for only 2 to 20 cycles during which DSI and VSI receive a tonic depolarization. When this tonic depolarization wanes, swimming stops. The tonic excitation of DSI arises from both afferent inputs and from mutual excitatory interactions among the DSI (Getting and Dekin, 1985).

The pyloric system of the lobster is thought to control the pumping and filtering of food in the foregut. The motor pattern which produces rhythmic contractions of the foregut muscles is generated by a restricted group of neurons in the stomatogastric and commissural ganglia (Selverston et al., 1983). The synaptic connectivity within the pyloric network is shown in Figure 1B along with the most common pattern produced by this network. With the exception of the AB neuron, all the other cells of the pyloric system are motor neurons; the AB cell is the only interneuron. Each cycle consists of three phases: An AB-PD burst; and LP-IC burst; and finally, a PY-VD burst. The pyloric rhythm is thought to be generated by the oscillatory membrane properties of some of the neurons working in concert with the multiple reciprocal inhibitory connections. The dependence of pattern generation on both network and cellular properties can be shown by selectively isolating different portions of the network (Miller and Selverston, 1979; Miller and Selverston, 1982a, b). If the AB cell is isolated from all synaptic interactions with other stomatogastric neurons, it continues to produce a burst pattern (Miller and Selverston, 1982a). Thus, one of the building blocks for this system is the intrinsic bursting capabilities of the AB neuron. The ionic basis for bursting in the AB neuron, however, is not known in detail. Other burster neurons, particularly in molluscs, rely heavily upon the interaction of inward calcium currents to produce depolarization and outward potassium currents to produce hyperpolarization (Berridge and Rapp, 1979; Meech, 1979). These two antagonistic processes are linked with a delay (1) because the currents are voltage dependent, and (2) because one of the potassium currents is activated by an increase in internal calcium concentration. If, however, the AB cell is "killed," the remainder of the network is capable of generating rhythmic activity but with an altered burst pattern and cycle period (Miller and Selverston, 1982b). Thus, the existence of pattern generation by this system does not depend upon a single mechanism, but rather on the combination of oscillatory membrane properties with multiple reciprocal inhibitory synaptic interactions.

In the intact pyloric system, the overall cycle period is determined primarily by the inherent oscillatory behavior of the AB neuron and its strong synaptic connections to the rest of the network (Selverston et al., 1983). Phase relationships, however, are derived primarily from the inhibitory synaptic interactions. Strong inhibitory connections from the AB and PD cells to the rest of the network prevent other cells from being activated during the AB-PD burst. The LP-IC bursts alternate with the PY-VD bursts in part because of reciprocal inhibitory connections. The form of the burst in each cell type is further shaped by the presence of PIR, plateau potentials, and intrinsic bursting properties. The pyloric system is self-sustaining in that once initiated, it can continue to run for hundreds of cycles. This property arises from both the endogenous bursting properties of the AB-PD group as well as the inherent oscillatory nature of the synaptic connectivity pattern.

These examples illustrate several important points which have emerged from the study of invertebrate CPGs. First, pattern generation results from cooperative interactions of many processes, some cellular, some synaptic, and other network interconnections. Second, although the networks generating particular patterns may not be conserved between different rhythmic behaviors, the building block mechanisms do appear to be conserved. Different motor patterns can be generated by different combinations of a common set of mechanisms. As the number of possible combinations is very large, so is the number of possible pattern generators and motor patterns.

5   WHERE WE GO FROM HERE

The concept that CPGs may be assembled from common building block mechanisms raises a number of interesting and potentially very important issues. In this section, I will deal with just two of them. First, are there any rules governing the assembly of the building block mechanisms into functional CPG networks. Second, are the building blocks within a CPG fixed, or are they subject to modification or modulation. These are two areas in which invertebrate systems are likely to make major contributions at both the mechanistic and conceptual levels.

Although the list of potential building block mechanisms presented above is extensive, it is probably not complete. As additional systems are characterized, the list will no doubt grow. Despite the incompleteness, the list would be more useful if relationships between various building blocks could be found. That is, can rules for the assembly of CPG networks from these building blocks be defined? At this point, the statement of firm rules

TABLE 1.

System Behavior	Class	Bursting Pacemaker Properties	Synaptic Balance	Number of Phases
1. Cardiac ganglion (Crust.)	Cont.	Yes	E	1
2. Respiratory Pumping (Aplysia)	Cont.	Yes(?)	E	1
3. Swimming (*Aequorea*)	Inter	Yes	E	1
4. Feeding (*Helisoma*)	Inter	Yes(?)	E	1
5. Pyloric system (lobster)	Cont.	Yes	I	3
6. Swimming (*Clione*)	Cont.	Yes	I	2
7. Heart control (leech)	Cont.	Yes	I	2
8. Ventilation (crabs)	Cont.	Yes(?)	I(?)	2
9. Feeding (*Lymnaea*)	Inter	Yes	I	3
10. Gastric system (lobster)	Inter	Yes	I	3
11. Swimming (leech)	Inter	?	I	2
12. Feeding (*Tritonia*)	Inter(?)	Yes(?)	?	2
13. Feeding (*Pleurobranchaea*)	Inter(?)	?	?	2
14. Swimmeret system (crayfish)	Inter	?	E/I(?)	2
15. Flight (locust)	Inter(?)	?	E/I(?)	2
16. Swimming (*Tritonia*)	Rare	No	E/I	3
17. Tailflip (crayfish)ₐ	Rare	No	E/I	NA
18. Jump (locust)ₐ	Rare	No	E/I	NA

[a]Although these motor responses are not rhythmic in nature, they are included because each involves the production of a stereotyped motor pattern requiring precise timing among synergists and antagonists. In addition, they provide a link between reflective responses and rhythmic motor patterns.

NA, not applicable.

is probably premature, but a number of interesting correlations have begun to emerge. The most straightforward and simplest correlation is that synergists (neurons which fire together and act as a group) tend to be coupled by excitatory connections. This interaction may be mediated by electrical or chemical synapses, or both. Conversely, antagonistic neurons within a CPG tend to be coupled by reciprocal inhibition. Although these two types of synaptic interactions may contribute to pattern generation, one of their major roles is to regulate phase relationships within the pattern.

Additional correlations may be seen by comparing rhythmic behaviors in a number of animals. Table 1 summarizes some of the better known invertebrate rhythmic motor systems. The first column lists the rhythmic behaviors. In the second column, behaviors have been classified into one of three goups. A rhythmic behavior is considered *continuous* (cont.) if it is expressed more than 90% of the time. *Intermittent* behaviors (inter.) are not performed all of the time, but when active, produce many cycles (hundreds or even thousands of cycles). A behavior is classified as *rare* if it occurs infrequently and is characterized by a small number of cycles. The third column indicates whether or not bursting pacemaker properties (BPP) are thought to be involved in pattern generation. Bursting pacemaker properties include endogenous or conditional bursting as well as the ability to produce plateau potentials. The fourth column estimates the relative importance of excitatory or inhibitory synaptic connections within the CPG network. An "E" or "I" means that the predominant synaptic interaction is either excitatory or inhibitory respectively. An "E/I" means that both excitation and inhibition are observed and are of about equal importance. Only those synaptic interactions between the CPG neurons have been considered. Synaptic connections from the CPG to motor neurons, although important for motor pattern formation, have been excluded unless the motor neurons are known to be members of the CPG. The fifth column indicates the number of active phases within the CPG pattern. In some systems, all the cells within the CPG tend to burst together, thus producing only one active phase even though a cycle consists of a burst plus a silent period.

Several correlations become apparent. First, rhythmic behaviors which are expressed for many cycles at a time (continuous and intermittent) are associated with one or more cells with bursting pacemaker properties within the CPG. At one extreme end of the scale are the rhythmic behaviors which are expressed nearly all the time. These include the cardiac rhythm in crustacea, respiratory pumping in *Aplysia*, swimming in *Clione*, heart rhythm control in leech, and the pyloric rhythm of lobsters. The generation of these rhythms appears to involve BPP in some or all of the CPG neurons. At the opposite end of the scale are behaviors such as swimming in *Tritonia*, which is performed rarely and only for a few cycles. The CPG for this behavior does not incorporate BPP but rather relies on network properties for pattern generation. Between these two extremes fall a large number of intermittent behaviors, ones that are not expressed continually but which may, when active, run for many, many cycles. Most of these behaviors also involve BPP within their CPG. Why systems which run for many, many cycles should rely heavily on intrinsic BPP remains unclear. Perhaps these intrinsic properties impart long-term stability or perhaps are metabolically efficient.

A second correlation which can be seem in Table 1 is that systems which are dominated by inhibitory synaptic interactions tend to rely heavily upon intrinsic BPP (Table 1, systems 5-10). For example, cycle period in the pyloric rhythm of lobster is determined largely (but not exclusively) by the bursting properties of the AB neuron. All the chemical synaptic interactions between the neurons within the stomatogastric ganglion are inhibitory (Figure 1B). The only excitatory synapses are mediated by the P cell located in the commissural ganglia. Although the P cell fires phasically, its effects are exerted tonically (Miller and Selverston, 1982b). Similarly, all the synaptic interactions between the HN interneurons of the leech heartbeat timing oscillator are inhibitory (Figure 1C) and some of the HN neurons appear to possess burster capabilities. Inhibitory synaptic interactions also dominate in the lobster gastric mill network (Selverston et al., 1983) and the leech swimming network (Friesen et al., 1976). For both these systems, network interactions have been proposed as the major basis for pattern generation. Recently, however, Russell and Hartline (1984) have described BPP in gastric mill neurons and suggest that BPP may play an important role in pattern generation. The mode of pattern generation in the leech swim system is not well understood (Kristan and Weeks, 1983). The correlation of inhibitory connections with BPP would suggest that some neurons within the leech swim CPG may possess BPP. As Russell and Hartline (1984) point out, it is necessary to test for BPP under conditions where they are likely to be expressed.

But what about systems that do not involve endogenous or conditional burster neurons? A good example is provided by the *Tritonia* swim CPG, which contains three groups of interneurons (Getting, 1981; Getting et al., 1980). None of these are thought to possess intrinsic bursting capabilities (Getting 1983b). In this system, chemically mediated excitatory synapses outnumber inhibitory ones 9 to 6 (Getting, 1981, 1983c.) Likewise, the flight system of locust is thought to involve a mix of excitatory and inhibitory synaptic connections (Robertson and Pearson, 1985). As yet, the participation of BPP in this system is not known. As stated earlier, an oscillatory system needs both excitatory and inhibitory processes linked by a delay. If a CPG is dominated by inhibitory synaptic interactions, the necessary excitation appears to be provided by intrinsic bursting properties. If, on the other hand, phasic synaptic excitation is present in a general balance with synaptic inhibition, then bursting pacemaker properties may not to be required.

One group of systems provides a notable exception to the correlation of BPP with a predominance of inhibitory connections. The first four systems listed in Table 1 rely on BPP, yet the dominant synaptic interaction within the CPG network is excitation. This group of systems, however, produces only one synchronous burst (or active phase) per cycle (Table 1, column 5). It would appear that in these systems, there is little need for synaptic inhibition, since inhibitory processes are inherent in bursting pacemaker properties. Phasic synaptic excitation serves to promote burst synchrony. Systems which produce two or more active burst phases per cycle apparently require inhibition to ensure proper phasing.

These correlations can be summarized as follows:

1. Synergists are coupled by synaptic excitation, antagonists by inhibition.

2. Systems which are active for many cycles at a time incorporate BPP

in their CPGs. Corollary: Systems which are used infrequently and produce only a few cycles rely heavily upon a balance of synaptic excitation and inhibition for pattern generation.

3. Inhibitory synaptic interactions dominate in systems that incorporate BPP and produce two or more active burst phases per cycle. Corollary: Single phase oscillators using BPP are dominated by excitatory synaptic interactions.

To be truly useful, these correlations should have predictive value, particularly for other systems where detailed knowledge of the cellular and synaptic organization may not be available. For example, the "scratch" response in cats and turtles (Stein, 1983) is not active very often and usually consists of only a few cycles. The above correlations would suggest that this rhythmic pattern would be generated by network oscillator involving a mix of synaptic excitation and inhibition. As another example, the respiratory rhythm in mammals is continuously active. The correlations would predict that the respiratory pattern generator would incorporate cells with bursting pacemaker properties. Although the respiratory pattern generator has been localized to the lower brain stem (see Cohen, 1979, for review), relatively little is understood about mechanisms of pattern generation or the involvement of bursting pacemaker properties (Feldman and Cleland, 1981). Recently, we have shown that neurons within the dorsal respiratory group of the guinea pig can become burster neurons in the presence of thyrotropin releasing hormone (Dekin et al., 1984). Although the role of dorsal respiratory group neurons in pattern generation has been questioned (Speck and Feldman, 1982), this observation raises the possibility that respiratory neurons may possess BPP.

These correlations should not become "blinders" in the sense of directing attention on only selected aspects of a particular system. We should learn from the study of invertebrates that CPGs operate by a cooperative interaction of many network, synaptic, and cellular properties. To focus on only a few of these to the exclusion of others would be a gross oversimplification. But I hope these correlations will be useful to focus our attention on gaps in our knowledge (note the numerous question marks in Table 1) and to guide experimental approaches to other systems. At the very least, these correlations suggest questions to be addressed experimentally, and, at best, may represent the emergence of general principles governing the organization of pattern generator networks.

As a final point, I would like to raise the possibility that the constituent building blocks and their assembly into functional networks are not fixed but may be altered and reorganized by inputs to the system. We now have clear examples where network, synaptic, or cellular properties within a CPG can be modified and changed. The swim system of *Tritonia* provides a good example where network connectivity can be altered. Due to the presence of multicomponent synaptic potentials, the sign of several connections within the swim CPG changes over the time course of a single cycle (Getting, 1983b). Early in the cycle, C2 neuron excites DSI and inhibits one of the VSI. Later in a cycle, this same presynaptic neuron, using the same monosynaptic pathways, inhibits DSI and excites VSI. This dynamic oscillation in the sign of the C2 synapses contributes to the generation of an oscillatory swim pattern. As another example, the sign of the synaptic interaction between the six DSI can also be altered (Getting and Dekin, 1985). These six synergists are interconnected by monosynaptic excitatory pathways. In addition, they are coupled by a polysynaptic inhibitory pathway. In a quiescent, nonswimming animal, the dominant synaptic interaction between the DSI is inhibition mediated by the polysynaptic pathway. In this state, the network is stable and will not produce the swim motor program, yet the DSI can be activated to participate as premotor cells controlling reflexive withdrawals. During the production of the swim pattern, however, the polysynaptic pathway is inhibited and the DSI become mutually excitatory via their monosynaptic connections. Under these conditions, the network produces the swim pattern. The "switch" in the sign of the DSI interactions is controlled by the C2 neurons. Any input which activates C2 will cause the DSI interactions to adopt their mutual excitatory interaction and promote generation of the swim pattern.

The lobster pyloric system provides additional examples of synaptic and cellular modifications by inputs to CPG networks. As summarized by Marder (1984), the relative strength of IPSPs produced by the AB and PD neurons can be dramatically altered by exogenous neurotransmitters or by stimulation of neuronal inputs. Alternations in the strength and time course of these IPSPs can produce phase shifts in the relative timing of the postsynaptic cells, thus altering not only the magnitude of the pattern produced by also its quality. Miller and Selverston (1982a) have shown that the cellular properties of pyloric neurons can also be altered. The two PD neurons when isolated from synaptic inputs fire tonically. Short, high-frequency stimulation of the stomatogastric nerve, however, elicits an episode of bursting in the PD cells, presumable by inducing in these cells bursting pacemaker properties. The PD neurons are conditional bursters in that their bursting properties can be "switched" on and off.

These examples and others provide illustration that all of the three major building block categories (network, synaptic, and cellular) may be under dynamic control. Command signals to CPG networks may, therefore, serve not only a "permissive" role in activating the CPG but also an "instructive" role by organizing the building block mechanisms into an appropriate configuration to generate a particular motor pattern. In the future, the mechanisms underlying the reorganization and modulation of neural circuits will be an area of considerable interest. Invertebrate motor systems will no doubt play a continuing important role in the quest for an understanding of how these functions are mediated.

ACKNOWLEDGMENTS

I thank Drs. M. Dekin, A. McClellan, and M. O'Donovan for their helpful comments on early drafts of this manuscript and to Michelle Lopez and Kathy Johnson for typing the manuscript. Supported in part by NIH research grants NS17328, NS15350, and HL32336.

REFERENCES

Adams, D. J., S. J. Smith, and S. H. Thompson, (1980). Ionic currents in molluscan soma. *Ann. Rev. Neurosci.*, **3**:141–167.

Alving, B. O. (1968). Spontaneous activity in isolated somata of *Aplysia* pacemaker neurons. *J. Gen. Physiol.*, **51**:29–45.

Anderson, W. W. and D. L. Baker, (1981). Synaptic mechanisms that generate network oscillations in the absence of discrete post-synaptic potentials. *J. Exp. Zool.*, **216**:187–191.

Arshavsky, Y. I., I. N. Beloozerova, G. N. Orlovsky, Y. V. Panchin, and G. A. Pavlova (1985a). Control of locomotion in marine mollusc, *Clione limacina*. III. On the origin of locomotry rhythm. *J. Exp. Brain. Res.*, **58**:273–284.

Arshavsky, Y. I., I. N. Beloozerova, G. N. Orlovsky, Y. V. Panchin, and G. A. Pavlova (1985b). Control of locomotion in marine mollusc, *Clione limacina*. IV. Role of type 12 interneurons. *J. Exp. Brain Res.*, **58**:285–293.

Benjamin, P. R. (1983). Gastropod feeding: Behavioral and neural analysis of a complex multicomponent system. In *Neural Origin of Rhythmic Movements*, A. Roberts and B. L. Roberts, eds. *Soc. Exp. Biol. Symp.* **37**. Cambridge University Press, Cambridge, pp. 159–193.

Berridge, M. J. and P. E. Rapp (1979). A comparative survey of the function, mechanism and control of cellular oscillators. *J. Exp. Biol.*, **81**:217–279.

Brown, D. A. and P. R. Adams (1979). Muscarinic suppression of a novel voltage-sensitive K-current in a vertebrate neuron. *Nature (Lond.)*, **283**:673–676.

Byrne, J. H. and J. Koester (1978). Respiratory pumping: Neural control of a centrally commanded behavior in *Aplysia*. *Brain Res.*, **143**:87–105.

Byrne, J. H., E. Shapiro, N. Dieringer, and J. Koester (1979). Biophysical mechanisms contributing to inking behavior in *Aplysia*. *J. Neurophysiol.*, **42**:1233–1250.

Byrne, J. H. (1980). Analysis of ionic conductance mechanisms in motor cells mediating inking behavior in *Aplysia californica*. *J. Neurophysiol.*, **43**:630–650.

Byrne, J. H. (1983). Identification and initial characterization of a cluster of command and pattern-generating neurons underlying respiratory pumping in *Aplysia californica*. *J. Neurophysiol.*, **49**:491–508.

Calabrese, R. L. and E. Peterson (1983). Neural control of heartbeat in the leech, *Hirudo medicinalis*. In *Neural Origin of Rhythmic Movements*, A. Roberts and B. L. Roberts, eds. *Soc. Exp. Biol. Symp.* **37**. Cambridge University Press, Cambridge, pp. 195–222.

Cohen, M. I. (1979). Neurogenesis of respiratory rhythm in the mammal. *Physiol. Rev.*, **59**:1105–1173.

Dekin, M. S. and P. A. Getting (1984). Firing pattern of neurons in the nucleus tractus solitarious: Modulation by membrane hyperpolarization. *Brain Res.*, **324**:180–184.

Dekin, M. S., G. B. Richerson, and P. A. Getting (1984). Thyrotropin-released hormone induces spontaneous bursting in neurons of the nucleus tractus solitarius. *Neurosci. Abstr.*, **10**:116.

Delcomyn, F. (1980). Neural basis of rhythmic behavior in animals. *Science*, **210**:492–498.

Dickinson, P. S. and F. Nagy (1983). Control of a central pattern generator by an identified modulatory interneuron in crustacea. II. Induction and modification of plateau potentials in pyloric neurons. *J. Exp. Biol.*, **105**:59–82.

Eisen, J. S. and E. Marder (1982). Mechanisms underlying pattern generation in lobster stomatogastric ganglion as determined by selective inactivation of identified neurons. III. Synaptic connections of electrically coupled pyloric neurons. *J. Neurophysiol.*, **48**:1392–1415.

Elliot, C. J. H. and P. R. Benjamin (1985). Interactions of pattern generating interneurons controlling feeding system of the snail, *Lymnaea stagnalis. J. Neurophysiol.*, **54**:1396–1412.

Feldman, J. L. and C. L. Cleland (1981). Possible role of pacemaker neurons in mammalian respiratory rhythmogenesis. In *Cellular Pacemakers*, D. O. Carpenter, ed. Wiley, New York.

Fentress, J. C., ed. (1975). *Simpler Networks and Behavior.* Edward Arnold, London.

Friesen, W. O. (1975). Physiological anatomy and burst pattern in the cardiac ganglion of the spiny lobster, *Panulirus interruptus. J. Comp. Physiol.*, **101**:173–189.

Friesen, W. O., M. Poon, and G. S. Stent (1976). An oscillatory neuronal circuit generating a locomotor rhythm. *Proc. Nat. Acad. Sci.* **73**:3734–3738.

Friesen, W. O. and G. S. Stent (1977). Generation of a locomotry rhythm by a neural network of recurrent cyclic inhibition. *Biol. Cyber.*, **28**:27–40.

Friesen, W. O. and G. S. Stent (1978). Neural circuits for generating rhythmic movements. *Ann. Rev. Biophys. Bioeng.*, **7**:37–61.

Friesen, W. O. and G. D. Block (1984). What is a biological oscillator? *Am. J. Physiol.*, **262**:847–851.

Getting, P. A., R. R. Lennard, and R. I. Hume (1980). Central pattern generator mediating swimming in *Tritonia.* I. Identification and synaptic interactions. *J. Neurophysiol.*, **44**:151–164.

Getting, P. A. (1981). Mechanisms of pattern generation underlying swimming in *Tritonia.* I. Neuronal network formed by monosynaptic connections. *J. Neurophysiol.*, **46**:65–79.

Getting, P. A. (1983a). Neural control of swimming in *Tritonia.* In *Neural Origin of Rhythmic Movements*, A. Roberts and B. L. Roberts, eds. Soc. Exp. Biol. Sym. **37**. Cambridge University Press, Cambridge.

Getting, P. A. (1983b). Mechanisms of pattern generation underlying swimming in *Tritonia.* II. Network reconstruction. *J. Neurophysiol.*, **49**:1017–1035.

Getting, P. A. (1983c). Mechanisms of pattern generation underlying swimming in *Tritonia.* III. Intrinsic and synaptic mechanisms for delayed excitation. *J. Neurophysiol.*, **49**:1036–1050.

Getting, P. A. and M. S. Dekin (1985). Mechanisms of pattern generation underlying swimming in *Tritonia*. IV. Gating of a central pattern generator. *J. Neurophysiol.*, **53**:466–479.

Glass, L. and R. E. Young (1979). Structure and dynamics of neural network oscillators. *Brain Research*, **179**:207–218.

Graubard, K. (1978). Synaptic transmission without action potentials: Input-output properties of a nonspiking presynaptic neuron. *J. Neurophysiol.*, **41**:1014–1025.

Graubard, K., J. A. Raper, and D. K. Hartline (1983). Graded synaptic transmission between identified spiking neurons. *J. Neurophysiol.*, **50**:508–521.

Grillner, S. 1977. On the neural control of movement—a comparison of different rhythmic behaviors. In *Function and Formation of Neural Systems*, G. S. Stent, ed. Dahlem Konferenzen, Berlin, pp. 197–224.

Hartline, D. K. (1979). Integrative neurophysiology of the lobster cardiac ganglion. *Amer. Zool.*, **19**:53–65.

Hodgkin, A. L. and A. F. Huxley (1952). A quantitative description of membrane current and its application to conduction and excitation in nerve. *J. Physiol. (Lond.)*, **117**:500–544.

Hume, R. I. and P. A. Getting (1982a). Motor organization of *Tritonia* swimming. II. Synaptic drive to flexion neurons from premotor interneurons. *J. Neurophysiol.*, **47**:75–90.

Hume, R. I. and P. A. Getting (1982b). Motor organization of *Tritonia* swimming. III. Contribution of intrinsic membrane properties to flexion neuron burst formation. *J. Neurophysiol.*, **47**:91–102.

Jones, B. R., J. W. Johnson, and S. H. Thompson (1983). Mechanisms of postinhibitory rebound in molluscan neurons. *Neurosci. Abstr.*, **9**:1187.

Kater, S. B. (1974). Feeding in *Helisoma trivolvis*: The morphological and physiological basis of a fixed action pattern. *Amer. Zool.*, **14**:1017–1036.

Kehoe, J. (1972). Three acetylcholine receptors in *Aplysia* neurons. *J. Physiol. (Lond.* **225**:115–146.

Kennedy, D. (1973). Control of motor output. In *Control of Posture and Locomotion*, vol.7, R. B. Stein, K. G. Pearson, R. S. Smith, and J. B. Redford, eds. Plenum Press, New York, pp. 429–436.

Kennedy, D. and W. J. Davis (1977). Organization of invertebrate motor systems. In *Handbook of Physiology: The Nervous System*. Vol. 1, Part 2, J. M. Brookhart, V. B. Montcastle, and E. R. Kandel, American Physiological Society, Williams eds. and Wilkins, Baltimore, pp. 1023–1087.

Koester, J. (1983). Respiratory pumping in *Aplysia* is mediated by two coupled clusters of interneurons. *Neuroscience Abstr.*, **9**:542.

Krasne, F. B. and J. J. Wine (1984). The production of crayfish tailflip escape responses. In *Neural Mechanisms of Startle Behavior*, R. C. Eaton, ed. Plenum Press, New York, pp. 179–211.

Kristan, W. B., Jr. (1980). Generation of rhythmic motor patterns. In *Information Processing in the Nervous System*, by H. M. Pinsker and W. D. Willis, Jr, eds. Raven Press, New York, pp. 241–261.

Kristan, W. B., Jr., and J. C. Weeks (1983). Neurons controlling the initiation, generation, and modulation of leech swimming. In *Neural Origin of Rhythmic Movements*, A. Roberts and B. L. Roberts, eds. *Soc. Exp. Biol. Symp.* **37**. Cambridge University Press, Cambridge, pp. 243–260.

Larimer, J. L. (1976). Command interneurons and locomotor behavior in crustaceans. In *Neural Control of Locomotion*. Vol. 18, R. Herman, S. Grillner, P. Stein, and D. Stuart, eds. Plenum Press, New York, pp. 293–326.

Lennard, P. R., P. A. Getting, and R. I. Hume (1980). Central pattern generator mediating swimming in *Tritonia*. II. Initiation, maintenance and termination. *J. Neurophysiol.*, **44**:165–173.

Levitan, I. B., A. J. Harman, and W. B. Adams (1979). Synaptic and hormonal modulation of a neuronal oscillator: A search for neuronal mechanisms. *J. Exp. Biol.*, **81**:131–151.

Marder, E. (1984). Mechanisms underlying neurotransmitter modulation of a neuronal circuit. *Trends Neurosci.* **7**:48–53.

Maynard, D. M. (1955). Activity in a crustacean ganglion. II. Pattern and interaction in burst formation. *Biol. Bull.*, **109**:420–436.

McClellan, A. D. (1982). Movements and motor patterns of the buccal mass of *Pleurobranchaea* during feeding, regurgitation and rejection. *J. Exp. Biol.*, **98**:195–211.

Meech, R. W. (1974). Calcium influx induces a post-tetanic hyperpolarization in *Aplysia* neurons. *Comp. Biochem. Physiol. A.*, **48**:387–395.

Meech, R. W. (1978). Calcium-dependent potassium activation in nervous tissue. *Ann. Rev. Biophys. Bioeng.*, **7**:1–18.

Meech, R. W. (1979). Membrane potential oscillations in molluscan "burster" neurons. *J. Exp. Biol.* **81**:93–112.

Mendelson, M. (1971). Oscillator neurons in crustacean ganglia. *Science*, **171**:1170–1173.

Merickel, M. and R. Gray (1980). Investigation of burst generation by the electrically coupled cyberchron network in the snail, *Helisoma*, using a single-electrode voltage clamp. *J. Neurobiol.*, **11**:73–102.

Miller, J. P. and A. I. Selverston (1979). Rapid killing of single neurons by irradiation of intracellularly injected dyes. *Science*, **206**:702–704.

Miller, J. P. and A. I. Selverston (1982a). Mechanisms underlying pattern generation in lobster stomatogastric ganglion as determined by selective inactivation of identified neurons. II. Oscillatory properties of pyloric neurons. *J. Neurophysiol.*, **48**:1378–1391.

Miller, J. P. and A. I. Selverston (1982b). Mechanisms of pattern generation in lobster stomatogastric ganglion as determined by selective inactivation of identified neurons. IV. Network properties of pyloric system. *J. Neurophysiol.*, **48**:1416–1432.

Mulloney, B. and A. I. Selverston (1974). Organization of the stomatogastric ganglion of the spiny lobster. III. Coordination of the two subsets of the gastric system. *J. Comp. Physiol.*, **91**:53–78.

Noble, D. (1983). Ionic mechanisms of rhythmic firing. In *Neural Origin of Rhythmic Movements*, A. Roberts and B. L. Roberts, eds. *Soc. Exp. Biol. Symp.*, **37**, Cambridge University Press, Cambridge, pp. 1–28.

Paul, D. H. and B. Mulloney (1985). Local interneurons in the swimmeret system of the crayfish. *J. Comp. Physiol.*, **156**:489–502.

Paul, D. H. and B. Mulloney (1985). Non-spiking local interneurons in the motor pattern generator for the crayfish swimmeret system. *J. Neurophysiol.* **54**:28–39.

Pearson, K. G., W. J. Heitler, and J. D. Steeves (1980). Triggering of a locust jump by multimodel inhibitory interneurons. *J. Neurophysiol.*, **43**:257–278.

Roberts, A. and B. L., Roberts, eds. (1983). *Neural Origin of Rhythmic Movements. Soc. Exp. Biol. Symp.* **37**. Cambridge University Press, Cambridge.

Robertson, R. M. and M. Moulins (1981). Firing between two spike thresholds: Implications for oscillating lobster interneurons. *Science*, **214**:941–944.

Robertson, R. M. and M. Moulins (1984). Oscillatory command input to the motor pattern generators of the crustacean stomatogastric ganglion. II. Gastric rhythm. *J. Comp. Physiol.*, **154**:473–491.

Robertson, R. M. and K. G. Pearson (1985). Neural circuits in the flight system of locusts. *J. Neurophysiol.*, **53**:110–128.

Russell, D. F. and D. K. Hartline (1978). Bursting neural networks: A reexamination. *Science*, **200**:453–456.

Russell, D. F. and D. K. Hartline (1984). Synaptic regulation of cellular properties and burst oscillations of neurons in gastric mill system of spiny lobsters, *Panulirus interruptus*. *J. Neurophysiol.*, **52**:54–73.

Satterlie, R. A. (1985a). Reciprocal inhibition and post-inhibitory rebound produce reverberation in locomotor pattern generator. *Science*, **229**:402–404.

Satterlie, R. A. (1985b). Central generation of swimming activity in the hydrozoan jellyfish, *Aequorea aequorea*. *J. Neurobiol.* **16**:41–55.

Selverston, A. I., D. F. Russell, J. P. Miller, and D. G. King (1976). The stomatogastric nervous system: Structure and function of a small neural network. *Prog. Neurobiol.*, **7**:215–290.

Selverston, A. I. and B. Mulloney (1974). Organization of the stomatogastric ganglion of the spiny lobster. II. Neurons driving the medial tooth. *J. Comp. Physiol.*, **91**:33–51.

Selverston, A. I., J. P. Miller, and M. Wadepuhl (1983). Cooperative mechanisms for the production of rhythmic movements. In *Neural Origin of Rhythmic Movements*. A. Roberts and B. L. Roberts, eds. *Soc. Exp. Biol. Symp.* 37. Cambridge University Press, Cambridge, pp. 55–88.

Simmers, A. J. and B. M. H. Bush (1980). Non-spiking neurons controlling ventilation in crabs. *Brain Res.* **197**:247–252.

Speck, D. F. and J. L. Feldman (1982). The effects of microstimulation and microlesions in the ventral and dorsal respiratory groups in medulla of cat. *J. Neurosci.*, **2**:744–757.

Stein, P. S. G. (1983). The vertebrate scratch reflex. In *Neural Origin of Rhythmic Movements*, A. Roberts and B. L. Roberts, eds. *Soc. Exp. Biol. Symp.*, **37**. Cambridge University Press, Cambridge, pp. 383–403.

Szekely, G. (1965). Logical network controlling limb movements in urodela. *Acta. Physiol. Acad. Sci. Hung.*, **27**:285–289.

Tazaki, K. and I. M. Cooke (1983). Neuronal mechanisms underlying rhythmic bursts in crustacean cardiac ganglia. In *Neural Origin of Rhythmic Movements*, A. Roberts and B. L. Roberts, eds. *Soc. Exp. Biol. Symp.*, **37**. Cambridge University Press, Cambridge, pp. 129–158.

Thompson, S. H. (1974). Pattern generator for rhythmic output in *Melibe. Neurosci. Abstr.*, **4**:450.

Usherwood, P. N. R., and D. R. Newth, eds. (1975). *"Simple" Nervous Systems*. Edward Arnold, London.

Wiersma, C. A. G. and K. Ikeda (1964). Interneurons commanding swimmeret movements in the crayfish, *Procambarus clarkii* (Girard). *Comp. Biochem. Physiol.*, **12**:509–525.

Willows, A. O. D. (1980). Physiological basis of feeding behavior in *Tritonia diomedia*. II. Neuronal mechanisms. *J. Neurobiol.* **44**:849–861.

Wilson, D. M. (1961). The central nervous control of flight in a locust. *J. Exp. Biol.*, **38**:471–490.

Wine, J. J. (1984). The structural basis of an innate behavioral pattern. *J. Exp. Biol.*, **112**:283–319.

Chapter Five

EVOLUTION OF THE VERTEBRATE CENTRAL PATTERN GENERATOR FOR LOCOMOTION

AVIS H. COHEN

Section of Neurobiology and Behavior
Cornell University
Ithaca, New York

1 INTRODUCTION

Locomotion is generally discussed as a single class of movements. Similarly, it is common to talk of the central pattern generator for locomotion as if it were a single neural system identifiable across the vertebrate phyla, albeit with some differences. In reality, however, locomotion includes such diverse forms as swimming, stepping, running, hopping, crawling, etc. Such diversity would strongly imply that the underlying CPGs were also strikingly different. Based on an analysis of the phylogenetic transitions in locomotor motor patterns, I will propose a possible evolutionary pathway which would link the vertebrate locomotor CPGs. The pathway will be such that the transformations among transitional species could have resulted from fairly simple changes. The evidence will be drawn from both phylogenetic and ontogenetic comparisons. Especially important will be the parallels between the two.

The motivation for attempting to formulate such a relatively direct pathway lies in the potential generality conferred by the evolutionary connections on results obtained in diverse animals. For example, the lamprey locomotor CPG is convenient to study because of its robustness and its relative anatomical simplicity. However, there is no certainty that results in the lamprey will generalize to CPGs in other vertebrates. A hypothetical evolutionary pathway does not guarantee that the underlying physiology has generality, but it would suggest that a search for mechanisms similar to those found in simpler vertebrates could be fruitful. Indeed, the hope is that a clear statement of the evolutionary connections might point to possible physiological differences as well as similarities one might expect to encounter when comparing unrelated species. During the course of the discussion, I will also point out the gaps in our knowledge required to make the path continuous and suggest experiments that could fill them.

In discussing intralimb interactions in locomotion I will concentrate on the hindlimb, since more information is known regarding its anatomy, physiology, and movements. Furthermore, because the forelimb has undergone greater evolutionary change, its relationships are apt to be less direct and the transformations, therefore, more obscure. Principles developed for the hindlimb should hold for the forelimb in outline if not in detail.

2   STATEMENT OF THE PROBLEM

As described by Grillner et al., (cf Chapter 1), the motor pattern seen in the swimming lamprey, is characterized by three features. First, the axial muscles are active sequentially with a phase delay averaging 1% of the period per segment (Wallén and Williams, 1984). Thus, in forward swimming, the average phase delay between contractions of ipsilateral adjacent segments is small but greater than zero. Second, the pair of axial muscles opposing each other within a single segment are active strictly out-of-phase; that is, the phase delay separating the onsets of their contractions is 50% of the period. Third, contractions of all the muscles in a given body region last about equal lengths of time and are a constant proportion of the period. There is little variability from this basic pattern in normal swimming, or during a range of similar undulatory movements lampreys use under somewhat controlled conditions. However, there can be a substantial increase in phase lag during larval burrowing* (Ayers et al., 1983). It should be noted that this relatively uncomplicated movement pattern is

---

*[1] The phase, which is delay divided by period, Ayers et al. (1983) stated as 0.015 per segment. However, on the basis of the period and delay provided in their table 1, it should be 0.0229, which is closer to the 0.03 delays observed in the activity of isolated larval cords (Cohen et al., 1986).

appropriate to lampreys which have an extremely uncomplicated anatomy. They lack joints or paired fins and have only a continuous notochord with soft vertebral arches and simple dorsal and anal fins.

Such anatomical simplicity is in contrast to land-dwelling quadrupeds such as cats with their multijointed limbs, complex articulations, and multifunctional muscles. The motor patterns observed during quadrupedal locomotion with the need to power jointed appendages is correspondingly more complex than in the lamprey. Synergists may either contract synchronously or nearly synchronously, but antagonists are no longer out-of-phase nor do they always strictly alternate. There is a strong tendency toward alternation between antagonists, but antagonists often co-contract to stabilize joints; moreover, multiarticular and multifunctional muscles often have multiple bursts, one alternating with the antagonist and one co-contracting with it. To lend even greater variability in the phase relations between muscle pairs, flexor bursts vary relatively little, while the length of extensor bursts varies considerably. This guarantees support during ground contact. Along with the changes in burst pattern, there have been changes in the spinal cord organization as well. Whereas motor pools to antagonistic muscle pairs in the lamprey lie on opposite sides of the cord, in quadrupeds motor pools to antagonists within a single limb are on the same side of the cord.

Lampreys lack limbs, paired fins, and any noticeable regional specialization of the axial muscles. As far as is known, they do not depart from the basic pattern of alternation between local opposing muscles. On the other hand, in many quadrupeds, comparable limb muscles at a single cord level can exhibit a range of both alternating or symmetrical (walk and trot) and non-alternating or asymmetrical (canter, gallop, etc.) phase relations. Another striking difference is that in the lamprey there is little or no variability in the phase delays between any given rostral and caudal pair of ipsilateral muscles, while in higher quadrupeds such as cats and horses, there is a considerable range of phase relations between the ipsilateral limb pairs and their accompanying muscles.

To simplify the discussion somewhat, I will often assume that the motor patterns of intact animals more or less accurately reflect the organization of the CPGs which give rise to them. In the lamprey, this raises no problems since the motoneurons are passively driven. In the isolated spinal cord they thereby reflect the activity of the underlying CPG quite well. Moreover, the motor pattern of the intact swimming fish and the isolated cord are essentially identical (Cohen and Wallén, 1980; Wallén and Williams, 1984). Similarly, in dogfish (Grillner et al., 1976; Grillner and Kashin, 1976), and young chicks (Jacobson and Hollyday, 1982a,b), the intact and the fictive patterns are very similar. In cats, the motor pattern of intact animals is more complex. It also reflects more complex modulation by sensory and descending control systems. Because of this there is a great deal of variability among preparations and there are some differences between

the motor patterns of intact, chronic spinal (Forssberg, 1979), and functionally "isolated" cords (Grillner and Zangger, 1979). Although the differences are more quantitative than qualitative, assertions about the CPG
based on intact cats should be made cautiously. The evidence in other animals is inadequate to judge, but I will assume a relatively close correspon-
dence especially in non-mammalian vertebrates. For many animals only
movements are available without details of the patterns of muscle activities
that drive them. In such cases, great caution is required, as it is extremely
difficult to deduce the motor activity without detailed knowledge of the
biomechanics, which has generally been unstudied (see e.g., Blight, 1977;
Gans, 1974).

Grillner (1981; Grillner and Kashin, 1976) has proposed a basic scheme
for the locomotor CPG in vertebrates. It consists of a chain of burst generators or oscillators, coupled to give the complete coordinated motor pattern. In the cat, Grillner's model consists of a pair of unit oscillators per
joint, a flexor oscillator and an extensor oscillator. The pairs of joint oscillators are coupled to make up limb oscillators, which in turn are coupled
across the girdles to produce the various gaits. This model fits the observations to date (cf Grillner, 1981 for a review of the evidence), but little is
known about the structure of the CPG or its component oscillators. In the
lamprey, the scheme consists of a double chain of oscillators coupled along
the cord to produce the traveling wave (cf. Rand et al. Chapt. 9). It is
known that each unit oscillator spans 1–4 segments (Cohen and Wallén,
1980). As far as is understood, the oscillators of the lamprey CPG differ
only to the extent that their frequency of bursting to a given concentration
of excitatory drug differs (Cohen, 1987) as does their response to bath applied serotonin (Harris-Warrick and Cohen, 1985). Most commonly, when
cut into rostral and caudal pieces the rostral group of oscillators will burst
at a higher frequency than will the caudal group. However, it is not rare
for the opposite to be seen, and in some cords the two pieces will burst
at comparable frequencies. In the present context, I will also assume that
the CPG is a chain of coupled unit oscillators. The structure of the unit
oscillators will remain unspecified; they could be truly discrete oscillatory
ensembles, or, they could be a single chain of essentially interlocking oscillatory neurons. For the purposes of the present discussion, both should
behave similarly (cf. Rand et al. Chapt. 9). There are some configurations
which will require a rethinking of the present ideas. Until there is more
known, however, the structure will be assumed as described, with the
understanding that some conclusions will be rethought if necessary.

The comparison between lamprey and quadruped CPGs can now be
restated using this terminology so that the necessary transformations become transparent (Fig. 1). In adult lampreys adjacent ipsilateral oscillators
are active with phase delays of about 1% of the period, while opposing
oscillators are active strictly out-of-phase (phase delay = 50%). The range
of the phase delays in larval lampreys appears to be greater (Cohen et al.,

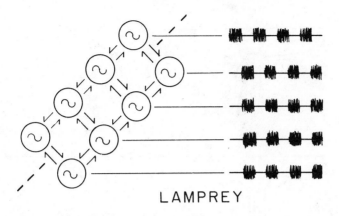

LAMPREY

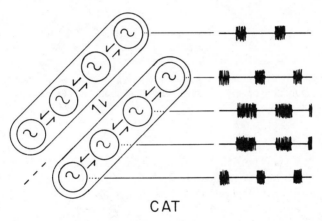

CAT

FIGURE 1. Diagrams of lamprey and cat CPGs based on coupled oscillator models. Above is detail of 4 segmental oscillators of the lampreys; below is a detail of oscillators to left and right flexors (outer oscillators) and extensors. See text for description.

1986; S. T. Alford, N. R. Burton, A. H. Cohen, and T. L. Williams, in preparation) but is too poorly characterized to be dealt with at this time. On the other hand, in cats and other mammalian quadrupeds, oscillators driving synergists which act on a single joint are active with phase delays at or near zero, while ipsilateral adjacent oscillators driving antagonists generally alternate their activity with phase delays considerably greater than zero, but these can vary depending on the muscles and on the period. The oscillators to the muscles of a single limb are active either out-of-phase with the corresponding oscillators of the opposing limb (walk and trot), or, depending on the gait, they are active with phase delays varying from less than 50% (canter and gallop) to zero (bound). Moreover, the phase relations between the groups of oscillators to ipsilateral pairs of fore- and

134   Avis H. Cohen

anterior   *posterior*

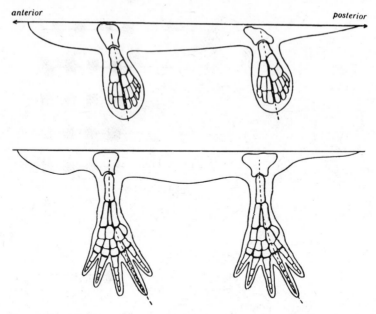

FIGURE 2. Diagrams illustrating comparison between a primitive aquatic fish-like form and a primitive tetrapod. Both have similar pectoral and pelvic appendages. (Adapted from Goodrich, 1930, Fig. 168.)

hindlimbs can vary considerably depending on the gait. In contrast, in lampreys, which have no paired fins, the evidence to date is that the phase delays between any two ipsilateral oscillators are very nearly invariant or have two possible phase relations.

3 CHANGES AMONG IPSILATERAL ADJACENT OSCILLATORS

3.1 Alternation Between Neighboring Motor Pools

From paired fins it is not difficult to envision the evolution of limbs and their neural control. Many fins have the necessary musculoskeletal elements and more complex fins even have a joint structure not dissimilar to that noted in weight bearing limbs (Rosen et al., 1981; Goodrich, 1958). Indeed, some fishes apparently do use their fins for weight bearing, although this has not been studied in detail. A beautiful general description of the phylogenetic transformation from fins to limbs (Fig. 2) appears in Goodrich's classic book, *Studies of the Structure and Development of Vertebrates* (1930, reprinted 1958). Unfortunately, little is known regarding the details of the muscle activity which drives fin movements, but it is clear that there are antagonistic fin muscles and these must be alternating at least to some degree for their activity to produce coordinated movements. The difficult step, then, is from lampreys which require only a simple traveling wave along axial and median fin muscles to fishes which have added fully coordinated pairs of pectoral and pelvic fins.

The first question one may ask is whether the specializations required for limb control are limited to only a few segments. I would suggest that the answer is no. Limbs and fins can occur at almost any segment with a highly variable number of segments intervening (Fig. 3 from Goodrich, 1913). A clear statement of the various interpretations of this fact were given by E. S. Goodrich himself in 1913. He collected evidence for several arguments in favor of the view that any segment could and did give rise to limbs or fins. His most compelling evidence was from fish. He noted that, for example, "the first dorsal fin is opposite the pectoral in *Lamna*, between the pectoral and pelvic in *Alopecias*, opposite the pelvic in *Scyllium* and behind the pelvic in *Raja*" (p. 236 but not illustrated). Thus, fins can be found on any segment and no evidence for intercalation or deletion of segments can account for the independent phylogenetic rearrangements the fins appeared to have undergone. Goodrich concluded that homologous organs such as limbs and fins can be derived from diverse segments and that, "In the segmental vertebrate, the material for the formation of muscular, nervous, and skeletal segments are distributed along the body; those particular segments which occur in appropriate positions are entrusted, so to speak, with the development of special organs" (p. 244). His arguments may be less compelling (although not disproven) for tetrapods, but in the present context they are also less important. If fins can be controlled appropriately by essentially any segment, then any group of segments must have had the evolutionary potential to give rise to limbs. Once the tetrapod ancestors separated off, it is conceivable that the equipotentiality of the spinal segments became increasingly limited as the specialization increased. In any case, the earlier events are more critical for the present argument, and they point to all segments having the potential to drive fins in a coordinated fashion.

To bridge the gap from lampreys to fish with paired fins, I will draw from recent observations in lampreys which have elaborated the fine structure of the swimming motor pattern and the neural control of motoneurons. In lampreys there appear to be at least two functional classes of motoneurons (unrelated to speed of their related muscle fiber contraction): those to the more dorsal myotomal fibers and those to the more ventral myotomal fibers (Wallén et al., 1985). Whether there is a third separate class of motoneurons to the lateral fibers is unclear. The two classes of motoneurons differ morphologically. Moreover, the drive from the locomotor CPG to the two classes to motoneurons also appears to differ to some greater or lesser degree. The motoneurons to the more dorsal fibers are similar morphologically to those found by Rovainen and Birnberger (1971) to innervate fin muscle fibers. Although one cannot, as yet, dem-

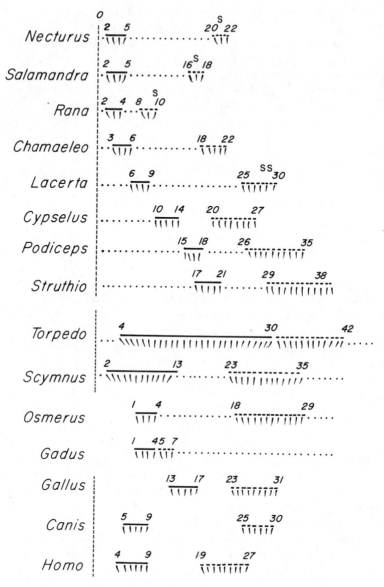

FIGURE 3. Diagram to the same scale indicating the nerve supply of the fin or limb segments of a range of vertebrates. The spinal nerves are represented by dots and strokes, the latter being those which share in the plexus. The solid line extends over those segments supplying the pectoral appendage and the broken line those segments which supply the pelvic appendage. (All but chick and mammal are from Goodrich, 1913.)

onstrate that the morphological similarity implies any deeper relationship, these observations become especially intriguing when they are related to the observation that motoneurons to the lamprey dorsal fin are active out-of-phase with the local ipsilateral axial muscles (Fig. 4, Buchanan and Cohen, 1982).

On the basis of these findings I suggest the following hypothesis. In lampreys, the locomotor CPG is not a simple uniform chain of oscillators. Rather, each muscle hemi-segment is driven by two (or more) oscillators which are normally tightly coupled. They must be separable to provide dorso-ventral flexions, but in straight lateral undulatory movements they are essentially coactive. In the caudal region, the coupling between a sub-set of the dorsal oscillators has undergone a greater degree of separation to provide independent control of the fin, thus allowing alternation be-tween fin and local axial muscles as observed by Buchanan and Cohen (1982). I leave aside for now the mechanism by which the concordance of muscle and oscillator is maintained as they both undergo changes in func-tion and morphology.

I am suggesting that lampreys have two or more functional classes of oscillators which could be homologous to those which drive alternating fin and limb muscles in more complex vertebrates. Unfortunately, beyond the demonstration by Wallén et al. described above, at present, it is extremely difficult to prove that the oscillators to the dorsal and ventral muscle fibers are, in fact, independent. It is also extremely difficult to prove that the fin oscillators have any relationship to the dorsal myotomal oscillators beyond the morphological similarity of their motoneurons. And, finally, proof that there is any relationship between the dorsal and ventral oscillators in lam-preys and the flexor and extensor oscillators of limbed vertebrates will also be difficult to obtain. However, in the light of early studies by Alfred Romer, there is reason to believe that such relationships could exist.

Based on comparative anatomical studies of primitive living and fossil mammals, Romer (1922) was led to the conclusion that "the limb muscles of tetrapods may be naturally arranged in two groups, homologous with and derived from, the two simple muscle masses present in the paired fins of fish"—the dorsal and ventral muscle masses. While examining the on-

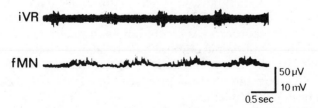

FIGURE 4. Lamprey root recording (upper trace) and fin motoneuron intracellular recording (lower trace) during fictive swimming by isolated cord. Motoneuron exited via ventral root to innervate dorsal fin. (Adapted from Buchanan & Cohen, 1982.)

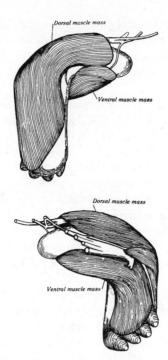

FIGURE 5. Right pelvic limb of the chick embryo, Stage I, "six days." Above external, below internal views. (Adapted from Romer, 1927.)

togeny of the chick, he further suggested that "the development of the chick pelvic musculature shows clearly the early establishment of two muscle masses seemingly homologous with those believed to have been present in primitive land forms, and the muscles differentiated from these two masses correspond closely with those believed to have been derived from each of the two primitive tetrapod groups" (pg. 348, Romer, 1927; cf Fig. 5). Romer hypothesized that the dorsal and ventral muscle masses were phylogenetically highly conservative. Indeed, modern studies have confirmed this conservatism. The two muscle masses and their associated mature homologues have been traced again in the frog, *Xenopus laevis* (Lamb, 1976), chick (Landmesser, 1978a), and mouse (Lance Jones, 1979). Landmesser (1978a,b) and Hollyday (1980) have also shown that the positions of the motoneuron pools of the hindlimb muscles can best be predicted from their embryonic origin. Quite reliably, motoneurons to dorsal muscles lie laterally and motoneurons to ventral muscles lie medially. However, this separation has not been seen in teleost fish, (Fetcho, 1983), nor has it been noted in lamprey.

Finally, and most important in the present context, Romer proposed a functional separation of the dorsal and ventral muscle masses of the hindlimb. He suggested that the dorsal mass gave rise to functional flexors and ventral muscle mass gave rise to extensors. However, the situation is apparently more complex. For example, as Landmesser (1978a) points out, in such a functional separation, if one uses as key criteria the ontogeny of the muscle and the position of its associated motoneuron pool, the iliofibularis of the chick is homologous to the gluteals of the cat, but the former functions primarily as a knee flexor while the latter functions primarily as a hip extensor. Which then is to be taken as the functional class of this muscle and its homologues? If the EMG pattern during locomotion is brought in, the functional separation between dorsal and ventral muscles is also complex, but not hopelessly so.

In chicks (Jacobson and Hollyday, 1982a,b), all the ventrally derived hindlimb muscles that have been examined are active during the exten-

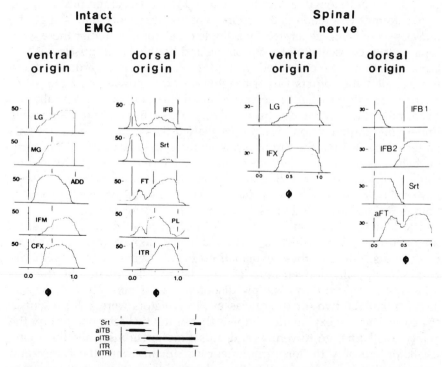

FIGURE 6. EMG and motor nerve recordings in intact (left) and fictive spinal (right) chick hindlimbs. Upper figures are histograms showing relative coordination of muscles with MG-off as the reference point for intact; Srt is the reference for the fictive prep. Abscissa, phase of EMG cycle. Ordinate, number of cycles. Lower figure is summary of EMG activity pooled from 16 chicks. Narrow bars denote standard deviations (adapted from Jacobson and Hollyday, 1982). Muscles are arranged by muscle mass origin (taken from Landmesser and Morris, 1975). Abbreviations are: MG, medial gastrocnemius; LG, lateral gastrocnemius; ADD, adductor; IFM, ischiofemoralis; CFX, caudilioflexorius; IFB, iliofibularis; Srt, sartorius; Ft, femorotibialis; PL, peroneus longus; ITR, iliotrochantericus; IFX, ischioflexorius; a,pITB, anterior, posterior iliotibialis.

sion, or stance phase of the locomotor cycle. The dorsally derived muscles are more variable. Some are active only during the swing phase, that is during lift off or while the limb is off the ground, some are largely active only during the stance phase, but most have two periods of activity, one during the swing and one during the stance (Fig. 6). Jacobson and Holly-day suggest that the "swing" activity be further classified into swing flex-ion and swing extension. The motor output during chick fictive locomotion is essentially the same but the data are somewhat less complete. Motoneu-rons to ventrally derived muscles are active together and motoneurons to dorsally derived muscles are more variable. Again the more common pat-tern for the latter is to exhibit both a stance and one or the other swing burst. The authors attempted to correlate burst timing with position of the motoneuron pool, but no relationship other than a dorsal/ventral separa-tion was found (Hollyday, unpubl. data and personal communication).

No attempt was made to determine whether the stance bursts of all the muscles were being generated by a single oscillator or whether there were separate stance oscillators for the single and double burst muscles. When burst duration was correlated with the cycle period regardless of the muscle, all stance bursts varied roughly linearly and all swing bursts re-mained roughly constant. Keeping in mind the fact that no ventrally de-rived muscle was active during the swing phase, there are three possible underlying configurations for the oscillators that could give rise to this pattern (Fig. 7). First, the simplest possibility is that regardless of the origin of their muscle all motoneurons producing stance bursts are driven by a single group of oscillators. Second, dorsally and ventrally derived muscles have separate extensor burst oscillators. Third, a single oscillator produces both flexor and extensor bursts for the double-bursting muscles.

The first two explanations would mean that pools of double bursting motoneurons, all of which innervate dorsally derived muscles, receive dual inputs. Either of these explanations could suggest that ventrally de-rived and dorsally derived muscles were being differentiated by the ner-vous system, but not in a simple dichotomous fashion. They could also suggest that the two (or three) classes of oscillators were still present in the cord. The first explanation implies that of the two sets, one group, the stance oscillators, go to ventral and dorsal motoneurons while the swing oscillators go only to dorsal motoneurons. In this view, the stance and swing oscillators are assumed to have changed their coupling to be essen-tially out-of-phase.

The second explanation also implies that motoneurons to dorsal and ventral muscles receive inputs from two classes of oscillators, possibly ho-mologous to those of the lamprey. However, in this case, the dorsal and ventral oscillators are not simply coupled, since some dorsal oscillators would be co-active with the ventral oscillators while others would be out-of-phase.

The third explanation requires the emergence of a novel oscillator. Such

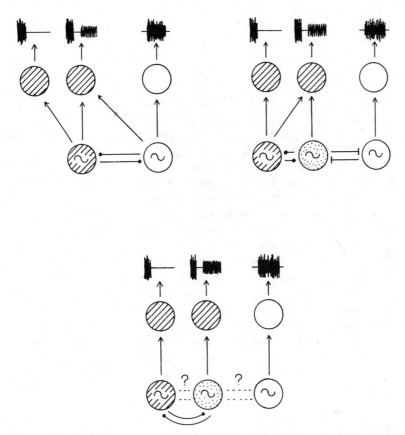

FIGURE 7. Three possible configurations which could generate extensor flexor and double-bursting hindlimb motor pattern in chick. The two types of flexor bursts are treated as one for convenience. See text for details. Upper left: (1) Flexor and extensor bursts are each generated by one type of oscillator. (2) Flexor bursts have common origin, but extensor bursts have different oscillators. (3) Each type of burst pattern has separate oscillator, with double-bursting pattern generated by more complex oscillator. Supported coupling is indicated (is inhibitory and excitatory). Cross-hatched are of dorsal origin, clear of ventral origin, stippled undertermined.

an oscillator must generate two bursts to the other's one, and in addition, the duration of one of the bursts must vary with period while the other does not. The swing and stance flexor bursts could be the short and long portions of the cycle of a relaxation oscillator (cf. Kopell, Chapt. 10) derived from the dorsal oscillators. The ventral oscillator could be the same but only give rise to bursting during one part of its cycle. Unfortunately, without more information it is impossible to differentiate between these three possibilities.

It is impossible to make such an analysis for cats. Complex needs have added a new level of complexity to the range of possible motor patterns manifested even in the reduced cat preparation. The resultant variability obscures the relationships which can be inferred in simpler systems. More information from functionally isolated cord preparations including the detailed activity patterns of more muscles should go far to fill this gap. Although all the components of the locomotor pattern have been demonstrated in the fictive or deafferented preparation, the precise relative timing of many muscle bursts is unclear and can vary considerably. Grillner and Zangger (1984) show quite clearly in the mesencephalic preparation that in the absence of sensory input the flexors and extensors do not simply alternate. They also show that in this simplified preparation no single pattern emerges. There was some evidence for alternation between some pairs of dorsal and ventral muscles, but it was inconsistent. Generally, in the mesencephalic as well as the decorticate curarized preparations (Perret and Cabelguen, 1980), the removal of sensory feedback destabilizes the coupling between the burst generators and leads to a deteriorated pattern. In view of these observations, at the level of mammals no conclusions can be drawn as yet with respect to the dorsal/ventral hypothesis.

The extreme phylogenetic conservatism of the embryological separation manifested in both early muscle development and motor pool position has led to the proposal that it plays a significant but obscure functional role (Landmesser, 1978a). Evidence of a different type that the muscle mass separation is, indeed, a major factor in development comes from Hollyday's (1983) observation that motoneuron outgrowth in chick embryos begins, but is then delayed until the two muscle masses have differentiated—suggesting that this separation is the critical factor required for their continued outgrowth.

Rather than posit a direct dichotomous connection between ventral muscle mass with extensors and dorsal muscle mass with flexors, I would propose the following. Phylogenetically, the ventral mass has consistently given rise to essentially one class of muscles driven by one class of oscillators. However, the history of the dorsal mass has been less well defined. For example, in primitive cyclostomes, such as the lamprey, the ventral mass gives rise to the ventral axial muscle and is driven by ventral oscillators. The dorsal muscle mass need give rise only to the dorsal axial muscle and dorsal fins. These muscles are driven by one or more classes of oscillators (Fig. 8). With the emergence of paired fins in other fishes and limbs in land-dwelling vertebrates, the ventral mass developed into one set of homologous muscles with a clearly defined functional role, while phylogenetic changes that occurred, occurred at the expense of the dorsally derived muscles. Thus, patterns of activity of dorsally derived muscles within and across animals are varied and complex. The dorsal muscles appear to be driven by both swing and stance and possibly more oscillators.

I will set aside the question of how many functional types of oscillators exist. There could be only two, but, as suggested by Jacobson and Holly-

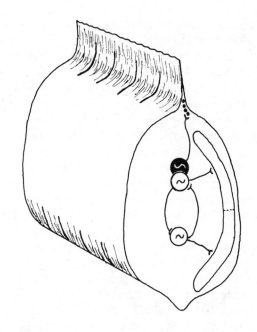

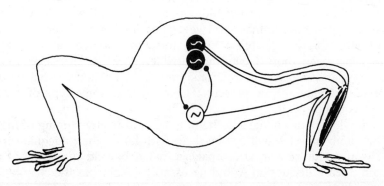

FIGURE 8. Diagram indicating hypothesized relationship between oscillators to dorsal and ventral muscle. In lamprey, one type of oscillator controls ventral muscle and one type controls dorsal axial muscle as well as dorsal fin muscle. In primitive tetrapod (after Goodrich, 1930), the "ventral" oscillators control ventral muscles and "dorsal" oscillators control dorsal muscles (see text for details).

day (1982a), more certainly could be present. In mammals it seems possible that the suggested dorsal/ventral relationship continues, but unfortunately no firm evidence exists. It can only be said that the muscle homologies can be traced (Lance Jones, 1979) and that there are separate oscillators to each muscle group, but the relations between the oscillators are variable and unclear. Such complexity should not be too surprising in view of the evolutionary distance between birds and mammals. Substantial phylogenetic changes have occurred as limbs have become increasingly complex. Most compelling would be a detailed examination of the motor patterns in relation to muscle origin in primitive reptilian, amphibian, and mammalian hindlimb muscles to determine whether or not the greatest differences are found among the dorsally derived muscles. Such work has been done for the shoulder (Jenkins and Goslow, 1983), but more on the hindlimb is needed.

Some additional support for the dorsal/ventral hypothesis presented here comes from other developmental studies in *Xenopus laevis*. One study (Lamb, 1976) found that there is a temporal separation in the innervation of dorsal and ventral muscle groups. More recently, Moody and Jacobson (1983; Jacobson, 1983) found that the cellular ancestry and developmental relationships for ventral and dorsal muscle masses are very different. Ventral muscle and all primary motoneurons are derived from the one ancestral cell line; the dorsal muscle and sensory neurons are derived from another. On the basis of their observations, they suggest that motoneurons apparently can recognize ventral muscle and its derivatives and "prefer" them. The effect of this special relationship between ventral muscle mass and motoneurons could be that, as phylogenetic changes have occurred, the more mutable muscles, that is, the dorsally derived muscles, have been those with a looser tie to their motoneurons. Thus, the phylogenetic tie between ventral muscle mass and ventral oscillators has been more consistent while the relationship between dorsal muscle mass and dorsal oscillators has been more labile and variable. With the increased role of descending and sensory control in mammals, the relationship has become obscured but may still be present. However, only some type of cellular analysis could prove it.

The phylogenetic changes in the function and relative timing of the individual limb muscles will not be dealt with here. Their adequate treatment would require a level of analysis that is beyond the scope of this chapter. Such a discussion would necessarily encompass the changes the joints and muscles have undergone as the limbs have rotated from the position retained by some reptiles and salamanders to that typical of mammals. In the former, the limbs project laterally out from the trunk, not unlike fins, whereas in mammals, the limbs have rotated to a position beneath the body where they can swing freely.

The transformation from quadrupedal mammals to bipedal humans has been examined by Forssberg (1982, 1985). The early human stepping motor pattern is remarkably different from either quadrupeds or adult humans. Infants begin with digitigrade stepping, more closely resembling that of cats than adult humans, but the stepping is produced by motor patterns which have distinctly unique characteristics. Most striking is the fact that the activity of the flexors is very close to tonic with only hints of a burst structure. A parametric analysis of joint angle changes demonstrated by the knee/ankle, and the toe/heel were similar to cat movements at birth. By 10 months of age, the movements become more akin to that of adult humans. On the other hand, the knee/hip and toe/body sway are never similar to either. The knee and hip begin tightly coupled in infants and only dissociate as in adult stepping by 6 months. Unfortunately, the role of descending control systems and sensory feedback cannot easily be evaluated even by comparisons with anencephalic children. Without more evidence from other primates to show evidence of intermediate patterns, it is difficult to know how to place these data in the present phylogenetic context.

3.2   Phase Relations Among Adjacent Ipsilateral Oscillators to Axial and Synergistic Limb Muscles

Next, I would like to trace the phylogenetic changes that have occurred in the phase relations among axial muscles. In aquatic vertebrates from cyclostomes to amphibians these muscles provide the bulk of the force needed for locomotion. Exceptions can be found among the elasmobranchs (e.g., rays; cf. Grillner et al., Chapt. 1; see below) and teleosts. Examples from the teleosts include short bodied fishes such as the *Chaetodon* which depends primarily on its median and paired fins (Webb, 1984a) while some species of electric fish (see below) utilize almost exclusively their median fins for locomotion (Lissman, 1961). Among limbed vertebrates the axial muscles have a more limited role to play in locomotion, but again there are some glaring counter examples (e.g., salamanders, snakes, cetaceans).

The use of the axial muscles reflects the phylogenetic divergence that occurred as vertebrates developed the capacity to live on land. A comparative examination of early ontogenetic development will be used to demonstrate the commonalities and the differences that have arisen in the neural control of the locomotor apparatus. It will be necessary to assume that movements performed by relatively undisturbed embryos are being produced by the locomotor CPG and reflect its general organization. Unfortunately, in the case of early embryonic movements it is more difficult than ever to prove. Moreover, the roles of the descending and sensory control systems can generally only be inferred since they cannot or have not been removed in the studies cited. With these caveats, I will try to demonstrate linkages between developmental stages that suggest continuous molding of a common underlying control system.

An extensive review of the work on embryonic movement patterns has been presented by Bekoff (1985). She noted that early embryonic myotomal muscle is used similarly by all vertebrates studied. The first clearly coordinated neurogenic trunk movements, C-coils, are characterized by simultaneous contraction of the myotomal muscle on one side of the embryo, with presumed relaxation on the other side. Bekoff finds examples of C-coils in every major class of vertebrates. C-shaped bends to either side can occur spontaneously, but the occurrence of a bend to one side has no apparent relationship to a bend to the other side. It is uncertain whether this very primitive use of the motor apparatus reflects activity of the locomotor CPG. If it is generated by the developing CPG, it suggests that the earliest state is one in which the segmental oscillators are coupled to produce zero stable phase lag or synchrony among segmental muscles. Some of the synchrony could be due to electrotonic coupling between either interneurons, motoneurons or muscles, which may or may not remain in more developed animals. At this early stage, left and right sides are still uncoordinated except in so far as they do not appear to be co-active.

The next ontogenic stage is alternating C-coils which combine to produce standing waves (cf. Fig. 9 for the distinction between standing and traveling wave motions). Such S-waves, with no traveling wave in evidence, are again common to all studied embryonic vertebrates. This stage reflects some degree of coordination via inhibitory coupling between the left and right sides of the cord, but still only the most restricted type of coordination down the cord so as to produce a phase lag of zero. It is unclear whether both concave zones of the S-wave are the result of active contractions, or whether the caudal is only passively generated. In larval salamanders there is apparently only one zone, alternating between the two sides (Blight, 1977). The caudal concavity is passively produced by tail flexures, but little more is known.

C-coils and S-waves are not restricted to embryonic fish. Adult fish exhibit C-coils as reflex responses to annoying stimuli or to Mauthner cell stimulation (Eaton et al., 1977). In lampreys the reflex may, but need not be, followed by undulatory swimming movements (McClellan and Grillner, 1983). C-coils are also used by several adult fish as "fast-starts" to catch prey fish (Webb, 1984a). Lampreys and longer bodied adult teleost fishes, such as pike, use S-waves for fast-starts (Webb, 1984b). However, it is uncertain that embryonic and adult S-waves are generated by the same neural control systems. The S-starts of lamprey reflex responses are known to have two zones of contraction (McClellan, 1984; McClellan and Grillner, 1983), but in fish it has not been demonstrated. Although the underlying control systems are unknown, but C-coils and S-waves point to the possibility that throughout the lives of these vertebrates there are segmental burst generators which may retain the coupling required to produce coordinated synchronous contractions of the myotomal muscles.

A major evolutionary fork becomes apparent with the next stage of em-

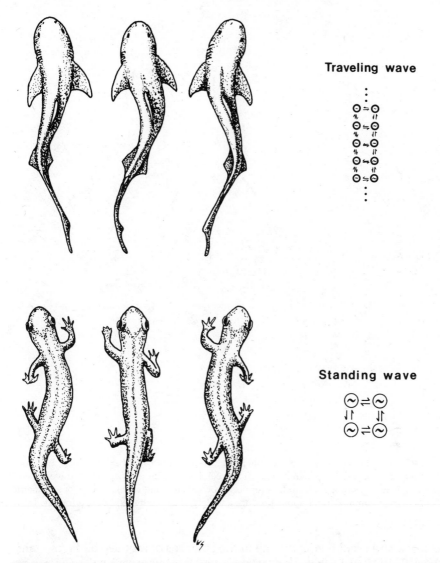

Traveling wave

Standing wave

FIGURE 9. Traveling versus standing wave motions. In fish, upper figure, wave propagates down the body. In salamanders, the body curve forms straightens and reforms to generate a standing wave motion.

bryonic development. Only those vertebrates which actually employ undulatory locomotion during some period of their life ever develop the ability to produce traveling waves. Bekoff sees no solid evidence for embryonic traveling waves in any vertebrate phylogenetically past amphibians. That is, there are confirmed traveling waves seen in all the lower aquatic embryos of vertebrates, such as cyclostomes, elasmobranchs,

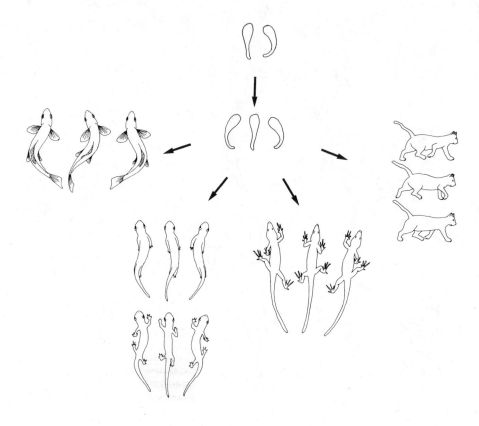

FIGURE 10. Ontogeny of motor movements across vertebrates. All exhibit Stage 1, C-coils and Stage 2, S-waves. They then diverge at Stage 3. Fish and amphibia produce traveling and standing waves. Tetrapods, including reptiles produce standing wave motions or symmetric gait patterns. Mammalian tetrapods produce a variety of gait patterns. See text for details.

teleosts, and amphibia, but none in the embryos of reptiles, birds, or mammals. Snakes and other elongated reptiles are discussed below as a possible special case; little is known regarding embryonic cetaceans. It would appear, as illustrated in Fig. 10, that the development of the intersegmental control up to that required for S-waves is shared by all vertebrates. But the controls needed for traveling waves are not acquired by the latter groups of vertebrates which will never make use of them.

The traveling wave pattern seen during adult swimming in lampreys and dogfish has been well characterized. There is good evidence that the fictive motor patterns of lampreys and dogfish do not differ from their respective intact motor patterns (cf. Grillner et al., chapt. 1). It would seem that in these two species the locomotor pattern is a product of both the isolated CPG and the CPG interacting with descending and sensory afferents. The patterns of the two species are also very similar to each other. It would be tempting in the presence of such similar swimming motor patterns to say that the lamprey and dogfish locmotor CPGs were the same. One apparent difference is that the local oscillators of lampreys, when separated from each other, burst at different frequencies. This has not been reported in dogfish. On the basis of this difference, Kopell (1986) has suggested that dogfish have greater descending control of the coordinating system and perhaps less control intrinsic to the cord than do lampreys. However, without more information on the oscillators, the coupling, and the possible range of movements in both species, the only statement that can be made is that between the lamprey and dogfish there is, at present, no firm evidence that there have been any significant changes in the CPG control of the axial muscles.

In newts, Blight (1977) found, in accord with the studies described above, that early embryos predominantly produce C-shaped bends. Using EMG recording, he confirmed that all axial muscles on one side contract simultaneously. Only later-stage embryos produce a true traveling wave of muscle activity. Waves of contraction are seen in later embryos during slow swims, but the phase lags disappear as the velocity increases. Thus, developing control systems are able to alter the phase lag in this amphibian. The bodies of adult salamanders execute sequences of standing waves to locomote on land (cf. Fig 9; Roos, 1964). It has been assumed that the adults use traveling waves in water, but whether they are actively or passively generated is not known, as no muscle recordings have been made to prove it. Since it is well documented that urodele amphibians have the capacity to generate traveling waves of contractions during larval stages, it seems likely that adults may, indeed, use them as well. However, direct evidence would be desirable.

Tadpoles of *Rana* have been observed to produce traveling waves of motor activity only in the presence of dorsal afferents (Stehouwer and Farel, 1980). If all the dorsal roots are cut in the otherwise intact tadpole, or if the CNS is removed completely, the CPG continues to have the capacity for rhythmic, alternating ventral root discharges, but with no apparent intersegmental phase delays. It is conceivable that, under some other conditions, phase delays could emerge, but this remains conjectural. Whether the input must be phasic is not known since no curarized preparation was used. Unfortunately, the comparable experiments of cutting the dorsal roots in *Xenopus* have not been done, but in these animals curarized larvae can produce traveling waves (Soffe and Roberts, 1982). Stehouwer and Farel (1981) have shown that even single pulses of dorsal root activity have a powerful impact on the frequency of fictive swimming, but they have not addressed the question of the intersegmental phase lag in such experiments. Thus, it remains uncertain exactly what role is played by sensory input with respect to the intersegmental coordination. As they stand, the observations suggest that the intersegmental coordinating systems in some frogs may depend on afferent input to produce a phase delay, but the critical experiments remain to be done.

The quadruped reptiles appear to locomote with standing wave patterns (Sukhanov, 1974), but no muscle recordings exist to prove it. Gans has evidence that the ancestors of elongated reptiles such as snakes have lost the intersegmental coordination of their aquatic and short-bodied ancestors (Gans, 1985, 1986). He hypothesizes that complex sensory regulation required for overground undulatory locomotion replaces a less flexible intrinsic inter-segmental coordinating system. The evolutionary stages he proposes are as follows (Gans, 1984). Tetrapody with force-generating limbs is the ancestral form for the reptiles. A so-called concertina movement (cf. Gans, 1974, for a description) is observed in some of the transitional elongated species with reduced limbs such as skinks and pygopodids. This is posited to be derived from the ancestral reptilian tetrapody by shifting force generation and control from the limbs to the segmental axial muscles. However, many such species still show limited control and such species are unable to generate the lateral propulsive force required for full-blown and fully functional concertina movements that can be seen in snakes. Because of this, he proposes that snakes represent one terminal condition in the evolution of limbless reptiles. Snakes and only a few elongated limbed reptiles improve this pattern of locomotion toward lateral undulations. According to Gans, such movements depend almost exclusively on sensory feed-back to govern local contractions. Highly elongated animals utilize the irregularities of the surface to generate propulsive locomotor forces. Thus, in the highly elongated reptiles, the waves of contractions differ in their amplitude and shape.

Gans's hypothesis would require that, in elongated reptiles, sensory input substitutes for, or supplements the intersegmental coordinating systems. Proof of his contention requires detailed analysis to demonstrate true independence of the wave motions along the body in the intact animal, as well as independent bursts in the "fictive" preparation. However, it is not hard to envision the phylogenetic addition of many trunk segments and the concomitant reduction and eventual loss of the connections between segmental oscillators. However, there is the observation that many snakes swim by means of regularly undulatory movements. Water is a uniform medium which should be inadequate to coordinate local propulsive waves. However, without EMG analysis, the motor patterns generating these waves remain open to interpretation. Perhaps spinal curvature detectors can provide the needed sensory cues to coordinate the regular bending.

Finally, in limbed mammals, including man, the axial muscles serve to support, stabilize, and bend the back dorsally and ventrally during locomotion. Their activity in man (Thorstensson et al., 1984) and walking cats (Carlson et al., 1979) has two components per step-cycle, one to coincide with the ipsilateral stance phase and one to coincide with the contralateral stance phase. Whether there are regional rostral-to-caudal differences which might correspond to a traveling wave is unknown but also unlikely. Thus, in mammals the oscillators to the axial muscles are 2:1 phase-locked with their ipsilateral limb muscle oscillators. 2:1 activity can be observed under abnormal conditions in lamprey (Rand et al., Chapt. 9), turtles (Stein, 1978), chick (Jacobson and Hollyday, 1982b), and cat (Kulagin and Shik, 1970; Forssberg et al., 1980;) but has not been noted in an intact animal for muscles other than the back. The exact phase relations of the trunk muscles relative to the limb muscles is difficult to specify, because it is not clear with which muscles they should be compared.

In chicks (Jacobson and Hollyday, 1982b) and cats (Grillner and Zangger, 1979) the synergistic limb muscles acting at a single joint generally tend to be co-active with little appreciable phase lag between them. The delays observed, especially in fictive preparations, cannot obviously be related to traveling waves of activation down the cord. Similarly, there are no consistent phase delays among proximal to distal muscles pairs that could be construed as a traveling wave motion. Phase delays exist, but they seem rather to have been shaped to conform to the needs of the more complex articulations of the limbed animals.

3.3 Phase Relations Among Neighboring Oscillators to Fin Muscles

So far the phase relations among limb and axial muscles have been considered. Now the phase relations among segmented fin muscles will be examined, as they can be considerably more complex. Traveling waves along the pectoral fins were reported by von Holst (1973) and Webb (1973), but no muscle recordings were made to confirm them. Nothing more is known about the patterns of muscular activity driving the paired fins except for the continuing work on the greatly enlarged pectoral fins of the stingray, *Dasyatis sabina*, by Leonard and his collaborators. In this elasmobranch, traveling waves of elevation and depression have been described in some detail (Droge and Leonard, 1983a,b). The same pattern of well coordinated activity can be observed in intact, decerebrate, and spinal animals both in the presence and absence of phasic sensory feedback. The phase delay they have recorded between adjacent fin segments is 3.4% of the cycle, much greater than that between adjacent segmental axial muscles of lampreys or dogfish. A consequence of this large phase delay is that one wavelength is less than the length of the fish. In fact, one wavelength extends roughly over only 80% of the body. However, although the authors have recorded muscle activity in the intact unrestrained fish, they were unable to obtain a range of movements because of the problems with movement. Therefore, it is not known whether the stingray is capable of a wider range of motor patterns and if so, what they may be and whether they require the presence of sensory and/or descending control. The decerebrate cur-

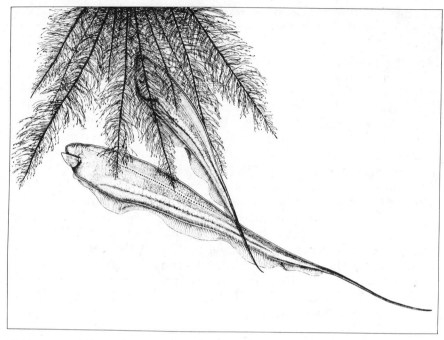

FIGURE 11. Male and female *Eigenmannia* in mating display. Note multiple waves in the ventral fins. (Drawn by Clara Yanez, from Hagedornand and Heiligenberg, 1985.)

arized stingray has episodes of 2:1 bursting between antagonists, but the source of the control for this is unknown.

There are highly complex wave motions along the median fins of some species of electric fish. Several species of these animals have a single elongated median fin which extends almost the entire length of the body. The dorsal fin of *Gymnarchus* and the ventral fin of *Eigenmannia* are two good examples. No EMG recordings have been made of the movements, but Lissman (1961) has used ciné analysis to describe those of *Gymnarchus*. They can be observed visually quite easily as the animals spontaneously move about catching fast-swimming prey fish or performing mating displays (Fig. 11). The movements of these fins during swimming are truly spectacular. Multiple waves of fin oscillations spread rostrally and caudally from a lead segment which can be seen to move up and down the body. The number of waves along the fin also seems to be able to vary considerably from one moment to the next, implying an ability to change phase delays rapidly. The fin movements apparently provide exquisitely precise changes in the speed and direction of movement.

It is believed that the body remains stationary to prevent distortion of the electric field the animal generates to detect surrounding objects (Lissman, 1961). Although the axial muscles appear superficially to be unused except for bending and very rapid swimming, this needs to be confirmed with EMG recording. Nor have recordings yet been made in a reduced preparation to prove that the complex fin undulations are spinally controlled. However, it seems likely in view of the fact that no new mechanisms need be invoked to explain them (see Sect. 5, later in Chapt.). The relationship between the undulations of the fin and body is unknown for those movements in which both axial and fin muscles are active. It would be of interest to know whether the wavelengths along the body and fin are equal. If so, are there more than one per body length, or is there only a single wavelength along the body? Alternatively, it is possible that the wavelengths of fin and body differ entirely or in some complex manner during fast swimming.

Especially noteworthy is the fact that *Gymnarchus* and *Eigenmannia* are totally unrelated species, one in the order Mormyriformes and the other in the order Gymnotiformes. They share only their use of an electric organ discharge, and this is believed to be an example of convergence, since the details of their systems are very different (Bass and Hopkins, 1982; Bass, 1986). Thus, their control of their median fins by the locomotor CPG is most likely also an example of convergent evolution. It seems somewhat more likely that such convergence should occur if the necessary transformations were not too drastic. On the basis of the arguments briefly developed later in this Chapter (see Section 5) and in Kopell (Chapter 10), I suggest that there are remarkably straightforward mechanisms which could produce the elegant movements of these animals. Moreover, they require very little change in the basic structure of the locomotor CPG proposed above.

3.4 Summary and Conclusions

Alternation in the activity of adjacent oscillators could have arisen simply from changed coupling between pairs of identical neighboring oscillators. However, there appear to exist in the lamprey two (or more) classes of oscillators which may have a special connection with the two (or more) functional muscle classes of higher vertebrates. Looking at only two for the sake of simplicity, I suggest that throughout vertebrate evolution homologues of the oscillators which drive the dorsal and ventral muscles of lampreys have continued to drive the muscles of the respective dorsal and ventral muscle masses. When necessary, phylogenetic changes could have occurred in the coupling between individual pairs of dorsal and ventral oscillators to accommodate functional needs.

In the lamprey, adjacent oscillators that drive a pair of dorsal and ventral muscles are nearly synchronous but are more loosely coupled than a pair that drive two muscles of the same type. Presumably, the need for control of the dorsal fin of the lamprey and the paired fins or limbs of other vertebrates, has led to a change in the coupling between dorsal and ventral oscillators from excitatory to inhibitory. This could have produced the required switch from in-phase to out-of-phase activity. With the added demands coming from weight-bearing, limb muscles have had to stabilize as well as to propel. As functions have been added, some muscles have begun to receive inputs from more than one class of oscillators. Small changes in phase delays that accompany the increased complexity of limbs have presumably been accomplished by a succession of small changes in the strength or details of the coupling between individual oscillators. Because neural changes leave no fossil record, it is difficult to test the hypothesis presented here. However, this functional approach fits all the observations to date while suggesting mechanisms which encompass a minimum of complicated or difficult ontogenetic or phylogenetic transformations.

The changes in the relationships among similar adjacent oscillators appear to have been fairly straightforward. It is believed that the vertebrate evolutionary chain was from fish to amphibians and then branched shortly before or at the origins of reptiles (Young, 1981). One path went from reptiles to birds and another gave rise to the mammals. These pathways are reflected to some degree in the ontogeny of the locomotor motor patterns (Fig. 10):

The first two stages of the ontogeny seem to be uniform in all phyla.

Stage (1) C-coils: The ipsilateral oscillators are first coupled to provide a synchronous wave of activity down the embryo.

Stage (2) S-waves: Next, the two sides become coupled, presumably via inhibitory coupling, to provide alternating C-coils which produce standing waves of motor activity. After this, there is divergence which is akin to the phylogenetic divergence:

Stage (3a): Fish develop the intersegmental coupling required to produce traveling waves down their bodies; the lamprey and the dogfish, as prototypical examples, require neither descending nor sensory control to generate a traveling wave of motor activity (except to start it or in the case of the lamprey, to keep it going). Many fishes retain the ability in some manner to produce synchronous C-coils or S-waves for fast starts of reflex responses. The wavelength for locomotor undulations tends to be nearly equal to the body length in the lamprey and dogfish. For many short-bodied fish, the wavelength is greater than the body length, and for some fish which employ median fins for their primary source of propulsive force, the wavelength may be much less than the length of the body and may vary greatly.

Stage (3b): Amphibia may or may not be somewhat different as befitting remnants of a transitional group. Embryonic and larval forms can all produce traveling waves of motor activity. Deafferented and functionally isolated cords of urodeles have not been tested to see if their locomotor CPGs have intrinsic intersegmental coupling capable of generating traveling waves, but the more evolved amphibia, the anurans, may be mixed in this capacity. *Rana* species seem to require sensory input to produce a phase lag between segments, while *Xenopus* does not.

Stage (3c): Embryonic reptiles use only standing waves, never displaying the control necessary for traveling waves. Adult limbed reptiles also use standing waves while elongated forms use more complex motions such as lateral undulations and concertina movements. Gans has argued that terrestrial snakes, which may be thought to utilize traveling waves akin to fish, in fact are almost strictly dependent on sensory feedback and, indeed, this may be more important than intrinsic intersegmental coordination. His suggestion deserves experimental test.

Stage (3d): Birds and mammals, as would be expected, are not observed to generate traveling wave motions at any stage of their development. Trunk muscles in mammals have not been studied in great detail, but the studies that have been done find two bursts of activity that are nearly synchronous with the extensors of the two limbs.

It is not difficult to envision the changes leading to stage 1 or those leading from stage 1 to stage 2. Stage 1 requires synchronizing coupling between the segmental oscillators. If the preferred, or natural, frequencies of the oscillators are similar, then the coupling need not be very strong. Stage 2 requires the addition of reciprocal *net* inhibitory or desynchronizing coupling between the left and right oscillators of each segment. I say "net" because the coupling could be a combination of inhibitory and excitatory so long as the total effective coupling is negative (cf. Rand et al., Chapt. 9; Cohen and Harris-Warrick, 1984). In the final section in this chapter (Section 5), I will deal with other mechanisms for effecting changes in the phase delays between oscillators which could explain the other transformations outlined here.

4 PHASE RELATIONS AMONG FINS AND LIMBS

To trace the changes in interlimb relations, I will begin with the behavior of the regional groups of embryonic oscillators. As in adjacent segmental oscillators, the phylogeny and the ontogeny of inter-regional and inter-limb relationships parallel each other nicely. The standing wave motions of embryonic vertebrates are most likely generated by synchronous contractions somewhere within the concave region of the body. One may argue about precisely where in the curve the muscles are active (Blight, 1977), but there is no dispute that there are muscles which are co-active. This means that the final vertebrate pattern of movement seen universally is that of two opposing and alternating zones of contraction. It is unknown whether during S-waves there are also simultaneous rostral and caudal zones of contraction. In adult lampreys, S-starts can result from simulta-

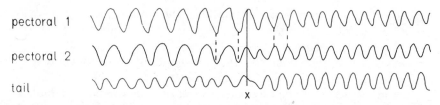

pectoral 1

pectoral 2

tail

x

FIGURE 12. Movement patterns of both pectoral fins and tail fin. Taken from *Sargus*, medulla-operated. Note spontaneous switch from synchrony to alternation at "x." (Adapted from von Holst, 1973.)

neous opposing rostral and caudal contractions (McClellan and Grillner, 1983), but the generality of this observation has not been established. Fish and amphibia develop additional intersegmental coordinating capacity along the trunk which allows a continuous traveling wave of activity down the entire chain of segmental oscillators. Limbed reptiles, birds, and mammals apparently do not.

As noted in Section 3.3, nothing is known of the coordination between fin and trunk musculature, so there is no indication as to how the fins interact with the axial muscles during either C-starts, S-starts, or traveling wave undulations. Von Holst (1973) only looked at fin:fin interactions using overall fin displacement. He did not describe the details of the fin or trunk movements, nor did he make it clear which segments generated the dorsal or tail fin movements he measured. As a result, detailed interpretations of the motor patterns of the segmental muscles are impossible and nothing more can be said about the coordination of the unpaired fins or any of the fins and the axial muscles.

With respect to coordination between paired fins it is possible to say from von Holst's studies that in the medullary fish with afferents intact the pectoral fins can have several patterns (Fig. 12). The fins can move synchronously, alternatively, or have 2:1 or 3:1 coupling. In-phase and out-of-phase paired fin movements have also been described in intact lungfishes (Rosen et al., 1981). Although detailed movement or EMG analysis has not been done, apparently, in lungfish, alternating pectoral and pelvic fin movements are superimposed on trunk movements akin to standing waves. Fin movements in spinal and/or deafferented fish have not been examined in any species except the stingray (see Sect. 3.3).

Walking salamanders appear to employ solely standing wave motions with their limbs strictly alternating between and within the pectoral and pelvic girdles (Fig. 9; Roos, 1964). Although detailed comparisons have never been made, the similarities between "walking" lungfish and salamanders have been noted by Rosen et al. (1981) in an evolutionary context. No one has recorded from salamander limbs during swimming, so it is impossible to compare limb use during standing and traveling wave patterns.

Frogs are more complex, as would be expected, given that they have a greater range of locomotor patterns. The isolated CNS of tadpoles with emerging limbs has been studied by Stehouwer and Farel (1983). They found that as the limbs developed, their activity was superimposed on myotomal activity. First, alternation with the local myotomal muscles was observed. With further development both in-phase and out-of-phase activity could occur. The same motor patterns can be evoked from chronic spinalized tadpoles (McClellan and Farel, 1985). Thus, presumably as the coordinating system of the developing tadpole is layed down, it is manifested in the interlimb interactions, forshadowing the adult patterns of stepping and jumping. The elongated trunk and tail in *Rana* are lost at metamorphosis making a traveling wave equivalent to that seen in the tadpole impossible. Whether phase relations among limbs can include patterns other than strict alternation and synchrony has not been examined.

Among intact-limbed reptiles, only symmetrical limb movements imposed on standing wave motions of the body have been described (Sukhanov, 1974), but only a few studies have been done. Therefore, it is unknown whether additional flexibility has emerged in these animals. And Sukhanov has emphasized the limited range of gait patterns for limbed reptiles. When induced to locomote by stimulation of descending fiber tracts, the spinal turtle—just as the intact—exhibits strict alternation within and between the limb pairs (Stein, 1978). Some points of stimulation produced 2:1 movement patterns (cf. Chapts. by Kopell and Rand et al. for possible interpretations of 2:1 patterns), but no other coordination patterns were observed, nor have such 2:1 patterns been observed in intact animals.

In other intact mammals, considerable variation in interlimb coordination patterns has been noted (Gambaryan, 1974; Hildebrand, 1976). However, in intact animals it is difficult to distinguish between the role played by descending and sensory control systems and intrinsic spinal CPG control mechanisms. Where possible, examination of functionally isolated spinal cords gives a more precise although perhaps less complete picture. Viala and Vidal (1978) have noted that in spinalized, curarized rabbits the coordination between fore- and hind-limbs can differ. Forelimbs can be either synchronized ($\varphi = 0.0$) or unsynchronized ($\varphi \neq 0.0$), while hindlimbs are only unsynchronized. Unfortunately, the phase values for "unsynchronized" patterns are not specified further then differing from $\varphi = 0$, making it difficult to say more or compare with other studies. Intergirdle coordination was observed as well. The coordination pattern illustrated included both a "trot" and a "pace", that is, the ipsilateral limbs were either in-phase ($\varphi = 0.0$) or out-of-phase ($\varphi = 0.5$). Whether other patterns could occur is not commented upon. The switch between these two patterns was spontaneous and was not induced by the experimenters. Grillner and Zangger (1979) found that during fictive locomotion the hindlimbs of spinal cats can either alternate ($\varphi = 0.5$) or they can have a phase difference more closely resembling a gallop ($\varphi = 0.25$). They can also exhibit 2:1 or 3:1 patterns. Unfortunately, it is extremely difficult to obtain a full range of possible phase relations because such preparations are unstable and not easily controlled. Those patterns described for rabbits were all obtained without sensory stimulation, but in cats, to evoke fictive locomotion dorsal columns, dorsal roots or sensory nerves generally must be tonically stimulated. Changes in phase relations between the limbs of the reduced cats can then be induced by changing the stimulation intensity or frequency.

In experiments with spinalized, curarized mammals the spinal cord is devoid of descending control other than the tonic drug stimulation which is generally not manipulated after application. The parameter that has been varied is sensory stimulation. Therefore in rabbits the phase changes noted are all caused by mechanisms intrinsic to the spinal cord or to dwindling titre of drug, while it is safe to conclude that the changes in phase relations described above in cats are a function of sensory control systems interacting with the coordinating mechanisms of the CPG. As will be described in Section 5, it is often impossible to determine whether a change in phase is brought about by a change in relative oscillator frequencies or by a change in coupling. In those cases presented here, it is more likely to be primarily a change in the coupling. In the case of the rabbit, the abrupt switch from in-phase to out-of-phase is unaccompanied by any changes in frequency or input. It seems most likely, therefore, to reflect a gradual drift from net excitatory to net inhibitory coupling due to changes in excitability (cf. Rand et al., Chapt. 9). The changes from alternating to non-alternating phase relations in cats can be interpreted similarly as reflecting a discontinuous change in coupling (from net inhibitory to net excitatory), but in this case induced by the gradually increasing sensory input to the CPG. Since in the cat, the change in phase is associated with a change in the frequency of the oscillators, the sensory input is probably also causing a gradual increase in the drive to the oscillators. The question as to whether the mechanism producing the change in coupling is the same as that producing the change in the frequency cannot be addressed without more evidence.

Changes from alternating (walk, trot) to more nearly in-phase (canter, gallop) gaits in intact animals are often similar to that described for the reduced preparation (e.g., "the animal *broke* into a gallop"). It seems most likely that in intact animals what varies is the descending control. It is known that descending control systems can affect the coordination. This has been demonstrated in mesencephalic cat preparations in which the cats propel the treadmill belt themselves (Fig. 13). These animals are induced to move by stimulation to the midbrain (Shik et al., 1966). As stimulation strength increases, the animal's step frequency increases until the gait abruptly switches from a trot to a canter, and occasionally even to a gallop. Thus, although the sensory inflow is changing, the causal element for changes in gait in these experiments is the variable descending input

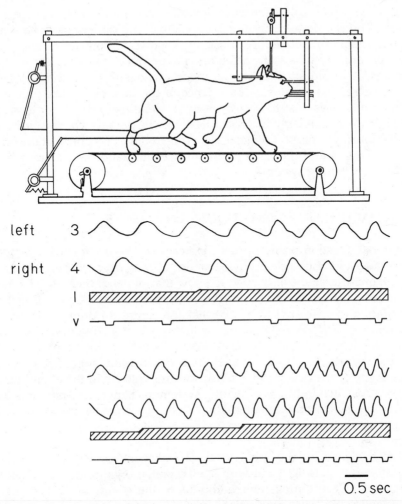

FIGURE 13. Mesencephalic cat walking on a treadmill belt which is free-wheeling (see diagram above), movement recording from left and right hindlimbs as strength of stimulation is increased (I). Note switch from alternating to non-alternating gait. (Adapted from Shik et al., 1966.)

to the cord. It is clear, therefore, that either descending or sensory control systems can accomplish gait transitions in mammals.

In summary, alternation is the only interlimb coordination pattern observed in all intact, reduced, or spinal animals studied. On this basis, it seems reasonable to conclude that it is the primitive or "default" coordination pattern for the vertebrate locomotor CPG. The data are too incomplete to say any more than that in-phase or non-alternating patterns have been observed in isolated spinal preparations of cats and rabbits; sensory or descending control systems can be responsible for inducing the changes in gait. The coordinating system, especially of the cat, seems to be somewhat unstable in isolation, exquisitely sensitive to both descending and sensory control and is easily acted upon to produce a wide variety of other patterns. It would appear that the major phylogenetic trend has been to increased separation and independence of the limb oscillators combined with an increased role to be played by descending and sensory systems which lend considerably increased flexibility. A possible conclusion could be that, during evolution, what is changing in the CPG control of the limbs is the access to and the need for extrinsic control and the general lability of the coordinating systems.

5   SUMMARY AND CONCLUDING COMMENTS

The initial question posed in this chapter was whether for the locomotor CPG one could trace a clear phylogenetic pathway from lampreys to mammalian quadrupeds. I have tried to show that, indeed, there is. The most tenuous step from lampreys and fish with paired fins is made firmer by the finding of Wallén et al. (1985) that the control of dorsal and ventral myotomal muscles is via separate oscillators. Combined with the conservatism of the dorsal and ventral muscle masses hypothesized and documented by Romer (1922, 1927), their observation suggests a neural homologue of the flexor and extensor control systems in fishes and quadrupeds. A switch in the coordinating system to change the phase relationship from synchrony to alternation between neighboring dorsal and ventral oscillators can then account for neighboring antagonistic motor pools.

The evidence for the universality of embryonic movements suggests that all vertebrates start out with similar spinal organization and similar locomotor CPGs. Ontogenetic additions to the coordinating systems of fishes and some larval amphibians have allowed undulatory movements. If the standing wave motions of embryos, amphibia, and reptiles are all generated by pairs of diagonal synchronous contractions, it would mean that all vertebrates (except perhaps birds) exhibit this coordination pattern at some point during ontogeny. The crossed diagonal stepping pattern appears to correspond to the same coordination scheme and is also seen universally among limbed vertebrates. Therefore, it is reasonable to posit that this pattern is the basic pattern, and that the instructions for it reside in the spinal cords in all vertebrates. With the evolution of more sophisticated and versatile vertebrates, more layers of control have been added to an increasingly more sensitive and labile CPG coordinating system.

There are two possible types of mechanisms which could account for the range and the changes in inter-muscle and inter-limb phase relationships found across vertebrates. The mechanisms are suggested by mathematical analysis of chains of coupled oscillators (cf. Chapt. 9 by Rand et al.; Chapt. 10 by Kopell). A robust relationship found in these studies is that the phase delay between oscillators coupled together in a chain is a function of the ratio $\omega_1 - \omega_2/\alpha$ where $\omega_1 - \omega_2$ is the frequency difference between oscillators a and b and α is the strength of their mutual coupling. (Cohen et al., 1982; see Chapts. 9 and 10 for a more complete treatment of this). This implies that changes in either relative frequencies of the oscillators (i.e., ω), or changes in the strength of the coupling (i.e., α) can alter the phase lag between them. That such a relationship can indeed exist under physiological conditions was shown in a study of the effects of serotonin on the isolated spinal cord of the lamprey (Harris-Warrick and Cohen, 1985). There it was noted that differential changes in the frequencies of the regional oscillators induced by bath-applied serotonin were correlated with changes in phase lag. It is not possible to prove, nor is it likely to be the case, that coupling was totally unaffected by serotonin, but the change in phase lag was clearly associated with an increase in $\omega_1 - \omega_2$.

One implication of this relationship between the phase lag and its determinants is that there are several straightforward possible physiological mechanisms underlying the hypothesized phylogenetic and ontogenetic transitions. For example, in tadpoles of *Rana*, sensory input could affect the coupling to produce a phase lag either via traditional phasic feedback mechanisms, or by altering the levels of excitability of the oscillators. Alternatively, it could affect the coordinating system by a more tonic mechanism. Sensory input does appear capable of such a tonic role in the tadpole (Steuhouwer and Farel, 1981). Moreover, tonic dorsal root input can stabilize the CPG in decorticate curarized cats (Perret and Cabelguen, 1980), suggesting that there are several diverse roles for the sensory control systems which remain to be elucidated. In the case of the electric fish, the wavelength of the fin oscillations is highly labile, as is the leading segment. The changes in phase lag implied by the varying wavelengths could be governed by descending control systems. The descending inputs could effect the changes in phase lag in either of two ways (cf Kopell, Chapt. 10). The inputs could vary the frequencies of the segmental oscillators via a gain control mechanism, or they could vary the strength of coordinating neuron synapses. Such mechanisms also make it easier to comprehend how two unrelated species were independently able to acquire the necessary control systems for such a complex behavior. In this view the basic locomotor CPG need change very little to accommodate the increasing demands natural selection placed on it. Overall, there are few phylogenetic or ontogenetic transitions which cannot be accounted for by moderately uncomplicated changes either in the relative frequencies of the oscillators or changes in the coupling. Changes in the coupling could include changes in the ratio of ascending to descending coupling as well as changes in the sign or changes in the strength of the coupling among the oscillators or groups of oscillators.

During the course of the discussion I have tried not only to point out phylogenetic continuity, but also to point to experiments which should help to prove or disprove that continuity. Although the fossils do not exist, the evidence should still be obtainable. The arguments have attempted to show that one need not posit dramatic change in the basic oscillator(s) of the CPG across the vertebrates. The most fundamental change in the CPG has been in the transition to weight-bearing limbs. But this could be achieved by the introduction of either greater sensory input or greater sensitivity to sensory input by the extensor oscillators. It is true that even defining the "unit" oscillator is not a simple task. Moreover, as the connections onto and between oscillators have undoubtedly changed substantially in different organisms, the separation between oscillator and inputs will be obscured and difficult to determine (cf. Harris-Warrick, Chapt. 8; Getting, Chapt. 4). Nonetheless, the discussion here suggests it should ultimately be possible.

ACKNOWLEDGMENTS

Discussions with many people were helpful in clarifying the ideas presented here. If I have failed it is entirely my failure. People I wish especially to thank are Nancy Kopell, Margaret Hollyday, Sally Moody and Ann Bekoff. Invaluable comments on the manuscript were provided by Jeff Dean, Carl Gans, and Ron Hoy. The figures were done by Wendy Sussdorf and Margy Nelson. Patient manuscript preparation was by Sally Mancil. The work was supported by NIH grant NS16803.

REFERENCES

Ayers, J. A., G. A. Carpenter, S. Currie, and J. Kinch (1983). Which behavior does the lamprey central motor program mediate? *Science*, **221**:1312–1314.

Bass, A. H. (1986). Species differences in electric organs of mormyrids: Substrates for species-typical electric organ discharge waveforms. *J. Comp. Physiol.*, **244**: 313–303.

Bass, A. H. and C. D. Hopkins (1982). Comparative aspects of brain organization of an African "wave" electric fish, *Gymnarchus niloticus*. *J. Morphol.*, **174**:313–334.

Bekoff, A. (1985). Development of locomotion in vertebrates: a comparative perspective. In *Comparative Development of Adaptive Skills: Evolutionary Implications*, Gallin, E. S., ed. Erlbaum, Hillsdale, pp. 57–94.

Blight, A. R. (1977). The muscular control of vertebrate swimming movements. *Biol. Rev.*, **52**:181–218.

Buchanan, J. T. and A. H. Cohen (1982). Activities of identified interneurons, motoneurons, and muscle fibers during fictive swimming in the lamprey and effects of reticulospinal and dorsal cell stimulation. *J. Neurophysiol.*, **47**:948–960.

Carlson, H., J. Halbertsma, and M. Zomlefer (1979). Control of the trunk during walking in the cat. *Acta Physiol Scand.*, **105**:251–253.

Cohen, A. H. (1987) Intersegmental coordinating system of the lamprey central pattern generator for locomotion. *J. Comp. Physiol.*, **160**: 181–193.

Cohen, A. H. and R. M. Harris-Warrick (1984). Strychnine eliminates alternating motor output during fictive locomotion in the lamprey. *Brain Res.*, **293**:164–167.

Cohen, A. H., P. J. Holmes, and R. H. Rand (1982). The nature of the coupling between segmental oscillators of the lamprey spinal generator for locomotion: A mathematical model. *J. Math. Biol.*, **13**:345–369.

Cohen, A. H., S. A. Mackler, and M. E. Selzer (1986). Functional regeneration following spinal transection demonstrated in the isolated spinal cord of the larval sea lamprey. *Proc. Natl. Acad. Sci.*, **83**:2763–2766.

Cohen, A. H. and P. Wallén (1980). The neuronal correlate of locomotion in fish: "Fictive swimming" induced in an in vitro preparation of the lamprey spinal cord. *Exp. Brain Res.*, **41**:11–18.

Droge, M. H. and R. B. Leonard (1983a). Swimming pattern in intact and decerebrated stingrays. *J. Neurophysiol.*, **50**:162–177.

Droge, M. H. and R. B. Leonard (1983b). Swimming rhythm in decerebrated, paralyzed stingrays: normal and abnormal coupling. *J. Neurophysiol.*, **50**:178–191.

Eaton, R. C., R. A. Bombardieri, and D. L. Meyer (1977). The Mauthner-initiated startle response in teleost fish. *J. Exp. Biol.*, **66**:65–81.

Fetcho, J. R. (1983). The organization of the motoneurons innervating the axial musculature of goldfish. *Soc. Neurosci. Abst.* 338.9.

Forssberg, H. (1979). On integrative motor functions in the cat's spinal cord. *Acta. Physiol. Scand., Suppl.* 474:1–56.

Forssberg, H. (1985). Ontogeny of human locomotor control. I. Infant stepping, supported locomotion and transition to independent locomotion. *Exp. Brain Res.*, **57**:480–493.

Forssberg, H., S. Grillner, J. Halbertsma, and S. Rossignol (1980). The locomotion of the low spinal cat. 2: interlimb coordination. *Acta. Physiol. Scand.*, **108**:283–295.

Forssberg, H. (1982). Spinal locomotor functions and descending control. In *Brain Stem Control of Spinal Mechanisms*, B. Sjölund and A. Björklund, eds. Elsevier Biomedical Press, Amsterdam, pp. 253–271.

Gambaryan, P. P. (1974). *How Mammals Run.* Halsted Press, New York.

Gans, C. (1974). *Biomechanics.* Lippincott, Philadelphia.

Gans. C. (1984). Slide-pushing—A transitional locomotor method of elongated squamates. *Symp. Zool. Soc. Lond.*, **52,** pp. 13–26.

Gans, C. (1985). Motor coordination factors in the transition from tetrapody to limblessness in lower vertebrates. In *Coordination of Motor Behaviour. Seminar Series 24, Soc. Exp. Bio.*, B. H. H. Bush and F. Clarac, eds. Cambridge University Press, Cambridge, pp. 183–200.

Gans, C. (1986). Limbless locomotion: A current overview. In *Functional Morphology of Vertebrates*, R. Duncker and G. Fleisher, eds. Gustav Fisher-Verlag, Stuttgart and New York, Series, Fortschritte der Zoologie, pp. 13–22.

Goodrich, E. S. (1913). Metameric segmentation and homology. *Quart. J. Microscop. Sci.*, **59**:227–248.

Goodrich, E. S. (1958). *Studies of the Structure and Development of Vertebrates*. Dover, New York.

Goslow, G. E. Jr., R. M. Reinking, and D. G. Stuart (1973). The cat step cycle: hindlimb joint angles and muscle lengths during unrestrained locomotion. *J. Morphol.*, **141**:1–41.

Grillner, S., C. Perret, and P. Zangger (1976). Central generation of locomotion in the spinal dogfish. *Brain Res.*, **109**:255–269.

Grillner, S. (1981). Control of locomotion in bipeds, tetrapods, and fish. In *Handbook of Physiology. Section 1. The Nervous System, Vol II, Part 2,* V. B. Brooks, ed. *Amer. Physiol. Soc.*, Bethesda, pp. 1179–1236.

Grillner S. and S. Kashin (1976). On the generation and performance of swimming in fish. In *Neural Control of Locomotion*, Vol. 18, R. Herman, S. Grillner, P. Stein, and D. Stuart, eds. New York, Plenum Press, pp. 181–202.

Grillner, S. and P. Zangger (1979). On the central generation of locomotion in the low spinal cat. *Exp. Brain Res.*, **34**:241–261.

Grillner, S. and P. Zangger (1984). The effect of dorsal root transection on the efferent motor pattern in the cat's hindlimb during locomotion. *Acta Physiol. Scand.*, **120**:393–405.

Hagedorn, M. and W. Heiligenberg (1985). Court and Spark: Electric signals used in the courtship and mating of gymnotoid fish. *Animal Behavior,* **33**:254–265.

Harris-Warrick, R. M. and A. H. Cohen. (1985). Serotonin modulates the central pattern generator for locomotion in the isolated lamprey spinal cord. *J. Exp. Biol.*, **116**:27–46.

Hildebrand, M. (1976). Analysis of tetrapod gaits: General considerations and symmetrical gaits. In *Neural Control of Locomotion*, Vol. 18, R. H. Herman, S. Grillner, P. Stein, and D. Stuart, eds. New York, Plenum Press, pp. 203–236.

Hollyday, M. (1980). Organization of motor pools in the chick lumbar lateral motor column. *J. Comp. Neurol.*, **194**:143–170.

Hollyday, M. (1983). Development of motor innervation of chick limbs. In *Limb Development and Regeneration*, Part A, J. F. Fallon and A. T. Caplan, eds. pp. 183–193.

Holst, E. von (1973). *The Behavioral Physiology of Animals and Man: The Collected Papers of Erich von Holst.* Vol. 1. University of Miami Press, Coral Gables, Florida.

Jacobson, M. (1983). Clonal organization of the central nervous system of the frog. III: Clones stemming from individual balstomers of the 128-, 256-, and 512-cell stages. *J. Neurosci.*, **3**:1019–1038.

Jacobson, R. D. and M. Hollyday (1982a). A behavioral and electromyographic study of walking in the chick. *J. Neurophysiol.*, **48**:238–256.

Jacobson, R. D. and M. Hollyday (1982b). Electrically evoked walking and fictive locomotion in the chick. *J. Neurophysiol.*, **48**:257–270.

Jenkins, Jr., F. A. and G. E. Goslow, Jr. (1983). The functional anatomy of the shoulder of the Savannah monitor lizard (*Varanus exanthematicus*). *J. Morph.*, **175**:195–216.

Kopell, N. (1986). Modeling CPGs: A robust approach. In *Neurobiology of Vertebrate*

Locomotion, S. Grillner, P. S. G. Stein, D. Stuart, H. Forssberg, and R. Herman, eds. Macmillian, London pp. 383–385.

Kulagin, A. S. and M. L. Shik (1970). Interaction of symmetrical limbs during controlled locomotion. *Biofiika*, 15:164–170. (Engl. transl. 171–178).

Lance Jones, C. L. (1979). The morphogenesis of the thigh of the mouse with special reference to tetrapod muscle homologies. *J. Morph.*, 162:275–310.

Lamb, A. H. (1976). The projection patterns of the ventral horn to the hindlimb during development. *Develop. Biol.*, 54:82–99.

Landmesser, L. and D. G. Morris (1975). The development of functional innervation in the hindlimb of the chick embryo. *J. Physiol.*, 249:301–327.

Landmesser, L. (1978a). The distribution of motoneurones supplying chick hindlimb muscles. *J. Physiol.*, 284:371–389.

Landmesser, L. (1978b). The development of the motor projection patterns in the chick hindlimb. *J. Physiol.*, 284:391–414.

Lissman, H. W. (1961). Zoology, locomotory adaptions and the problem of electric fish. In *The Cell and the Organism*, J. A. Ramsey and V. B. Wigglesworth, eds. Cambridge University Press, Cambridge, pp. 301–317.

McClellan, A. D. (1984). Descending control and sensory gating of 'fictive' swimming and turning responses elicited in an in vito preparation of the lamprey brainstem/spinal cord. *Brain Res.*, 302:151–162.

McClellan, A. D. and P. B. Farel (1985). Pharmacological activation of locomotor patterns in larval and adult frog spinal cords. *Brain Res.*, 332:119–130.

McClellan, A. D. and S. Grillner (1983). Initiation and sensory gating of 'fictive' swimming and withdrawal responses in an in vitro preparation of the lamprey spinal cord. *Brain Res.*, 269:237–250.

Moody, S. A. and M. Jacobson (1983). Compartmental relationships between anuran primary motoneurons and somitic muscle fibers that they first innervate. *J. Neurosci.*, 3:1670–1682.

Perret, C. and J. M. Cabelguen (1980). Main characteristics of the hindlimb locomotor cycle in the decorticate cat with special reference to bifunctional muscles. *Brain Res.*, 187:333–352.

Romer, A. S. (1922). Locomotor apparatus of certain primitive and mammal-like reptiles. *Bull. Amer. Mus. Nat. His.*, 46:517–606.

Romer, A. S. (1927). The development of the thigh musculature of the chick. *J. Morph. Physiol.*, 43:347–385.

Roos, P. J. (1964). Lateral bending in newt locomotion. *Koninklijke Nederlands Akademie van Wetenschappen Proceedings C.* 67:223–232.

Rosen, D. E., P. L. Forey, B. G. Gardiner, and C. Patterson (1981). Lungfishes, tetrapods, paleontology, and plesiomorphy. *Bull. Amer. Mus. Nat. Hist.*, 167: 163–275.

Rovainen, C. M. and K. L. Birnberger (1971). Identification and properties of motoneurons to fin muscle of the sea lamprey. *J.Neurophysiol.*, 34:974–982.

Shik, M. L., F. V. Severin, G. N. Orlovskii (1966). Control of walking and running by means of electrical stimulation of the mid-brain. *Biofizyka*, 11:659–666.

Soffe, S. R. and A. Roberts (1982). Activity of myotomal motoneurons during fictive swimming in frog embryos. *J. Neurophysiol.*, 48:1279–1288.

Stehouwer, D. J. and P. B. Farel (1980). Central and peripheral controls of swimming in anuran larvae. *Brain Res.*, **195**:323–335.

Stehouwer, D. J. and P. B. Farel (1981). Sensory interactions with a central motor program in anuran larvae. *Brain Res.*, **218**:131–140.

Stehouwer, D. J. and P. B. Farel (1983). Development of hindlimb locomotor activity in the bullfrog (*Rana catesbeiana*) studied in vitro. *Science*, **219**:516–518.

Stein, P. S. G. (1978). Swimming movements elicited by electrical stimulation of the turtle spinal cord: the high spinal preparation. *J. Comp. Physiol.*, **124**:203–210.

Sukhanov, V. G. (1974). *General System of Symmetrical Locomotion of Terrestrial Vertebrates and Some Features of Movement of Lower Vertebrates.* Amerikind Publ. Co., New Delhi, India.

Thorstensson, A., J. Nilsson, H. Carlson, and M. Zomlefer (1984). Trunk movements in human locomotion. *Acta Physiol. Scand.*, **121**:9–22.

Viala, D. and C. Vidal (1978). Evidence for distinct spinal locomotion generators supplying respectively fore- and hindlimbs in the rabbit. *Brain Res.*, **155**:182–186.

Wallén, P., S. Grillner, J. Feldman, and S. Bergelt (1985). Dorsal and ventral myotome motoneurones in lamprey. *J. Neurosci.*, **5**:654–661.

Wallén, P. and T. L. Williams (1984). Fictive locomotion in the lamprey spinal cord *in vitro* compared with swimming in the intact and spinal animal. *J. Physiol.* **347**:225–239.

Webb, P. W. (1973). Kinematics of pectoral fin propulsion in *Cymatogaster aggregata*. *J. Exp. Biol.*, **59**:697–710.

Webb, P. W. (1978). Fast-start performance and body form in seven species of teleost fish. *J. Exp. Biol.*, **74**:211–226.

Webb, P. W. (1984a). Body and fin form and strike tactics of four teleost predators attacking fathead minnow (*Pimephales promelas*) prey. *Can. J. Fish. Aquat. Sci.*, **41**:157–165.

Webb, P. W. (1984b). Body form, locomotion, and foraging in aquatic vertebrates. *Amer. Zool.*, **24**:107–120.

Wortham, R. A. (1948). The development of the muscles and tendons in the lower leg and foot of chick embryos. *J. Morph.*, **83**:105–148.

Young, J. Z. (1981). *The Life of Vertebrates.* Oxford University Press, New York.

Chapter Six

LOCOMOTION AND SCRATCHING IN TETRAPODS

ISRAEL M. GELFAND
GRISJA N. ORLOVSKY
MARK L. SHIK

Moscow State University and
Institute of Information Transmission
Academy of Sciences of the USSR
Moscow, Soviet Union

1 INTRODUCTION

In this paper, some neuronal mechanisms controlling limb movements during the scratch reflex and locomotion in tetrapods are considered. During the scratch reflex, one of the hindlimbs performs rhythmic movements while the three others maintain the body at an appropriate posture. During locomotion, all four limbs perform rhythmic stepping movements. The rhythms of the limbs' movements are usually the same while the phase relations between the limbs can vary over a wide range determining the type of gait (trot, gallop, etc.).

Each limb is controlled by a separate nervous mechanism, the main part of which is located in the spinal cord. This mechanism, which we term a spinal generator (Fig. 1), determines the main characteristics of rhythmic limb movement, i.e., the cycle duration, phases of activity of various muscles in the cycle, etc. During the scratch reflex, only one of the generators is active, while during locomotion, all four are active.

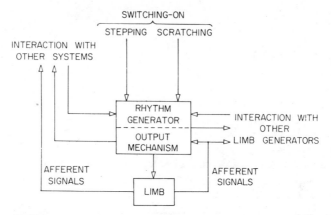

FIGURE 1. Spinal generator for stepping and scratching (see text).

In both kinds of movements, afferent signals from the receptors located in a moving limb are unnecessary for producing the rhythmic activity in the control system. This is proved by the facts that (1) stepping and scratching movements can be observed in animals with the limbs deafferented, and (2) efferent activity in muscle nerves, similar to that during locomotion or scratching, can be observed in animals immobilized with curare or other myorelaxants. This activity has been termed "fictive" locomotion or scratching. In the spinal generator, therefore, one can distinguish a central part (termed the "central pattern generator" or CPG) which produces the efferent pattern for fictive locomotion and scratching. Thus, the central pattern generator is the spinal generator deprived of the sensory feedback. Afferent signals arriving at a spinal generator can modify its efferent pattern. The afferent input is more significant for locomotion than for scratching, since stepping movements must be coordinated not only in relation to the body position (as in the case of scratching) but also in relation to the supporting surface.

The spinal generator can be arbitrarily divided into two parts—the rhythm generator and the output mechanism. Such a division is possible because a portion of the spinal neurons (in particular, the motoneurons) influence neither the cycle duration nor the duration of flexor and extensor parts of the cycle, although they exhibit the rhythmic discharge modulation during stepping and scratching.

A spinal generator controlling an individual limb is, in principle, an autonomous system since it can operate separately from other limb generators. However, during locomotion, this autonomy is restricted, because stepping movements of individual limbs must be mutually synchronized and properly phased. This coordination is achieved through an interaction between spinal generators. Each generator sends signals concerning its current state to the others. These signals come both from intraspinal mechanisms (which is proved by the coordinated activity of all four generators during fictive locomotion) and from the sensory receptors of the moving limbs.

Activity of spinal generators must also be coordinated with the activity of a number of brain mechanisms which determine the behavior of an animal, its position in the field of gravity, and its relation to external objects, etc. For this purpose, information concerning the current state of the spinal generators, the limb positions, the muscle contractions, etc., is sent to corresponding brain centers. From these centers the spinal generators receive the requisite correcting signals.

Finally, each spinal generator has inputs for its "switching-on" and for the control of its level of activity. Switching-on of the spinal generator of one hindlimb during the scratch reflex occurs in response to irritation of a definite area of the skin, depending on the efficiency of the stimulus (i.e., if it evokes a reflex or not), and depending on some higher brain centers. During locomotion, the spinal generators of all four limbs are switched on simultaneously. Their activation is closely linked to definite kinds of the animal's behavior (e.g., searching for food, running away from predatory animals) and is produced by higher brain centers.

In the present paper, primarily two problems are considered: (1) organization of the central part of a spinal generator (i.e., the CPG), and (2) organization of the system which activates the CPG. The questions concerning interaction between spinal generators and other systems, as well as those concerning the role of sensory feedback, are considered only minimally (however, cf. Rossignol et al., Chapt. 7).

2 ORGANIZATION OF SPINAL GENERATORS FOR STEPPING AND SCRATCHING

2.1 Efferent Patterns of Stepping and Scratching

We shall consider here the nervous mechanisms controlling rhythmic movements of hindlimbs since they have been investigated in more detail. Most data have been obtained in experiments on cats (decerebrate, decorticate, or spinal) in which stepping or scratching movements can be evoked by various kinds of stimulation. Fictive movements are also observed in these preparations after immobilizing them with gallamine triethiodide (Flaxedil). The main features of the efferent patterns of actual and fictive stepping or scratching are similar. Figure 2 schematically shows the activity of hindlimb motoneurons during stepping (A) and scratching (B). Each of these movements can be considered as consisting of two components—the tonic (postural) and rhythmic (phasic) ones. The tonic component of stepping can be observed (at least, in intact animals) before stepping movements begin, i.e., when an animal is standing. At this time,

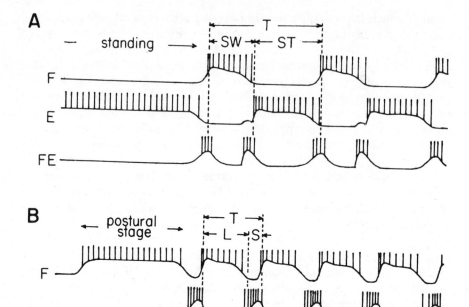

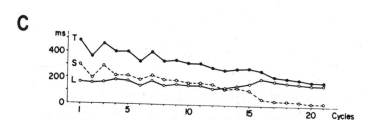

FIGURE 2. Efferent pattern of stepping (A) and scratching (B). There are shown schematically the activities of a flexor (F) and extensor (E) motoneurons, as well as that of a motoneuron of two-joint muscle (FE). Rhythmic movements are preceded by the corresponding postures: standing for stepping and "postural stage" for scratching. A cycle of stepping consists of the swing (SW) and stance (ST) phases with dominating flexor and extensor activities correspondingly. A scratch cycle consists of the long, flexor phase (L) and short, extensor phase (S). (C) smooth transition from long to short cycles observed at the beginning of fictive scratch reflex. There are shown durations of successive cycles (T) and of flexor and extensor phases (L and S). (Berkinblit et al., 1978b.)

170

a tonic discharge of extensor motoneurons (the left part of Fig. 2A) evokes excitation of limb extensors which counteract the force of body weight. The tonic component of scratching can be observed in pure form during the initial (postural) stage of the scratch reflex, when a tonic discharge of flexor motoneurons (the left part of Fig. 2B) evokes excitation of the limb flexors (mainly those of the hip and foot). As a result, the limb protracts far forward and reaches the irritated area of the skin. When rhythmic limb movements begin, periodic pauses appear in the tonic activity of corresponding "postural" groups of motoneurons (extensor motoneurons in stepping and flexor motoneurons in scratching). During these pauses, the antagonistic motoneurons discharge (right parts of Figs. 2A and 2B).

The cycle duration in actual stepping can vary over a wide range depending on the speed of locomotion. In the cat, at low speed it is 1–2 sec, at high speed, 0.3–0.5 sec. These changes are almost completely determined by the changes of the stance (extensor) phase of the cycle (ST in Fig. 2A). However, the swing (flexor) phase (SW) is of rather constant duration (0.2–0.3 sec). In fictive stepping, the range of cycle durations is smaller than in normal locomotion.

In contrast to stepping, the cycle duration in scratching (both actual and fictive) is rather constant (about 0.25 sec), and decreases only slightly with more intense movements. The duration of the flexor (L) phase is about 0.2 sec, i.e., similar to that in stepping. The duration of the extensor (S) phase is very short, about 0.05 sec.

The behavior of two-joint limb muscles (which flex one joint and extend another) is usually more complicated than that of "pure" flexors and extensors. Their motoneurons may have two waves of depolarization per cycle and two bursts of discharges, respectively (Deliagina et al., 1975; Engberg and Lundberg, 1969; Gambarian et al., 1971; Perret, 1983; Perret and Cabelguen, 1980). These bursts may not coincide with those in flexor and extensor motoneurons (Figs. 2A and 2B, the lower curves).

Thus, efferent patterns of stepping and scratching have common features: (1) activities of flexor and extensor motoneuron pools alternate, and (2) the durations of the flexor phase in these two movements are almost the same. The main differences are as follows: (1) the cycle periods for scratching are considerably shorter than those of stepping because of the very short extensor phase, and (2) the postural component in stepping is the extensor activity, while in scratching, it is the flexor activity. In spite of these differences, we think that essentially the same nervous mechanisms are used to generate the efferent patterns in these two movements. This suggestion is based, in particular, on the fact that, in a few cases, when evoking the fictive scratch reflex, one could observe a smooth transition from long cycles with dominating extensor phase (which is typical of stepping) to short cycles with dominating flexor phase (typical of scratching; Fig. 2C). Spinal interneurons, recorded during such transitions, preserved the phase of their activity in the cycle (Berkinblit et al., 1978b). This fact

A

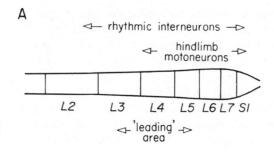

B

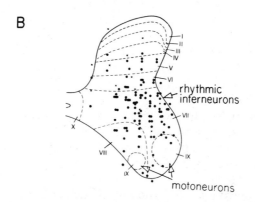

FIGURE 3. Location of the generator for stepping and scratching in the lumbosacral enlargement of the spinal cord. (A) Location of the hindlimb motoneurons as well as of interneurons having the rhythmic activity related to the scratch (step) cycle. The "leading" area with mostly pronounced generatory properties is indicated. (B) Distribution of interneurons, having the rhythmic activity related to the scratch cycle, over the cross-section of the L5 segment (dots and crosses: deep and weak rhythmic modulation of a neuron discharge, correspondingly). (Berkinblit et al., 1978a.)

would be difficult to explain if the "stepping" and "scratching" cycles were generated by different mechanisms. It seems more likely that there is a common generator admitting considerable changes in the regime of its operation.

2.2   Capacity for Rhythmic Generation Is Distributed Along the Spinal Cord

The spinal generators for hindlimbs are located in the lumbosacral enlargement of the spinal cord (segments L3–S1, Fig. 3A). Neurons of the generators of each limb are located mainly on the ipsilateral side of the cord. Motoneuron pools of the hindlimb are distributed over the length of the enlargement, the pools of hip muscles being located mainly in L4–L5, those of knee muscles in L5–L6, and those of ankle and digit muscles in L7–S1. During stepping and scratching, all these pools exhibit rhythmic activity. A great number of interneurons, situated over the whole length of the enlargement, also exhibit rhythmic activity related to that of moto-neurons. Mapping of the spinal cord during fictive scratching has shown that most of the rhythmically modulated cells are located in the lateral part of the intermediate area of the spinal gray matter, as well as in the ventral horn (Fig. 3B; Bayev et al., 1981; Berkinblit et al., 1978a). Corresponding results have been obtained for stepping (Bayev et al., 1979; Orlovsky and Feldman, 1972).

The capacity for rhythmic generation is also distributed along the lumbosacral enlargement. This was proven for the scratch reflex by function-ally "switching-off" various parts of the cord (by means of cooling) or by destruction of a part of the spinal gray matter (Deliagina et al., 1983). Fig-ure 4A shows the efferent activity in nerves to the sartorius (Sart) and gastrocnemius (G) muscles during fictive scratching, as well as the activity of a spinal interneuron from L4. Then, by cooling L5 (Fig. 4B), the caudal part of the spinal hindlimb center (started from L5) was disconnected from its rostral part, which was demonstrated by termination of activity in the G motoneuron pool located caudal to the cooling probe, in L7–S1 (Fig. 4C).

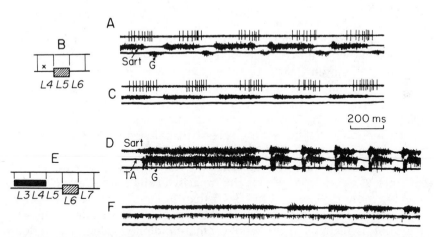

FIGURE 4. Generation of the scratch rhythm by the intact spinal cord and by its limited parts. (A) The rhythmic activity in nerves to m. sartorius (Sart) and m. gastrocnemius (G), as well as the activity of a spinal interneuron from L4 (a site of the microelectrode insertion is shown by the cross in (B) during fictive scratching. Then cooling the L5 segment was started (position of the cooler on the lateral surface of the cord is shown in B). (C) Activity of the Sart and interneuron 60 s after the beginning of cooling, when the L5 and lower segment were switched-off from the rhythmical process (which is proved by terminating the G rhythmic activity). (D–F) Generation of the scratch rhythm in the isolated L5 segment. Initial fictive scratching is shown in D. Then the gray matter in L3–L4 segments was destroyed, and the L6 segment was cooled (E). Rhythmic activity in the Sart nerve under these conditions, evoked by pinna stimulation, is shown in F. (Deliagina et al., 1983.)

Nevertheless, L3 and L4 continued to generate the normal scratch rhythm, which was demonstrated by rhythmic activity of Sart motoneurons (the Sart motoneuron pool is located in L4–L5), and by rhythmic bursts in an interneuron from L4. Figure 4E shows a scheme of the experiment with "isolation" of L5. For this purpose, the gray matter of L3–L4 was destroyed and the caudal part of the hindlimb center was "switched off" by cooling L6. While destroying the gray matter, spinal pathways responsible for activation of generator were preserved. The "isolated" L5 segment was capable of generating the scratch rhythm which is demonstrated by rhythmic activity of Sart motoneurons from L5 (Fig. 4F). Elicitation of rhythmic generation in caudal segments (L6 and lower) after destroying the L3–L5 gray matter was difficult, but it became much easier when the excitability of neurons in L6–S1 was raised by slight cooling (Brooks, 1983).

Thus, the rhythm generator that controls limb movements during scratching is a distributed system. The question as to whether separate parts of the lumbosacral enlargement can also generate slow (locomotor) rhythms remains to be answered. What is the principle of coordination of generator elements of these various segments? This question is difficult to answer since the lumbosacral enlargement is rather short (5–6 segments) and, therefore, the phase shift between oscillations in the rostral and caudal segments, if it existed, would be small. Besides, to reveal the phase shift, one must compare the activities of analogous parts of the generators from the rostral and caudal segments. However, it is difficult to say which elements are analogous since the interneuron organization of the generator is not known, and connections between interneurons of the rhythm generator and motoneurons are not known either. Nevertheless, it is interesting to note that, during scratching, there is a phase shift between the flexor motorneuron pools from the L4–L5 segments (Sart) and from L6–L7 (tibialis anterior—TA) (Fig. 4D). This may suggest a "sequential" principle of coordination with the leading role of rostral segments in determining the rhythm of the whole system.

There is another fact which implies the leading role of the more rostral segments. As mentioned above, the capacity of rhythm generation is considerably more pronounced in L3–L5 than in L6–S1. It seems, therefore, very likely that it is the generator mechanism of L3–L5 that determines the rhythm of oscillations in the whole spinal hindlimb center. Such a dominance of rostral segments correlates well with the fact that it is in these segments that the neuron mechanism controlling hip muscles, i.e., the muscles of the "leading" joint of the limb (see Berkenblit et al., 1978b), is located.

The hypothesis that the spinal limb center may contain several rhythm generators was first advanced by Grillner (1981). In his model, each joint is controlled by a separate generator with the generators affecting each other. The facts that the limb musculature is to some extent presented somatotopically along the lumbosacral spinal cord, and that the capacity for

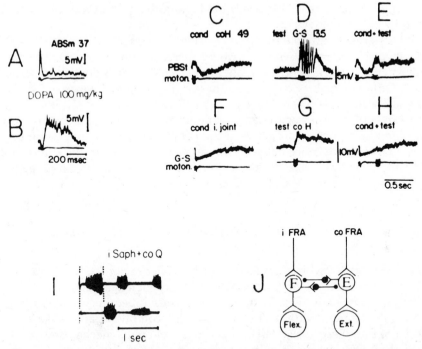

FIGURE 5. Elements of the generatory mechanisms revealed by L-dopa in acute spinal cat. (A,B) Drastic changes of the state of the spinal cord evoked by L-dopa. Before L-dopa injection, a flexor motoneuron of the posterior biceps–semitendinosus (PBSt) muscle group responded by a short EPSP to stimulation of the ipsilateral anterior biceps–semimembranosus (ABSm) muscle nerve. The strength of stimulation (indicated in A) was sufficient to excite flexor reflex afferents (FRA). after the L-dopa injection, the same stimulation evokes the long-latency, long-duration EPSP (B) instead of the short-latency one shown in A. (C–H) Demonstration of the inhibitory interaction between the interneuron groups which are responsible for excitation of motoneurons observed after L-dopa injection. Recordings were performed from a PBSt, i.e., flexor, motoneuron (C–E) and from an extensor gastrocnemius–soleus (GS) motoneurons (F–H). In the flexor motoneuron (C–E) a train of volleys in high threshold muscle afferents evoked the characteristic long-lasting EPSP (D), which was effectively inhibited (E) by a preceding train of volleys in contralateral high threshold afferents (H, hamstring). Conversely, in the extensor motoneuron (F–H) the long-lasting EPSP was evoked from contralateral high threshold muscle afferents (H) and inhibited from the ipsilateral joint nerve (H). (I) Alternating discharges in flexor (sartorius) and extensor (vastus) muscle nerves (upper and lower traces, correspondingly) after injection of L-dopa and Nialamid. Acute spinal cat was pretreated with Nialamid (10 mg) and given L-dopa (100 mg/kg). Ipsilateral saphenus and contralateral quadriceps nerves were stimulated (marked by dotted lines). (J) The half-center organization of the interneuronal network released after L-dopa (see text). (Jankowska et al., 1967a,b.)

rhythmic oscillations is also distributed along this part of the cord, correspond well to Grillner's idea.

It is interesting to note that the "distributed" generator is typical for the spinal cord of animals which move by means of undulatory body or fin movements, i.e., in lamprey (Cohen and Wallén, 1980) dogfish (Grillner, 1974; Grillner et al., Chapt. 1), stingray (Droge and Leonard, 1983a,b; Leonard et al., 1979), and frog embryo (Roberts et al., 1981; Stehouwer and Farel, 1983). The segmental generators are coordinated in such a way that there is a phase shift between their oscillations, this shift being proportional to the distance between the segments. Moreover, the shift is not dependent on the cycle duration (i.e., on the speed of swimming) (cf. Grillner et al., Chapt. 1; Cohen, Chapt. 5).

2.3   Elements of Generatory Mechanisms Revealed by Means of L-dopa

It was demonstrated by Lundberg and his colleagues that, in spinal cats, intravenous injection of L-dopa (L-dihydroxyphenylalanine) resulted in dramatic changes in the state of the spinal cord: it became capable of generating the efferent pattern similar to that of locomotion (Jankowska et al., 1967 a,b; Lundberg 1969, 1981). This activity of spinal mechanisms can be evoked by stimulation of high-threshold cutaneous and muscle afferents called "the flexor reflex afferents". Before L-dopa administration they evoke only the short-term excitation of flexor motoneurons of the ipsilateral limb (Fig. 5A). By contrast, after L-dopa administration, stimulation of an ipsilateral nerve evokes the long-lasting depolarization and late discharge of flexor motoneurons resembling the flexor phase of the step cycle (Fig. 5B), while stimulation of a contralateral nerve evokes the similar pattern of activity in extensor motoneurons (Fig. 5G). A short train of stimuli applied to the nerve can even evoke several successive cycles with alternating activity of flexor and extensor motoneurons (Fig. 5I). Analysis of this phenomenon (see the legend to Fig. 5C–H) has shown that the excitation of flexor and extensor motoneurons is produced by two groups of interneurons (F and E in Fig. 5J) which convert a short stimulus into the long-lasting EPSP. It has also been found that these groups of interneurons exert strong inhibitory actions upon each other, i.e., excitation of one group causes activity of another group to terminate. Besides, each group exerts some inhibitory action upon the antagonistic motoneurons.

The existence of F and E groups with properties described above was demonstrated in an indirect way, by analyzing synaptic potentials in motoneurons and recording the corresponding activity in interneurons with unknown connections (Jankowska et al., 1967a,b). Nevertheless, the fact that the periodic excitation to flexor and extensor motoneurons during stepping is delivered by two groups of interneurons with strong mutual inhibitory interaction seems to be of great importance for understanding the organization of the spinal generator.

In relation to the data obtained in animals treated with L-dopa, a question arises: do F and E groups constitute the rhythm generator, or do they only mediate influences of the true generator upon motoneurons? If one supplements the F and E groups or their interconnections with no properties depending on time, the system shown in Figure 5J is stable. In the absence of tonic excitatory inflow, the F and E groups are not active. With tonic excitatory inflow, one of the groups is active while the other is inhibited. Thus, the above question concerning F and E groups can be reformulated in the following way: can the excitation transit from one group to another, and what are the reasons for the transition? Lundberg's point of view is that the F and E groups do constitute the rhythm generator, and that the excitation transits from one group to another because neurons of the groups cannot be active for a long time, i.e., they possess a property of "fatigue." Such a model of a stepping generator was first proposed by Brown and called "the model of two half centers" (Brown, 1911,1914; see also Lundberg, 1971). We agree with Lundberg's point of view that the F and E groups constitute the rhythm generator but we think that the main reason for transition of excitation is not "fatigue" but the excitatory interaction between F and E groups which supplements the inhibitory interaction and is delayed in relation to it (see also Euler, 1983). The suggestion is based on observations of the activity of spinal interneurons during scratching and stepping.

2.4 Activity of Spinal Interneurons During Scratching and Stepping

As mentioned in Section 2, small "pieces" of the spinal cord (1–2 segments) from the region of L3–L5, are capable of generating the scratch rhythm. With further decrease of the volume of "generating tissue," the rhythm becomes unstable and then disappears (Deliagina et al., 1983). Thus, a region of the cord with a length of 1–2 segments contains neuronal mechanisms sufficient and seemingly necessary for both generating the rhythm and producing the almost normal efferent pattern in those motoneuron pools which are contained in this region. Taking into account the data concerning the density of neurons in the cord, (Gelfan and Rapisarda, 1964) one may estimate that such a region contains 10^4–10^5 neurons. To date, the functions of most of these cells, their properties and connections, are not known. The means of identification or knowledge about their connections has been developed for only a few small groups (mainly by their responses to stimulation of peripheral nerves). To this group belong, besides motoneurons, the Renshaw cells, "la interneurons" of the system of reciprocal inhibition, a few groups of propriospinal neurons, and a few groups of neurons giving rise to ascending tracts (e.g., to spinocerebellar tracts).

Both the Renshaw cells and Ia inhibitory interneurons exhibit rhythmical modulation of their discharge during fictive scratching and stepping (Deliagina and Feldman, 1981; Deliagina and Orlovsky, 1980; Feldman and Orlovsky, 1975; Jordan et al., 1981). But they do not belong to the rhythm generator since considerable changes of their activity with stimulation of ventral roots do not influence the cycle duration (Feldman and Orlovsky, 1975; Jordan et al., 1981). The Renshaw cells and Ia interneurons exert inhibitory action upon motoneurons, but they are not the neurons responsible for the basic pattern of rhythmic changes of the motoneuron membrane potential shown in Figure 2A and 2B, since in some cases, the depolarization appears in motoneurons just at the moment of maximum inhibitory drive from Renshaw cells and Ia interneurons (Deliagina and Feldman, 1981; Feldman and Orlovsky, 1975).

Since identified neurons appeared not to be responsible for producing the basic pattern of motoneuron discharges, unidentified interneurons (i.e., the cells which were met by chance when introducing the microelectrode into the cord) were recorded during fictive scratching (Bayev et al., 1981; Berkinblit et al., 1978a) as well as during stepping (Bayev et al., 1979; Orlovsky and Feldman, 1972). During scratching, neurons were recorded from the segments with the most pronounced generatory properties (L4–L5), and during stepping, L6 was also explored. A great number of recorded cells exhibited rhythmic modulation of their activity, i.e., they fired a burst in a definite phase of the cycle (see, for example the neuron in Fig. 4A). Phases of activity were different for different neurons. Figure 6 shows the distribution of neuron discharges over the normalized cycle during scratching (A) and stepping (B). The beginning of the flexor phase was taken as the cycle beginning. One can see that there are populations of interneurons firing in-phase with motoneurons. Group 1 neurons are active during the flexor phase both during scratching and during stepping. Because of the shortness of the extensor (S) phase of the scratch cycle, it is difficult to distinguish the units whose activity coincides with that of extensor motoneurons, while in the step cycle such neurons are clearly seen (group 3).

However, it was also found that activity of a great part of the interneurons were co-active neither with the flexor nor with the extensor motoneurons. In the L-phase of the scratch cycle, soon after the activation of group 1 neurons, successive activation of neurons of group 2 (and, partly, of group 3) starts; their recruiting continues for the whole L-phase (Fig. 6). These neurons stop firing by the end of the L-phase or at the beginning of the S-phase. A similar picture can be seen for stepping (Fig. 6B): new neurons were recruited throughout the flexor phase, while some of them terminate their discharge only in the subsequent (extensor) phase.

Because of the shortness of the S-phase of the scratch cycle, it is difficult to say if, in this phase, there is successive excitation of neurons whose activity does not correspond with that of extensor motoneurons. In the

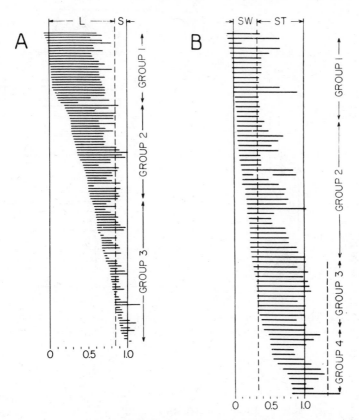

FIGURE 6. Phase distribution of spinal interneurons obtained for fictive scratching (A) and for locomotion of the cat with deafferented hindlimbs (B). Neurons were recorded from the L4–L5 segments (A) and L4–L6 segments (B). Solid vertical lines indicate the cycle borders, interrupted lines indicate borders between flexor and extensor phases of the cycle. Horizontal lines show phases of activity of individual neurons in the normalized cycle. Main groups of interneurons are indicated.

step cycle, there are such neurons in the extensor phase though their number is smaller than in the flexor phase.

The interneurons, whose discharge starts in one phase and terminates in the other, would be well suited for transmitting the excitation from one phase to the other, i.e., they would make the model of two half-centers capable of rhythmic generation. Let us consider such a model.

2.5   Model of Two Centers with Inhibitory–Excitatory Connections

The model shown in Figure 7A can generate the efferent pattern of both scratching and stepping. Neuron groups F_1 and E_1 correspond to groups F and E discovered by Lundberg and his colleagues (Fig. 5J), i.e., they are mutually linked by strong inhibitory connections, and they control respec-

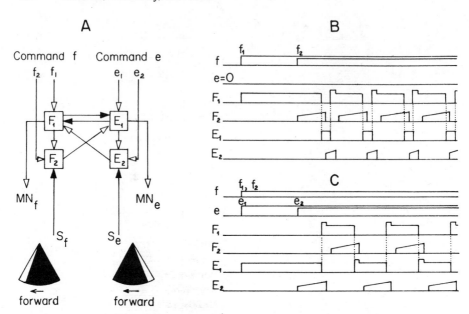

FIGURE 7. Model of the spinal generator consisting of two centers with inhibitory-excitatory connections (A), and processes in it during scratching (B) and stepping (C) (see text).

tively the flexor and extensor motoneurons by sending excitation to them. Besides groups F_1 and E_1, the model contains groups F_2 and E_2 which are activated by groups F_1 and E_1, correspondingly, and, in turn, excite neurons of the opposite phase, groups F_2 and E_2. These correspond to those neuron groups found for scratching and stepping, whose activity is delayed in relation to groups F_1 and E_1. The inputs and outputs of groups F_2 and E_2 have not been determined experimentally; they are postulated for the model.

Regulation of the generator is performed by means of tonic commands coming from higher brain centers. Command f coming to the flexor center consists of two components, f_1 and f_2. Command f_1 excites group F_1 of the flexor center and, thus, evokes tonic activation of flexor motoneurons which is observed during the postural stage of the scratch reflex (Fig. 2B). Command f_2 does not affect the postural component of movement, rather it enhances the excitation of group F_2 of the flexor center, i.e., the group responsible for transition of activity from the flexor center to the extensor one. In other words, command f_2 promotes the initiation of rhythmic oscillations in the model. The existence of the two commands has been demonstrated for the scratch reflex: one of them is responsible for excitation of flexor motoneurons, the other one switches on the rhythm generator (see Section 2.1).

The control of the extensor center is performed by command e that also consists of two components, e_1 and e_2. Command e_1 excites group E_1 which is responsible for the postural extensor activity observed, for instance, in a standing animal (Fig. 2A). Command e_2 promotes excitation of group E_2, through which the activity transits from the extensor to the flexor center.

The model with inhibitory-excitatory connections between two anti-phase centers was used to explain the operation of locomotor generators in molluscs *Tritonia* (Getting, 1983a,b; Chapt. 4) and *Clione* (Arshavsky et al., 1985a,b). The quantitative analyses and computer simulation have shown that it is essential for the model operation that the excitatory influences between the centers be delayed in relation to the inhibitory ones (Getting, 1983a). In *Tritonia*, one of the reasons for such a delay is the organization of synapses which initially hyperpolarize the postsynaptic membrane, and then depolarize it. In *Clione*, the delay of excitation is determined by the fact that the neurons of a center have different thresholds, and the high-threshold neurons begin to discharge later. These "late" neurons produce excitation of the antagonistic center through a special interneuron. In our model, a delay of excitation, addressed to the antagonistic center, is determined by a delay of activation of groups F_2 and E_2 in relation to F_1 and E_1, respectively. A reason for the delay may be, for example, the successive (polysynaptic) excitation of neurons within groups F_2 and E_2. In a system of neurons with mutual excitatory connections, it is possible, at least theoretically, to obtain great time delays. Such a mechanism was proposed by various authors for explaining the generation of slow rhythms in the nervous system (Dunin-Barkovsky and Jacobson, 1971; Rashevsky, 1972; Wilson and Waldron, 1968). However, we cannot exclude other reasons for the delay of excitation of the reciprocal center, for example, due to complex inhibitory-excitatory synapses as in *Tritonia* (Getting, 1983b; Chapt. 4).

We set a hypothesis of delayed excitation of the antagonistic center above that of "fatigue" (adaptation) of the active center because there are no indications of fatigue in the activity of interneurons controlling flexor and extensor motoneurons during stepping and scratching. For example, the duration of the extensor phase of that step can exceed a second; the rhythmic extensor activity can even be transformed in the postural activity. Correspondingly, tonic activity of flexor motoneurons during scratch reflex can continue indefinitely provided the limb is kept at the hind position (Deliagina et al., 1975). In this case, all the interneurons whose activity is coincident with that of flexor motoneurons (group 1 in Fig. 6A) exhibit tonic discharge (Berkinblit et al., 1978b). Thus, in those groups of interneurons which, presumably, control motoneurons, we found no reasons for temporal changes for their activity. The reasons for such changes seem to be outside these groups.

2.5.1 Generation of Scratching

Operation of the generator in the regime of scratching is illustrated in Figure 7B. To put the generator in operation in this regime, a tonic command f must be addressed to the flexor center. Suppose its component f_1 arrives earlier than f_2. A tonic excitation of F_1, evoked by f_1, results in a tonic activation of flexor motoneurons; this is a postural stage of the scratch reflex. Excitatory drive from F_1 to F_2 is not sufficient for activation of F_2, and F_2 activity starts only after arrival to F_2 of the tonic command f_2. Activity of F_2 increases gradually. When this activity becomes high enough, the excitatory input from F_2 to E_1 exceeds the inhibitory one from F_1 to E_1, and E_1 comes to an active state. Being excited, E_1 immediately inhibits groups F_1 of the flexor center. At the same time, E_1 excites extensor motoneurons. After a definite delay, "late" neurons of the extensor center (E_2) are also excited. As a result of inhibition of group F_1, excitatory drive from F_1 to F_2 terminates, and activity of F_2 soon terminates also. This means that the only source of excitation of groups E_1 (as well as an extensor burst) terminates. After this, the antagonistic group F_1 becomes active for two reasons: termination of the inhibitory drive from E_1 and an excitatory drive still coming from E_2 group is not necessary for the operation of the generator in the regime of scratching, since transition of activity to the antagonistic (flexor) center can take place simply as a result of termination of the inhibitory drive from E_1 to F_1. Remember that F_1 has a tonic excitatory input, f_1.

2.5.2 Generation of Stepping

Operation of the generator in this regime is illustrated in Figure 7C. Activation of the rhythm generator is produced against a background of tonic discharge by extensor motoneurons determinated by tonic command e_1 that excites group E_1 of the extensor center. To evoke a rhythmic process, tonic command e_2 must be addressed to group E_2. As a result of the convergence of excitatory inputs from E_1 and e_2, activity of E_2 begins to increase. When it becomes adequate, the excitatory drive from E_2 to F_1 exceeds the inhibitory drive from E_1 and F_1, and F_1 comes to an active state. Being excited, F_1 immediately inhibits E_1. Thus, the transition of activity from the extensor to the flexor center is finished. An opposite process was considered above, in describing the regime of scratching.

2.5.3 Control of Two-Joint Muscles

Motoneuron pools of some two-joint muscles during stepping and scratching exhibit a more complicated pattern of activity than pools of "pure" flexors or extensors; for instance, they may have two bursts of discharges per cycle, at the borders between the flexor and extensor phases (Fig. 2). In our model, there are two groups of neurons (F_2 and E_2) active at the borders between these phases; they are well suited for the control of two-joint muscles. One could also "add" the output signals from F_2 and E_2 to the input signals of flexor and extensor motoneurons (delivered from F_1 and E_1) and thus obtain some of the more complicated patterns of the discharge from these motoneurons as are sometimes observed. For example, extensor motoneurons during stepping can exhibit an increase of the activity towards the end of the extensor phase (Perret, 1983). To obtain such a picture, it is sufficient to address the E_2 output signal to them.

Our suggestion concerning the control of the two-joint muscles may supplement that of Perret. He supposed that the two-joint muscle motoneurons are controlled by the same signals as flexor and extensor motoneurons, these signals being added to one another in accordance with definite rules (Perret, 1983).

2.6 Afferent Influences upon the Rhythm Generator

Different sensory inputs exert considerable influence on the efferent patterns of stepping and scratching (cf. Rossignol et al., Chapt. 7). They can exert their influence by acting upon the output spinal mechanism (e.g., motoneurons, Ia interneurons). In such a case, they can change the level of activity of different motoneuron pools but not affect the duration of the cycle and its phases. For example, impulses from muscle spindles belong to such a class of spinal inputs (Deliagina and Orlovsky, 1980; Feldman and Orlovsky, 1975). If the afferent signals reach the rhythm generator, they can influence the duration of the cycle and its flexor and extensor components. Here we shall consider only such sensory inputs.

Rhythmical activity of the generator during fictitious scratching can be abolished by deflecting the hindlimb backward (Deliagina et al., 1975). This fact is reflected in Fig. 7A (the bottom left corner): limb positions required for generation are shown as a white sector ("zone of generation"), while those in which generation is impossible are shown as a black sector. If the limb is deflected backward, stimulation of the receptive field of the scratch reflex evokes only tonic excitation of flexor motoneurons (postural component of the reflex). In the framework of our model, this means that the F_1 group is excited while F_2 cannot be excited, and therefore, the activity cannot transit to the extensor center. Thus, inhibitory influences from the limb (S_f) should be addressed to F_2.

When not fictive, but actual, scratching is evoked, a descending tonic command evokes excitation of flexor motoneurons. Due to the contraction of the hip flexors, the limb moves foward and into the zone of generation. The rhythm generator comes into operation and sends rhythmical signals to flexor and extensor motoneurons. As a result, the limb begins to oscillate. It is worth noticing that the amplitude of oscillations at the ankle and knee joints is great while that at hip joint is small (Deliagina et al., 1975). Therefore, during actual scratching the limb never leaves the zone of generation.

What would happen if the contraction of hip extensors during the S-phase was great and the limb deflected far backward, as can occur, for example, during the jump when the hip angle rapidly changes by 100° (Gambarian et al., 1971)? Such deflection will immediately abolish activity of the rhythm generator. A tonic activity of flexors will appear, and the limb will move forward until it gets into the zone of generation; then a new extensor burst will be produced, etc. Thus, periodic oscillations arise, the rhythm of oscillations differing from the "proper" rhythm of the central pattern generator. The difference in rhythm is accounted for by the fact that the subsequent burst of activity is triggered only after the limb fulfills a cycle of mechanical oscillations evoked by the preceding burst. Such a regime could be used by galloping animals. This kind of locomotion can be considered as a periodically repeated jump (Gambarian et al., 1971). During the gallop, amplitudes of oscillations at the ankle and knee joints are closer to those during scratching, while oscillations at the hip joint are very great (70° or more) (Gambarian et al., 1971). This regime could also be used for a single jump provided the central command terminates soon after triggering the generator.

Now we shall consider the role of sensory input, not for jumping or galloping, but for normal stepping. It is known that hampering the limb movement during the stance (extensor) phase of the step cycle results in prolongation of this phase; the swing (flexor) phase begins only after the limb has reached a certain caudal position (Grillner and Rossignol, 1978; Shik and Orlovsky, 1965). In addition, Sherrington (1910a) found that in the spinal dog, stepping movements of the hindlimbs began spontaneously when an animal was suspended in the vertical position with its hindlimbs deflected backward. Thus, deflection of the limb backward promotes activation of the generator of stepping, and it will seem that receptors signalling the limb position (mainly, position of the hip) are responsible for this effect. On the other hand, Pearson and Duysens (1976) have demonstrated that the rhythm generator also has an inhibitory input from load-detecting limb receptors. This input prevents activation of the generator till the limb becomes unloaded: that happens when the limb is deflected backward at the end of a step. The afferent influences on the generator for stepping are schematically shown in Fig. 7A (the bottom right corner). In contrast to scratching, the zone of generation is situated at the caudal limb position. When the limb gets into this zone (which happens by the end of the stance phase of the step cycle), the rhythm generator comes into operation, and its activity begins with transition of excitation from the extensors to flexors. In the framework of our model this means that the E_2 group is excited and, through it, the activity transits to the flexor center. Thus inhibitory influences from the limb (S_2) should be addressed to E_2 but not to F_2 as it was during scratching. With excitation of the flexor center, the limb moves forward (the swing phase of the cycle) and then touches the ground. Since the limb is then out of the zone of generation, the afferent input inhibits the rhythm generator. A similar kind of the generator was proposed for stepping by Pearson (1976).

Thus, we suppose that the same principle is used while generating the temporal pattern of stepping and galloping; the generator is active in the

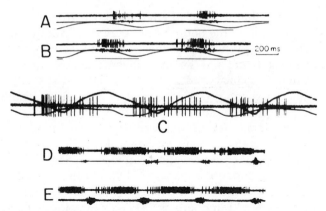

FIGURE 8. The DSCT conveys messages about the activity of the peripheral motor apparatus. The neuron of the DSCT presented in this figure was excited by afferents from ankle extensors(s). It fired in bursts during locomotion (A), and its activity increased with more intense locomotion (B). The middle trace is the gastrocnemius EMG, the lower one the angle of the ankle (flexion-up). Horizontal lines indicate the stance phases. Such a rhythmic activity of DSCT neurons disappeared after deafferentation of the hindlimbs (Arshavsky et al., 1972). (C–E) The VSCT conveys messages about intraspinal processes. (C) Activity of a VSCT neuron during locomotion (the hindlimbs of the cat were deafferented): the upper and lower traces are movements of the contralateral shoulder joint and of the ipsilateral hip joint. (D,E) Activity of a VSCT neuron recorded initially during actual scratching (D) and then during fictive scratching (E) after the animal had been immobilized with Flaxedil. The lower trace is the gastrocnemius EMG (D) or electroneurogram (E).

monocyclic regime, each burst of activity being triggered by signals from limb receptors. This is why the rhythm of oscillations differs from the "proper" rhythm of the central pattern generator. During walking, for example, the limb movement in the stance phase can be very slow, and thus, the cycle can be very long, up to several seconds.

2.7   Interaction Between Spinal Generators and Other Systems

During operation, spinal generators for stepping and scratching send signals to various parts of the nervous system. In response, they receive commands which can modify their activity. The interaction between the spinal generators and the cerebellum has been studied most extensively.

Signals from the spinal generator of a hindlimb reach the cerebellum via the dorsal and ventral spinocerebellar tracts (DSCT and VSCT) and the spinoreticulocerebellar pathway (SRCP). The DSCT transmits detailed information about the operation of the peripheral motor apparatus such as the phase and strength of contraction of single muscles, the joint angles, the time at which the stepping limb touches the ground, etc. (Arshavsky et al., 1972a). Figure 8A and 8B shows the activity of a DSCT neuron during locomotion. The analysis of the neuron's responses to passive limb movements showed that it received afferent signals from the ankle extensor(s). During locomotion the neuron fired periodically in the stance phase of the step (Fig. 8A,B). When the extensor activity increased (cf. the electromyograms in Fig. 8A,B) and the limb movements become more forceful, the neuron activity also increased.

The rhythmical activity of DSCT neurons is determined by afferent signals from the peripheral motor apparatus rather than from central structures; and during locomotion of cats with deafferented hindlimbs, as well as during fictitious scratching, any rhythmical modulation in DSCT neurons is absent. In contrast, information conveyed by the VSCT and SRCP is of central origin. Lundberg advanced a hypothesis that the VSCT conveys information about the activity of central spinal mechanisms but not about peripheral events (Lundberg, 1971). This hypothesis has been confirmed experimentally by a demonstration that the activity of VSCT neurons is rhythmically modulated during locomotion after deafferentiation of the hindlimbs (Fig. 8C; Arshavsky et al., 1972b). Also, comparison of the activity of VSCT neurons during actual and fictive scratching has shown that cessation of the rhythmical afferent inflow from limb receptors (after an animal has been immobilized) does not affect the pattern of modulation of VSCT neurons (Fig. 8D,E) (Arshavsky et al., 1978b). This persistent modulation after immobilization and deafferentation shows that intraspinal processes are the main source of rhythmic activity of these neurons. The same result has been obtained for neurons of the SRCP (Arshavsky et al., 1978a). Thus, the VSCT and SRCP transmit to the cerebellum the signals about activity of intraspinal mechanisms. Apparently these signals monitor mainly the activity of the rhythm generator rather than that of the output spinal mechanisms. This has been demonstrated by experiments with cooling and lesions of the spinal cord (Fig. 9; Arshavsky et al., 1984). While cooling the L5 segment, the rhythmicity of that and more caudal segments containing the major portion of the hindlimb motoneurons and interneurons was switched off. In spite of this, the activity of a reticulocerebellar neuron (belonging to the SRCP) did not change its pattern of activity (Fig. 9A,C). The same result has been obtained for neurons of VSCT. Thus, to produce a normal rhythmic modulation in the VSCT and SRCP neurons, it is sufficient to evoke rhythmic oscillations in a portion of the generator segments. The rhythmic bursting by reticulocerebellar neurons cannot be attributed to a rhythmic process in any particular segment. Figure 9 shows that a neuron exhibited normal rhythmic activity when oscillations were generated by the L5 and more caudal segments (Fig. 9F). From these results a hypothesis has been advanced that the VSCT and SRCP convey to the cerebellum a "generalized picture" of operation of the spinal generator (Arshavsky et al., 1983, 1984). This picture ignores such details as the relative contribution of various spinal segments to generation of oscillations, but, rather, reflects some essential data concerning the op-

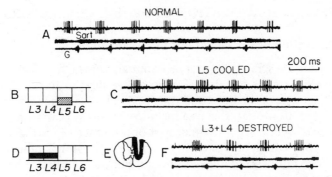

FIGURE 9. Neurons of the SRCP have inputs from various parts of the spinal generator. (A) Activity of a reticulo-cerebellar neuron during fictive scratching under normal conditions. Then the lower part of the spinal cord was switched-off by cooling the L5 segment (B), and rhythm generation persisted only in the L3–L4 segments. Under these conditions, the neuron exhibited a normal rhythmic pattern (C). Then the L5 segment was rewarmed, and the gray matter of the L3–L4 segments was destroyed by thermocoagulation (D,E). Under these conditions, the rhythm generator persisted in the L5 and more caudal segments, and the reticulo-cerebellar neuron continued to fire in bursts (F).

eration of the generator. First of all, it conveys the fact that a rhythmic process in the spinal cord has arisen, as well as conveying information about the frequency of oscillations. It was also demonstrated that activity of each VSCT or SRCP neuron is strictly related to a definite phase of the cycle, with VSCT neurons preferably active in the flexor phase and SRCP ones in the extensor phase (Arshavsky et al., 1978,a,b). This suggests that signals transmitted by the VSCT and SRCP neurons at a given moment indicate that at that moment the extensor center of the generator is active.

Thus, two kinds of messages come from the spinal cord to the cerebellum: those concerning the operation of the rhythm generator (through the VSCT and SRCP) and those concerning the current state of the peripheral motor apparatus (through the DSCT). It is on the basis of these signals that the activity of cerebellum and other brain centers, related with it, is organized. While studying rhythmic signals coming from the brain stem to the spinal cord through the reticulo-, vestibulo-, and rubro-spinal tracts, it was demonstrated that they are produced on the basis of a "generalized picture" of operation of the spinal generator(s) which is conveyed to the cerebellum through the VSCT and SRCP (Arshavsky et al., 1978a,b, 1983, 1984; Orlovsky, 1982a,b). In this connection a hypothesis has been advanced that while interacting with one another, each motor center considers only the essential data concerning the state of the other centers. The "essentiality" of data depends on the concrete motor and behavioral task (Arshavsky et al., 1983, 1984).

3 SYSTEMS FOR ACTIVATION OF SPINAL GENERATORS

3.1 Activation of the Generator for Scratching

The generator for scratching in intact animals comes into operation when a definite skin area is irritated. The receptive field in the dog covers the sides, neck, a part of the head and the proximal part of the forelimbs (Sherrington, 1906). In the cat, the area includes the neck, pinnas, and adjacent skin areas, as well as the proximal part of forelimbs (Sherrington, 1910b). Impulses from cutaneous afferents excite propriospinal neurons. These neurons have not been identified to date, but their existence has been established by various experimental facts. For example, if a number of pharmacological substances that affect synaptic transmission are applied to the spinal cord near the entrance of afferent neurons, it considerably facilitates the elicitation of the scratch reflex in decerebrate animals (Feldberg and Fleischhauer, 1960; Panchin and Skryma, 1978). Apparently, propriospinal neurons are under the inhibitory influences from higher brain centers, and elicitation of the scratch reflex is possible only when these influences are decreased.

By a method of partial transections of the spinal cord, the central pathway of the scratch reflex was traced to the lumbosacral enlargement where the generator of scratching is located (Deliagina, 1977). However, it remains unknown whether this pathway is formed by the axons of "primary" propriospinal neurons or whether there are relays within it. Existence of relays is indicated by the fact that, in the cat's thoracic cord, there are propriospinal neurons with long descending axons which are activated with pinna stimulation (Berkinblit et al., 1977). It was also found that, with stimulation of the receptive field of the scratch reflex, two kinds of signals come to the spinal generator of scratching; one of them is responsible mainly for the postural component of scratch movements, and the other, is for the switching-on of the rhythm generator. This finding suggests that the pathways of these two signals in the spinal cord coincide incompletely (Deliagina, 1977). Thus, for the scratch reflex, the existence of two command signals was demonstrated experimentally: commands f_1 and f_2 in our model (Fig. 7A) correspond to these signals.

3.2 Subthalamic and Mesencephalic Locomotor Regions

It was shown that electrical stimulation (30–60 pps) of certain regions in the brain elicits locomotion in animals which are not capable of stepping following administration of anesthesia or brain damage (Hinsey et al., 1930). One of these regions is located in the hypothalamus ("subthalamic locomotor region"; Waller, 1940), the other is in the midbrain ("mesencephalic locomotor region"; Shik et al., 1966, Fig. 10A). In chronic experiments, lesions of these regions produce different effects. After bilateral

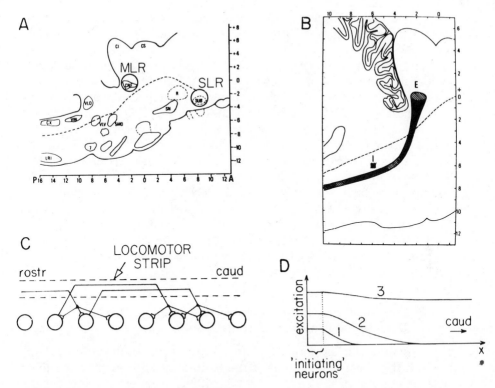

FIGURE 10. Locomotor regions of the brain stem and a scheme of the arrangement of the medullary locomotor column. (A) Subthalamic (SLR) and mesencephalic (MLR) locomotor regions are indicated by circles on a scheme of the parasagittal section of the brain stem. Abbreviations: 5MD, motor trigeminal nucleus, dorsal division; 7, facial nucleus; CI and CS, inferior and superior colliculi; CNF, cuneiform nucleus; CX, external cuneate nucleus; LRI, lateral reticular nucleus, internal division; R, red nucleus; SN, substantia nigra, SUB, subthalamic nucleus; VIN, inferior vestibular nucleus; VLD and VLV, lateral vestibular nucleus, dorsal and ventral division. (B) Pontomedullary locomotor strip (E) and midsagittal pontine inhibitory region (I) are shown on a scheme of the brain stem. (C) Scheme of interneuron connections in the medullary locomotor column. (D) Increasing of the strength and (or) frequency of locomotor strip stimulation (ordinate) is followed by increasing the distance of propagation of activity in rostrocaudal direction (abscissa).

lesion of the subthalamic locomotor region, the cat cannot walk spontaneously for 7–10 days, and neither nociceptive stimuli nor food evoke locomotion, although the animal responds by aggression to pain and eats food which it can reach without making a step. Nevertheless, stimulation of the mesencephalic locomotor region during this period elicits locomotion, and the animal walks or runs depending on strength of stimulation without bumping the walls of the room. It can also bypass or jump over obstacles (Sirota and Shik, 1973). However, a lesion of the mesencephalic region does not interfere essentially with motor activity and locomotion in the cat provided the subthalamic locomotor region is intact (Sirota and Shik, 1973).

These observations may be explained as follows. The subthalamic region elicits locomotion by projecting to spinal generators for stepping not directly, but through an intercalated center. The latter is located in the midbrain (mesencephalic locomotor region; Melnikova, 1977) and in the lower brain stem (see Section 3). Since the mesencephalic locomotor region is only a part of this system, its removal does not produce any dramatic effect. On the contrary, the subthalamic locomotor region is necessary for locomotion in chronic experiments because it can act through locomotor regions of the brain stem to generate the locomotor component of behavior. Tonic activity of the subthalamic region also allows the cereberal cortex to control more caudal locomotor regions through corticofugal fibers (Shik et al., 1968; Tower, 1936). Meanwhile, direct stimulation of the mesencephalic and more caudal locomotor regions can elicit locomotion even after decerebration caudal to the subthalamic region.

3.3 Pontomedullary Locomotor Strip and Stepping Strip in Dorsolateral Funiculus of Spinal Cord

The mesencephalic locomotor region is a rostral part of the strip passing through the lateral tegmentum of the brain stem and reaching the first cervical segment of the spinal cord (Fig. 10B). Points of this strip, when stimulated, elicit locomotion (Mori et al., 1977; Shik and Yagodnitsyn, 1977). The diameter of the strip is about 200 μm, i.e., it may consist of hundreds of axons. However the strip seems not to be a continuous tract: after electrolytic lesion of one site of the strip, one can elicit locomotion stimulating its other site or the mesencephalic locomotor region (Budakova and Shik, 1980). Somas of neurons sending axons in the strip are situated medial to it, in the lateral tegmentum of the lower brain stem (Fig. 10C). These cells, whose axons form the locomotor strip and which respond synaptically to a stimulus applied to the strip, were called the "locomotor column". Electrophysiological data suggest that passing some millimeters along the strip (usually in a caudal direction) axons leave the strip and form synapses (mainly excitatory) on other neurons of the column (Selionov and Shik 1981, 1983; Fig. 10C). Correspondingly, excitation of a certain portion of the system (by a single stimulus applied through the microelectrode introduced into the locomotor strip) is followed by activities of more caudal neurons (Fig. 10D, 1). By increasing the strength and frequency of repetitive stimulation one can observe oligo- or polysynaptic responses of more and more remote neurons. It was proposed that when the strength and frequency of stimulation is sufficient to evoke locomotion, the whole pontomedullary locomotor column becomes excited (Fig. 10D, 3). In other words, the column is capable of transmitting activity for

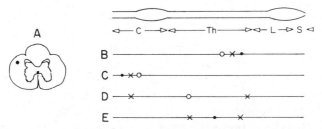

FIGURE 11. Stepping strip. (A) Location of the strip on the coronal section of the spinal cord. (B–E) Effects of lesion of the stepping points in the dorsolateral funiculus of the spinal cord. Stepping point destroyed by electrolytic coagulation is designated by cross (x). Stepping point which remained effective after destruction of other points(s) is shown by a circle (o), and the point which became ineffective is indicated by a point (.). Location of stepping points corresponds to the inset above B.

long distances, considerably exceeding the length of axons of neurons of the locomotor column (Shik, 1983). This polysynaptic pathway might be employed for activation of stepping generators. Indeed, polysynaptic responses to single stimuli applied to the medulary locomotor strip can be recorded in neurons of the C2–C3 spinal segments (Kazennikov et al., 1979). When the frequency of stimulation reaches 20–40 pps., the probability of the responses increases (Kazennikov et al., 1983b).

There is also a strip in the spinal cord similar, in some (but not all) respects, to the pontomeduallary one. Stimulation of a certain site in the dorsal part of the lateral funiculus (Fig. 11A) elicits stepping of the ipsilateral hindlimb in the cat (Kazennikov et al., 1983a; Roaf and Sherrington, 1910; Sherrington, 1910, 1931; Yamaguchi, 1981). Stepping can be evoked by stimulation of the appropriate points at levels from C2 to L2 (Kazennikov et al., 1983a). The stepping spinal strip, like the locomotor pontomedullary strip, is about 200 μm in diameter.

The stepping strip does not activate the hindlimb generator for stepping directly. This was proved in experiments with interruption of the strip (Kazennikov et al., 1983a; Fig. 11, B–E). After the lesion at the low thoracic level (B), stimulation of the strip caudal to the lesion became ineffective while stimulation rostral to the lesion produced stepping of the ipsilateral hindlimb as it did before coagulation. After the lesion at the cervical level (C), stimulation rostral to the lesion failed to elicit stepping while more caudal stimulation was effective. When interruptions were made at two sites (D,E), stimulation of the intermediate point evoked stepping provided the distance between the two lesioned sites was large (D), and became ineffective when the distance was small (less than 120 μm; E). Thus, stimulation remains effective in those cases when the length of uninterrupted strip (including the stimulation point) is great enough.

Currently, the origin of axons forming the stepping strip is unknown. However, it is known that the collaterals of the axons synapse with propriospinal neurons throughout the nerve axis. These propriospinal neurons, in their turn, send axons which descend outside the strip (in contrast to relations between the medullary strip and column) to the stepping generator of the hindlimb. To activate the generator for stepping, excitation of a great number of propriospinal neurons is necessary. When the propriospinal neurons are excited only within a short interval of the nerve axis, they can neither activate the generator nor excite propriospinal neurons in those sites which are protected from "direct" excitation by the interruption of the strip. Thus, although the pontomedullary and spinal columns (and, possibly, strips) are probably homologous structures, they clearly differ in the strength of excitatory interaction, the characteristic length of axons, and, perhaps, by some other features.

It is necessary to note that the stepping spinal strips are not necessary for elicitation of locomotion by stimulation of the mesencephalic locomotor region, since the stimulation was effective after interruption of both (left and right) strips at any level of the spinal cord (Kazennikov et al., 1983a).

3.4   Three Descending Systems

There are three putative activators for the spinal generators of stepping. One of them was considered in Section 3: the polysynaptic pathway of the bulbospinal column. The second candidate is the reticulospinal tract originating in the medial reticullar formation of the lower brain stem. Neurons of this tract become active during locomotion (Orlovsky, 1970) but not scratching (Pavlova, 1977) whereas activity of the vestibulo- and rubrospinal tracts is increased and cyclically modulated in both types of cyclical movements (Arshavsky et al., 1978a,b; Orlovsky, 1972 a,b). In addition, it was shown by partial transections of the spinal cord that activation of stepping generators is possible provided that ventrolateral funiculus (where the reticulospinal tract is located) is spared (Eidelberg, 1981, Eidelberg et al., 1981; Steeves and Jordan, 1980). However, one should keep in mind that this funiculus also contains axons belonging to other types of neurons, in particular, propriospinal neurons. There is also another objection against the crucial role of the reticulospinal tract in activation of the stepping generators. After the lesion of the gray matter at the level of C2–C3 segments, provided the length of destruction is more than 5–6 mm, it is impossible to evoke locomotion by stimulating the mesencephalic locomotor region, even though lateral and ventral spinal funiculi are intact (Kazennikov et al., 1980). This observation suggests that propriospinal neurons are of importance for the activation of stepping generators.

The third candidate is the monoaminergic descending system. Investigations of Lundberg and his colleagues (Jankowska et al., 1967a,b; Lundberg, 1981; and Viala and Buser, 1971), have shown that L-dopa and 5-hydroxytryptophan, especially together with monoaminoxidase inhibitors, evoke a "stepping state" in the spinal cord. It was suggested that these precursors imitate the activity of noradrenergic, serotoninergic, and also, possibly, dopaminergic neurons of the brain stem, respectively. It is known that descending axons of these neurons terminate in the spinal cord, and there are no monoaminergic cell bodies in the mammalian spinal cord. However, Steeves et al. (1980) have shown that after treatment with 6-hydroxydopamine which is followed by the almost total disappearance of noradrenaline from the spinal cord, the stimulation of the mesencephalic locomotor region remains effective in elicitation of locomotion. Evidently, the descending noradrenergic system is not necessary for evoking locomotion.

We believe that the effects of the three descending systems supply one another. Possibly, each of them is addressed to its own targets in the spinal cord and supplies locomotion with a certain "color" by changing, for example, the tonic component of stepping, or influencing different types of neurons in the stepping generator, or affecting those inhibitory neurons which tonically repress activity of the generator. In particular, the reticulospinal tract, by projecting monosynaptically to certain flexor motoneurons (Shapovalov, 1975), could enhance their excitability without interfering with the rhythm generator. The vestibulospinal tract could play a similar role in relation to extensor motoneurons (Orlovsky, 1972).

There are parts of the brain stem (the rostroventral portion of the midbrain, as well as dorsal and ventral midsagittal areas of the pons) which do not elicit locomotion themselves but influence, essentially, the possibility of its elicitation (Mori et al., 1977, 1982; Shik and Orlovsky, 1976). The corresponding descending pathways for these influences are not yet identified.

4   CONCLUSION

Investigation of the nervous system of vertebrates is difficult because a great number of neurons are active when the brain is solving any problems, including the task of controlling rhythmic limb movements. A common approach used by experimenters under such conditions is to ignore the fact that the number of involved neurons is large. Large populations of neurons with similar activity or with similar connections are implicitly substituted by a single element. This approach is often effective. For example, the efferent patterns of stepping and scratching can be described, as a first approximation, as the activity of "typical" motoneurons. The command tonic signal, activating the spinal generator of cyclic movements, can be represented by two parameters, although this command, in reality, is a flow of impulses in a great number of descending fibers, and the effect of this flow depends, for example, on the degree of synchronization between neurons, projecting to the common targets.

In this paper there are also some examples demonstrating that certain nervous mechanisms are explainable provided one takes into account a large number of neurons involved. One example is "the distributed rhythm generator": the definition itself means that the generator consists of many neurons, and this is its essential feature. Another example is the group of spinal neurons which are recruited in a proper order during the cycle (group 2 in Fig. 6A). A third example is a polysynaptic system of propagation of activity from the locomotor region of the brain stem to spinal stepping generators. Moreover, one can suggest that this propagation is only one of several operations which the fundamental arrangement of the vertebrate neuroaxis can produce, depending on some parameters (number of neurons, distribution of connections and of thresholds, etc.). Unfortunately, at this time we have neither the experimental methods for simultaneous recording of events in large populations of neurons nor a theoretical approach to their analysis.

REFERENCES

Arshavsky, Yu. I., I. N. Beloozerova, G. N. Orlovsky, Yu. V. Panchin, and G. A. Pavlova (1985a). Control of locomotion in marine mollusc *Clione limacina*. III. On the origin of locomotory rhythm. *Exp. Brain Res.*, **58**:272–289.

Arshavsky, Yu. I., I. N. Beloozerova, G. N. Orlovsky, Yu. V. Panchin, and G. A. Pavlova (1985b). Control of locomotion in marine mollusc *Clione limacina*. IV. Role of type 12 interneurons. *Exp. Brain Res.*, **58**:290–301.

Arshavsky, Yu. I., M. B. Berkinblit, O. I. Fukson, I. M. Gelfand, and G. N. Orlovsky (1972a). Recordings of neurons of the dorsal spinocerebellar tract during evoked locomotion. *Brain Res.*, **43**:272–275.

Arshavsky, Yu. I., M. B. Berkinblit, O. I. Fukson, I. M. Gelfand, and G. N. Orlovsky (1972b). Origin of modulation in neurons of the ventral spinocerebellar tract during evoked locomotion. *Brain Res.*, **43**:276–279.

Arshavsky, Yu. I., I. M. Gelfand, and G. N. Orlovsky (1983). The cerebellum and control of rhythmical movements. *Trends Neurosci.*, **6**:417–422.

Arshavsky, Yu. I., I. M. Gelfand, and G. N. Orlovsky (1984). *The Cerebellum and Control of Rhythmical Movements*, Nauka, Moscow, p. 165.

Arshavsky, Yu. I., I. M. Gelfand, G. N. Orlovsky, and G. A. Pavlova (1978a). Messages conveyed by spinocerebellar pathways during scratching in the cat. I. Activity of neurons of the lateral reticular nucleus. *Brain Res.*, **151**:479–491.

Arshavsky, Yu., I., I. M. Gelfand, G. N. Orlovsky, and G. A. Pavlova (1978b). Messages conveyed by spinocerebellar pathways during scratching in the cat. II. Activity of neurons of the ventral spinocerebellar tract. *Brain Res.*, **151**:493–506.

Arshavsky, Yu. I., I. M. Gelfand, G. N. Orlovsky, and G. A. Pavlova (1978c). Messages conveyed by descending tracts during scratching in the cat. I. Activity of vestibulospinal neurons. *Brain Res.*, **159**:99–110.

Arshavsky, Yu. I., G. N. Orlovsky, G. A. Pavlova, and C. Perret (1978). Messages conveyed by descending tracts during scratching in the cat. I. Activity of rubrospinal neurons. *Brain Res.*, **159**:111–123.

Arshavsky, Yu. I., I. M. Gelfand, G. N. Orlovsky, G. A. Pavlova, and L. B. Popova (1984). Origin of signals conveyed by the ventral spinocerebellar tract and spino-reticulo-cerebellar pathway. *Exp. Brain Res.*, **54**:426–431.

Bayev, K. V., A. M. Dekhtyarenko, T. V. Zavadskaya, and P. G. Kostyuk (1979). Activity of lumbar interneurons during fictitious locomotion of thalamic cats. *Neurophysiology (Kiev)*, **11**:329–338.

Bayev, K. V., A. M. Dekhtyarenko, T. V. Zavadskaya, and P. G. Kostyuk (1981). Activity of lumbosacral interneurons during fictitious scratching. *Neurophysiology (Kiev)*, **13**:57–66.

Berkinblit, M. B., T. G. Deliagina, A. G. Feldman, I. M. Gelfand, and G. N. Orlovsky (1978a). Generation of scratching. I. Activity of spinal interneurons during scratching. *J. Neurophysiol.*, **41**:1040–1057.

Berkinblit, M. B., T. G. Deliagina, A. G. Feldman, I. M. Gelfand, and G. N. Orlovsky (1978b). Generation of scratching. II. Nonregular regimes of generation. *J. Neurophysiol.*, **41**:1058–1068.

Berkinblit, M. B., T. G. Deliagina, G. N. Orlovsky, and A. G. Feldman (1977). Activity of propriospinal neurons during scratch reflex in the cat. *Neurophysiology (Kiev)*, **9**:504–511.

Brooks, V. B. (1983). Study of brain function by local, reversible cooling. *Rev. Physiol. Biochem. Pharmacol.*, **95**:1–109.

Brown, T. G. (1911). The intrinsic factors in the act of progression in the mammal. *Proc. Roy. Soc. Ser. B*, **84**:308–319.

Brown, T. G. (1914). On the nature of the fundamental activity of the nervous centres, together with an analysis of the conditioning of rhythmic activity in progression, and a theory of evolution of function in the nervous system. *J. Physiol. (London)*, **48**:18–46.

Budakova, N. N. and M. L. Shik (1980). Walking does not require continuity of the medullar "locomotor strip". *Bull. Exp. Biol. Med. (Moscow)*, **89**, No. 1:3–6.

Cohen, A. H. and P. Wallén (1980). The neuronal correlate of locomotion in fish: "Fictive swimming" induced in an in vitro preparation of the lamprey spinal cord. *Exp. Brain Res.* **41**: 11–18.

Deliagina, T. G. (1977). Central pathway of the scratch reflex in the cat. *Neurophysiology (Kiev)*, **9**:619–621.

Deliagina, T. G. and A. G. Feldman (1981). Activity of Renshaw cells during fictive scratch reflex in the cat. *Exp. Brain. Res.*, **42**:108–115.

Deliagina, T. G., A. G. Feldman, I. M. Gelfand, and G. N. Orlovsky (1975). On the role of central program and afferent inflow in the control of scratching movements in the cat. *Brain Res.*, **100**:297–313.

Deliagina, T. G. and G. N. Orlovsky (1980). Activity of Ia inhibitory interneurons during fictitious scratch reflex in the cat. *Brain Res.*, **193**:439–447.

Deliagina, T. G., G. N. Orlovsky, and G. A. Pavlova (1983). The capacity for generation of rhythmic oscillations is distributed in the lumbrosacral spinal cord of the cat. *Exp. Brain Res.*, **53**:81–90.

Droge, M. H. and R. B. Leonard (1983a). Swimming pattern in intact and decerebrated stingrays. *J. Neurophysiol.*, **50**:162–177.

Droge, M. H. and R. B. Leonard (1983b). Swimming rhythm in decerebrated paralyzed stingrays: normal and abnormal coupling. *J. Neurophysiol.*, **50**:178–191.

Dunin-Barkovsky, V. L. and V. S. Jacobson (1971). Analysis of transient processes and oscillations in net of "counting" neurons. *Biophysics (Moscow)*, **16**:1080–1084.

Duysens, J. and K. G. Pearson (1980). Inhibition of flexor burst generation by loading ankle extensor muscles in walking cats. *Brain Res.*, **187**:321–332.

Eidelberg, E. (1981). Consequences of spinal cord lesions upon motor function with special reference to locomotor activity. *Progr. Neurobiol.* **17**:185–202.

Eidelberg, E., J. L. Stiry, J. G. Walden, and B. L. Meyer (1981). Anatomical correlates of return of locomotor function after partial spinal cord lesions in cats. *Exp. Brain Res.*, **42**:81–88.

Engberg, I. and A. Lundberg (1969). An electromyographic analysis of muscular activity in the hindlimb of the cat during unrestrained locomotion. *Acta Physiol. Scand.* **75**:614–630.

Euler, C. von (1983). On the central pattern generator for the basic breathing rhythmicity. *J. Appl. Physiol. Respirat. Environ. Exercise Physiol.*, **55**:1647–1659.

Feldberg, W. and K. Fleischhauer (1960). Scratching movements evoked by drugs applied to the upper cervical cord. *J. Physiol. (London)*, **151**:502–517.

Feldman, A. G. and G. N. Orlovsky (1975). Activity of interneurons mediating reciprocal Ia inhibition during locomotion. *Brain Res.*, **84**:181–194.

Gambarian, P. P., G. N. Orlovsky, T. G. Protopopova, F. V. Severin, and M. L. Shik (1971). Muscular activity of different kinds of cat locomotion, and adjusting changes of the organs of movements in the family *Felidae*. *Proc. Zool. Inst. USSR*, **48**:220–239.

Gelfan, S. and A. F. Rapisarda (1964). Synaptic density of spinal neurons of normal dogs and dogs with experimental hindlimb rigidity. *J. Comp. Neurol.*, **123**:73–96.

Getting, P. A. (1983a). Mechanisms of pattern generation underlying swimming in *Tritonia*. II. Network reconstruction. *J. Neurophysiol.*, **49**:1017–1035.

Getting, P. A. (1983b). Mechanisms of pattern generation underlying swimming in *Tritonia*. III. Intrinsic and synaptic mechanisms for delayed excitation. *J. Neurophysiol.*, **49**:1036–1050.

Grillner, S. (1974). On the generation of locomotion in the spinal dogfish. *Exp. Brain Res.*, **20**:159–170.

Grillner, S. (1981). Control of locomotion in bipeds, tetrapods, and fish. In *Handbook of Physiology*, Sect. 1, v. II: *Motor Control*, V. B. Brooks, ed., Amer. Physiol. Soc., Bethesda, Maryland, pp. 1179–1236.

Grillner, S., A. McClellan, K. Sigvardt, P. Wallén, and T. Williams (1982). On the neural generation of "fictive locomotion" in a lower vertebrate nervous system, *in vitro*. In *Brain stem control of spinal mechanisms*, B. Sjölund and A. Björklund, eds. Elsevier Biomedical Press, pp. 273–295.

Grillner, S. and S. Rossignol (1978). On the initiation of the swing phase of locomotion in chronic spinal cats. *Brain Res.*, **146**:269–277.

Hinsey, J. C., S. W. Ranson, and R. F. McNattin (1930). The role of the hypothalamus and mesencephalon in locomotion. *Arch. Neurol. Psych.*, **23**:1–43.

Jankowska, E., M. Jukes, S. Lund, and A. Lundberg (1967a). The effect of L-dopa on the spinal cord. 5. Reciprocal organization of pathways transmitting excitatory action to alpha-motoneurons of flexors and extensors. *Acta Physiol. Scand.*, **70**:369–388.

Jankowska, E., M. Jukes, S. Lund, and A. Lundberg (1967b). The effect of L-dopa on the spinal cord. 6. Half-centre organization of interneurones transmitting effects from the flexor reflex afferents. *Acta Physiol. Scand.*, **70**:389–402.

Jordan, L. M., C. A. Pratt, and J. E. Menzies (1981). Intraspinal mechanisms for the control of locomotion. *Adv. Physiol. Sci.*, **1**:183–185.

Kazennikov, O. V., V. A. Selionov, M. L. Shik, and G. V. Yakovleva (1979). Neurons of upper cervical segments responding to stimulation of the bulbar "locomotor strip". *Neurophysiology (Kiev)*, **11**:245–253.

Kazennikov, O. V., M. L. Shik, and G. V. Yakovleva (1980). Two pathways for the brain stem "locomotor influence" on the spinal cord. *Sechenov Physiol. J. (Leningrad)*, **66**:1260–1263.

Kazennikov, O. V., M. L. Shik, and G. V. Yakovleva (1983a). Stepping movements elicited by stimulation of the dorsolateral funiculus in the cat spinal cord. *Bull. Exp. Biol. Med. (Moscow)*, **96**, No. 8:8–10.

Kazennikov, O. V., M. L. Shik, and G. V. Yakovleva (1983b). Responses of neurons of upper spinal cervical segments in cat to stimulation of brain stem locomotor region with different frequencies. *Neurophysiology (Kiev)*, **15**:355–361.

Kazennikov, O. V., M. L. Shik, and G. V. Yakovleva (1985). Synaptic responses of propriospinal neurons to stimulation of the stepping strip in the dorsolateral funiculus. *Neurophysiology (Kiev)*, **17**:281–289.

Lennard, P. R. and P. S. G. Stein (1977). Swimming movements elicited by electrical stimulation of turtle spinal cord. 1. Low-spinal and intact preparations. *J. Neurophysiol.*, **40**:768–778.

Leonard, R. B., P. Rudomin, M. H. Droge, A. E. Grossman, and W. D. Willis (1979). Locomotion in the decerebrate stingray. *Neurosci. Lett.*, **14**:315–319.

Lundberg, A. (1969). Convergence of excitatory and inhibitory action on interneurones in the spinal cord. In *The Interneuron*, M. A. B. Brazier, ed. University California Press, Los Angeles, pp. 231–265.

Lundberg, A. (1971). Function of the ventral spinocerebellar tract—a new hypothesis. *Exp. Brain Res.*, **12**:317–330.

Lundberg, A. (1981). Half-centres revisited. *Adv. Physiol. Sci.*, **1**:155–167.

Melnikova, Z. L. (1977). Study of relations between subthalamic and midbrain "locomotor regions" in rats. *Neurophysiol. (Kiev)*, **9**:275–280.

Mori, S., K. Kawahara, T. Sakamoto, M. Aoki, and T. Tomiyama (1982). Setting and resetting of level of postural muscle tone in decerebrate cat by stimulation of brain stem. *J. Neurosphysiol.*, **48**:737–748.

Mori, S., M. L. Shik, and A. S. Yagodnitsyn (1977). Role of pontine tegmentum for locomotor control in mesencephalic cat. *J. Neurophysiol.*, **40**:284–295.

Orlovsky, G. N. (1970). Work of the reticulospinal neurons during locomotion. *Biophysics*, **15**:728–737.

Orlovsky, G. N. (1972a). The effect of different descending systems on flexor and extensor activity during locomotion. *Brain Res.*, **40**:359–371.

Orlovsky, G. N. (1972b). Activity of vestibulospinal neurons during locomotion. *Brain Res.*, **46**:85–98.

Orlovsky, G. N. (1972c). Activity of rubrospinal neurons during locomotion. *Brain Res.*, **46**:99–112.

Orlovsky, G. N. and A. G. Feldman (1972). Classification of lumbosacral neurons according to their discharge patterns during evoked locomotion. *Neurophysiology (Kiev)*, **4**:410–417.

Panchin, Yu. V. and R. N. Skryma (1978). Scratch reflex evoked by strychnine application to the spinal cord. *Neurophysiology*, **10**:622–624.

Pavlova, G. A. (1977). Activity of the reticulospinal neurons during scratch-reflex. *Biophysics*, **22**:740–742.

Pearson, K. G. (1976). The control of walking. *Sci. Amer.*, **235**, No. 6:72–86.

Pearson, K. G. and J. Duysens (1976). Function of segmental reflexes in the control of stepping in cockroaches and cats. In *Neural Control of Locomotion*, R. M. Herman, S. Grillner, P. S. G. Stein, and D. G. Stuart, eds. Plenum Press, New York, pp. 519–537.

Perret, C. (1983). Centrally generated pattern of motoneuron activity during locomotion in the cat. In *Neural origin of rhythmic movements*, A. Roberts and B. Roberts, eds. Soc. Exp. Biol. Symp., vol. 37, pp. 405–422.

Perret, C. and J. M. Cabelguen (1980). Main characteristics of the hindlimb locomotor cycle in the decorticate cat with special reference to bifunctional muscle. *Brain Res.*, **187**:333–352.

Rashevsky, N. (1972). Neural circuit which exhibits some features of epileptic attacks. *Bull. Math. Biophys.*, **34**:71–78.

Roaf, H. E. and C. S. Sherrington (1910). Further remarks on the spinal mammalian preparation. *Quart. J. Physiol.*, **3**:209–211.

Roberts, A., J. A. Kahn, S. R. Soffe, and J. D. W. Clarke (1981). Neural control of swimming in a vertebrate. *Science*, **213**:1032–1034.

Selionov, V. A. and M. L. Shik (1981). Responses of medullary neurons to microstimulation of the "locomotor strip" in cat. *Neurophysiology (Kiev)*, **13**:275–282.

Selionov, V. A. and M. L. Shik (1983). Synaptic responses of neurons of the lateral medullary reticular formation in cats to stimulation of the "locomotor strip". *Neurophysiology (Kiev)*, **15**:195–197.

Selionov, V. A. and M. L. Shik (1984). Medullary locomotor strip and column in the cat. *Neuroscience* **13**:1267–1278.

Shapovalov, A. I. (1975). Neuronal organization and synaptic mechanisms of supraspinal control in vertebrates. *Rev. Physiol. Biochem. Pharmacol.*, **72**:1–54.

Sherrington, C. S. (1906). Observations on the scratch-reflex in the spinal dog. *J. Physiol. (Lond.)*, **34**:1–50.

Sherrington, C. S. (1910a). Flexion reflex of the limb, crossed extension reflex, and reflex stepping and standing. *J. Physiol. (Lond.)*, **40**:28–121.

Sherrington, C. S. (1910b). Notes on the scratch-reflex of the cat. *Quart. J. Exp. Physiol.*, **3**:213–220.

Sherrington, C. S. (1931). Quantitative management of contraction in lowest level coordination. *Brain*, **54**:1–28.

Shik, M. L. (1983). Action of the brain stem locomotor region on spinal stepping generators via propriospinal pathways. In *Spinal Cord Reconstruction*, C. C. Kao, R. P. Bunge, and P. J. Reier, eds. Raven Press, New York, pp. 421–434.

Shik, M. L. (1985). Locomotor region of the brain stem and hypothesis on "the locomotor column." *Uspechi fiziol. nauk*, **16**:76–95 (in Russian).

Shik, M. L. and G. N. Orlovsky (1965). Co-ordination of the limbs during running of the dog. *Biophysics* **10**:1037–1047.

Shik, M. L. and G. N. Orlovsky (1976). Neurophysiology of locomotor automatism. *Physiol. Rev.*, **56**:465–501.

Shik, M. L., G. N. Orlovsky, and F. V. Severin (1968). Locomotion of the mesencephalic cat elicited by stimulation of the pyramids. *Biophysics*, **13**:127–135.

Shik, M. L., F. V. Severin, and G. N. Orlovsky (1966). Control of walking and running by means of electrical stimulation of the midbrain. *Biophysics*, **11**:659–666.

Shik, M. L. and A. S. Yagodnitsyn (1977). The pontobulbar "locomotor strip". *Neurophysiology (Kiev)*, **9**:95–97.

Sirota, M. G. and M. L. Shik (1973). The cat locomotion elicited through the electrode implanted in the midbrain. *Sechenov Physiol. J. (Leningrad)*, **59**:1314–1321.

Steeves, J. D. and L. M. Jordan (1980). Localization of a descending pathway in the spinal cord which is necessary for controlled treadmill locomotion. *Neurosci. Lett.*, **20**:283–288.

Steeves, J. D., B. J. Schmidt, B. J. Skovgaard, and L. M. Jordan (1980). Effect of noradrenaline and 5-hydroxytryptamine depletion on locomotion in the cat. *Brain Res.*, **185**:349–362.

Stehouwer, D. J., and P. B. Farel (1983). Development of hindlimb locomotor activity in the Bullfrog (*Rana catesbeiana*) studied in vitro. *Science*, **219**:516–518.

Stein, P. S. G. (1978). Swimming movements elicited by electrical stimulation of the turtle spinal cord: the high spinal preparation. *J. Comp. Physiol.*, **124**:203–210.

Tower, S. S. (1936). Extrapyramidal action from the cat's cerebral cortex: motor and inhibitory. *Brain*, **59**:408–444.

Viala, D. and P. Buser (1971). Modalité's d'obtention de rythmes locomoteurs chez le lapin spinal par traitments pharmacologiques (L-dopa, 5-HTP, d-amphetamine). *Brain Res.*, **35**:151–165.

Waller, W. H. (1940). Progression movements elicited by subthalamic stimulation. *J. Neurophysiol.*, **3**:300–307.

Wilson, D. M. and J. Waldron (1968). Models for generation of the motor output in flying locusts. *Proc. IEEE*, **56**:1058–1064.

Yamaguchi, T. (1981). Fictive stepping evoked by electrical stimulation of the white matter of the cervical cord in decerebrate cats. *J. Physiol. Soc. Jpn.*, **43**:303, Abstract. No. 108.

Chapter Seven

THE ROLE OF SENSORY INPUTS IN REGULATING PATTERNS OF RHYTHMICAL MOVEMENTS IN HIGHER VERTEBRATES

A Comparison Between Locomotion, Respiration, and Mastication

SERGE ROSSIGNOL*
JAMES P. LUND†
TREVOR DREW*

Center for Research in the Neurological Sciences
**Department of Physiology, Faculty of Medicine*
†Department of Stomatology, Faculty of Dental Medicine
University of Montreal
Montreal, Quebec, Canada

GENERAL INTRODUCTION

This chapter is devoted to the role of sensory feedback in the regulation of three centrally generated rhythmic movements in higher mammals, namely locomotion, respiration, and mastication. The reader is referred to the chapter by Grillner et al. (this volume) for a review of the mechanisms in lower vertebrates.

Different approaches can be taken to study the role of afferent feedback and this review has been subdivided according to the three methods most generally used: first, the recording of the discharge of the primary afferents themselves during movement; second, the removal of the afferent feedback either through deafferentation (or more specific procedures) and paralysis; and, third, the stimulation of the afferents themselves.

Following the description of different reflex mechanisms in the three systems, we have attempted to generalize some of the mechanisms by which the afferent feedback may interact with centrally patterned movements so that they are best adapted to the demands and the real circumstances in which they are performed.

1   ACTIVITY OF AFFERENTS

If one is to understand the role that sensory inputs play in the control of rhythmical movements, the first requirement is a knowledge of their patterns of afferent activity during the movements. As will be shown, there are three basic patterns of afferent activity: (1) continuous activity that is

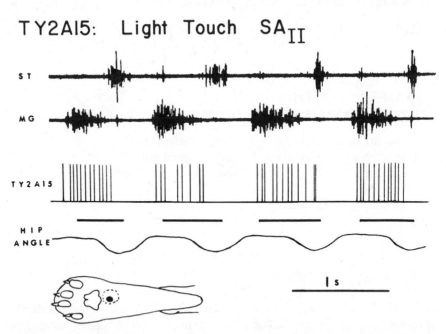

FIGURE 1. Activity of a slowly adapting, cutaneous mechanoreceptor recorded during walking in an intact cat together with EMGs from semitendinosus (ST) and medial gastrocnemius (MG). Ty2A15, Output pulses from window discriminator. Black bars signal foot contact. The dotted line around the receptive field indicates the approximate area of skin stretch sensitivity (From Loeb, 1981).

unrelated or weakly related to the phase of movement; (2) rhythmical activity that waxes and wanes in phase with the cycle of movement; and (3) receptors that fire only occasionally. In this section, we will summarize studies of the behavior of spinal and cranial primary afferent neurons during locomotion, respiration, and mastication, and from this we will make some suggestions about what parts they can and cannot play in the control system.

1.1 Epithelial Receptors

1.1.1 Locomotion

Although many cutaneous afferents have been recorded during locomotion in chronic cats (Loeb, 1981, mentions having studied more than 200), there are few descriptions of their patterns of activity, due most probably to the fact that they behave as expected by the observer, and that most low threshold mechanoreceptors are stimulated by contact with their receptive fields. Thus, receptors on the toes or footpads are phasically active during stance (Fig. 1). However, some fire during locomotion even though their fields are not touched, particularly those located on or near folds of skin that open and close during movement (Loeb, 1981). Some hair receptors fire two bursts per cycle (Loeb et al., 1977). Unfortunately, there has been no attempt to correlate the discharge frequency of primary afferents to the parameters of movement in locomotion.

1.1.2 Respiration

There is almost no data on the patterns of activity of hair and skin receptors of the chest wall. In his study of respiratory cutaneous reflexes, Sumi (1963) reported that one touch unit "was so sensitive that it exhibited intermittent trains of spontaneous discharges, presumably produced by slight movement of the skin of the thoracic area during respiration." We presume that no other touch fibers, hair, or pressure-sensitive receptors were rhythmically active. However, it is premature to conclude that cutaneous afferents provide no significant information during normal respiration, because an extensive laminectomy had been done by Sumi to record from the dorsal roots. In addition, trigeminal sensory neurons that receive inputs from cutaneous receptors with fields around the nares fire in phase with respiration (Olsson and Lund, unpublished observations).

The richly innervated larynx is a critical point in the airway. Among its receptors (which are the source of a number of reflexes), many are rhythmically active in eupneic, or normal, breathing (Sant'Ambrogio et al., 1983). These authors divided the primary afferents recorded from the recurrent laryngeal nerve into three groups: pressure, flow, and drive. A common feature of the response patterns was that the greatest firing frequency usually occurred in inspiration. Flow receptors appear to be mucosal, while drive receptors probably include proprioceptors in the ligaments and joints that are activated by contraction and movements during eupnea (Martensson, 1963).

1.1.3 Mastication

The behavior of skin and hair follicle receptors has been described for anesthetized rabbits that chewed either when a stiff rubber tube was put in the mouth, or in response to stimulation of the motor cortex (Appenteng et al., 1982a; Lund et al., 1982). In those experiments, the discharge patterns of the primary afferent neurons were recorded from the mandibular division of the trigeminal ganglion. All of the *hair afferents* studied were rapidly adapting, whereas approximately equal numbers of rapidly and slowly adapting skin afferents were found. The stretching and relaxing of the skin during movement was enough to excite 60% of hair afferents. These were distributed over the whole of the lower face, although the most active were located close to the corner of the mouth. The firing frequency of the hair afferents was linearly related to the velocity of movement in all directions, so that when the jaw was opened and closed by hand in one plane, there were two bursts of activity, corresponding to the velocity peaks. During mastication, the frequency of firing was proportional to the velocity of the movement vector (Fig. 2D) and was highest during early jaw closure (Fig. 2B).

Only a few *skin afferents* (8/80) were active, and all of them had receptive fields close to the corner of the mouth, where the greatest stretching of the skin occurs during movement. Most of the skin receptors discharged only in the closing phase (Fig. 2A), but only one had a firing frequency related to a parameter of movement (Fig. 2C). The firing pattern of skin receptors, but not hair receptors, seemed to be easily changed by moving the rubber tube into and out of the cheek behind their receptive fields. Skin and hair afferents with receptive fields on the lower lip, that were inactive during rhythmical movements with the mouth empty, would fire during the closing phase if the lips contacted the rubber tube.

The behavior of primary afferents innervating the *oral mucosa* is similar to those from the skin: none of them appear to respond during mastication unless their receptive fields are touched (Appenteng et al., 1982b). No afferents were tonically active; they usually began to fire during closure and, for the majority that were rapidly adapting, the burst was of short duration, although the firing of some slowly adapting receptors continued into early opening. There was no correlation between the firing frequency of these neurons and displacement or velocity. Those receptors that discharged during movements made with an empty mouth fired more readily during chewing on the tube. Others that were silent could be made to fire bursts by putting the tube in the area of their receptive field.

In summary, the data gathered during mastication show that many hair

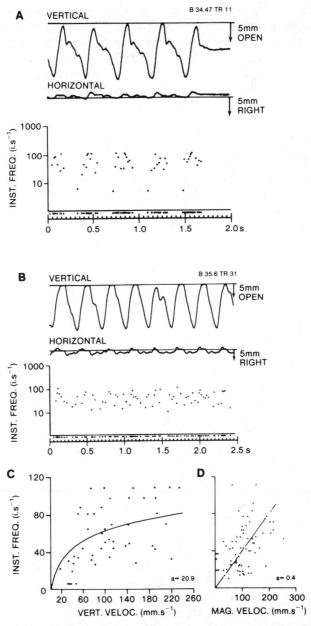

FIGURE 2. Activity of skin (A) and hair (B) afferents during mastication. Both units had rapidly adapting receptive fields just behind the corner of the mouth. The skin afferent fired strongly during jaw closure and its instantaneous firing frequency was weakly correlated with the vertical velocity during the burst (C). The hair afferent fired continuously during the movements. Maximum frequency occurred during jaw closure and firing rate was proportional to the velocity of the movement vector (D).

205

afferents are continuously active during movements. In addition, their firing frequency, as well as that of a small population of skin afferents, is proportional to the velocity of movement, and, like cutaneous receptors in the hand (Gandevia and McCloskey, 1976), could play a part in kinesthesia. However, most skin and all mucosal afferents signal pressure on their receptive fields caused either by contact with an object or by distention.

1.2 Muscle Spindle Afferents

Unlike the limbs, muscle receptors are unequally distributed between the main antagonist muscle groups in the masticatory and respiratory systems. The diaphragm and the muscles that open the jaw contain few spindles or tendon organs (Kubota et al., 1974; Dubner et al., 1978), although they are numerous in the major jaw closing (Kubota et al., 1974; Lund et al., 1978) and intercostal muscles (Jung-Caillol and Duron, 1976). The lack of receptors in certain muscles is probably related to a lack of need for postural activity (Euler, 1970) and for a significant load-compensating reflex (Corda et al., 1965; Lamarre and Lund, 1975).

1.2.1 Locomotion

Spindle afferents from the hindlimb muscles were first recorded during locomotion by Severin et al. (1967). They recorded from dorsal root filaments innervating flexors and extensors of the ankle of mesencephalic cats that walked on a treadmill during stimulation of the MLR. Local electrical stimulation of the muscle in which the receptor was thought to lie was used to distinguish between spindle afferents and tendon organs, but there was no attempt to subdivide the primary and secondary afferents. The pattern of activity of the spindle receptors is simply described—they were most active during contraction of the muscle of origin. These results favor the hypothesis that there is strong fusimotor activity during the alpha motoneuron burst.

Fusimotor Activity. This was confirmed by Perret (1976), who recorded from fusimotor neurons of decorticate cats during spontaneous locomotion. Furthermore, Sjostrom and Zangger (1975, 1976) and Perret (1976) showed that a strong alpha-gamma linkage is part of the rhythmic pattern generated in the spinal cord by L-dopa, clonidine or dorsal root stimulation, and that it results in strong bursts of firing in extensor and flexor primary afferents.

Although all reports agree that muscles spindles contract during the EMG burst of the extrafusal fibers, the pattern of firing recorded from primary and secondary afferents in awake cats cannot usually be accounted for by the simple coactivation model that was first suggested. This prompted Murphy et al. (1984) to examine the differences between static and dynamic fusimotor input to a hindlimb ankle extensor, triceps surae.

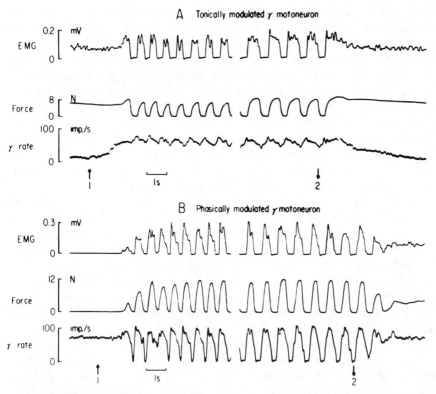

FIGURE 3. Firing patterns of tonically (A) and phasically (B) modulated medial gastrocnemius fusimotor neurons recorded during walking in decerebrate cat. Force and EMG, integrated activity and tension of soleus muscle. Arrows, onset and offset of treadmill. (From Murphy et al., 1984.)

Working in the premamillary cat, they dissected axons from the muscle nerves of a fixed, partially denervated leg, identified the fusimotor neurons, measured their conduction velocity and recorded their activity while the other limbs walked on a treadmill. In complementary experiments, fusimotor axons were stimulated, and the effects on spindle afferents were used to classify the dynamic and static fusimotor populations. They found that dynamic fusimotor neurons had a high rate of discharge at rest that was deeply modulated during locomotion, with peak firing occurring during the EMG burst (Fig. 3A). In contrast, the tonic activity of static fusimotor neurons was low at rest, rose at the start of locomotion, but was only slightly modulated in phase with the cycle (Fig. 3B).

Spindle Afferent Sensitivity to Stretch. These results explain many of the features of the responses of spindle afferents of hindlimb ankle extensors to stretch that were reported by Perret and Berthoz (1973) and Cabelguen (1981). The responses were recorded in a preparation similar to the one used by Murphy et al. (1984), except that the distal tendons of extensor and flexor muscles of the ankle were cut and connected to a stretcher, so that ramp and sinusoidal length changes could be applied. The static sensitivity of the extensor spindles was low when the muscles were at rest (no static drive). It rose at the start of locomotion (start of tonic static activity), but the sensitivity of secondary endings, which are innervated only by static fusimotor neurons (Appelberg et al., 1966), rose little during the EMG burst. On the other hand, the dynamic sensitivity of the primary endings was high before movement (tonic dynamic drive), low during the flexion phase of locomotion and very high during the muscle contraction, when the phasic dynamic sensitivity is highest (Fig. 3B). These results have recently been confirmed by Taylor et al. (1985).

However, we cannot assume that the pattern of fusimotor organization described for the hindlimb ankle extensor muscles applies elsewhere, not even to other muscles acting about the same joint, because Perret and Berthoz (1973) and Cabelguen (1981) showed that, although the stretch response of pure ankle extensor receptors was dominated by dynamic fusimotor action, static action was strongest in flexors. Loeb (1984) suggests that it is the dynamic gammas that are tonically active in flexor muscles, and that the static fusimotor neurons fire during the muscle burst. Furthermore, bifunctional muscles, such as semitendinosus, seemed to receive a balance of static and dynamic drive.

When the fusimotor fibers of knee extensor and biarticular muscles are blocked with lidocaine during walking, the firing rate of primary and secondary afferents falls during extrafusal contraction and during lengthening, adding to the evidence that some fusimotor neurons are active at all phases of the locomotor cycle (Loeb and Hoffer, 1985).

Spindle Afferent Activity. Muscle spindle afferents have been recorded from dorsal root filaments of decorticate cats, and from the dorsal roots or ganglia of awake cats through implanted microwires. Indwelling cuff electrodes around muscle nerves, length gauges, and strain gauges on muscle tendons are usually used as aides in the interpretation of the complex patterns of spindle activity that occur. It has also been possible to classify primary and secondary spindle afferents by comparing either their conduction velocities (Loeb and Duysens, 1979), or their response to vibration and their sensitivity to passive stretch before and after injections of succinylcholine (Prochazka et al., 1976).

The first studies of the hindlimb of the intact cat described the behavior of primary afferents (Prochazka et al., 1976, 1977). They reported that ankle extensor (triceps surae) spindle primaries were most active during the passive stretch that occurs in the F phase of the swing (Fig. 4A). There was often a pause in firing just after the onset of the EMG burst in E_1, after which firing resumed during muscle contraction, presumably in response to a fusimotor input. More recently, Prochazka (1980) reported that the firing frequency of some ankle extensor primary afferents was greater dur-

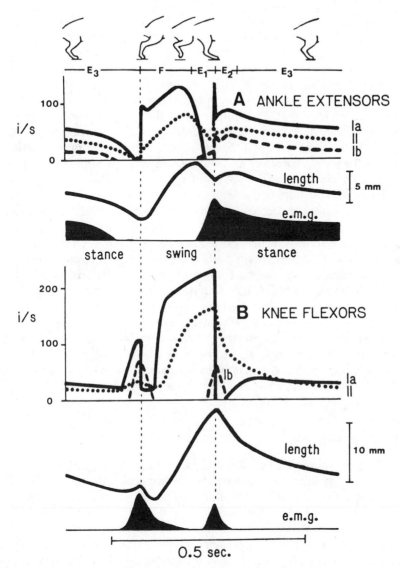

FIGURE 4. Diagram showing average patterns of activity of primary (Ia), secondary (II) and tendon organ (Ib) afferents from ankle extensors (A) and knee flexor (B) muscles. Muscle length and EMG activity are shown for comparison. The average step cycle is shown at the top. (Figure provided by A. Prochazka.)

ing the slow lengthening contraction in E_2 than during the F phase or during manual stretch of the muscle when the cat was anesthetized. This is the pattern predicted by the fusimotor studies (Loeb, 1984). Knee flexor primaries are most active at the end of F and during E_1, again, in the phases during which the parent muscle is stretched (Fig. 4B).

Loeb and his colleagues [Loeb and Duysens (1979), Loeb (1981), and

Loeb and Hoffer (1981), Loeb et al., (1985)] agree that the pattern of firing of spindle primary afferents of ankle and knee extensor muscles is dominated by their sensitivity to stretch, but found that functional flexor spindle primaries fire more strongly during contraction than has been reported by Prochazka (Fig. 4B). They suggest that these receptors are powerfully driven by gamma static motoneurons during rapid extrafusal contraction (Loeb, 1984). The spindle primaries of bifunctional muscles respond in a mixed way to stretch and there is a lot of variability in the population (Loeb et al., 1985). Spindle secondaries of all muscles studied appear to be length-sensitive and show small increases in firing frequency during active shortening (Fig. 4A and B).

The period of activity of forelimbs spindle afferents from a flexor (biceps brachii), and extensor (triceps brachii) and two bifunctional muscles (subscapularis and teres major) coincided with that of the parent muscle. This included two bursts of firing of the bifunctional groups (Cabelguen et al., 1984). Another finding that supports the existence of a strong coupling of fusimotor output to the alpha command was the relationship of spindle firing frequency to EMG burst amplitude. In contrast to the hindlimb, there was no evidence that the balance of static and dynamic fusimotor drive was different in the three muscle groups. Cabelguen et al. (1984) found, as did Perret and Berthoz (1973) and Taylor et al. (1981), that spindle afferents sometimes fire in rhythmical bursts without any apparent extrafusal contraction. This has been interpreted as evidence that the fusimotor neurons are more sensitive to the central command than alpha motoneurons (Perret, 1976).

1.2.2 Respiration

Fusimotor Activity. The external intercostals are active during inspiration, together with the diaphragm and levator costae muscles, while their antagonists, the internal intercostals, act in expiration. Sears (1964) recorded from axons in nerve filaments to these muscles of anesthetized cats, and found that the firing frequency of fusimotor neurons was strongly modulated by the respiratory rhythm. Inspiratory and expiratory fusimotor neurons fired reciprocally and in-phase with their corresponding alpha motoneurons. Many were recruited earlier than alpha motoneurons and fired at higher frequency. Eklund et al. (1964), using a similar preparation, confirmed the existence of rhythmic fusimotor neurons, and found a second population that fired tonically throughout the cycle. The blockage of gamma fibers with lidocaine almost abolished inspiratory afferent activity (Critchlow and Euler, 1963, Fig. 5). As in the hindlimb (Loeb and Hoffer, 1985), the response to stretch also fell, most probably due to the removal of tonic gamma activity.

As elsewhere in the body, the fusimotor neurons can be reflexly excited by scratching the skin of the thoracic wall and twisting the ear, and they

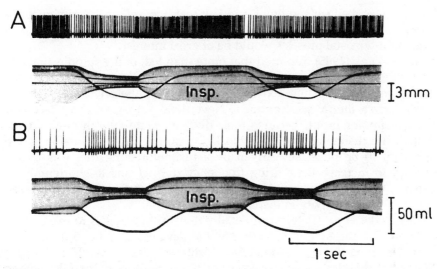

FIGURE 5. Discharge of a muscle spindle afferent from the intercostal muscles before (A) and 3.2 min after (B) the application of lignocaine to the intercostal nerve. The shaded record represents the intercostal width and the single trace is a measure of tidal volume. (From Critchlow and von Euler, 1962.)

are sensitive to succinylcholine. A comparison of the two groups showed that the tonic group are the more responsive to proprioceptive, spinal, and supraspinal inputs (Corda et al., 1966). An examination of spindle activity under tonic stretch and vibration led to the conclusion that the tonic group contains both static and dynamic fusimotor neurons (Corda et al., 1966); likewise, Euler and Peretti (1966) found that rhythmic gamma activation of the external intercostal spindles is performed by both groups.

Spindle Afferent Activity. In the earliest study of muscle spindle afferents, Siebens and Puletti (1961) showed that the muscles of the chest wall contained receptors that were excited by inspiration or expiration. However, there are indications that the two groups are not controlled as a simple reciprocal pair. Twenty of the 22 inspiratory spindles recorded by Critchlow and Euler (1963) discharged at the highest rate during inspiration. This was taken as evidence that there was strong fusimotor drive during the extrafusal contraction (Fig. 5). In contrast, the alpha-linked rhythmic gamma effects on expiratory spindles seems to be weak, because only three of nine expiratory units were most active during the burst. The same may pertain to their agonists, the levator costae muscles. Hilaire et al. (1983) recorded from the spindle afferents of an unclassified type from these muscles. They were silent in early inspiration when the receptors were presumably unloaded. They began to fire late in the EMG burst and were most active in expiration. In view of the different patterns of spindle activity described for the limbs and jaw that may reflect fundamental differences in fusimotor control, more comparative data on the internal and external intercostal muscles would be of great interest.

Corda et al. (1965), reported that more than half of the spindle afferents from the few spindles that are in the diaphragm behave in a passive way during respiration. Their activity is decreased or abolished during inspiration, when the muscle contracts. Nevertheless, they probably receive a tonic fusimotor input, because their discharge rate falls throughout the cycle if the fusimotor fibers are blocked with lidocaine. A smaller group appeared to be phasically driven by a fusimotor burst that was strong enough to increase their firing frequency during muscle shortening. In general, increasing the respiratory load by blocking the trachea increased spindle afferent activity in inspiration.

Prochazka et al. (1979) formulated a general hypothesis to explain the patterns of firing of spindle afferents that have been recorded in mastication, locomotion, respiration, and voluntary movements. They suggest that when muscles shorten or lengthen at a rate of more than 0.2 resting lengths per second, the firing pattern of the spindle afferents is dominated by the length changes. Fusimotor action is a major determinant at slower velocities. It is evident that the cut-off velocity can only be an approximation that varies to some extent with the level of fusimotor drive and between some muscle groups e.g., hindlimb flexors and extensors.

1.2.3 Mastication

The unique location of the cell bodies of the spindle primary and secondary afferents in the trigeminal mesencephalic nucleus, (Jerge, 1963; Cody et al., 1975) has allowed their activity to be recorded during movements with relative ease through implanted chambers. Such experiments have been performed on monkeys during isometric biting (Lund et al., 1979; Larson et al., 1981a and b), voluntary tracking (Larson et al., 1983), mastication (Matsunami and Kubota, 1972; Goodwin and Luschei, 1975;) and on cats that were eating and lapping (Taylor, and Cody, 1974; Cody et al., 1975; Taylor et al., 1981; Gottlieb and Taylor, 1983).

Lund et al. (1979) described the activity patterns of a small number of spindle afferents and fusimotor neurons. Fusimotor neurons began to fire 200–300 ms before the beginning of isometric biting was sensed by the force transducer (Fig. 6A), but the spindle afferents increased their firing frequency much later (Fig. 6B). The spindle afferents reached firing frequencies of up to 300 impulses per second early in the task and maintained this level of activity until the monkey began to release the bar, whereafter the frequency increased again as the jaw opened (Fig. 6C and 6D). However, there was little or no relationship between the rate of firing and the biting force. During the series of rhythmical movements that were subsequently made to lick the fruit juice off the dispensing tube, the spindle

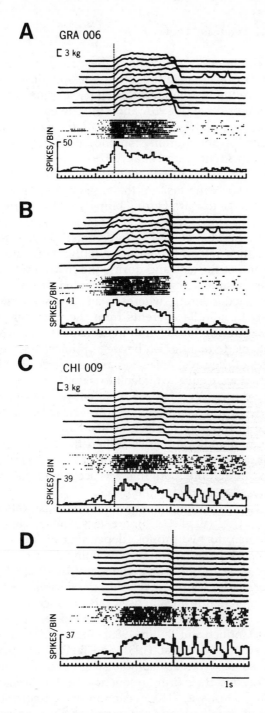

FIGURE 6. Comparison of masseteric fusimotor neuron (A and B) and spindle afferent firing (C and D) during biting on a strain gauge. Force records, rasters, and histograms (bin width 50 ms) are aligned at force onset (A and C) and offset (B and D). The activity that follows the offset coincides with the rhythmic ingestive movements that follow the fruit juice reward that sometimes produced small force changes. (From Lund et al., 1979.)

afferents fired rhythmically, with the highest frequency occurring in the opening phase. However, as in the biting, the spindle afferent activity increased well above the resting level during jaw closure, due, no doubt, to the phasic fusimotor drive (Fig. 6A and 6B). The coupling between alpha and gamma motoneurons seemed to change during the switch to rhythmical movements, because gamma motoneuron output per unit of biting force dropped at this time (Lund et al., 1979).

Larson et al. (1981a and b) subdivided the spindle afferents that they recorded in a similar biting task on the basis of their sensitivity to sinusoidal displacements of the jaw. During biting and during rhythmical ingestive movements, neurons classified as primary afferents behaved in the way described by Lund et al. (1979). In contrast, the low sensitivity units did not increase their rate of firing during biting, but were excited by jaw opening at the end of the task and during the rhythmical movements. On the basis of these results, Larson et al. concluded that dynamic fusimotor neurons are activated in biting, whereas static fusimotor neurons are not.

In their study of spindle afferents from the masseter and temporalis muscles recorded during mastication in monkeys, Goodwin and Luschei (1975) were not able to distinguish between primary and secondary afferents on the basis of their responses to passive stretch. The firing patterns during mastication were equally difficult to classify, ranging from units that were only active during opening, to units that were obviously responding to fusimotor drive during shortening. However, some of the latter had a strong response to the initial stretch at the start of opening, suggesting that they must be spindle primaries. When the monkeys ate brittle biscuits, there was a sudden unloading of the jaw closing muscles each time the teeth broke through the food; this was accomplished by a fall in afferent activity and a silent period in the EMG.

The results from experiments conducted on awake cats by Taylor and Cody, (1974), and Cody et al. (1975), are very similar. These authors classified the afferents into two groups, depending on the maximum firing frequency that was attained during jaw opening. They proposed that low frequency units were secondary afferents and that high frequency units were spindle primaries. Support for this classification was provided by later experiments on lightly anesthetised cats in which succinylcholine was used to increase the dynamic sensitivity of the primary endings (Appenteng et al., 1980, Gottlieb and Taylor, 1983). Some additional data on awake cats was provided by Taylor et al. (1981) and Taylor and Appenteng (1981). Neurons classified as secondary spindle afferents usually fire throughout the cycle (Fig. 7B) and their firing frequency can be correlated to jaw displacement during all phases. The maximum firing frequency of 80 to 200 spikes per second usually occurs at the end of the opening phase, when the major closing muscles are longest. Primary afferents show evidence of some length sensitivity (Fig. 7A), and primary and secondary spindle afferents can increase their discharge rate during muscle contraction, espe-

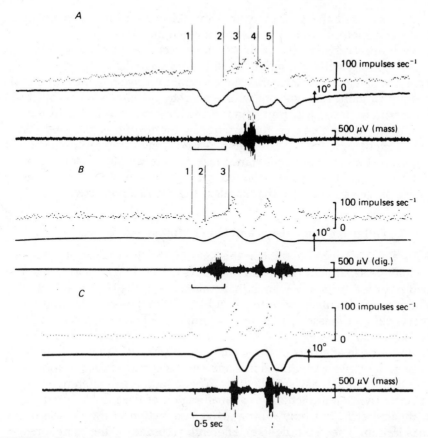

FIGURE 7. Responses of primary (A) and secondary (B) endings of jaw closing muscle spindles and (C) a modulated (probably static) fusimotor axon during reflex movements of the jaw in the lightly anesthetized cat. Upper traces, instantaneous firing frequency. Middle traces, jaw movement (opening upwards) and lower trace, masseter or digastric EMGs. (From Appenteng et al., 1980.)

cially when the food is tough and closure is slow. The spindle primaries are highly sensitive to the velocity of stretch, and fire at rates of up to 600 spikes per second in the burst of activity that comes at the start of opening.

Recordings from fusimotor fibers of the masseter nerve of lightly anesthetised cats by Appenteng et al. (1980), Taylor et al. (1981b), and Gottlieb and Taylor (1983) have shown that the dynamic sensitivity of the primary endings appears to be increased by tonic dynamic gamma activity that continues throughout the whole sequence of movements (cf. Grillner, 1981b). Likewise, the phasic activity of static fusimotor neurons, that begins just before jaw closure, seems to cause the primary afferent burst and maintain the firing of both groups during muscle contraction (Fig. 7C).

We discussed the possibility that the relationship between fusimotor and alpha motorneuron drive changes when monkeys switch from biting to rhythmical movements. A similar thing occurs as cats change from eating to lapping, when the length sensitivity of secondary afferents goes up. This was taken as evidence that static fusimotor drive had increased in the passage from the one type of rhythmical act to the other (Cody et al., 1975). Furthermore, feedback from spindles fluctuates with changes in the pattern of movement, caused for instance by the texture of the food (Taylor and Appenteng, 1981). Although increased firing during muscle shortening against an increased resistance may be due simply to slowing of the movement, Grillner (1981b) pointed out that there could be an increase in phasic static gamma drive that parallels the rise in alpha activity.

1.3   Golgi Tendon Organs and Other Muscle Afferents

Since there is very little data on this subject, the three types of movement will not be separated. Lund and Matthews, (1979; 1981) reported that they had recorded from a few jaw muscle afferents in the Gasserian ganglion. These were identified by probing and local stimulation within the medial pterygoid and masseter muscle and temporalis tendon region. Although conscious that local electrical stimulation is not a foolproof method of identifying muscle afferents in these complex muscles (Cody et al., 1972), the authors tentatively identified five afferents as coming from tendon organs and the remainder as "spindle-like". The tendon organ afferents were excited by twitch contractions of a small region of the muscle, fired during manual stretch, but only during active contraction of the muscle during mastication. The "spindle-like" afferents recorded in the ganglion were silenced by local twitches and their response to passive stretch was purely static. During mastication induced by cortical stimulation, they fired during opening when the mouth was empty, but could be induced to fire in the closing phase by putting a rubber tube in the mouth. The size of the extracellular action potentials of these "spindle-like" afferent neurons was small, suggesting that they could be Group III primary afferent neurons.

Larson et al. (1983) recorded from some position-sensitive muscle afferents in the trigeminal mesencephalic nucleus which substantially increased their firing rate during jaw closure. They tentatively identified them as tendon organ afferents because they exhibited a saw-tooth modulation of their instantaneous firing frequency that was thought to reflect the firing of a motor unit that inserted into the receptor. However, Appenteng and Prochazka (1984) point out that tendon organ afferents from the ankle extensors fire smoothly during muscle contraction, despite segmentation of the EMG burst. They compared the patterns of activity during imposed stretches and locomotion, and were able to show that the firing frequency of the tendon organ afferents increased in stepwise fashion during slow, smooth increases in whole muscle force. They attributed this to the recruitment of motor units inserting into the tendon of the receptor. Only 1a afferents showed saw-tooth modulation.

During locomotion, the firing pattern of these receptors, studied by Appenteng and Prochazka (1984) in intact cats, was exactly that described by Severin et al. (1967) who recorded from five tendon organ afferents from ankle extensor muscles and two from flexors of the decerebrate cat. The latter fired during ankle flexion, and the authors show a recording from an extensor tendon organ afferent that began to fire strongly at the beginning of the lengthening contraction of the muscle at the start of E_2 during stance. In their 1976 paper, Prochazka et al. identified two tendon organ afferents in flexor digitorum longus, a physiological extensor. These became active at the end of E_1, just before foot contact, and they continued to fire until the end of stance (Fig. 4). As can be seen in the figure, the period of activity of the receptors corresponds to that of the muscle. Loeb and Duysens (1979) described one hamstrings 1b afferent that fired in the swing phase, late in the semitendinosus burst, and Loeb (1981) discusses three others from medial gastrocnemius, tibialis posterior, and flexor digitorum brevis. Each appeared to fire during the period of activity in the parent muscle.

As in the other two systems, the few reports on tendon organs in the respiratory muscles agree that the maximum rate of firing occurs during the contraction of the muscle. Levator costae receptors fired a high frequency burst in the inspiratory phase, and stopped briefly as the muscle relaxed at the beginning of expiration (Hilaire et al., 1983). There seem to be more tendon organ afferents than spindle afferents coming from the diaphragm, and they fire as predicted, with the highest frequency occurring during the contraction of the muscle (Corda et al., 1965).

1.4 Joint Afferents

1.4.1 Locomotion

Before discussing the results of experiments using the walking animal, it is well to remember the controversy surrounding the properties and identity of these afferents. The authors of most early studies of afferent fibers, dissected from the articular nerves of the cat knee joint, described a large population of slowly adapting receptors that were most active at intermediate joint angles (Boyd and Roberts, 1953; Skoglund, 1956). This was contradicted by Burgess and Clark (1969), who found few receptors of this type. Later, it came to be accepted that most midrange receptors were muscle afferents (McCloskey, 1978), because they were found to respond to intravenous injections of succinylcholine (Burgess and Clark, 1969), and to be silenced by twitch contractions of the popliteus muscle (McIntyre et al., 1978). The fact that many midrange receptors are excited by stimulation of popliteus fusimotor neurons is proof that spindle afferents do travel in the posterior articular nerve (McIntyre et al., 1978). However, the situation has become complicated again since Ferrell (1980) reported that there are many full range afferents in the posterior articular nerve that remain after removal of the popliteus muscle. Furthermore, their response to joint rotation is enhanced by succinylcholine. So, while it seems that receptors in knee and hip joint (Carli et al., 1979) can be expected to signal the joint angle throughout the locomotor cycle, the identification of movement-sensitive afferents that travel in the posterior articular nerve of the knee is still uncertain.

Loeb et al., (1977) reported that they were able to record three knee joint afferents from the dorsal roots of freely moving cats which they identified (under general anesthesia) by stimulation of the posterior articular nerve. All of them were midrange receptors, one was not active during locomotion, one was smoothly modulated during stance, and the last one, illustrated in their Figure 2, fired during all phases of extension. At the time, the authors admitted that it was possible that this primary afferent came from a popliteus spindle secondary, but Loeb suggested afterwards that Ferrell's findings make this unlikely. A few more receptors with similar properties have been added to the sample (Loeb, 1981). Shimamura et al. (1984) recorded from dorsal root afferents of the thalamic cat during walking. They classified an unspecified number of afferents as forelimb joint receptors and stated that they discharged during stance. However, until descriptions of well-identified neurons are available, it is not possible to draw firm conclusions from their data.

1.4.2   Respiration

Godwin-Austin (1969) studied afferent neurons that responded to manual movement of the ribs after all peripheral nerve branches had been cut, except those to the joints and adjacent muscles. The articular receptors were classified by the elimination of units that fired when the muscles were briefly stimulated. All but 10% were slowly adapting and their firing frequency was proportional to the displacement of the rib. Most were active throughout the range of movement that the ribs make in spontaneous breathing, and some had a dynamic response that increased with the velocity of manual displacement. About 70% were excited when the ribs were in an expiratory position. This is in contrast to pulmonary stretch receptors that are more commonly sensitive to inflation than deflation (Knowlton and Larrabee, 1946; Widdicombe, 1954).

An approximation of the normal pattern of firing was obtained by restoring the mechanical linkage between the ribs that was lost when the muscles were denervated. When this had been done, it was found that receptors sensitive to manual displacement of the rib in the caudal direction fired at their highest frequency in expiration, those sensitive to rostral movement were most active in inspiration. Hilaire et al. (1983) have recently confirmed Godwin-Austin's findings.

1.4.3   Mastication

Injections of horseradish peroxidase into the temporomandibular joint capsule (Romfh et al., 1979) and single unit recording (Lund and Matthews, 1979, 1981) have shown that the cell bodies of the articular receptors of the cat and rabbit are in the mandibular division of the Gasserian ganglion. None of the afferents recorded in the rabbit fire when the jaw is in the resting position, but all but one fired during manual displacement of the jaw within the boundaries of normal movements (Lund and Matthews, 1981). When it could be tested, the pattern of firing was similar during mastication (Lund et al., 1982, Fig. 8). Based on the responses to passive movement, the population is capable of signalling the displacement and velocity of the condyle in all directions (Lund and Matthews,

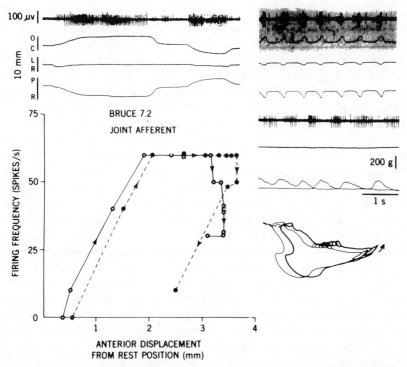

FIGURE 8. Response of a temporomandibular joint afferent during passive movement of the jaw (top left) and mastication (top right). Mastication was produced by cortical stimulation and the stimulus artifact partially obscures the record. The afferent was identified by moving the articular socket with a strain gauge, the output of which has replaced the horizontal transducer in the middle record on the right. The receptor was located in the caudal wall of the capsule (diagram) and was excited by opening (1st trial, upper left) or protusion (2nd trial). Mean firing rate is plotted against anterior displacement during 2 trials. O–C, opening and closing; L–R, left and right; P–R, protrusion and retrusion. (From Lund et al., 1982.)

1981). Each member had a preferred direction of movement that seemed to be determined by stretch of the region of the capsule that contains the receptor.

In agreement with the general principle that the largest concentration of joint receptors is found in those parts of the capsule most subjected to mechanical change during movement (Gardner, 1948), almost all receptors in the temporomandibular joint and in the costovertebral joints are in the rostral or caudal aspects (Lund and Matthews, 1981; Godwin-Austin, 1969).

1.5 Special Receptors

1.5.1 Respiration

Pulmonary Receptors. The tracheobronchial tree is supplied with parasympathetic (vagal) and sympathetic afferent fibers, but only the former have been studied in any detail. Vagal myelinated fibers innervating stretch receptors are thought to be located in the smooth muscle of the bronchi and trachea (Bartlett et al., 1976; Pack, 1981), but the density of receptors in a particular structure varies between species (Sant 'Ambrogio, 1982). In the dog, the slowly adapting receptors are most densely distributed in the trachea, while rapidly adapting receptors predominate in the bronchi (Sant 'Ambrogio, 1982). The former discharge tonically at constant intrapulmonary pressure and adapt very slowly, whereas the latter, rapidly adapting group, has an irregular discharge pattern that rapidly fades (Knowlton and Larrabee, 1946). Although the sensitivity of the receptors in the bronchi is modified by changes in airway CO_2 concentration, this is not likely to be important under normal physiological conditions (Pack, 1981; Sant 'Ambrogio, 1982). However, the patterns of activity of most of these receptors is modified by congestion and chemical irritants (Paintal, 1973; Pack, 1981; Sant 'Ambrogio, 1982).

Adrian (1933) was the first to describe the discharge of individual vagal afferent fibers during respiration. He showed that a population of fibers that probably arose from the pulmonary stretch receptors is stimulated by expansion of the lungs. Activity in these fibers is proportional to lung volume and, therefore, the maximum firing frequency (50–100 spikes/s in quiet breathing) occurs during inspiration. About 60% have low thresholds and are active during the respiratory pause of artificial respiration; the others are recruited as inspiration progresses (Paintal, 1973). It is now known that this pattern only describes the behavior of slowly adapting receptors in the intrathoracic trachea. The increase in rate of extrathoracic receptors occurs in expiration because the transmural pressure across the membranous posterior wall, in which the receptors are located, is positive only during this phase (Scarpelli et al., 1965).

Rapidly adapting stretch receptors appear under a number of other descriptive names such as "deflation receptors, irritant receptors, and cough receptors" (Paintal, 1973; Sant 'Ambrogio, 1982). In the trachea, they are located around the circumference of the wall, and are not confined to the trachealis muscle of the posterior wall, as are the slowly adapting group. (Sant 'Ambrogio et al., 1978). There is good evidence that the receptors are located in the mucosa. The discharge frequency of these neurons is not smoothly modulated during the respiratory cycle; bursts of spikes occur during inspiration and expiration and/or at peak inspiration (Fillenz and Widdicombe, 1971).

The last major type of pulmonary receptor, the J receptors of Paintal (1969, 1973, 1977) and other C-fiber endings do not have a discharge pattern that is related to respiratory movements (Sant 'Ambrogio, 1982).

Another group of mechanoreceptive myelinated afferent fibers that fire in phase with respiration have been recorded from the sympathetic nerves (Kostreva et al., 1975). These appear to have some of the properties of both types of vagal stretch receptors. They are slowly adapting and fire irregularly at a mean frequency that is related to the transpulmonary pressure.

Chemoreceptors. The main drive that maintains respiration is furnished by the central and peripheral chemoreceptors. If this input is sufficiently decreased by hypocapnia and hyperoxia, respiration ceases (Euler, 1981). CO_2 acts through peripheral and medullary chemoreceptors to stimulate respiration. Although they did not record directly from central chemoreceptors, Euler and Söderberg (1952) found both rhythmical and continuous discharges in respiratory areas of the denervated brain stem that were dependent on PCO_2.

Individual chemoreceptor afferents have been studied in the periphery. Carotid body chemoreceptors are activated by increases in either arterial $H+$ or arterial PCO_2, and by decreases in PO_2 (Biscoe et al., 1970), and aortic chemoreceptors have similar properties (Paintal, 1973). Since the stimuli to the receptors vary with the phase of respiration and the receptors respond to changes in alveolar gas concentrations with a latency of about 0.5 s, it is not surprising that the discharge rate varies with the respiratory cycle when the rate is slow (Hornbein et al., 1961; Leitner and Dejours, 1968). However, at natural respiratory rates, the combination of small oscillations in the stimulus, slow adaptation, and phase lags, means that the discharge frequency of chemoreceptors is relatively constant (Leitner and Dejours, 1968).

1.5.2 Mastication

The periodontal ligament that anchors the teeth to the alveolar bone contains receptors that respond to the pressure or rate of change of pressure applied to the teeth. The sense organs appear to be free nerve endings and Ruffini-type terminals that are closely applied to collagen bundles of the ligament (Byers, 1985). Some of the latter have processes that penetrate

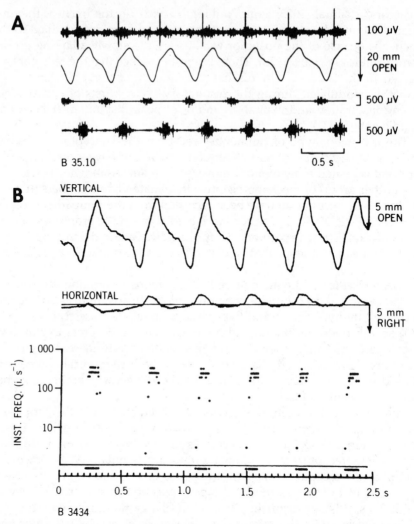

FIGURE 9. Pattern of firing of rapidly adapting (A) and slowly adapting (B) incisor periodontal receptors during chewing on a rubber tube. In A, the microelectrode recording, together with digastric and masseteric EMGs and vertical movement are shown. The traces in B are described in Fig. 2. (From Appenteng et al., 1982b.)

between the fibers of the bundles in a way that resembles Golgi tendon organs. Each primary afferent innervates one, or, at the most, three roots (Ness, 1954; Hannam, 1969; Linden, 1978). The cell bodies of these afferents are located in the Gasserian ganglion and in the mesencephalic nucleus. As one would expect, these receptors can code the magnitude of biting force (Larson et al., 1981a, b), and they are active in mastication (Appenteg et al., 1982b). The large majority of periodontal afferents from the molar teeth recorded in the ganglion of the rabbit are rapidly adapting, and these fire a single spike, or short burst in the transition from the fast-closing to the slow-closing phase (Fig. 9A). Slowly adapting receptors predominate around the incisors. These increase their discharge rate throughout the occlusal phase as pressure increases on the teeth that they supply (Fig. 9B).

1.6 Summary

Most of the types of sensory afferents that we have discussed in this section are phasically active during locomotion, respiration, or mastication. They come from receptors in the skin, mucosa, joint capsules, ligaments, and muscles, and they have low thresholds to mechanical stimulation. Their patterns of activity sometimes suggest possible roles in kinesthesia and in motor control. Those that fire short bursts seem to do so at critical points in the cycle, for instance when a foot contacts the ground. They often signal the transition from one phase to another, and could, perhaps, participate in phase switching. Others tend to fire throughout a phase, and their firing frequency is sometimes proportional to a parameter of movement. This type of feedback could be used to control some feature of that phase, such as EMG amplitude or burst duration.

Some afferents, notably chemoreceptors, baroreceptors, and hair follicle afferents, fire in a tonic or continuously modulated way throughout a series of movements. Their output could drive or alter pattern generating circuits or reflex arcs.

2 INACTIVATION OF AFFERENTS

2.1 Introduction

The preceding section indicated that the pattern of discharge of most primary afferents is linked to specific aspects of the rhythmic movements. On the basis of such recordings, some inferences can be made regarding the possible contribution of the afferents to the control of these movements. However, supplementary insights can be gained through two other experimental approaches. One which will be reviewed in the present section consists of inactivating the afferents by different means and observing the resulting changes in the pattern of movement. The complementary approach of stimulating the afferents and recording the resultant modifications of the pattern will be treated in the next section.

Different procedures have been used to inactivate the afferents. First, for the locomotor system, observations have been made after a complete lumbosacral or cervical *deafferentation* achieved by dorsal rhizotomy. This removes all types of afferents from one limb or one limb girdle except those few afferents which travel in the ventral root and which can be severed by a ganglionectomy. Second, *nerve section* has been used to study the contribution of afferents of a certain type, or afferents from a circumscribed region (e.g., bilateral vagotomy or section of a cutaneous limb nerve). Third, *local anesthesia* has been utilized to reversibly eliminate the feedback from a restricted area such as periodontal pressoreceptors of the lower jaw, cutaneous receptors from the foot pads or from joint afferents.

Finally, all movement-related feedback from all parts of the body can be removed by a chemical *neuromuscular blockade (paralysis)*. In such "fictive," motionless preparations, organized rhythmical patterns are recorded from the nerves themselves instead of the muscles. Because there is no movement, the afferent feedback is tonic and is thus incongruous with the centrally generated rhythmic pattern. These preparations are thus particularly useful for studying how controlled tonic or phasic peripheral inputs may interact with a centrally generated pattern.

2.2 Locomotion

2.2.1 Rhizotomy:Deafferented Preparations

Acute Deafferentation. In early studies designed to investigate the general consequences of chronic deafferentation on the control of movements in cats, it was reported that there was a period of excitation during recovery from anesthesia where the deafferented leg moved rhythmically in coordination with the other limbs. The movements of the deafferented limb were, however, more feeble than the movements of the others (Sprong, 1929; Hnik, 1956; Wetzel et al., 1976).

From more detailed recent studies, the effects of an acute lumbosacral deafferentation on the locomotor pattern of the hindlimbs can be summarized under three broad categories: (1) effects on muscle force; (2) effects on the timing of the various events within the step cycle, and (3) effects on the interlimb coordination.

First, Shik et al. (1966) described that the hindquarters of acute decerebrate cats, which can usually bear their weight during MLR-induced locomotion, needed to be suspended after deafferentation. In contrast, Grillner and Zangger (1984) have recently reported that such preparations were capable of supporting their own weight, although there could be a decrease in amplitude of the movements and sometimes a decrease in EMG amplitude. This may account for the tendency of the knee and ankle to yield towards the end of stance (Fig. 10C).

Second, deafferentation may reduce the precision in the timing of activation and inactivation of muscles at the transition phases, such as between extension and flexion. In an early account of acute deafferentation experiments, Grillner and Zangger (1975) reported that, occasionally, either the EMG activity recorded from hip flexors overlapped for a short period the EMG activity recorded in ankle extensors, or, the activity recorded in ankle extensors overlapped the activity in the ankle flexors. This

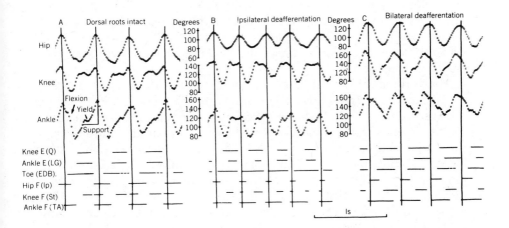

FIGURE 10. Kinematic and electromyographic study of acute deafferentation in cats. Joint angles measured from a limb during walking, before (A), after ipsilateral (B) and bilateral (C) transection of all dorsal roots caudal to L2 in a pre-collicular, postmammillary decerebrate cat in which locomotion was induced by electrical stimulation of the MLR. The angle displacements were measured from film sequences taken at 64 frames/s, synchronized with simultaneously recorded EMG records from selected hindlimb muscles. The onset of the swing phase of each cycle is indicated by the vertical bars. The horizontal bars indicate the EMG activity of some muscles acting on the hindlimb. Abbreviations: Q, quadriceps; LG, gastrocnemius lateralis; EDB, extensor digitorum brevis; Ip, iliopsoas; St, semitendinosus; TA, tibialis anterior. (From Grillner and Zangger, 1984.)

was not a constant feature (see the timing studies in Grillner and Zangger, 1984). Furthermore, it is quite clear from the records that, apart from these transitional periods, the muscles which were normally active during one phase were silenced in the opposite phase. This suggests that the major part of this reciprocal inhibition is indeed of central origin.

In general, the duration of flexor and extensor bursts becomes somewhat more variable after deafferentation, and the whole locomotor pattern is more unstable. Nevertheless, the relative timing relationships with respect to the groups of flexor muscles on the one hand, and the groups of extensor muscles on the other, are preserved, although minor changes in this order may occur for the knee and ankle extensors (EMGs in Fig. 10). The characteristic timing of certain muscles is also retained. For example, the extensor digitorum brevis, indicated as "toe (EDB)" in Figure 10, is still activated before the ankle extensor and the knee extensor, even after bilateral deafferentation.

Third, the deafferented limbs are coordinated with the other limbs in the usual order (HL-FL-HR-FR). Although this coordination may be achieved centrally (see section on fictive locomotion), the movements of the deafferented hindlimbs appear to depend more on the movements of the forelimbs than is usually the case. Thus, when locomotion is initiated by MLR stimulation, the hindlimbs may start walking only after the forelimbs and stop when the movements of the forelimbs are prevented from moving (Shik et al, 1966). The forelimbs may also provide timing cues to account for the reported speed adaptation of the deafferented limbs (Grillner and Zangger, 1984).

Movements of the forelimbs are, however, not essential for the generation of hindlimb walking in the deafferented preparation. Indeed, Grillner and Zangger (1979) showed that after an acute bilateral deafferentation in an acutely spinalized cat, or even in a chronic spinal cat, tonic stimulation of the L6 dorsal root or of the dorsal column can elicit a rhythmic locomotor pattern in both hindlimbs.

Thus, it is clear that the acutely deafferented limb can produce the basic sequence of muscle activity, including complex EMG patterns (Grillner and Zangger, 1984; Székely, Czéh and Vörös, 1969). This point has been convincingly reviewed by Delcomyn (1980) for many types of patterns in many species. However, the fact that afferent feedback is not essential for the genesis of the basic locomotor pattern should not overshadow the essential role that the elaborate feedback information carried by the afferent discharges described in the previous section undoubtedly plays in the control and adaptation of this pattern.

In effect, after deafferentation, the movements are not as precise, nor are they as well adapted and coordinated, and they are generally weaker. It should also be pointed out that Szekely et al. (1969) reported that deafferented newts could produce a quite complex EMG pattern resembling that found in normal animals, even though the locomotor movements themselves could show significant anomalies. Deficits such as a reduction in weight support or a decrease in amplitude of joint excursion may only represent defects in the output pattern due to an acute loss of motorneu-ronal excitability. They need not imply an inadequate timing of the central pattern, but it remains true that the overall locomotor performance is "de-graded" after deafferentation, as emphasized by Grillner and Zangger (1984). Thus, an apparently normal EMG pattern in a restricted number of muscles should not be equated to a normal pattern of movement of the whole limb. Indeed, even the slightest alteration in the usual balance of force produced by the different antagonistic muscle groups acting at dif-ferent joints could lead to abnormal movements.

Chronic Deafferentation. The interpretation of the results obtained in studies of chronic deafferentation may be complicated by at least three factors. First, it should be made clear that the reduced usage or the non-use of a deafferented limb in a given movement does not signify that affer-ents are needed for the execution of that movement. The animal may choose not to use a limb in the first few days after surgery because of pain or, after some time, if the same task can be accomplished using the other limbs. Second, plastic compensatory changes do occur (sprouting, for ex-ample) and these can conceal the specific deficits due to the deafferenta-tion. It is not easy to differentiate an abnormality due to the absence of afferents from an abnormality due to behavioral substitution. However, these substitutions are only partial and never completely replace the miss-ing afferents, a point clearly made by Goldberger and Murray (1978). In other words, the afferent limb of specific reflexes never returns and the role that these might play is permanently lost. These studies may then indicate if the afferents have unique roles which cannot be compensated by other systems. Third, chronic deafferentation experiments have often been performed in cats and monkeys to study various spinal reflexes rather than to evaluate the importance of the afferents in locomotion. Therefore, the description of the locomotor deficits themselves are often incomplete.

Mott and Sherrington (1895) reported that, after unilateral section of cervical or lumbar sensory roots, monkeys did not use the deafferented limb during walking (see discussion in Grillner, 1975). The work of Taub has, however, convincingly shown that the non-use during locomotion of a single deafferented forelimb is more a strategy adopted by the monkey than an absolute impossibility to use the limb. Indeed, after bilateral de-afferentation of the forelimbs the monkey has to use the limbs and does so in a remarkable manner so that "it is often difficult to distinguish an intact monkey from a bilaterally deafferented monkey in slow ambulation" (Taub, 1976).

Sprong (1929) reports that, while recovering from the anesthesia for a unilateral deafferentation, cats performed rhythmic coordinated movements with all four legs although the movements of the leg with the lesion were of smaller amplitude. In the following days, the tonus of the deafferented leg decreased and, during walking, the leg was often misplaced, being either hyperextended and contacting ground with the dorsum of the paw or being abducted. After a bilateral deafferentation, some cats did not use the limbs at all for walking; others showed progression movements which were maximal during the first 24 hours and disappeared after two days. During that period, the hindlegs dragged along and made large excursions of alternate flexion and extension at the hip. Similar movements resembling the "butterfly style of swimmers" were described by Hnik (1956).

After a unilateral deafferentation, Ranson (1929) described the operated limb as useless, the limb being dragged during walking with incomplete flexion movements. Incoordinated movements resembling those found in clinical sensory ataxia were reported by Teasdall and Stavraky (1955). Deafferentation of the forelimbs in kittens also led to an hyperextension and a misplacement of the foot on the dorsum (Lassek and Moyer, 1953).

A more precise description of locomotor behavior after unilateral deafferentation of a hindlimb was given by Wiesendanger (1964). Overground, the flexion-extension movements occured mainly at the hip whereas the distal part, especially the ankle, was kept extended. In "quick locomotion," the deafferented limb was dragged behind and performed paddling movements. EMG recordings in cats performing locomotor movements while suspended in a sling showed a greater background activity and periods of overlapping activity in antagonistic ankle muscles, suggesting reduced reciprocal inhibition.

The first detailed gait study (analysis of footfall patterns) in chronically deafferented cats was performed by Wetzel et al. (1976). Two weeks after an extradural and unilateral lumbosacral ganglionectomy, several defects were described. It was noted that there was an irregular usage, and a disorganized footfall pattern of the deafferented limb. Some cats could lift the limb above the belt, while other cats could not, and in some cases even "walked on their knees" although the limbs performed alternating forward-backward movements. The limb was "malpositioned" either too far forward or too far back during the steps. This led to a relative incoordination with the contralateral hindlimb as well as with the forelimbs. There was a decrease in force and a shorter stance duration which reduced the utilization of the operated limb. There was also an improper adaptation of the stance duration to the increasing speed of the treadmill, the stance being either too short or too long. It is difficult to say, however, if these deficits in speed adaptation are worse or similar to those of the acutely deafferented cats. Finally, angular measurements indicated that the cats did not completely extend the hip joint at the end of stance.

In another study on partial unilateral deafferentation (L6 spared), kinematic studies indicated that the ankle yielded much more during stance and that this was compensated by a less pronounced yield in the knee to ensure an approximately constant leg length (Rasmussen et al., 1986).

The most detailed behavioral description of locomotion after unilateral deafferentation in cats was made by Goldberger (Goldberger 1977; Goldberger and Murray, 1978; Goldberger, 1983). The sequence of recovery was divided into four periods. In the acute period (1–2 days) the cats did not use the deafferented limb during locomotion and it was kept extended. In the following period of uncontrolled locomotion (2–9 days), the limb was hyperflexed during swing and then, after a pause, briskly extended in stance. The positioning of the paw was haphazard, often landing on the dorsum of the foot and the leg was adducted or abducted. It was thus impossible for these animals to cross a 2-inch runway. In the third period of controlled locomotion (9–18 days), the animals could cross the 2-inch runway and were able to maintain a position of normal adduction. The limb landed under the animal's center of gravity and was thus capable of sharing the weight of the body (although some deficit in weight bearing was observed in some animals). Other animals walked along the runway with three legs only, keeping the deafferented leg flexed. In the last period of stabilized recovery (18–21 days), the cats displayed an almost normal pattern while walking on a narrow walkway. However, less weight was borne by the deafferented limb and it exhibited a shorter stance. Recent studies using [^{3}H]-fluorodeoxyglucose as a metabolic indicator have reported that muscles of the deafferented leg, especially the extensor muscles, are much less used during walking than those of the contralateral limb which was taken as the control (Eidelberg and Miller, 1985).

Thus, compensatory mechanisms are quite efficient and may, in the best of cases, allow the cat to use the deafferented limb to walk properly. This compensation appears even clearer when structures that may participate in this compensation are also lesioned. For instance, additional deafferentation of the contralateral limb may lead to more severe deficits (see, however, Taub, 1976 for the monkey). A lumbosacral deafferentation produces more severe deficits when combined with a previous unilateral trunk deafferentation (Goldberger and Murray, 1980). Spinal hemisection on the side of a unilateral hindlimb deafferentation (Goldberger, 1977) or extirpation of the motor cortex contralateral to a unilateral forelimb deafferentation (Lassek and Moyer, 1953) may render useless the operated limb even though such spinal or cortical lesions on their own are reported to have only minor consequences, at least in undemanding locomotion.

2.2.2 Paralysis: Fictive Locomotion

The preceding section suggested that some characteristic timing features were maintained after deafferentation of the hindlimbs. It could be argued, especially in decerebrate preparations in which the forelimbs are walking, that these timing features are derived from cues originating outside the lesioned limb. The evidence showing that this is not the case comes from paralyzed preparations in which there can be no phasic afferent inputs.

After decortication and paralysis in the cat, a spontaneous, well-organized rhythmic locomotor activity can be recorded in the nerves of the hindlimbs (Perret, 1976; Perret and Cabelguen, 1980; Perret, 1983) and the forelimbs (Cabelguen et al., 1981). The same can be observed in paralyzed thalamic cats decerebrated at A13 (Bayev, 1978). Similarly, stimulation of the MLR in paralyzed and decerebrate cats can induce locomotion in the hindlimbs (Jordan et al., 1979) as well as in the forelimbs (Arshavsky et al., 1986; Amemiya and Yamaguchi, 1984). Finally, after acute spinalization and paralysis, chemical activation such as narcosis (Graham-Brown, 1911; Viala and Buser, 1969a), L-dopa potentiated by nialamide (Jankowska et al., 1967; Grillner and Zangger, 1979) or other monoamines (Viala and Buser, 1971) can induce rhythmical activity with locomotor-like properties in the hindlimbs. Such coordinated activity can also be found in the forelimbs and hindlimbs of high spinal cats (Miller and Van der Meché, 1976; Zangger, 1978) and in the forelimbs of high spinal rabbits after a section at C1 and T12 (Viala and Vidal, 1978).

Although the rhythm is usually slower, the assymetrical structure of the step cycle (more or less invariant period of flexor activity and variable duration of extensor activity) is retained. The coordination between the two hindlimbs can be one of alternation, or can be in-phase (Grillner and Zangger, 1979). The coordination between the forelimbs and the hindlimbs is also usually present (see Fig. 11A) but can be rather loose (Cabelguen et al., 1981).

Under these conditions, the pattern of rhythmical activity in one limb can be rather complex with the characteristic timing of certain groups of motoneurons retained. For example, the bifunctional semitendinosus and posterior biceps (knee flexors and hip extensors), which normally discharge a much shorter burst than the ankle flexor, tibialis anterior, preserve this characteristic in fictive locomotion (Grillner and Zangger, 1979). An example taken in an acutely spinalized cat pretreated with L-dopa, nialamide and 4-aminopyridine is shown in Fig. 11B (Rossignol et al., 1985). The fine characteristics of the discharges found in the normal cats are retained (see Engberg and Lundberg, 1969). For instance, semitendinosus discharges a sharp burst prior to the hip flexor sartorius and there may be some activity during the opposite phase when the hip extensor, semimembranosus, is active. The knee extensor and hip flexor, rectus femoris, discharges during late swing and has a second burst during stance.

The muscles acting at the toes also preserve their particular timing under the conditions of fictive locomotion. Extensor digitorum brevis, which was shown to discharge at a characteristic time in the deafferented state (Grillner and Zangger, 1984), also discharges before the extensors in the fictive state (Bayev, 1978). Similarly, O'Donovan et al., (1982) have shown that the two long toe muscles, flexor hallucis longus and flexor

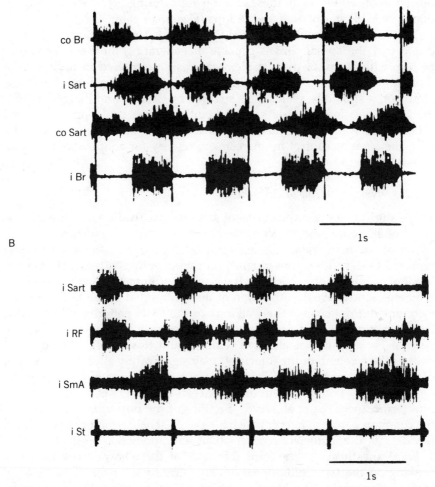

A

co Br

i Sart

co Sart

i Br

1s

B

i Sart

i RF

i SmA

i St

1s

FIGURE 11. Fictive locomotion in the cat. (A) Recordings of the efferent activity in a flexor muscle nerve of each of the four limbs of a decorticate and paralysed cat showing the timing relationships between the forelimb and hindlimb motor commands. The vertical lines indicate the onset of activity in the contralateral (right) brachialis and the figure demonstrates that there is a well-coordinated pattern of activity between the fore- and hindlimbs. (B) shows electroneurographic recordings from a decorticate, paralysed and spinalized cat (T13) which was pre-treated with Nialamide (50mg/kg), L-dopa (50mg/kg) and 4-aminopyridine (20 mg/kg). The pattern of activity recorded from some of the bifunctional muscles of one hindlimb closely resembles that observed during normal locomotion. Of particular note is the pattern of activity in the knee flexor and hip extensor, semitendinosus, and the hip flexor and knee extensor, sartorius. Abbreviations: Br, brachialis; Sart, sartorius; RF, rectus femoris; St, semitendinosus; i, ipsilateral; co, contralateral. (A) modified from Cabelguen et al, 1981; (B) modified from Rossignol et al, 1985.

digitorum longus, which are anatomical synergists differentially utilized during locomotion, retain these relationships during fictive locomotion induced by MLR stimulation and L-dopa (Fleshman et al., 1984).

The findings presented here for the paralyzed preparations clearly indicate that the spinal cord is capable of generating the basic locomotor pattern with many of the complex features encountered in normal locomotion in the absence of all phasic, movement-related afferent feedback. However, it should be realized, as stressed by Grillner and Zangger (1979), that the activation of these spinal circuits "at best could produce a bad caricature of walking" because, as was seen in the section on deafferentation, the afferent control mechanisms necessary for adaptation and compensation are missing.

2.2.3 Nerve Section or Anesthesia

A few studies mention the effects of selective inactivation of some specific types of afferents, and the conclusions are sometimes confusing. The removal of cutaneous afferents achieved by cutting cutaneous nerves was reported to have little consequence on the stepping pattern of either the hindlimbs (Sherrington, 1910) or the forelimbs (Shimamura et al., 1984). In Engberg's study (1964), infiltration of the central pad of the hindfoot with xylocaine did not change the walking nor the EMG patterns of intact cats. However, unpublished observations suggest that anesthesia of the foot pads of the chronic spinal kitten (Grillner and Rossignol), or of the foot pads of the forelimb of the intact cat, may significantly alter the placement of the foot on the treadmill. Anesthesia of the foot dorsum has little effect on the walking pattern in chronic spinal cats (Forssberg et al., 1977) or the intact cat (Prochazka et al., 1978). Sections of the posterior tibial nerve or the common peroneal nerve, which are mixed sensory-motor nerves, leave few deficits after sufficient recovery (Duysens and Stein, 1978).

Local anesthesia of the joint receptors of the elbow in thalamic cats walking on the treadmill appears to significantly alter the forelimb locomotor movements. The angle at which swing is initiated appears to be increased. There is also some degree of overlap of flexor and extensor EMG activity at transitional phases. Anesthesia of the shoulder, elbow, and wrist on one side was reported to abolish stepping on that side (Shimamura et al., 1984).

In intact cats, anesthesia of the knee joint may lead to anomalies in posture and gait such as limping, outward rotation of the leg, and misplacement of the foot (Ferrell et al., 1985). To further study the effects on proprioception, a trolley was designed to impose backward movements of the leg and measure the distance at which the leg normally swings forwards. It was found that this distance was significantly increased after anesthesia of the knee joint. These observations emphasize that joint afferents may play an important role in controlling the timing of the cycle (see also later).

2.2.4   Conclusion

In conclusion, afferents are essential for the execution of the full range of locomotor movement at all joints (more specifically the distal ones), the precise coupling between the different joints, the fine coordination between the legs, the exact force that the limb must exert to bear its share of the weight, the exact position that the limb must have in relation to the center of gravity, and the precise adaptation of the cycle to speed, slope, and terrain. The failure to adequately fulfill even one of these conditions leads to an abnormal and maladapted locomotor function.

2.3   Respiration

2.3.1   Vagotomy and Paralysis

Very similar experimental approaches have been taken for studying the respiratory system. This system offers certain advantages over the locomotor system in that key control elements lie at different levels of the CNS and, thus, can be selectively isolated. The phrenic and intercostal motoneurons, which innervate, respectively, the diaphragm and the intercostal muscles, are located in the cervical cord, whereas the driving premotoneurons are located mainly in the medulla. In decerebrate cats it is possible to study "fictive" respiration by curarization and artificial ventilation using a cycle-triggered pump which inflates the lungs at a rate and amplitude determined by the simultaneously recorded activity in a phrenic nerve. The effects on medullary mechanisms of afferent inputs from the chest walls can be minimized by a pneumothorax or a low cervical spinal section. Finally, the influence of pulmonary stretch receptors (PSRs) can be eliminated by a bilateral vagotomy (see Feldman et al., in this volume and a review by Cohen, 1979, for further methodological details on such studies).

If the vagi are cut in a paralyzed animal the spontaneous rate of breathing (Fig. 12D) slows down. An analogous situation is found in locomotion where the "fictive" rhythm is usually slower than real walking. In the face of an increased respiratory demand (increasing CO_2), the depth of each breath increases (Fig. 12B and C), whereas the respiratory frequency stays largely the same (Fig. 12D). In paralyzed animals with intact vagi, the integrated phrenic nerve activity during the inspiratory (I) phase increases as a ramp which abruptly declines at the onset of the expiration (E) phase (Fig. 12A). If the cycle-triggered pump is inactivated for only one cycle so that inspiration occurs without lung inflation and without the consequent activation of the PSRs, the I phase is significantly prolonged in that cycle only. The slope of the integrated phrenic activity during I is the same whether or not the lungs are inflated, at least under these conditions of anesthesia. This will be important in a later section when the physiological role of the Breuer-Hering reflex will be discussed.

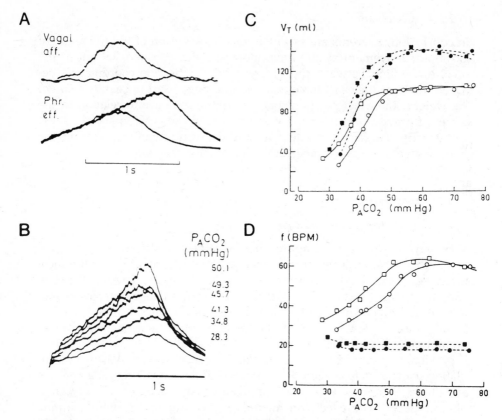

FIGURE 12. The effects of vagotomy on respiration. (A) Superimposed records from two breaths with and without cyclic, volume-related, vagal feedback from PSRs. Upper tracing: moving average of vagal afferent activity, mainly from PSRs. Lower tracings: moving average of inspiratory phrenic activity. The figure illustrates that the phrenic nerve activity, in the absence of vagal input, continues at the same rate until the inspiration is "switched-off". There is no sign of inhibition of the inspiratory activity in advance of this ispiratory "off-switch." (B) Superimposed records of a moving average of inspiratory phrenic nerve activity at different levels of $PaCO_2$ in the absence of cyclic volume-related feedback from PSRs, showing that increased respiratory drive increases the slope of the phrenic nerve activity and thus results in an increased tidal volume without changing the frequency. (C) and (D) show quantitatively the effect of increasing $PaCO_2$ on the tidal volume of each breath (C) and on the frequency of the respiratory rhythm (D), before (open symbols) and after (filled symbols) vagotomy. Vagotomy decreases the spontaneous respiratory rate which remains relatively constant when $PaCO_2$ is increased; tidal volume shows a greater increment to the increased $PaCO_2$ than in the intact cat. Increasing the temperature of the animal (squares) caused an increase in respiratory frequency and tidal volume for any given CO_2 concentration. The cat was decerebrated at a precollicular level and the increased $PaCO_2$ was achieved through a rebreathing procedure. A and B from von Euler, 1985; C and D from von Euler et al, 1970.

Thus, as in the locomotor system, in the absence of afferent feedback the basic fundamental respiratory rhythm can still be generated (see the chapter by Feldman et al. in this volume for other aspects of coordination between different components of the respiratory system).

2.4 Mastication

2.4.1 Paralysis, Deafferentation, and Anesthesia

Several species of animals have been shown to produce masticatory rhythmic activity after paralysis. Since this topic has been detailed in the chapter by Lund and Enomoto (this volume), only some specific points will be treated here. The basic structure of the rhythm appears to be similar to the normal pattern although a detailed analysis of the specific timing of different muscles is not available. The frequency of the chewing rhythm evoked by cortical stimulation is the same before and after paralysis in the rabbit (Dellow and Lund 1971), and only about 10% slower in the cat (Nakamura et al., 1976).

The anatomical organization of the masticatory system is such that some specific classes of afferents can be removed. For example, a lesion of the mesencephalic nucleus of the fifth cranial nerve (MES V) eliminates the feedback from spindles as well as from some periodontal receptors. In such a study, Goodwin and Luschei (1974) reported that monkeys chewed preferentially on the side opposite the deafferentation. However, the basic frequency of the rhythm and the timing of individual muscle discharges were virtually unchanged, even after bilateral lesions of MES V.

Using short-acting local anesthetics, it has also been possible to selectively remove the feedback from periodontal pressoreceptors. In humans, such a procedure reduces the force output of maximal voluntary biting by as much as 40%, suggesting that these afferents may be the source of an important positive feedback action on closure motoneurones (Lund and Lamarre, 1973). Since these pressoreceptors are among those which can excite the jaw-opening motoneurons and inhibit jaw-closure motoneurons in the jaw-opening reflex (JOR), it is possible that this excitatory action is mediated separately through a cortical pathway which could override the effects of the brain stem pathway (Lund and Lamarre, 1974).

3 ACTIVATION OF AFFERENTS

3.1 Locomotion

3.1.1 Introduction

The preceding sections have considered the ability of the mammalian CNS to generate locomotor, respiratory, and masticatory rhythms in the absence of peripheral feedback. It was concluded that a central pattern, closely resembling that seen in the intact animal, is present after deafferentation, but that afferent feedback is essential for the production of normal movements. The exact manner in which afferent input interacts with rhythmic processes under normal circumstances is, however, unknown. There is no information concerning the efficacy with which normally generated afferent impulses affect the motor output. Due to the technical and analytical problems involved in recording and tracing the "functional" path of the afferent input, the indirect method of afferent stimulation has been usefully employed to study the role of peripheral input.

In this section we will consider the effects of two different approaches to the problem: first, the effect of changing tonic inputs, and second, the effect of giving a short phasic perturbation at different times in the step cycle. In general, afferent inputs to the various systems have phase-dependent effects. This expression is often used to describe quite different phenomena and it is perhaps useful to list these different meanings. In some cases the expression means that the response to a given input may vary in amplitude but not in character as the stimulus is delivered progressively later in one phase of the cycle. Alternatively, it may mean that the effects are different in the two opposing phases (flexion-extension, inspiration-expiration, opening-closure). These different effects in turn can either consist of the excitation of one group of muscles in one phase and the excitation of the antagonist group in the opposite phase, or the excitation of a group in one phase and the inhibition of the same group in the opposite phase.

3.1.2 Tonic Stimulation

In reduced preparations, some degree of afferent activity is usually needed to induce or strengthen the rhythmic activity either in terms of the output amplitude, the frequency, or to stabilize the cycle structure (Orlovsky and Feldman, 1972). In decerebrate preparations, this can be provided by tonic, non-specific, cutaneous stimulation of different areas such as the forelimbs (Viala and Buser, 1969b), the sacral region (Viala and Buser, 1971), hindlimb cutaneous nerves (Grillner and Zangger, 1979; Fleshman et al., 1984), dorsal roots or dorsal columns (Grillner and Zangger, 1979), or the trigeminal afferents of the face (Viala and Buser, 1974) or the pinna (Aoki and Mori, 1981). Activation of both cutaneous myelinated afferents (except A-delta), and C-fibers, are generally excitatory (Viala et al., 1978). The same applies to small group III and IV muscle fibers chemically activated by local intra-arterial injectin of bradykinin or KCl (Kniffki et al., 1981).

Other inputs from specific cutaneous fibers (A-delta) in specific areas such as the dorsal lumbar region of the rabbit (Viala and Buser, 1974; Viala et al., 1978) can inhibit fictive locomotion without producing an inhibition of the motoneurons, and, thus, presumably by an action through interneurones closely linked to the generator mechanism (Viala et al., 1978). Group

III and IV muscle afferents can sometimes inhibit the rhythmical process by tonically co-activating both antagonistic muscle groups (Kniffki et al., 1981).

Rather unspecific skin stimulation of the hindlimb or stimulation of cutaneous nerves can change the discharge pattern of certain bifunctional muscles such as semitendinosus or posterior biceps. In the decorticate cat, it was reported that semitendinosus generally discharged as an extensor during fictive locomotion (see, however, Grillner and Zangger, 1979), and that this discharge could be changed to a flexor discharge by skin stimulation (Perret and Cabelguen, 1976, 1980). Similar changes were seen for other types of bifunctional muscles acting, for example, as hip flexors and knee extensors (rectus femoris), and for more distal limb muscles. The same also applies to bifunctional muscles of the forelimbs (Cabelguen et al., 1981). In the rabbit, semitendinosus discharges as a flexor with a tonic ipsilateral skin nerve stimulation or as an extensor when the contralateral homologous skin nerve is stimulated (Vidal et al., 1979).

The lumbar back muscles usually discharge two bursts per cycle during locomotion in intact (Carlson et al., 1979), decerebrate, and spinal cats (Zomlefer et al., 1984). In fictive preparations, these motoneurons have one main burst per step cycle although a second burst can also appear when cutaneous afferents are stimulated (Koehler et al., 1984). As for bifunctional muscles it is possible that lumbar back muscles receive one central command during one phase of the step cycle and that a second command, in the opposite phase, is facilitated by peripheral inputs, a model suggested by Perret and Cabelguen (1976, 1980; Perret, 1976, 1983; see, however, Vidal et al., 1979).

The fictive locomotor output can also be changed by passively manipulating the position of a limb and thus activating muscular, joint, and skin afferents. Extreme flexion or extension of the limb favors a strong rhythmicity, whereas intermediate positions have been reported to favor sometimes a coactivation of antagonists (Viala and Buser, 1969b). Again, bifunctional muscles can discharge in one or the other phase of the step cycle, as judged from the activity in simple monoarticular muscles. In rabbits, if a limb is passively placed in extreme extension, the bifunctional semitendinosus may discharge in the flexion period. If the limb is placed in flexion it may discharge during the extension period (Vidal et al., 1979).

In real locomotion of the chronic spinal kitten, the locomotion of one limb can be blocked by holding it in a semi-flexed position (Fig. 13A). When the hip is slowly extended to the point it normally reaches at the end of stance, a new step cycle, coordinated with the opposite limb, is initiated (Grillner and Rossignol, 1978). This appears to be a simple mechanism by which the limb may adapt to the speed of the treadmill: when it reaches a certain angle the limb starts a new swing phase. This could be controlled by receptors signaling the limb position (Grillner and Rossignol, 1978) or the unloading of extensor muscles (Pearson and Duysens, 1976;

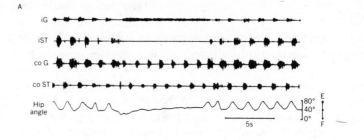

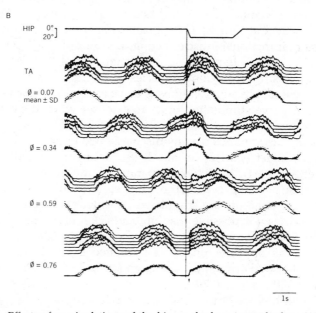

FIGURE 13. Effects of manipulations of the hip on the locomotor rhythm. (A) Emphasizes the importance of afferent input from the hip in initiating the flexor phase of locomotion. EMGs were recorded from flexor and extensor muscles of each hindlimb of a chronic spinal cat walking on a treadmill. The hip joint angle (lower trace) was continuously monitored with a Selspot system. When the ipsilateral limb was lifted and held during the stance phase, the initiation of the next flexor burst was prevented and the extensor EMG continued. A new flexion of the limb was initiated by extending the hip to the point at which swing was normally initiated in the steps preceeding this. The contralateral limb continued to walk throughout this period. (B) Records obtained from a decorticate, paralysed, and spinalized cat in which most muscles of the hindlimb were denervated and the nerves prepared to allow the fictive locomotor pattern to be recorded. The lower limb (below the knee joint) was removed and a stepping motor, attached to the distal femur, permitted ramp movements of the limb to be superimposed upon the locomotor rhythm. In the figure, ramp movements in the flexion direction were applied at four different phases of the locomotor cycle with respect to the onset of activity in TA (0.07, 0.34, 0.59, and 0.76). Each group of records shows, for each phase value, the consecutive bursts of TA-cycles, together with the associated mean and standard deviation (SD) curves obtained from the cycles shown above. A ramp movement imposed just after the onset of activity in TA (0.07) slightly increased the amplitude of the burst but shortened its duration. Later in the burst (0.34) stimulation reinforces and prolongs the TA activity. In the interburst period, stimulation may either produce a small "extra burst" (0.59), or may phase advance the next burst and thus reset the step cycle (0.76). Abbreviations: TA, tibialis anterior; G, gastrocnemius; St, semitendinosus; i, ipsilateral; co, contralateral. (A) modified from Grillner and Rossignol 1978. (B) from Andersson and Grillner, 1981.

Duysens and Pearson, 1980). Such mechanisms could be very important in the fine adjustments and coordination between limbs during turning, a situation mimicked by walking on two belts set at different speeds (Forssberg et al., 1980; see also Kulagin and Shik, 1970).

3.1.3 Phasic Stimulation

Muscle and Joint Receptors

Stretch Reflex. Stretch reflexes might be expected to play an important role in regulating the force output of different muscles during stepping. Monosynaptic reflexes elicited by stimulation of the cut dorsal root L5 and recorded in the knee extensor, vastus lateralis, and the hip flexor, iliopsoas, were modulated in amplitude during locomotion, and were largest during the period of activity of the respective muscles (Shik et al., 1966).

A detailed study of stretch reflexes was made in the decerebrate cat by Akazawa et al. (1982). One limb was denervated except for the soleus muscle which could be stretched briefly (1 mm stretch) in different parts of the cycle. The nerve to soleus could also be stimulated to evoke monosynaptic H-reflexes, thus by-passing the spindles. In agreement with the result of Shik et al. (1966), it was found that the amplitude of the stretch reflex was greatest during the muscle discharge period, and that the increase in reflex amplitude slightly led the EMG itself. Although the participation of fusimotor activity cannot be excluded (see later), it is unlikely to be the sole source of the phasic increase in the amplitude of the stretch reflex because the H-reflex was also similarly modulated.

How can this modulation be explained? It has been suggested that during fictive locomotion there might be an increase in transmission in IA pathways leading to an increase in EPSP amplitude in motoneurones and even to the appearance of polysynaptic IA EPSPs (Schomburg and Behrends, 1978a). However, a more complete study showing only small variations of IA EPSP amplitude during fictive locomotion (Shefchyk et al., 1984) suggests that the amplitude modulation of the stretch reflex can be largely explained by the cyclical modulation of the membrane potential of motoneurons. Other types of studies also indicate that there might be some presynaptic modulation of IA muscle afferent fibers from ankle extensor muscles (Bayev and Kostyuk, 1982).

Undoubtedly, the fusimotor system is active in all locomoting preparations and it must modify the gain of the stretch reflex pathways during locomotion. However, as summarized in the previous section on recordings of afferents, the pattern of fusimotor drive seems to differ from one muscle group to another, presumably in relationship to function. For instance, the secondary muscle afferents of hindlimb extensor muscles controlled by tonically firing static gamma-motoneurons would have a high sensitivity to muscle length change throughout the step cycle. On the other hand, the sensitivity of muscle spindle primaries in extensors would phasically change, being high when it would be needed in stance and low during swing, where a stretch reflex could be disruptive (Taylor et al., 1985). This is in keeping with suggestions made by Shik et al. (1966). In fact, Severin (1970) has shown that there is a reduction in EMG amplitude of the medial gastrocnemius when novocaine is applied to the nerve, before there is any block of conduction in the alpha range. However, similar experiments by Loeb and Hoffer (1985) have failed to confirm this observation.

Joint Afferents. Little is known about the effects of specific joint afferent stimulation during locomotion. Shimamura et al. (1984) reported that electrical stimulation of elbow joint afferents, through electrodes inserted in the joint cavity induced marked responses in elbow flexor muscles only when the limb reached its near-maximal extension; the effects were minimal in intermediate positions.

Entrainment. One global approach to studying the role of afferents in the control of locomotion is to perturb the whole limb during real locomotion, or to impose movements at certain joints during fictive locomotion.

In decerebrate cats, if hip flexion is delayed mechanically by blocking the limb at the onset of swing, then the onset of flexion is also delayed in the more distal joints. Similarly, if the hip flexion is accelerated during swing, knee flexion is also accelerated but ankle flexion is retarded (Orlovsky, 1972). This suggests that the timing of the program at any one joint may partly depend on signals originating from other joints. Although such intralimb coordination can be achieved by central mechanisms (as detailed in earlier sections) it is reasonable to suggest that, when present, afferents actively participate in the coordination between all the joints of a limb. Similarly, it should be recalled that locomotion of the whole limb can be blocked in the spinal cat by maintaining the hip joint in a flexed or semiflexed position, and that the locomotor pattern of the whole limb is reinitiated by extending the hip (Grillner and Rossignol, 1978). The hip afferents then appear to play a particularly important role on the overall pattern of the whole limb.

In fictive preparations (Andersson and Grillner, 1981), it was shown that ramp-formed movements imposed on the hip have different effects depending on their time of occurrence in the cycle (Fig. 13B). Ramp movements in the flexion direction, imposed in the early part of the tibialis anterior nerve activity, enhanced the amplitude but reduced its duration. The same ramp applied later, but still in the period of flexor activity, increased both its amplitude and duration. The same flexion ramp imposed in late extension tended to curtail the extension and phase-advance the next flexion phase. Thus, such flexion-directed movement will exert a positive feedback and promote the flexor activity when imposed during the flexion.

On the other hand, it will exert a negative feedback on extensors when occurring during the extension and thus will favor a phase-switching. Extension-directed ramp movements imposed in the late flexor period tended to reduce the flexor burst amplitude (negative feedback) and, when occurring somewhat later during the early part of extensor activity, tended to increase the extensor activity (positive feedback). The receptors involved are not known but are likely to be muscle or joint afferents because these effects can be obtained even after the skin has been removed.

Afferents from the hip can be powerful enough to entrain the rhythm, as was done with manual (Andersson et al., 1978b) or motor-driven sinusoidal displacements of the hip at different frequencies (Andersson and Grillner, 1983). Nerves of muscles acting at various levels, including the knee and ankle, were placed in an oil pool and arranged so as to allow the recording of the nerves while the hip was moved. The lower leg was removed below the knee. The oscillatory movements entrained the rhythm so that displacements in the flexion direction were accompanied by activity in flexors and vice versa. The recruitment order of muscles acting at the knee and ankle was kept so that the oscillation of the hip effectively influenced muscles acting below the hip and the knee. When entrained in a 1:1 coordination, the muscle bursts could increase in amplitude but were decreased at higher or lower oscillation frequencies.

Such feedback would act to adapt the central network to the peripheral events. Thus, if the the movements are slower than "expected," the efferent bursts will be longer and occur earlier; but if they proceed faster, the burst will occur somewhat earlier in the movement cycle.

Perturbations of Limb Movements in Humans. A number of studies in humans have also dealt with compensatory responses to more complex limb perturbations that may also involve the activation of receptors other than those in the limbs. In the experiments of Nashner (1980), these perturbations took the form of a disturbance of a platform incorporated in a runway. During walking, a backward acceleration or an increased dorsiflexion of the ankle, resulted in a marked increase in amplitude of activity in the ankle extensor, gastrocnemius. The amplitude of these responses, which occurred 95–110 ms after the onset of the platform movement, also varied markedly as a function of the time in stance when the disturbance was applied and were virtually absent at the end of stance. On the other hand, a forward acceleration or a plantarflexion of the ankle activated the ankle flexor, tibialis anterior. Because of the pattern of activation of certain muscles, it was suggested that these patterns represented global muscle synergies which can be incorporated in the locomotor pattern and modified by it in a phase-dependent manner. This point is particularly well developed in Forssberg (1985), who also considered other, more complex, types of corrections including anticipatory postural programs and visual corrections.

In other studies, the perturbation consists of acceleration or deceleration pulses to the treadmill or, in a sudden twitch of the triceps surae induced by tibial nerve stimulation (Dietz et al., 1984a; Berger et al., 1984). As in many other examples given before, the responses are phase-dependent. The latencies of the responses are compatible with a spinal trajectory, but the presence of early cortical potentials related to these disturbances could imply a supra-spinal contribution (Dietz et al., 1984b; Dietz et al., 1985). On the basis of ischemia experiments, these authors have suggested that group II muscle receptors are probably involved.

Cutaneous Receptors

Low Threshold Cutaneous Afferents

INTRODUCTION. Applying a brief stimulus during the rhythmical cycle, be it locomotor, respiratory, or masticatory, allows one to examine two issues. First, how do reflex responses vary as a function of time of the cycle and, second, how is the timing of the cycle changed by the reflex responses?

The responses evoked by cutaneous afferents have been most commonly examined by applying an electrical stimulation to either a cutaneous nerve or to the skin of the distal limb. Such experiments permit a thorough quantitative examination of the effects of the stimuli but have the disadvantage that the reflex responses are not evoked naturally. For this reason, we will begin this section with an examination of the responses that are evoked by a more natural stimulation of cutaneous afferents, either by means of air jets or by mechanical perturbation of a limb. Only the effects on the ipsilateral (stimulated) limb will be discussed here, as low threshold afferents affect only weakly the contralateral limb (Duysens et al., 1980; Duysens and Loeb, 1980; Rossignol and Drew, 1985).

MECHANICAL STIMULATION. Such experiments were first performed by Forssberg et al. (1975) on chronic spinal kittens walking on a treadmill. When the dorsum of one foot hit a rod, the cat moved the limb away from—and then over—the obstacle. Examination of this response in both spinal (Forssberg et al., 1975, 1976, 1977) and intact animals (Forssberg, 1979; Prochazka et al., 1978; Rossignol and Drew, 1985, 1986; Wand et al., 1980) has led to detailed descriptions of the reaction of the cat to such a stimulus. The basic mechanical response is demonstrated by the stick figures and joint angles of Figure 14A, where the movement of the limb is shown for an unstimulated cycle (1 and 3) and for the subsequent perturbed cycle (2 and 4). The initial response to the stimulus is a flexion of the knee caused by flexors, such as the semitendinosus. While the knee flexes, there is no change in the angles subtended at the hip and ankle, presumably because of a cocontraction of certain extensor muscles, such as the lateral gastrocnemius (Prochazka et al., 1978; Wand et al., 1980). The

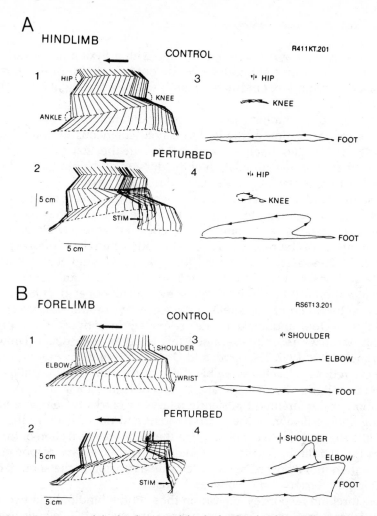

FIGURE 14. Responses of the hind- (A) and forelimbs (B) of a chronically implanted intact cat, to a mechanical perturbation applied during swing. Spots of light-reflective material were positioned over bony landmarks and the movements of the animal were recorded on video tape (60 frames/sec) using a shutter video camera. The X-Y coordinates of the spots were used to reconstruct the movement in the form of stick diagrams (1 and 2, swing phase only) or the trajectory of various spots (3 and 4, complete step cycle). Note, that since in 1 and 2 each point has been displaced relative to the preceding frame by the value of the foot displacement between two consecutive frames, that the horizontal calibration is twice that of the vertical one. The same scale was used for 3 and 4 to allow a direct comparison between the stick figures and the trajectories. Contact of the hindlimb with the rod causes a flexion principally at the knee which moves the foot above and over the obstacle (A: 2 and 4). The same stimulation at the forelimb causes not only flexion at the elbow but also a strong flexion at the shoulder which causes both the elbow and the foot to be moved above the obstacle (B: 2 and 4). In 1 and 2, the arrows pointing to the left indicate the direction of the movement of the limb. In 2, STIM indicates the exact video field on which contact with the rod was observed. In 3 and 4, the small arrows on the trajectories indicate the direction of the movement; note that the hip is fixed to zero in the X axis so that it only moves along the Y axis. All values were filtered with a moving window average of five consecutive points. From Rossignol and Drew, 1985.

result of this locking of the hip and ankle with a flexion of the knee is to move the foot away from and above the obstacle. Once in this position, the ankle and hip flex (and then extend) to bring the leg above and over the obstacle.

Although the stimulus will act on many different types of receptors, it appears that activation of the low threshold cutaneous receptors suffices to evoke this ordered sequence of activity. In the first place, Forssberg (1979) has shown that stimulation of the dorsum of the hindlimb with a jet of air causes short latency responses in knee and ankle flexors and similar movements to those described above. Second, the subcutaneous application of local anaesthetic to the dorsum of the foot abolishes the ordered mechanical response and some of the reflex responses, while decreasing the amplitude of the responses evoked in other muscles (Forssberg et al., 1975, 1977; Forssberg, 1979; Prochazka et al., 1978; Wand et al., 1980).

The responses evoked in the forelimbs by such stimuli have received scant attention until recently. A report by Matsukawa et al. (1982) showed that a perturbation of the forelimb during swing produced large changes in limb trajectory and evoked reflex responses in both triceps and biceps brachii. We have recently examined this issue in more detail (Drew and Rossignol, 1985, 1987; Rossignol and Drew, 1986) and have found that the forelimb reflexes closely ressemble those of the hindlimbs. As illustrated in Figure 14B, and by the joint angle plots of Figure 15, a mechanical perturbation of the forelimb transiently retards or blocks the elbow while inducing a hyperflexion of the shoulder joint and dorsiflexion of the wrist. This lifts the foot above the obstacle in the same way as flexion of the knee raises the hindlimb. By means of long latency secondary responses, the limb is then moved over the obstacle by an extension of the shoulder with concomitant flexion of the elbow and wrist.

The forelimb responses differ from those of the hindlimbs in two ways. First, in the forelimbs, large responses are evoked in elbow extensor muscles, such as triceps brachii, at the same latency as in flexor muscles (Fig. 15), whereas in the hindlimbs, the reflex responses occur mainly in flexor muscles. This apparent difference may be due only to the small number of extensor EMGs recorded in the hindlimbs in the earlier experiments. The second, related, difference is the strong cocontraction evident at the elbow and lacking at the knee. This is probably explained by the different anatomical arrangements of the two limbs with respect to the body, as suggested by Cabelguen et al. (1981). One should perhaps consider the shoulder to be functionally analogous to the knee and the elbow functionally analogous to the ankle, at least in locomotion (for further discussion of this point, see Drew and Rossignol, 1987).

ELECTRICAL STIMULATION. The consensus from experiments in which cutaneous afferents have been electrically stimulated during locomotion is that the evoked responses are qualitatively similar, if not identical, to those

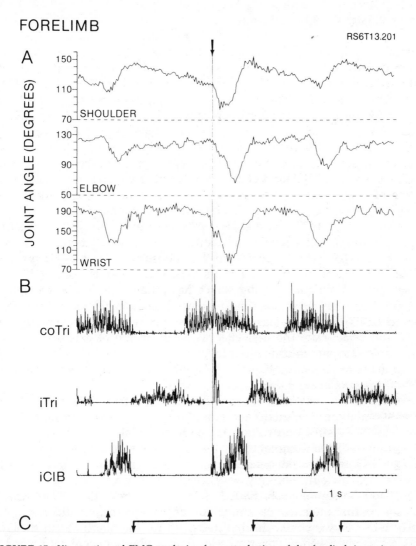

FORELIMB

RS6T13.201

FIGURE 15. Kinematic and EMG analysis of a perturbation of the forelimb in an intact cat. Angular traces and EMGs corresponding to Fig. 14b. In (A) the X-Y coordinates of the points were used to reconstruct the angular movements of the shoulder, elbow, and wrist. Three continuous cycles are displayed. The thin vertical line indicates the moment when the foot briefly made contact with the metal rod. Flexion is indicated by a downward deflection of the traces. Note that the initial effect of the perturbation is a hyperflexion of the shoulder together with retardment of elbow flexion and wrist ventroflexion. (B) shows simultaneously recorded and synchronized EMGs from ipsilateral elbow flexor (iClB) and extensor (iTri) muscles and from a contralateral elbow extensor (coTri). Note the short latency burst evoked in both iClB and iTri by the stimulation, and the somewhat longer latency response in coTri. In (C) the duty graph indicates the periods of contact of the ipsilateral foot with the belt (stance, solid line). Downward and upward arrows indicate respectively, the moment of contact and lift of the foot. Abbreviations: ClB, cleidobrachialis; Tri, Triceps brachii, long head; i, ipsilateral; co, contralateral. From Rossignol and drew, 1985.

produced by mechanical stimulation. For instance, weak electrical stimulation during swing of either the skin of the dorsum of the cat hindlimb (Abraham et al., 1985; Duysens and Loeb, 1980; Forssberg et al., 1976, 1977; Rossignol et al., 1986; Forssberg 1979; Prochazka et al., 1978; Wand et al., 1980) or of the cutaneous nerves which innervate this region (Duysens, 1977b) leads to a well-ordered and repeatable sequence of events. As with mechanical stimulation, there is early activation of the knee flexors, such as the semitendinosus (mean latency 9–10 ms; Forssberg et al., 1976, 1977; Forssberg, 1979; Wand et al., 1980) together with a slightly later activation of ankle flexors, such as the tibialis anterior (Duysens and Loeb, 1980; Forssberg, 1979; Wand et al., 1980), and occasionally ankle extensors (Prochazka et al., 1978; Wand et al., 1980). The flexor muscles, such as the semitendinosus, often display a second response at a latency of 25 ms (Forssberg, 1979). The longest latency responses (mean of 28–33 ms) are seen in muscles acting at the hip (Forssberg et al., 1976, Forssberg, 1979).

A similar stimulation during stance has little effect. In chronic spinal kittens, there may be strong, short-latency excitatory responses in extensors (circa 10–15 ms; see Fig. 6B in Forssberg et al., 1977) while in decerebrate and intact cats, the first effect is an inhibition of extensor activity (latency 10–15 ms) which is often followed by an excitation at latencies of 25–35 ms (Duysens and Stein, 1978; Duysens and Loeb, 1980; Forssberg, 1979; Prochazka et al., 1978).

As with mechanical stimulation little is known about the effects of electrical stimulation of forelimb afferents during locomotion. Studies in the decerebrate walking preparation (Halbertsma et al., 1976; Miller et al., 1977) reported that stimulation of the skin overlying the dorsum of the forepaw evoked phase-dependent responses in antagonistic muscles acting at the elbow joint. Recently, we have undertaken a more detailed study (Drew and Rossignol, 1985, 1987; Rossignol and Drew, 1985, 1986) which has shown that the effect of stimulation of the superficial radial nerve on flexor muscles was similar to that described for the hindlimbs in that responses were evoked in flexor muscles only when they were naturally active in the locomotor cycle (Fig. 16). However, as with the mechanical stimulation, differences were observed with respect to the extensor muscles. Stimulation during swing, at best evoked only very small, short-latency effects in extensors of the hindlimbs (Forssberg, 1979; Prochazka et al., 1978; Wand et al., 1980) whereas, as shown in Figure 16, in the forelimb, elbow extensors are strongly excited at times when they are quiescent in the locomotor cycle (Drew and Rossignol, 1985). Notably, the same stimulus during stance, when the extensors are normally active, failed to evoke any short-latency excitation, but, rather elicited an inhibition of activity which was often followed by excitation (Drew and Rossignol, 1985; 1987). These responses are not dependent on movement and can also be recorded in the paralyzed animal, although the relative amplitude of each response does not vary exactly in the same way as in the intact animal (Cabelguen et al., 1981; Saltiel et al., 1986).

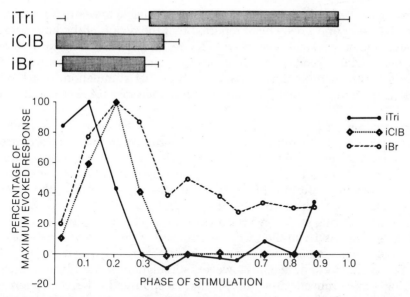

FIGURE 16. Responses in forelimb muscles of an intact cat to electrical stimulation of a cutaneous nerve during locomotion. The amplitude of the responses to stimulation of the superficial radial nerve (3.2XT) are plotted as a function of the phase of the step cycle in which the stimulus was applied. To quantify the excitatory responses elicited in different periods of the step cycle, the EMG activity was averaged, and those areas surpassing 90% of the average background level were integrated. These responses (n = 114) were expressed as a percentage of the maximal response amplitude observed in any one muscle. Each point corresponds to the mean amplitude of 6–17 responses. The shaded rectangles above the graph indicate the mean duration ($\pm$ 1SD) of the locomotor EMG burst of each muscle taken from 30 to 45 control cycles. Abbreviations: Tri, triceps brachii, long head; ClB, cleidobrachialis; Br, brachialis; i, ipsilateral. From Drew and Rossignol, 1985.

Unfortunately, similar experiments on human subjects are rare (see Forssberg, 1985). A report by Nashner et al. (1979) indicates that, during stepping-like movements on two platforms that can be alternately moved in the vertical direction, responses elicited by weak electrical stimulation of the dorsum of the foot in humans elicited flexor responses during the up-going movement and extensor responses during the down-going movements. A short report by Kanda and Sato (1983) shows that the responses obtained to a nonnoxious stimulation of the sural nerve, applied at different times in the step cycle while the subject was stepping on the spot, are similar to those found in cats. The hamstrings showed no responses during early stance but were inhibited and, subsequently, excited by a stimulation applied in late stance. The same stimulation in swing sometimes excited them at short latency (L = 50 ms). The quadriceps femoris did not respond during swing, but stimulation during stance evoked a similar inhibition and excitation to that seen in the hamstrings.

The effect of the location of the electrical stimulation (with respect to the dorsal or ventral surface of the foot, for example) on the reflex effects is relatively little studied and the few results available are rather contradictory. Duysens and Loeb (1980) reported that the region of the limb stimulated made only a small difference to the reflex responses evoked. Indeed, the only real difference was a tendency for a short-latency excitation of the medial gastrocnemius during stance with plantar stimulation, which was lacking with the stimulation of anterior skin margins (see also Abraham et al., 1985).

In our own experiments on the forelimb (Rossignol and Drew, 1986), stimulation to the plantar and dorsal surfaces of the forepaw produced very different effects. In particular, the lowest threshold responses (during swing) to dorsum stimulation were the activation of the wrist dorsiflexors and activation of the brachialis, while to plantar stimulation the lowest threshold effects were activation of wrist and digit ventroflexors. Dorsum stimulation during stance evoked no response in the wrist dorsiflexors and inhibited the activity of the triceps brachii and of the wrist ventroflexors, a situation analogous to that seen in the hindlimbs (Duysens and Loeb, 1980; Abraham et al., 1985). However, stimulation of the plantar surface during stance caused large short-latency responses in the ventroflexors, which were of the same latency and amplitude as those evoked during swing (see Fig. 4 of Rossignol and Drew, 1986). There was no activation of shoulder or elbow extensors during stance, and the elbow flexors were activated much more weakly during swing by plantar stimulation than by dorsum stimulation (unpublished observations). It would seem that such differences should not be unexpected and that the question of local sign in the hindlimb could be usefully reinvestigated.

The ensemble results from this section show some of the ways in which afferent inputs may be modulated according to the time in the step cycle in which a stimulus is delivered. The major, and most universal, finding is that a stimulation will generally evoke excitatory responses in flexor muscles when the stimulation is applied during the swing phase of locomotion, but may evoke a mixture of excitatory and inhibitory responses in extensor muscles when applied during stance. These reflex responses are probably relayed through several different pathways, as is evidenced by the different latencies of the responses. For example, flexor muscles may be excited at 10 or 25 ms; while extensor muscles may be either excited or inhibited at 10 ms and excited at 25–35 ms. The relative excitability of each pathway may also depend on the type of preparation. Finally, it should be emphasized that maximal short-latency reflex responses in certain muscles (e.g., the lateral gastrocnemius and triceps brachii) are evoked at different times from their period of activation by the central pattern generator, according to the reflex requirements of the animal.

EFFECT ON LOCOMOTOR RHYTHM.   The effect of mechanical or low threshold electrical stimulation on the locomotor rhythm is again dependent upon the phase of the step cycle in which the stimulus is delivered. Forssberg et al. (1976, 1977) showed that an electrical stimulation of the dorsum of the foot of the chronic spinal cat during flexion (F) increased the step cycle by about 100 ms (normal cycle duration 1–1.2 s), while stimulation in early to mid-stance (E_2 and early E_3) had no effect on cycle duration, even though there were large changes in the EMG amplitude and in joint angles. Stimuli given during E_1 and late E_3 were the most potent; the former caused a prolongation of the step cycle, while the latter shortened it by about 200 ms.

Similar large changes in cycle duration were observed by Duysens (Duysens and Pearson, 1976; Duysens 1977a; Duysens and Stein, 1978) in decerebrate animals. Low threshold cutaneous stimulation during swing of either the plantar skin, the foot pad, or of the posterior tibial nerve increased flexor EMG amplitude and duration, as well as the overall cycle duration. The same stimulation during stance increased extensor EMG amplitude and duration and again also increased cycle duration. It was also reported that the increased duration of the swing or stance phases of locomotion were proportionately greater than those of the overall cycle duration due to a shortening of the subsequent phase. For example, a stimulus which, applied during flexion, prolonged the swing phase would shorten the following period of stance.

Electrical stimulation applied to the skin or nerves of the hindlimb of chronically implanted, intact animals was less effective in causing changes in the step cycle. Forssberg (1979) showed that electrical stimulation of the dorsum only evoked significant changes in cycle duration when applied during swing. A similar finding was reported by Duysens and Stein (1978) for stimulation of the posterior tibial nerve, which increased flexor muscle and swing duration, but had little effect on overall cycle duration because the subsequent stance period was shortened. Weak stimulation of other hindlimb nerves, such as the sural and common peroneal, were also without marked effect on the composition of the locomotor cycle and rhythm.

Again, little information is available concerning the effect of forelimb afferents on the step cycle. Matsukawa et al., (1982) studied the effects of a mechanical perturbation of the forelimb in decerebrate and intact cats. They reported that stimulation during stance shortened the duration of that period by about 10%, whereas stimulation during swing increased its duration by up to 55%. No data on the total cycle duration was given.

In our own experiments, we have examined the effects of both mechanical and electrical stimulation on the step cycle (Drew and Rossignol, 1987). The effects of a mechanical perturbation of the forelimb during the swing phase were studied with respect to the timing of the EMG and to the timing of the swing and stance phases. Such stimuli markedly increased the duration of brachialis and lengthened the swing phase by about 10%. The subsequent stance phase was shortened by about the same amount so that the overall duration of the step cycle was unchanged. Electrical stimuli also provoked increases in the brachialis duration when applied during swing, again without changes in step cycle duration. Electrical stimulation during stance caused no significant change in EMG or cycle timing.

Nociceptive Afferents

The short latency effects of a noxious stimulation of the limbs during locomotion have been little examined: for this reason the effects of the rhythm on the stimulus and the effects of the stimulus on the rhythm will be combined into one section.

As described above, low intensity stimulation of the distal skin of the hindlimb in the intact animal prolonged swing by activating flexor muscles, but caused little change in the stance period, even though excitatory responses were evoked in extensor muscles (Forssberg 1979). When a noxious stimulus was applied in the same animal and in the same locus, the stimulation during swing increased both the EMG amplitude and the flexion of the limb. Noxious stimulation during stance evoked a large, short-latency activation of flexor muscles which caused the foot to be raised prematurely from the treadmill belt. This occurred at the same time as the unstimulated, contralateral limb was being transferred forwards. Thus, there was also a concommitant and premature placement of this limb to prevent falling. These responses caused widespread disruption of the locomotor rhythm and the animal did not recover its normal pattern of activity for another 2 or 3 cycles. It seems that under these circumstances, the priority for the animal is to avoid the stimulus rather than to maintain the locomotor rhythm.

A similar finding was made by Duysens (1977a and 1977b) in spontaneously walking, premammillary cats in which the stimulated limb was fixed in position. A strong electrical stimulus (75 times T) of the tibial or sural nerves caused a prolongation of the activity of flexor muscles when applied during swing and curtailed the activity of extensor muscles when applied during stance. Such stimuli also caused large changes in the step cycle duration; in general, stimulation during the swing phase and early stance shortened the step cycle while stimulation in mid or late stance lengthened it (Duysens 1977b).

As Gauthier and Rossignol (1981) demonstrated, strong noxious stimulation of a pure cutaneous nerve (superficial peroneal) in a decerebrate cat which is free to move all four limbs evoked well-coordinated responses on both sides of the body. In spinal and decerebrate cats (Gauthier and Rossignol 1981; Rossignol et al., 1981a, 1981b), stimulation during ipsilateral swing augments and prolongs the ipsilateral flexors and the contralateral extensor muscles, while stimulation during ipsilateral stance curtails the activity of the extensors of the stimulated side and prolongs the activity in contralateral flexors. Similar findings were made in acute spinal and paralyzed cats pretreated with L-dopa and nialamide, showing that a great part of the transmission is due to central mechanisms although, for these contralateral reflexes, there also appears to be a contribution from peripheral mechanisms (Rossignol et al., 1981 a, b)

There is little information on the responses evoked in human subjects by noxious stimuli. An early study by Lisin et al. (1973) showed that the amplitude of the reflex response evoked in the tibialis anterior by a strong stimulation of the sural nerve with the subject at rest, was decreased when the same stimulation was applied during the stance period of locomotion. Interestingly, in hemiparetic patients, although the response at rest was the same as in normal subjects, stimulation during stance evoked responses in extensor muscles and not in flexors. Belanger and Patla (1984) have reported that strong stimulation delivered through a copper ring on the second toe at different times during the step cycle evokes flexor responses during swing and some extensor responses during stance. Stimulation of the sural nerve in humans also yields phase-dependent responses in extensor and flexor muscles acting at the knee joint (Crenna and Frigo, 1984).

3.2   Respiration

3.2.1   Tonic Stimulation

The tonic activation of chemoreceptors, thermoreceptors, and baroreceptors influences the characteristics of the respiratory pattern and constitutes the basis of the homeostatic role played by the respiratory system. The details of these homeostatic control mechanisms, even though they implicate the activation of peripheral and central receptors, are considered to be out of the scope of this review, although the phasic activation of these receptors is treated in the next section. However, the work of von Euler et al. (1970) represented in Figure 12 shows how increasing CO_2 leads to an increase in breathing frequency (Fig. 12D) as well as an increase in tidal volume (Fig. 12C). Likewise, changes in temperature will cause an upward shift in these functions (Fig. 12C and D) so that the respiratory volume and the respiratory frequency will be both higher for a given CO_2 level.

3.2.2   Phasic Stimulation

Inflation and Deflation Reflexes

During Inspiration. When the lungs are inflated to a certain volume during the inspiration phase, inspiration is abruptly terminated and expiration initiated (the Breuer-Hering reflex: Head, 1889; Adrian, 1933). This control of inspiration duration by the PSRs has been extensively studied using well-defined lung inflations at different times after the onset of inspiration as detected from the integrated activity of the phrenic nerve (Clark and von Euler, 1972; Larrabee and Hodes, 1948; Cohen, 1975; Feldman and Gautier, 1976). Inflation volumes needed to terminate inspiration

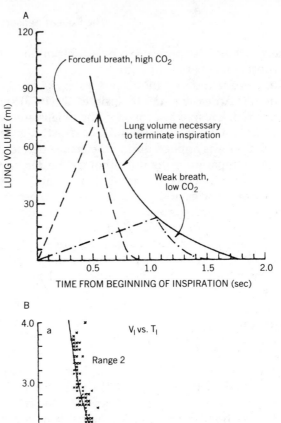

A

LUNG VOLUME (ml)

Forceful breath, high CO_2

Lung volume necessary
to terminate inspiration

Weak breath,
low CO_2

120

90

60

30

0.5   1.0   1.5   2.0

TIME FROM BEGINNING OF INSPIRATION (sec)

B

4.0

a V_I vs. T_I

Range 2

3.0

2.0

1.0

Range 1

1.0   2.0   3.0   4.0

sec

FIGURE 17. Relationship between tidal volume and respiratory frequency. (A) Lung volume threshold depends on the time from onset of inspiration. In a normal breath inspiration is terminated when the activity from PSRs reaches a certain threshold level. With increased CO_2 the diaphragm contracts more forcefully and more rapidly. This causes an increased tidal volume and the inspiration reaches the threshold lung volume earlier, and thus results in an increased respiratory rate. When CO_2 is decreased, the lung volume threshold is reached much later in the inspiration and respiratory rate is thus decreased. (B) In humans there are two distinct ranges (1 and 2). With a low respiratory drive, small increases in lung volume change only the tidal volume (range 1). Further increases in lung volume cause a shift into range 2 where the control of respiration is as shown in part A, ie. increases in CO_2 decrease the duration of the inspiration and increase the tidal volume. (A) from Wyman, 1977. (B) from Clark and von Euler, 1972.

252

depend on the time of inflation in relation to the onset of the inspiration phase. Early in inspiration, small volumes do not significantly affect the duration of the period of inspiration although large volumes may suddenly terminate inspiration and initiate expiration. Later on, during the inspiration period, progressively smaller volumes suffice to terminate inspiration.

The lung volume at which inspiration is terminated varies as an hyperbolic function (Fig. 17A) of time after the onset of inspiration (Clark and von Euler, 1972).

Because of the fact that the slope of integrated phrenic activity does not change when the PSRs are activated (Fig. 12A and later) but terminates abruptly at a certain threshold it was suggested that the negative afferent feedback operated through a trigger mechanism. Since the amount of PSR activation needed to trigger this mechanism decreases with time (Fig. 17A), it was suggested that the peripheral input from PSRs as well as the central inspiratory drive (from medullary neurons) converge on interneurons (the so-called R-beta neurons in the nucleus of the solitary tract) which would, in turn, trigger an "off-switch mechanism" terminating the inspiration phase. Furthermore, the threshold of this off-switch mechanism can be modified by the pneumotaxic center (the nucleus parabrachialis medialis and Kolliker-Fuse complex) and by respiratory drive (details of these models are given in Cohen and Feldman, 1977; von Euler, 1985).

In humans, the respiratory time-volume relationship, i.e., the curve relating the frequency of breathing and the tidal volume, has two distinct ranges (Fig. 17B). In range 1, the respiratory volumes vary below the threshold level at which PSRs play a significant role. This normal shallow breathing rate, controlled essentially by central mechanisms, is set at a more or less fixed frequency. This range 1 can also be seen in cats under urethane anesthesia but not pentobarbitone except when the animals are vagotomized. Range 2 is the hyperbolic relationship already described above and can only be seen when the afferents are intact. In this range the tidal volumes attain the threshold values at which the PSRs become operative.

Thus, in the respiratory system, a low respiratory drive (low CO_2) can induce small variations in tidal volumes without significantly changing the frequency (range 1). This can be achieved by central mechanisms because the lung volumes needed to meet the demand are below the threshold values at which PSRs are effective. With a high respiratory drive (high CO_2), the large volumes needed to meet the ventilation requirements reach the volume threshold and, therefore, in this situation (range 2), the afferents play an essential role in optimizing the rate and depth of breathing, perhaps to minimize energy expenditure (von Euler et al., 1970).

Positive feedback effects have also been described with inflation occurring during inspiration. Initially known as Head's paradoxical reflex, it was obtained when the vagi nerves were warmed after having been cooled, and these excitatory inspiratory responses were initially considered as artifacts (see Paintal, 1973). Larrabee and Knowlton (1946) showed that inflations of increasing magnitude induced progressively larger inhibition (negative feedback) of the phrenic motoneurones recorded in phrenic nerve filaments. At inflation volumes greater than 50 ml an excitatory component was also evoked, breaking through that inhibition for a short period. Because of the somewhat larger inflation volumes needed to evoke this effect, this reflex was not thought to be operative in eupneic conditions.

More recently, however, it was found that volumes of lung inflation even smaller than those of eupneic conditions could facilitate inspiratory activity (Dimarco et al., 1980, 1981; Fig. 18A). This low-threshold facilitatory reflex is completely abolished by cervical vagotomy and can be mimicked by electrical stimulation of the vagus nerve. Finally, it is more sensitive to anesthesia than the Breuer-Hering reflex, perhaps one of the main reasons why it was missed for so long. This reflex, originating from vagal afferents, is graded in amplitude with the inflation volumes used. However, its responsiveness does not vary with inspiration time, contrary to its inhibitory counterpart (the Breuer-Hering reflex), so it is presumably not transmitted through the previously mentioned R-beta neurons. It is postulated that the same PSRs are involved in mediating the negative and the positive feedback reflexes. The specific role of this reflex could be to determine the relative contribution of different inspiratory muscle groups since the external intercostal motoneurons are more facilitated than phrenic motoneurons.

Expiration. If the lungs are inflated during expiration, the expiration phase is prolonged and, consequently, the next inspiration is delayed (Fig. 18B). This component of the Breuer-Hering reflex also varies in a phase-dependent manner, i.e., the prolongation effect gets larger as the expiration phase progresses. This is true up to about 70% of the cycle. Lung inflations produced in the last 30% of the cycle, even if they are 3 times larger than eupneic volumes, are ineffective (Knox, 1973; Fig. 18B) as if inspiration was then inevitable.

Lung deflation reflexes, presumed to result at least in part from the activation of irritant receptors (see Paintal, 1973; earlier sections of this Chapter) are also phase-dependent. Deflations applied during inspiration will prolong I (see Koller and Ferrel, 1970), whereas deflations in the first 85% of the expiration phase will shorten expiration (Knox, 1973). Whether or not this reflex is used during eupnoea is not clear (Koller and Ferrel, 1970).

Since vagal stretch receptors have such powerful influences, it is to be expected that periodic lung inflations in paralyzed animals would entrain

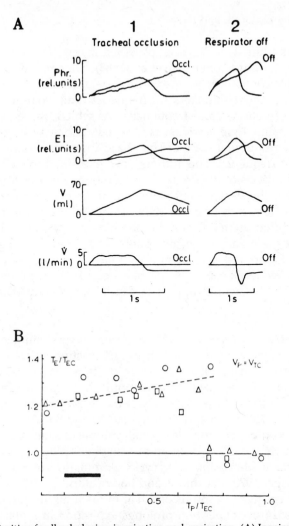

FIGURE 18. Positive feedback during inspiration and expiration. (A) Inspiration facilitating, and "off-switch" effects, of volume related feedback obtained in a spontaneously breathing cat (1) and in a paralysed animal ventilated by a servo-respirator (2). Superimposed records with and without volume changes. In 1, volume changes were prevented by tracheal occlusions (occl) and, in 2, by switching off the servo-respirator (off). From above: Phrenic activity (Phr), external intercostal activity (EI), volume (V), and airflow (V̇). Computer averaged records ($n = 5$). In the presence of lung expansion, the rate of rise of the inspiratory activity is facilitated (positive feedback) and the inspiratory duration is shortened (negative feedback). (B) shows expiratory prolongation produced by small lung inflations in three lightly anesthetised cats. The pulses had durations of 0.2 s (as approximately indicated by the heavy bar) and were of control tidal volume size, VTC. Points were obtained by averaging groups of two to nine individual data points, and the dashed line represents a linear regression on these points. The results show that expiration is prolonged by inflations given during the first 73% of the expiratory phase but that inflations given later are ineffective so that the next inspiration arrives at the predicted time. Abbreviations: T_{EC} expiratory duration during control cycle; TE, expiratory duration in following cycle when lung inflation applied. T_p/T_{EC} gives the phase of the stimulation with respect to the expiratory portion of the cycle. (A) from Dimarco et al, 1981; (B) from Knox, 1973.

the central rhythm. This has been observed many times but has been best quantified in the study of Petrillo et al. (1983). They found that the phrenic nerve activity could be entrained in different simple or complex ratios, depending on the parameters of frequency and volume utilized. The boundaries of volumes and frequencies for which phase-locked entrainment was obtained were widest for the 1:1 ratio, which constituted the most stable entrainment regime. The phase angle of entrainment varied as a function of frequency. The authors have explained this entrainment by the different aspects of the Breuer-Hering reflex since the entrainment disappears when the vagi are cut. With entrainment frequencies below the spontaneous frequency (measured by turning off the pump for one cycle), the lung inflation occurs during the phrenic activity and inhibits it. When the frequency is greater than the spontaneous one, the lung inflation arrives in expiration and prolongs it. No mention is made of the possibility that positive feedback could also participate in such entrainment phenomena, although this would appear a distinct possibility (Dimarco et al., 1981).

Baroreceptor and Chemoreceptor Reflexes. Several studies have shown that chemoreceptor as well as baroreceptor stimulation causes phase-dependent effects. The initial interest in studying brief phasic stimulation of chemoreceptors was that this could mimic the naturally occurring phasic variation of pH level at the frequency of the respiratory rhythm (see, however, Purves, 1979). Black and Torrance (1971) and Band et al. (1970) found that chemoreceptor activation by a small volume of saline equilibrated with 100% CO_2 increased either inspiration or expiration depending on the time of application in the respiratory cycle. Stimulation of the carotid sinus nerve (Eldridge, 1972a) or the carotid body (Eldridge, 1972b) increases inspiration when given in the second half of inspiration. Stimulation of the same nerves during expiration prolongs expiration in a phase-dependent manner up to 80% of the expiratory phase (Eldridge, 1976). These responses are typical examples of stimuli which exert excitatory effects in both phases and thus would serve to promote or stabilize each individual phase.

On the other hand, how this end result is achieved is undoubtedly complex. Indeed, Lipski et al. (1977) have shown that both R-alpha and R-beta cells in the nucleus tractus solitarius are excited by carotid body stimulation during inspiration. However, when these cells are made to fire during expiration, either by inflating the lungs or by iontophoretically injecting glutamate, the carotid body input exerts an inhibitory effect. Thus, as is the case for lung inflation during expiration, there must be separate pathways carrying the peripheral receptor inputs to the different types of motoneurons responsible for each phase, and these pathways must be differentially controlled.

3.3   Mastication

3.3.1   *Tonic Stimulation*

Tonic stimulation of afferents has potent effects on both the initiation and control of mastication. Bremer (1923), for example, showed that mastication in the decerebrate rabbit can be initiated by touching the teeth, and that the exact pattern of chewing depending upon the region of the buccal cavity which was stimulated. In anesthetised rats, van Willigen and Weijs-Boot (1984) have shown that mastication can be initiated by a long-lasting mechanical stimulation of the hard palate. In decerebrate, or lightly anesthetized rabbits, distension of the mouth by a balloon is sufficient to induce mastication. With deeper anesthesia, distension needs to be coupled to subthreshold stimulation of certain effective CNS sites (Lund and Dellow, 1971). Similarly, in anesthetised cats, cortical stimulation which is subthreshold for the initiation of mastication when given alone, evokes regular masticatory movements when coupled with tonic depression of the lower jaw (Nakamura et al, 1976). Tonic stimulation of afferents may not only aid in the initiation of mastication, but may also exert inhibitory effects. Lund and Dellow (1971) have shown, for example, that strong pinching of the forelimbs and rectal distension are both capable of inhibiting mastication.

Tonic stimulation may also cause marked changes in an already extant masticatory rhythm. Thus, light pressure on the labial surface of a maxillary incisor changes the pattern of chewing so that wide lateral excursions precede each opening phase. In the paralyzed cat, if the mandible is tonically depressed during mastication evoked by stimulation of the cortex, there is an increase in the amplitude of the rhythmical efferent activity and an acceleration of the masticatory rhythm (Nakamura et al., 1976). These effects were attributed to the stretch of masseter spindles and not to periodontal receptors since stimulation of the latter has no effect when the jaw is not depressed. In the guinea pig, a recent report has shown that the loading of the mandible increased the amplitude of the jaw closing muscle EMG, but did not affect the frequency of the rhythm even though the duration of the masseter burst was increased (Chandler et al., 1985). It is possible that this difference is due to the fact that the latter study examined spontaneous rhythmical jaw movements while Nakamura examined cortically induced mastication.

3.3.2   *Phasic Stimulation*

The results from stimulating cutaneous afferents from the jaws during different phases of the mastication cycle resemble very closely those obtained in the other systems. As cutaneous afferents from the limbs influence the motor output differently in the various phases of the step cycle, so affer-

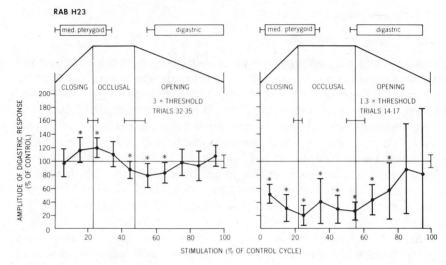

FIGURE 19. Phase dependency of the responses evoked in the digastric muscle by high and low threshold electrical stimulation of the gingiva during mastication. The amplitude of the responses (expressed as a percentage of the control values) are plotted against the time in the masticatory cycle when the stimulation was given (expressed as a percentage of the normalised control cycle) for stimulation at $3 \times T$ in (A) and $1.3 \times T$ in (B). With electrical stimulation at $3 \times T$ the largest responses in the digastric muscle were obtained during jaw closing, while for the low threshold stimulation ($1.3 \times T$) the largest responses were obtained during jaw opening. Note that the amplitude of the responses obtained with stimulation at $1.3 \times T$ was less than that of the control levels for all phases of the masticatory cycle (control values represented by the horizontal line; $\pm 1SD$). Vertical lines (± 1 SD) mark the end of closing and the beginning of jaw opening; the occlusal phase is between. The periods in which the medial pterygoid and digastric muscles were active in the control cycle are shown by the open rectangles (± 1 SD) and a simplified trace of the movement is shown above. Asterisks (*) indicate significant deviations from control ($P<0.05$). From Lund et al. 1981.

ents from the face excite the jaw opener and closer muscles in specific phases of the masticatory cycle.

This was first shown by Chase and McGinty (1970) who examined the effects of chewing (evoked by stimulation of the orbital gyrus) on the amplitude of the digastric and masseteric reflexes evoked by stimulation of the inferior alveolar nerve. It was found that the amplitude of the digastric reflex was facilitated (with respect to the control) during jaw opening and inhibited during jaw closure. The reverse was observed for the masseteric reflex, namely, facilitation during jaw closure and inhibition during opening.

More detailed experiments in both the anesthetized rabbit (Lund and Rossignol, 1981; Lund et al., 1981, 1983) and the intact cat (Lund et al., 1984) have shown that the modulation of the reflex pathway from cutaneous afferents of the jaw to the digastric muscles depends critically on both the strength of the stimulation and the phase of the masticatory cycle in which the stimulus is applied (Fig. 19). With low strength, nonnoxious stimulation of the gingiva or hard palate, the amplitude of the reflex evoked in the digastric muscle was largest during the phase of jaw opening and smallest during the period of jaw closing. In all cases, the reflex was smaller during chewing than that evoked when the rabbit was at rest. Such a reflex organization might provide a positive feedback signal which would tend to accelerate the opening of the mouth. However, if the strength of the stimulation was increased so as to activate high threshold afferents, then the amplitude of the digastric reflex was now maximal during the phase of jaw closure, and was sometimes larger than during the control, pre-masticatory period. Assocciated with the large excitatory digastric response, the stimulus caused a strong inhibition of masseter activity that had an average duration of 50 ms. At the transition from opening to closing, the stimulation was sometimes potent enough to completely abolish the jaw closing burst (Lund et al., 1981).

It should also be emphasized that this modulation of reflex activity is not dependent on the phasic afferent feedback produced by the mastication. Lund et al. (1983) have shown that qualitatively the same phasic modulation is obtained in the fictive rabbit preparation in which all phasic feedback is prevented by curarization, showing that the modulatory mechanisms are central in origin (see also Olsson et al., 1986).

The importance of the JOR is probably in protecting the soft tissues of the mouth during chewing when a particularly painful stimulus would necessitate a rapid jaw opening at a time of the cycle when the opening muscles are inactive. This out-of-phase reflex is very similar to that observed in the elbow extensor muscles of the forelimbs, which are also activated out of phase in order to serve the requisite locking of the elbow needed to negotiate the unexpected impediment to the flexion of the limb (see Fig. 15).

Effects on the Masticatory Rhythm. Such stimuli, as in locomotion, caused not only short latency reflex effects in muscles of the jaw, but also produce changes in the duration of the masticatory cycle. As Lund et al. (1981, 1983) have shown, although a low strength stimulus has minimal effects on the masticatory cycle, a stronger stimulus can effect both the opening and closure phases of the cycle. Briefly, a stimulus which arrives during the occlusal or opening phase of the cycle will either delay the time of onset of activity in the digastric muscle or will prolong its duration. In either case, the duration of the occlusal or opening phases is increased, as is the cycle duration. The same stimulus applied during jaw closing increases the activity in the digastric muscles and inhibits the activity of the masseter muscles, thus curtailing this period of activity and shortening the cycle.

More natural stimulation can also cause large changes in EMG amplitude and duration as well as in the pattern of the cycle. When a hard

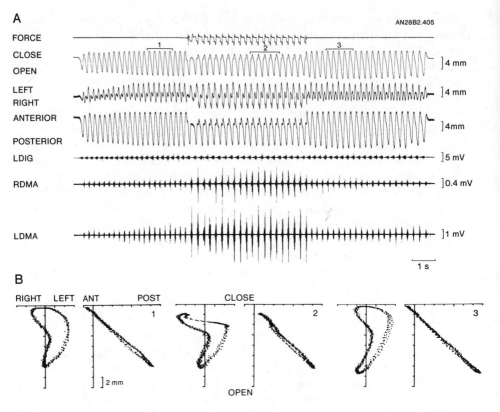

FIGURE 20. Spontaneous rhythmical mastication obtained from an anesthetized rabbit before, during, and after the insertion of a hard object between its teeth. (A) The traces show from top to bottom, the force measured from a strain gauge on the steel ball, the output of a phototransducer which permitted the movement of the lower jaw to be recorded in all three planes: close/open, left/right and anterior/posterior, and the EMGs recorded from opener, digastric (DIG), and closer, deep masseter (DMA), muscles of the jaw. The time when the object was introduced is shown by the downward deflections of the force transducer. The ball obstructed the closing of the teeth and caused a marked deviation of the teeth to the right as well as a markedly increased amplitude of activity in the jaw closer muscles. (B) plots the trajectory of the phototransducer which was attached to the lower jaw and shows in detail the lateral deviation caused by the ball (2) compared to the previous (1) and subsequent (3) periods of activity. from Lavigne et al., in press.

object, such as a steel ball, is introduced between the teeth, there is sometimes a jaw opening reflex (together with inhibition of the closer muscles)
when the object first strikes the teeth. Thereafter, the JOR appears to be
suppressed. Contact with the ball now markedly increases the amplitude
of jaw closing muscles and significantly prolongs the slow closure phase
(see Fig. 20). Thus, the presence of an object between the teeth radically
alters the chewing frequency. As can be seen from Figure 20, it also
changes the pattern of chewing movements which is now characterized by
large sideways movements—the type of movements needed to grind hard
pieces of food. When the sensory nerves to the maxillary and mandibular
molar teeth were cut, most of these adaptive responses were much reduced.

One study, involving electrical stimulation of cutaneous afferents, has
been performed in humans (Hannam and Lund, 1981) but it examined
only the effects on the cycle duration. Low threshold stimulation had very
little effect on the cycle duration as was found for the animal experiments.
High threshold stimulation on the other hand was found to increase the
duration of the cycle, but only if given during the phase of jaw closing.

4   SUMMING UP: ROLES, ANALOGIES, AND MODEL

4.1   Analogies and Differences

From the review of the literature on afferent recordings, deafferentation,
and afferent stimulation, a number of analogies and differences can be
outlined which may help to better define the roles played by afferent feedback in any one of the three systems which were examined, and which
may be usefully extended to the others.

Some of these analogies in control mechanisms have already been
drawn for locomotion and respiration (Grillner, 1977, 1979b; Feldman and
Grillner, 1983; von Euler, 1981; Cohen, 1981) and for locomotion and mastication (Lund and Rossignol, 1980; Lund et al., 1981, 1984; Lund and Olsson, 1983).

4.1.1   Rhythmical Patterns Generated in Absence of Afferent Feedback

The first analogy between the systems is that the basic pattern of all these
rhythmical processes can occur, sometimes with a surprising amount
of complexity, in the absence of afferent feedback. The evidence for
this comes both from curarization experiments, in which there are no
movement-related afferent feedback signals, as well as from experiments
in which the afferent systems are removed by deafferentation or denerva-
tion. The generality of this observation was best reviewed by Delcomyn
(1980) for different systems. That these rhythmical processes do occur in

such conditions certainly suggests that they are generated in the central nervous system by sets of specially wired neuronal networks which have been called central pattern generators (CPGs).

It is important to know as much as possible about the nature of these CPGs as their behavior represents, more or less, the operation of the system in open-loop conditions. It also helps to clarify which components of the system are of purely central origin—or built into the system—and which are due to afferent feedback mechanisms. The issue of whether or not a particular feature of the output pattern depends essentially on the presence of some afferent system has sometimes overshadowed the, perhaps more important point, that the output of the systems in open-loop situations does not predict the output in closed-loop conditions. Indeed, looking at a system with and without afferent feedback is really looking at a system operating in two radically different modes. In the *open-loop* mode, the system is internally calibrated from data that have been incorporated in neural elements as a result of evolution and learning. In the *closed-loop* mode, the system is continuously recalibrated (adapted) by feedback so that it can work with more accuracy, more stability, and with a greater range of frequencies (bandwith). It is thus adapted to take into account the non-linearities of the motor system and the continuously changing conditions in which the movements have to be executed.

Open-loop operation might be sufficient in some undemanding conditions, such as walking on an infinitely smooth surface, chewing gum, or breathing quietly. However, closed-loop operation is essential when there are demands to change the frequency of the pattern, or the timing of elements within the pattern, or when the amplitude of the movement (depth of breath, step length, mouth opening) must be altered to accommodate particular demands. It is also necessary when the coordination between limbs, or between simultaneously functioning rhythmic systems must be adjusted, or when there are unexpected perturbations which require a swift and useful correction of the pattern. In other words, when these rhythmic movements have to be adapted to the real-world demands for which they are intended, then the afferents are an essential part of the system which now operates in a closed-loop manner. Similar arguments can also be given for the interactions between descending controls in the various systems (see final section).

4.1.2   The Influence of Tonic and Phasic Afferent Feedback

In the next sections, the different types of afferent feedback will be summarized briefly, drawing analogies and differences when possible. We will then address the question of the mechanisms by which afferent feedback and central patterns can interact to modify the pattern or to superimpose corrective responses.

Tonic Afferent Inputs. Sensory pathways must participate in the detection of particular demands and allow the system to operate in the proper range—either faster or slower. Detection of high CO_2 by central and peripheral chemoreceptors will lead to a higher frequency of respiration and deeper breathing. The distention of the mouth by an intraoral device mimicking food will increase masticatory rhythm. The presence of an object between the teeth will favor a chewing pattern with more or less lateral grinding components. Pinching the tail or the paw, or changing the posture of the limbs, may increase the frequency of locomotion and change the relative amplitude of muscle activity. Other receptor inputs may reduce respiration (such as high O_2), inhibit locomotion (pressure on the skin of the lumbosacral region), or reduce mastication frequency (pressure on the forefoot, rectal distention, vocalization).

Thus, tonic peripheral afferent feedback may contribute in setting the frequency of the pattern, perhaps by summating with other control sources such as descending inputs. One evidence for this is that when the afferents or the descending inputs are removed, the "fictive" pattern is generally slower. Other evidence of such a summation are found in the various systems. For instance, subthreshold cortical stimulation combined with oral distension will evoke mastication, and loading the jaw will increase the masticatory rhythm evoked by the cortex. Similar observations are often made with decerebrate animals: the position of the limbs may enhance or inhibit the overall rhythm. The sum of central inspiratory drive and inputs from the lung stretch receptors will also set the frequency (moving upwards along the curve of Fig. 17A).

Phasic Afferent Inputs. How do phasic afferent inputs interact with the CPGs? The afferents may participate in setting the frequency of the rhythm by promoting one phase, and thus, prolonging it (phase promoting-reflexes, or positive feedback). Or, it could terminate the ongoing phase and thus switch to the opposite phase (phase switching reflexes or negative feedback; see Grillner, 1979a).

Positive Feedback: Phase Promoting Reflexes. Different kinds of studies have indicated the possibility of positive feedback from cutaneous, muscle, or joint receptors. In the *locomotor system* for instance, imposed ramp movements in the flexion direction increase flexor activity when they occur during the flexor activity of the fictive cycle (Fig. 13B). Similarly, electrical stimulation of the skin during swing may enhance the ongoing flexor burst. Ramps in the extension direction, applied during the period of extensor activity, can also increase the activity of extensors. Electrical stimulation of cutaneous afferents of the foot pads can prolong the stance phase. In the *respiratory system*, it was shown that lung inflation can increase the amplitude of inspriation when applied during inspiration, but may also increase expiration if applied during expiration. Finally, in the *masticatory system*, activation of pressoreceptors of the teeth enhances the force produced by jaw-closing muscles and reduces the overall masticatory frequency by prolonging the duration of the slow-closing phase.

In all systems it has been shown that gamma-motoneurons are co-activated with alpha-motoneurons, and that the fusimotor drive is such that the gain of the stretch reflexes during stance would be high and may thus servo-assist some extensor muscles in this phase of the movement.

Negative Feedback: Phase Switching Reflexes. Generally, negative feedback reflexes have received more attention because they seem to play a more obvious role in the switch between the two antagonist phases in a rhythmic movement.

During *mastication*, the jaw opening reflex pathway, which may be activated when the force applied on pressoreceptors attain a given threshold, may participate in terminating the jaw-closure phase. The stretch reflex evoked in jaw-closer muscles during opening would also tend to promote phase switching from opening to closing.

In *locomotion*, several afferent systems may participate in the control of the stance phase. It was reported that extension of the hip (which activates muscle and joint afferents) could play a role in terminating the stance phase and in initiating the swing phase. It can be expected that the stretch of other flexor muscles during stance or the activation of receptors at different joints may also participate. Finally, the unloading of extensor muscles at the ankle has also been claimed to be a separate mechanism to promote phase switching.

In *respiration*, the Breuer-Hering reflex is, par excellence, the negative feedback reflex whose obvious role is to contribute to terminate inspiration. Similarly, deflation reflexes elicited during expiration act to promote inspiration by curtailing expiration.

It is interesting here to compare how the afferent feedback in the respiratory and the locomotor systems might contribute to the adaptation of the output when there is an increased demand.

In the respiratory system, because the lung volume threshold at which the Breuer-Hering reflex is operative is greater at higher frequencies (see Fig. 17A), an increased respiratory drive will induce an increase in both frequency (Fig. 12D) and depth of breath (Fig. 12C). Assuming that the central inspiratory drive has a constant rate and that the vagal afferent feedback is intact, the sum of their combined input will reach the threshold for terminating inspiration earlier than if only the inspiratory drive was present (as is the case in vagotomized animals). Since the subsequent expiration is linearly related to the previous inspiration, it follows that both the afferent feedback and respiratory drive participate in determining the frequency. A high respiratory demand in a vagotomized animal will be met only by changing the depth of breath at a frequency which is set centrally at a lower value (see Fig. 12B) and would thus provide a much slower adaptation to the respiratory demand.

The locomotor equivalent would be a demand for higher speed. At least in cats, speed adjustments over a limited range of walk and trot (for example, doubling the speed from 0.7–1.5 m/s) can be achieved by mainly changing the step frequency and not the stance length which in these conditions change by about 10% (Grillner, 1981a). The hip angular excursion is in the order of 50 degrees in walk, trot, and gallop, and the initiation of flexion always occur at a similar angle value (Goslow et al., 1973). Afferent mechanisms related to critical hip position or unloading of ankle extensor muscles could thus participate in the determination of step frequency by providing fixed cues to terminate the stance phase.

Modulation of Sensory Feedback (Gating). The various feedback pathways that have been considered appear to be phasically modulated by the central pattern generators. The result of such a modulation may be that the stimulation of an afferent pathway excites or inhibits one group of motoneurones in one phase and has no effect in the opposite phase. If, however, the same afferent system projects to antagonistic motoneurons, the effects on one group may be seen in one phase while the effect on the antagonistic group will only be apparent in the opposite phase. There is also another interesting possibility, in which the same input can be used as a source of positive and negative feedback in one phase, but at different times within that phase. To account for this, it is necessary to postulate that afferent information is routed through different pathways whose excitability is differentially controlled in the different phases of the movement and in the different parts of any given phase.

Some of these mechanisms have been studied in the respiratory system. It has been suggested that the vagal afferents depolarize R-beta interneurons in the nucleus tractus solitarius which, when sufficiently excited, would trigger other so-called "off-switch" neurons responsible for turning off the inspiratory neurons. The same vagal afferents would, in parallel, project to other interneurons (unknown) which continuously excite the inspiratory neurons. In this system, then, the afferent input has a continuously increasing excitatory effect (positive feedback) on inspiratory neurons whereas the negative feedback circuit can only influence the inspiratory neurons through a trigger circuit after a certain time has elapsed.

In mastication, the pressoreceptors appear to exert a positive feedback as well as a negative feedback on the slow-closing phase. Although both effects might be carried through bulbar pathways, there is evidence pointing to the possibility that the positive feedback also involves a cortical loop.

It is not at all clear how cutaneous inputs can enhance the extensors for a certain portion of stance and then, towards the end, facilitate their termination and induce flexion. The same reasoning applies to ramp movements of the hip joint in different parts of the locomotor cycle.

Interactions Between Reflex Pathways and Pattern Generators. How are the various feedback pathways modulated by the circuits generating the rhythmic pattern? It seems that the major controls of this phase-dependent behavior can be explained by a combination of cyclic excitability changes of motoneurons and interneurons as well as the primary afferents themselves.

MODULATION OF MOTONEURON EXCITABILITY. The fact that some reflex responses are larger during the activity of certain muscles and absent in the reciprocal phase when the same muscles are silent may in part be attributed to the cyclical excitability changes of the motoneurons themselves. Thus, the stretch reflex of the jaw-closing motoneurons during opening, is prevented by concomitant central inhibition of the jaw-closure motoneurons. A similar mechanism could be invoked for the absence of a stretch reflex in extensor muscles during the swing phase of locomotion, since these have also been shown to be actively hyperpolarized during that period.

However, the motoneuronal excitability changes cannot explain why some reflexes are induced out of phase with the period of activation of the muscles. For instance, in the triceps brachii which is an extensor of the elbow that is active during stance, the largest reflex responses occur during swing, when the motoneurons are inactive, and not during stance, as would have been predicted if the reflex responsiveness were governed by the excitability changes of motoneurons. Similarly, the jaw-opening reflex is maximal during jaw closing, when normally the digastric motoneurons are silent. Such observations require that the modulation of responses, or even the selection of pathways, be made well before the motoneuronal stage.

MODULATION OF INTERNEURON EXCITABILITY. In the *respiratory system*, intracellular recordings of R-beta neurons have shown that the monosynaptic EPSPs, induced by single pulse stimulation of vagal afferents, decrease in amplitude as a function of time after the onset of inspiration and are absent when the stimuli arrive in expiration. This gating of vagal afferent input was explained by the concomitant postsynaptic inhibition of the R-beta neurons during expiration. Because of this inhibition, one has to postulate that inflation reflexes promoting expiration should be routed through other pathways not involving these R-beta interneurons. Similar reasoning should be applied to chemo- and baroreceptor pathways.

In the *masticatory system*, it appears that interneurons in the rostral trigeminal sensory nuclei which receive inputs from low-threshold mechanoreceptors are tonically depressed, whereas other interneurons receiving high threshold inputs are strongly phase-modulated (Olsson et al., 1986). This was taken to suggest that the reduced transmission in low-threshold pathways would prevent these movement-related stimuli from interfering with the movement, while maintaining those protective responses which could prevent damage caused by stimuli which excite high threshold afferents.

In *locomotion*, intracellular recordings of motoneurons in paralyzed cats using low threshold stimulation of the dorsum of the foot have indicated that the transmission in several pathways leading to motoneurons is modulated as a function of the step cycle (Andersson et al., 1978a; Forssberg, 1981; Schomburg and Behrends, 1978b). The study of Andersson et al. (1978b) indicated that there are several pathways involved in the responses of different latency ranges in the same or different muscle groups which are differentially modulated so that each pathway transmits maximally in one phase and minimally in another phase. The finding that the response amplitudes in the different latency ranges were not all modulated in the same phase strongly suggest that the amplitude of the responses is not a function of the motoneuronal excitability, but rather of premotoneuronal elements.

MODULATION OF PRIMARY AFFERENT EXCITABILITY. Whereas, it would appear that a great deal of the modulation of sensory transmission is bound to occur in interneurons in all systems, it is also probable that transmission in certain sensory pathways may be gated at a presynaptic level by a modulation of the primary afferents themselves, as some recent studies have indicated.

In the *respiratory system*, there is contradictory evidence on presynaptic mechanisms occurring at the level of vagal afferents (see Hildebrandt, 1977, for discussion of the positive evidence; and Camerer et al., 1979, for negative evidence). Evidence for presynaptic control of afferent inputs is also provided by Goldberg and Nakamura (1977) for the *masticatory system*.

During *locomotion*, presynaptic mechanisms would also appear to be significant. Phasically related dorsal root potentials (DRPs) have been recorded during fictive locomotion (Bayev and Kostyuk, 1982; Dubuc et al., 1986), and Wall's technique has shown that there are indeed changes in the excitability of various groups of afferents fibers (Bayev and Kostyuk, 1982). It is possible that the CPG might regulate the excitability of primary afferents in a rather precise way, since antidromic discharges of primary afferents, recorded in cut dorsal roots during fictive locomotion, may occur in different parts of the step cycle (Dubuc et al., 1985). However, the relationship between these presynaptic events and the phasic modulation of specific reflexes still has to be established.

4.2 General Scheme

Figure 21 is an attempt to define some simple concepts that may be derived from the above review of the literature.

First, one should consider that there appears to be, for all systems, a

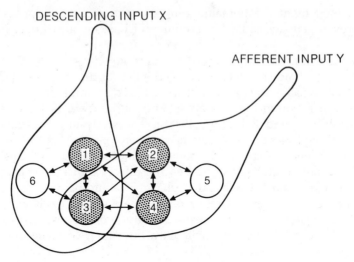

DESCENDING INPUT X

AFFERENT INPUT Y

FIGURE 21. General Schema representing one concept of the manner in which descending and afferent input may interact with the CPG.

network which can generate complex rhythmic patterns. In the model described here, elements 1 to 4 are considered to form the generating network with elements 1 and 3 being active roughly out of phase with elements 2 and 4. This system could operate in an open-loop manner in some conditions, and satisfy the demands based on predictions provided by evolution and learning which set internal calibrations (basic frequency, relative duration of each phase). The operating range of this system would, necessarily, be limited and the system would be unadaptable.

However, in normal conditions this system functions in a closed-loop manner. For a given movement, system-specific and movement-related afferents (labelled afferent input Y to highlight the specificity), as well as other inputs which affect the CPG through specific descending systems (descending input X), will become an integral part of the closed-loop system. Through positive and negative feedback mechanisms occurring in those elements under the sphere of influence of each input (see Fig. 21), the frequency, as well as the structure of the pattern itself, may be changed. This feedback will extend the operating range and will, moreover, increase its accuracy and stability.

It is most likely that both types of control mechanisms summate on some of the same key elements constituting the CPG (cf. element 3). Thus, if descending inputs or afferent inputs are removed, some adaptation of the CPG can still be achieved by the remaining system because the different control systems are additive.

When the system functions normally, the descending and peripheral inputs exert their effects in a phase-dependent manner as a number of the elements through which they normally exert their action are part of the generating system (elements 1 to 4). However, not all the elements influenced by these inputs are part of the CPG (elements 5 and 6), but can be influenced by it in a number of ways. For example, imagine that the motoneurons of the triceps brachii can be excited both by elements 3 and 5. The motoneurons would be driven in stance by element 3 as part of the central generator. If an afferent input arrives during swing when element 5 is excitable, because of inputs from elements 2–4, which are out of phase with element 3, then the triceps motoneurons will also be activated. Thus, specific sets of muscles can be activated in a different order than the one determined by the CPG to specifically compensate for certain perturbations. This would appear to be a rather specific role of the afferents.

Although grossly oversimplifying all the detailed interactions we have outlined in the previous sections, this diagram suggests that networks centrally producing a complex pattern may be incorporated in various closed-loop systems which adapt their operating range to all kinds of conditions or perturbations. In this mode of operation, these networks with their afferent feedback and their descending inputs constitute indivisible entities. When the control feedback is removed or when the descending controls are lesioned, the remaining reduced system operates in an open-loop mode which makes it altogether a different entity. Therefore, it will be of great importance to continue studying the complex mechanisms through which the afferent feedback and descending inputs normally interact with the central rhythmic networks to generate purposeful movements.

ACKNOWLEDGEMENTS

The authors wish to thank the Medical Research Council of Canada for continuing research support to the Group in Neurological Sciences. T. Drew is a chercheur-boursier from Le Fonds de la Recherche en Santé du Québec (FRSQ).

REFERENCES

Abraham, L. D., W. B. Marks, and G. E. Loeb (1985). The distal hindlimb musculature of the cat. Cutaneous reflexes during locomotion. *Exp,. Brain Res.*, **58**: 594–603.

Adrian, E. D. (1933). Afferent impulses in the vagus and their effect on respiration. *J. Physiol.*, **79**: 332–358.

Akazawa, K., J. W. Aldridge, J. D. Steeves, and R. B. Stein (1982). Modulation of stretch reflexes during locomotion in the mesencephalic cat. *J. Physiol.*, **329**: 553–567.

Amemiya, M. and T. Yamaguchi (1984). Fictive locomotion of the forelimb evoked by stimulation of the mesencephalic locomotor region in the decerebrate cat. *Neurosci. Lett.*, **50**: 91–96.

Andersson, O. and S. Grillner (1981). Peripheral control of the cat's step cycle. I. Phase dependent effects of ramp-movements of the hip during "fictive locomotion." *Acta Physiol. Scand.*, **113**: 89–101.

Andersson, O. and S. Grillner (1983). Peripheral control of the cat's step cycle. II. Entrainment of the central pattern generators for locomotion by sinusoidal hip movements during "fictive locomotion." *Acta Physiol. Scand.*, **118**: 229–239.

Andersson, O., H. Forssberg, S. Grillner, and M. Lindquist (1978a). Phasic gain control of the transmission in cutaneous reflex pathways to motoneurons during "fictive" locomotion. *Brain Res.*, **149**: 503–507.

Andersson, O., S. Grillner, M. Lindquist, and M. Zomlefer (1978b). Peripheral control of the spinal pattern generators for locomotion in cat. *Brain Res.*, **150**: 625–630.

Aoki, M. and S. Mori (1981). Locomotion elicited by pinna stimulation in the acute precollicular-postmammillary decerebrate cat. *Brain Res.*, **214**: 424–428.

Appelberg, B., P. Bessou, and Y. Laporte (1966). Action of static and dynamic fusimotor fibres on secondary endings of cat's spindles. *J. Physiol,* **185**: 160–171.

Appenteng, K., and A. Prochazka (1984). Tendon organ firing during active muscle lengthening in awake, normally behaving cats. *J. Physiol.*, **353**: 81–92.

Appenteng, K., J. P. Lund, and J. J. Seguin (1982a). Behavior of cutaneous mechanoreceptors recorded in mandibular division of Gasserian ganglion of the rabbit during movements of lower jaw. *J. Neurophysiol.*, **47**:151–166.

Appenteng, K., J. P. Lund, and J. J. Seguin (1982b). Intraoral mechanoreceptor activity during jaw movement in the anesthetized rabbit. *J. Neurophysiol.*, **48**: 27–37.

Appenteng, K., K. Morimoto, and A. Taylor (1980). Fusimotor activity in masseter nerve of the cat during reflex jaw movement. *J. Physiol.*, **305**:415–431.

Arshavsky, Y. I., G. N. Orlovsky, G. A. Pavlova, and L. B. Popova (1986). Activity of C3–C4 propriospinal neurons during fictitious forelimb locomotion in the cat. *Brain Res.*, **363**:354–357.

Band, D. M., I. R. Cameron, and S. J. G. Semple (1970). The effect on respiration of abrupt changes in carotid artery pH and Pco_2 in the cat. *J. Physiol.*, **211**:479–494.

Bartlett, D. Jr., P. Jeffery, G. Sant'Ambrogio, and J. C. M. Wise (1976). Location of stretch receptors in the trachea and bronchi of the dog. *J. Physiol.*, **258**:409–420.

Bayev, K. V. (1978). Central locomotor program for the cat's hindlimb. *Neurosci.*, **3**:1081–1092.

Bayev, K. V. and P. G. Kostyuk (1982). Polarization of primary afferent terminals of lumbosacral cord elicited by the activity of spinal locomotor generator. *Neurosci.*, **7**:1401–1409.

Belanger, M. and A. E. Patla (1984). Corrective responses to perturbation applied during walking in humans. *Neurosci. Lett.*, **49**:291–295.

Berger, W., V. Dietz, and J. Quintern (1984). Corrective reactions to stumbling in man: neuronal co-ordination of bilateral leg muscle activity during gait. *J. Physiol.*, **357**:109–125.

Biscoe, T. J., M. J. Purves, and S. R. Sampson (1970). The frequency of nerve impulses in single carotid body chemoreceptor afferent fibres recorded in vivo with intact circulation. *J. Physiol.*, **208**:121–131.

Black, A. M. S. and R. W. Torrance (1971). Respiratory oscillations in chemoreceptor discharge in the control of breathing. *Resp. Physiol.*, **13**:221–237.

Boyd, I. A. and T. D. M. Roberts (1953). Proprioceptive discharges from the stretch-receptors in the knee-joint of the cat. *J. Physiol.*, **122**:38–58.

Bremer, F. (1923). Physiologie nerveuse de la mastication chez le chat et le lapin. Réflexes de mastication. Réponses masticatrices corticales et centre cortical du goût. *Arch. Int. Physiol.*, **21**:308–352.

Burgess, P. R. and F. J. Clark (1969). Characteristics of knee joint receptors in the cat. *J. Physiol.*, **203**:317–335.

Byers, M. R. (1985). Sensory innervation of periodontal ligament of rat molars consists of unencapsulated ruffini-like mechanoreceptors and free nerve endings. *J. Comp. Neurol.*, **231**:500–518.

Cabelguen, J-M. (1981). Static and dynamic fusimotor controls in various hindlimb muscles during locomotor activity in the decorticate cat. *Brain Res.*, **213**:83–97.

Cabelguen, J-M., D. Orsal, and C. Perret (1984). Discharge of forelimb spindle primary afferents during locomotor activity in the decorticate cat. *Brain Res.*, **306**:359–364.

Cabelguen, J-M., D. Orsal, C. Perret, and M. Zattara (1981). Central pattern generation of forelimb and hindlimb locomotor activities in the cat. In *Regulatory Functions of the CNS, Motion and Organisation Principles*, Szentagothai, J., M. Palkovits, and J. Hamori, eds. Akademiai Kiado, Budapest, pp. 199–211.

Camerer, H., D. W. Richter, N. Rohrig, and M. Meesemann (1979). A model for "respiratory gating." In *Central Nervous Control Mechanisms in Breathing*, Euler, C. von and H. Lagercrantz, eds. Pergamon Press, New York, pp. 261–266.

Carli, G., F. Farabollini, G. Fontani, and M. Meucci (1979). Slowly adapting receptors in cat hip joint. *J. Neurophysiol.*, **42**:767–778.

Carlson, H., J. Halbertsma, and M. Zomlefer (1979). Control of the trunk during walking in the cat. *Acta Physiol. Scand.*, **105**:251–253.

Chandler, S. H., L. J. Goldberg, and R. W. Lambert (1985). The effects of orofacial sensory input on spontaneously occurring and apomorphine-induced rhythmical jaw movements in the anesthetized guinea pig. *Neurosci. Lett.* **53**:45–49.

Chase, M. H. and D. J. McGinty (1970). Modulation of spontaneous and reflex activity of the jaw musculature by orbital cortical stimulation in the freely moving cat. *Brain Res.*, **19**:117–126.

Clark, F. J. and C. von Euler (1972). On the regulation of depth and rate of breathing. *J. Physiol.*, **222**:267–295.

Cody, F. W. J., L. M. Harrison, and A. Taylor (1975). Analysis of activity of muscle spindles of jaw-closing muscles during normal movements in the cat. *J. Physiol.*, **253**:565–582.

Cody, F. W. J., R. W. H. Lee, and A. Taylor (1972). A functional analysis of the components of the mesencephalic nucleus of the fifth nerve in the cat. *J. Physiol.*, **225**:249–261.

Cohen, M. I. (1975). Phrenic and recurrent laryngeal discharge patterns and the Hering-Breuer reflex. *Am. J. Physiol.*, **228**:1489–1496.

Cohen, M. I. (1979). Neurogenesis of respiratory rhythm in the mammal. *Physiol. Rev.*, **59**:1105–1173.

Cohen, M. I. (1981). Pulmonary afferent and central influences on respiratory phase-switching in the cat. *Can. J. Physiol. Pharmacol.*, **59**:675–682.

Cohen, M. I. and J. L. Feldman (1977). Models of respiratory phase-switiching. *Fed. Proc.*, **36**:2367–2374.

Corda, M., C. von Euler, and G. Lennerstrand (1965). Proprioceptive innervation of the diaphragm. *J. Physiol.*, **178**:161–177.

Corda, M., C. von Euler, and G. Lennerstrand (1966). Reflex and cerebellar influences on "rhythmic" and "tonic" activity in the intercostal msucles. *J. Physiol.*, **184**:898–923.

Crenna, P. and C. Frigo (1984). Evidence of phase-dependent nociceptive reflexes during locomotion in man. *Exp. Neurol.*, **85**:336–345.

Critchlow, V. and C. von Euler (1962). Rhythmic control of intercostal muscle spindles. *Experientia*, **18**:426–427.

Critchlow, V. and C. von Euler (1963). Intercostal muscle spindle activity and its motor control. *J. Physiol.*, **168**:820–847.

Delcomyn, F. (1980). Neural basis of rhythmic behavior in animals. *Science*, **210**:492–498.

Dellow, P. G. and J. P. Lund (1971). Evidence for central timing of rhythmical mastication. *J. Physiol.*, **215**:1–13.

Dietz, V., J. Quintern, and W. Berger (1984a). Corrective reactions to stumbling in man: functional significance of spinal and transcortical reflexes. *Neurosci. Lett.*, **44**:131–135.

Dietz, V., J. Quintern, and W. Berger (1984b). Cerebral evoked potentials associated with the compensatory reactions following stance and gait perturbation. *Neurosci. Lett.*, **50**:181–186.

Dietz, V., J. Quintern, W. Berger, and E. Schenck (1985). Cerebral potentials and leg muscle EMG responses associated with stance perturbation. *Exp. Brain Res.*, **57**:348–354.

Dimarco, A. F., C. von Euler, J. R. Romaniuk, and Y. Yamamoto (1980). Low threshold facilitation of inspiration by lung volume increments. *Acta Physiol. Scand.*, **109**:343–344.

Dimarco, A. F., C. von Euler, J. R. Romaniuk, and Y. Yamamoto (1981). Positive feedback facilitation of external intercostal and phrenic inspiratory activity by pulmonary stretch receptors. *Acta Physiol. Scand.*, **113**:375–386.

Drew, T. and S. Rossignol (1985). Forelimb responses to cutaneous nerve stimulation during locomotion in intact cats. *Brain Res.*, **329**:323–328.

Drew, T. and S. Rossignol (1987). A kinematic and electromyographic study of cutaneous reflexes evoked from the forelimb of unrestrained walking cats. *J. Neurophysiol.*, **57**:1160–1184.

Dubner, R., B. J. Sessle, and A. T. Storey (1978). *The Neural Basis of Oral and Facial Function*, Plenum Press, New York.

Dubuc, R., J-M. Cabelguen, and S. Rossignol (1985). Rhythmic antidromic discharges in cut dorsal roots during locomotion. *Brain Res.*, **329**:375–378.

Dubuc, R., J-M. Cabelguen, and S. Rossignol (1986). Dorsal root potentials and antidromic discharges of primary afferents during fictive locomotion in the cat. In *Neurobiology of Vertebrate Locomotion,* Grillner, S., H. Forssberg, P. S. G. Stein, and D. Stuart, eds. McMillan, London, pp. 535–538.

Duysens, J. (1977a). Fluctuations in sensitivity to rhythm resetting effects during the cat's step cycle. *Brain Res.,* **33**:190–195.

Duysens, J. (1977b). Reflex control of locomotion as revealed by stimulation of cutaneous afferents in spontaneously walking premammillary cats. *J. Neurophysiol.,* **40**:737–751.

Duysens, J. and G. E. Loeb (1980). Modulation of ipsi- and contralateral reflex responses in unrestrained walking cats. *J. Neurophysiol.,* **44**:1024–1037.

Duysens, J. and K. G. Pearson (1976). The role of cutaneous afferents from the distal hindlimb in the regulation of the step cycle of thalamic cats. *Exp. Brain Res.,* **24**:245–255.

Duysens, J. and K. G. Pearson (1980). Inhibition of flexor burst generation by loading ankle extensor muscles in walking cats. *Brain Res.,* **187**:321–332.

Duysens, J. and R. B. Stein (1978). Reflexes induced by nerve stimulation in walking cats with implanted cuff electrodes. *Exp. Brain Res.,* **32**:213–224.

Duysens, J., G. E. Loeb, and B. J. Weston (1980). Crossed flexor reflex responses and their reversal in freely walking cats. *Brain Res.,* **197**:538–542.

Eidelberg, E. and A. L. Miller (1985). Effects of sensory deafferentation on glucose metabolism of muscles during locomotion. *Brain Res.,* **327**:316–318.

Eklund, G., C. von Euler, and S. Rutkowski (1964). Spontaneous and reflex activity of intercostal gamma motoneurons. *J. Physiol.,* **171**:139–163.

Eldridge, F. L. (1972a). The importance of timing on the respiratory effects of intermittent carotid sinus nerve stimulation. *J. Physiol.,* **222**:297–318.

Eldridge, F. L. (1972b). The importance of timing on the respiratory effects of intermittent carotid body chemoreceptor stimulation. *J. Physiol.,* **222**:319–333.

Eldridge, F. L. (1976). Expiratory effects of brief carotid sinus nerve and carotid body stimulations. *Resp. Physiol.,* **26**:395–410.

Engberg, I. (1964). Reflexes to foot muscles in the cat. *Acta. Physiol. Scand.,* **62**(suppl. 235):1–64.

Engberg, I. and A. Lundberg (1969). An electromyographic analysis of muscular activity in the hindlimb of the cat during unrestrained locomotion. *Acta Physiol. Scand.,* **75**:614–630.

Euler, C. von (1981). The contribution of sensory inputs to the pattern generation of breathing. *Can. J. Physiol. Pharmacol.,* **59**:700–706.

Euler, C. von (1985). Central pattern generation during breathing. In *The Motor System in Neurobiology,* Evarts, E. V., S. P. Wise, and D. Bousfield, eds. Elsevier Biomedical Press, New York, pp. 47–51.

Euler, C. von and G. Peretti (1966). Dynamic and static contributions to the rhythmic gamma activation of primary and secondary spindle endings in external intercostal muscles. *J. Physiol.,* **187**:501–516.

Euler, C. von and U. Soderberg (1952). Medullary chemosensitive receptors. *J. Physiol.,* **118**:545–554.

Euler, C. von, F. Herrero, and I. Wexler (1970). Control mechanisms determining rate and depth of respiratory movements. *Resp. Physiol.,* **10**:93–108.

Feldman, J. L. and H. Gautier (1976). Interaction of pulmonary afferents and pneumotaxic centre in control of respiratory pattern in cats. *J. Neurophysiol.*, **39**: 31–44.

Feldman, J. L. and S. Grillner (1983). Control of vertebrate respiration and locomotion: a brief account. *The Physiologist*, **26**:310–316.

Ferrell, W. R. (1980). The adequacy of stretch receptors in the cat knee joint for signalling joint angle throughout a full range of movement. *J. Physiol.*, **299**: 85–99.

Ferrell, W. R., R. H. Baxendale, C. Carnachan, and I. K. Hart (1985). The influence of joint afferent discharge on locomotion, proprioception, and activity in conscious cats. *Brain Res.*, **347**:41–48.

Fillenz, M. and J. G. Widdicombe (1971). Receptors of the lungs and airways. In *Handbook of Sensory Physiology*, Neil, E., ed. Springer-Verlag, Heidelberg, pp. 81–112.

Fleshman, J. W., A. Lev-Tov, and R. E. Burke (1984). Peripheral and central control of flexor digitorum longus and flexor hallucis longus motoneurons: the synaptic basis of functional diversity. *Exp. Brain Res.*, **54**:133–149.

Forssberg, H. (1979). Stumbling corrective reaction: a phase-dependent compensatory reaction during locomotion. *J. Neurophysiol.*, **42**:936–953.

Forssberg, H. (1981). Phasic gating of cutaneous reflexes during locomotion. In *Muscle Receptors and Movement*, Taylor, A. and A. Prochazka, eds. Macmillan, London, pp. 403–412.

Forssberg, H. (1985). Phase-dependent step adaptations during human locomotion. In *Feedback and Motor Control in Invertebrates and Vertebrates*, Barnes, W. J. P. and M. H. Gladden, eds. Croom Helm Ltd., London, pp. 451–464.

Forssberg, H., S. Grillner, J. Halbertsma, and S. Rossignol (1980). The locomotion of the low spinal cat: II. Interlimb coordination. *Acta Physiol. Scand.*, **108**:283–295.

Forssberg, H., S. Grillner, and S. Rossignol (1975). Phase dependent reflex reversal during walking in chronic spinal cats. *Brain Res.*, **85**:103–107.

Forssberg, H., S. Grillner, and S. Rossignol (1977). Phasic gain control of reflexes from the dorsum of the paw during spinal locomotion. *Brain Res.*, **132**:121–139.

Forssberg, H., S. Grillner, S. Rossignol., and P. Wallen (1976). Phasic control of reflexes during locomotion in vertebrates. In *Neural Control of Locomotion*, Herman, R. M., S. Grillner, P. Stein, and D. Stuart, eds. Plenum Press, New York, pp. 647–674.

Gandevia, S. C. and D. I. McCloskey (1976). Joint sense, muscle sense, and their combination as position sense measured at the distal interphalangeal joint of the middle finger. *J. Physiol.*, **260**:387–407.

Gardner, E. (1948). The innervation of the knee joint. *Anat. Rec.*, **101**:109–130.

Gauthier, L. and S. Rossignol (1981). Contralateral hindlimb responses to cutaneous stimulation during locomotion in high decerebrate cats. *Brain Res.*, **207**:303–320.

Godwin-Austin, R. B. (1969). The mechanoreceptors of the costovertebral joints. *J. Physiol.*, **202**:737–753.

Goldberg, L. J. and Y. Nakamura (1977). Production of primary afferent depolarization in group Ia fibers from the masseter muscle by stimulation of trigeminal cutaneous afferents. *Brain Res.*, **134**:561–567.

Goldberger, M. E. (1977). Locomotor recovery after unilateral hindlimb deafferentation in cats. *Brain Res.*, **123**:59–74.

Goldberger, M. E. (1983). Recovery of accurate limb movements after deafferentation in cats. In *Spinal cord reconstruction*, Kao, C. C., R. P. Bunge, and P. J. Reier, eds. Raven Press, New York, pp. 455–463.

Goldberger, M. E. and M. Murray (1978). Recovery of movement and axonal sprouting may obey some of the same laws. In *Neuronal Plasticity*, Cotman C. W., ed. Raven Press, New York, pp. 73–96.

Goldberger, M. E. and M. Murray (1980). Locomotor recovery after deafferentation of one side of the cat's trunk. *Exp. Neurol.*, **67**:103–117.

Goodwin, G. M. and E. S. Luschei (1974). Effects of destroying spindle afferents from jaw muscles on mastication in monkeys. *J. Neurophysiol.*, **37**:967–981.

Goodwin, G. M. and E. S. Luschei (1975). Discharge of spindle afferents from jaw-closing muscles during chewing in alert monkeys. *J. Neurophysiol.*, **38**:560–571.

Goslow, G. E. Jr., R. M. Reinking, and D. G. Stuart (1973). The cat step cycle: hindlimb joint angles and muscle lengths during unrestrained locomotion. *J. Morphol.*, **141**:1–42.

Gottlieb, S. and A. Taylor (1983). Interpretation of fusimotor activity in cat masseter nerve during reflex jaw movement. *J. Physiol.*, **345**:423–438.

Graham Brown, T. (1911). Studies in the physiology of the nervous system. VII. movements under narcosis in the pigeon. Movements under narcosis in the rabbit—progression—scratching—flexion. *Quart. J. Exp. Physiol.* **4**:151–182.

Grillner, S. (1975). Locomotion in vertebrates: central mechanisms and reflex interaction. *Physiol. Rev.*, **55**:247–304.

Grillner, S. (1977). On the neural control of movement—a comparison of different basic rhythmic behaviors. In *Function and Formation of Neural Systems*, Stent, G. S., ed. Life Sciences Research Report 6, Dahlem Konferenzen, Berlin, pp. 197–224.

Grillner, S. (1979a). Interaction between central and peripheral mechanisms in the control of locomotion. In *Reflex Control of Posture and Movement*, Granit, R. and O. Pompeiano, eds. Elsevier Press, *Prog. Brain Res.*, **50**:227–235.

Grillner, S. (1979b). Analogies between pattern generation in locomotion and breathing. In *Central Nervous Control Mechanisms in Breathing*, Euler, C. von and H. Lagercrantz, eds. Pergamon Press, New York, pp. 307–310.

Grillner, S. (1981a). Control of locomotion in bipeds, tetrapods and fish. In *Handbook of Physiology*, Brookhart, J. M. and V. B. Mountcastle, eds. Amer. Physiol. Soc., Maryland, pp. 1179–1236.

Grillner, S. (1981b). A critique of the papers by Ellaway, Murphy, and Trott; Appelberg, Hulliger, and Sojka; Rymer, Post, and Edwards; and Taylor and Appenteng. In *Muscle Receptors and Movement*, Taylor, A. and A. Prochazka eds. Macmillan, London, pp. 193–198.

Grillner, S. (1985). Neural control of vertebrate locomotion—central mechanisms and reflex interaction with special reference to the cat. In *Feedback and Motor*

Control in Invertebrates and Vertebrates, Barnes W. J. P. and M. H. Gladden, eds. Croom Helm Ltd., London, pp. 35–56.

Grillner, S. and S. Rossignol (1978). On the initiation of the swing phase of locomotion in chronic spinal cats. *Brain Res.,* **146**:260–277.

Grillner, S. and P. Zangger (1975). How detailed is the central pattern generation for locomotion. *Brain Res.,* **88**:367–371.

Grillner, S. and P. Zangger (1979). On the central generation of locomotion in the low spinal cat. *Exp. Brain. Res.,* **34**:241–261.

Grillner, S. and P. Zangger (1984). The effect of dorsal root transection on the efferent motor pattern in the cat's hindlimb during locomotion. *Acta Physiol. Scand.,* **120**:393–405.

Halbertsma, J., S. Miller, and F. G. A. van der Meche (1976). Basic programs for the phasing of flexion and extension movements of the limbs during locomotion. In *Neural Control of Locomotion,* Herman, R. M., S. Grillner, P. Stein, and D. Stuart, eds. Plenum Press, New York, pp. 489–517.

Hannam, A. G. (1969). The response of periodontal mechanoreceptors in the dog to controlled loading of the teeth. *Arch. Oral. Biol.,* **14**:781–791.

Hannam, A. G. and J. P. Lund (1981). The effect of intra-oral stimulation on the human masticatory cycle. *Arch. Oral. Biol.,* **26**:865–870.

Head, H. (1889). On the regulation of respiration. *J. Physiol.,* **10**:1–70.

Hilaire, G. G., J. G. Nicholls, and T. A. Sears (1983). Central and proprioceptive influences on the activity of levator costae motoneurons in the cat. *J. Physiol.,* **342**:527–548.

Hildebrandt, J. R. (1977). Gating: a mechanism for selective receptivity in the respiratory center. *Fed. Proc.,* **36**:2381–2385.

Hnik, P. (1956). Motor function disturbances and excitability changes following deafferentation. *Physiol. Bohemoslovenica.,* **5**:305–315.

Hornbein, T. F., Z. J. Griffo, and A. Roos (1961). Quantitation of chemoreceptor activity: interrelation of hypoxia and hypercapnia. *J. Neurophysiol.,* **24**:561–568.

Jankowska, E., M. G. M. Jukes, S. Lund, and A. Lundberg (1967). The effect of L-dopa on the spinal cord. 5. Reciprocal organization of pathways transmitting excitatory action to alpha motoneurons of flexors and extensors. *Acta Physiol. Scand.* **70**:369–388.

Jerge, C. R. (1963). Organization and function of the trigeminal mesencephalic nucleus. *J. Neurophysiol.,* **26**:379–392.

Jordan, L. M., C. A. Pratt, and J. A. Menzies (1979). Locomotion evoked by brain stem stimulation: occurrence without phasic segmental afferent input. *Brain Res.,* **177**:204–207.

Jung-Caillol, M. C. and B. Duron (1976). Number of neuromuscular spindles and electrical activity of the respiratory muscles. *Coll. Inst. Nat. Sante Rech. Med.,* **59**:165–173.

Kanda, K. and H. Sato (1983). Reflex responses of human thigh muscles to non-noxious sural stimulation during stepping. *Brain Res.,* **288**:378–380.

Kniffki, K. D., E. D. Schomburg, and H. Steffens (1981). Effects from fine muscle and cutaneous afferents on spinal locomotion in cats. *J. Physiol.,* **319**: 543–554.

Knowlton, G. C. and M. G. Larrabee (1946). A unitary analysis of pulmonary volume receptors. *Am. J. Physiol.*, **147**:100–114.

Knox, C. K. (1973). Characteristics of inflation and deflation reflexes during expiration in the cat. *J. Neurophysiol.*, **36**:284–295.

Koehler, W. J., E. D. Schomburg, and H. Steffens (1984). Phasic modulation of trunk muscle efferents during fictive spinal locomotion in cats. *J. Physiol.*, **353**:187–197.

Koller, E. A. and P. Ferrel (1970). Studies on the role of the lung deflation reflex. *Resp. Physiol.*, **10**:172–183.

Kostreva, D. R., E. J. Zuperku, G. L. Hess, R. L. Coon, and J. P. Kampine (1975). Pulmonary afferent activity recorded from sympathetic nerves. *J. Appl. Physiol.*, **39**:37–40.

Kubota, K., T. Masegi, and K. Quanbunchan (1974). Muscle spindle distribution in the masticatory muscle of the tree shrew. *J. Dent. Res.*, **53**:538–546.

Kulagin, A. S. and M. L. Shik (1970). Interaction of symmetrical limbs during controlled locomotion. *Biophysics USSR.*, **15**:171–178.

Lamarre, Y. and J. P. Lund (1975). Load compensation in human masseter muscles. *J. Physiol.*, **253**:21–35.

Larrabee, M. G. and R. Hodes (1948). Cyclic changes in the respiratory centres revealed by the effects of afferent impulses. *Am. J. Physiol.*, **155**:147–164.

Larrabee, M. G. and G. C. Knowlton (1946). Excitation and inhibition of phrenic motoneurons by inflation of the lungs. *Am. J. Physiol.*, **147**:90–99.

Larson, C. R., D. V. Finocchio, A. Smith, and E. S. Luschei (1983). Jaw muscle afferent firing during an isotonic jaw-positioning task in the monkey. *J. Neurophysiol.*, **50**:61–73.

Larson, C. R., A. Smith, and E. S. Luschei (1981a). Discharge characteristics and stretch sensitivity of jaw muscle afferents in the monkey during controlled isometric bites. *J. Neurophysiol.*, **46**:130–142.

Larson, C. R., A. Smith, and E. S. Luschei (1981b). Response characteristics of jaw muscle spindle and tooth mechanoreceptor afferents in monkeys during a controlled isometric biting task. In *Oral-FacialSensory and Motor Functions*, Kawamura, Y., ed. Quintessence, Tokyo, pp. 175–185.

Lassek, A. M. and E. K. Moyer (1953). An ontogenetic study of motor deficits following dorsal brachial rhizotomy. *J. Neurophysiol.*, **16**:243–251.

Lavigne, G., J. S. Kim, C. Valiquette, and J. P. Lund (1987). Evidence that periodontal pressoreceptors provide positive feedback to jaw closing muscles during mastication. *J. Neurophysiol.*, **58**:342–358.

Leitner, L. M. and P. Dejours (1968). The speed of response of chemoreceptors. In *The Proceedings of the Wates Foundation Symposium on Arterial Chemoreceptors*, Torrance, R. W., ed. Blackwell Scientific Publications, Oxford, pp. 79–90.

Linden, R. W. A. (1978). Properties of intraoral mechanoreceptors represented in the mesencephalic nucleus of the fifth nerve of cat. *J. Physiol.*, **279**: 395–408.

Lipski, J., R. M. McAllen, and K. M. Spyer (1977). The carotid chemoreceptor input to the respiratory neurons of the tractus solitarius. *J. Physiol.*, **269**:797–810.

Lisin, V. V., S. I. Frankstein, and M. B. Rechtmann (1973). The influence of locomotion on flexor reflex of the hindlimb in cat and man. *Exp. Neurol.*, **38**:180–183.

Loeb, G. E. (1981). Somatosensory unit input to the spinal cord during normal walking. *Can. J. Physiol. Pharmacol.*, **59**: 627–635.

Loeb, G. E. (1984). The control and responses of mammalian muscle spindles during normally executed motor tasks. In *Exercise and Sport Physiology*, R. L. Terjung, ed. The Collamore Press, Toronto, pp. 157–203.

Loeb, G. E. and J. Duysens (1979). Activity patterns in individual hindlimb primary and secondary muscle spindle afferents during normal movements in unrestrained cats. *J. Neurophysiol.*, **42**:420–440.

Loeb, G. E. and J. A. Hoffer (1981). Muscle spindle function during normal and perturbed locomotion in cats. In *Muscle Receptors and Movement*, Taylor A. and A. Prochazka, eds. Macmillan, London, pp. 219–228.

Loeb, G. E. and J. A. Hoffer (1985). Activity of spindle afferents from cat anterior thigh muscles. II Effects of fusimotor blockade. *J. Neurophysiol.*, **54**:565–577.

Loeb, G. E., M. J. Bak, and J. Duysens (1977). Long-term unit recording from somatosensory neurons in the spinal ganglia of the freely walking cat. *Science*, **197**:1192–1194.

Loeb, G. E., J. A. Hoffer, and C. A. Pratt (1985). Activity of spindle afferents from cat anterior thigh muscles. I. Identification and patterns during normal locomotion. *J. Neurophysiol.*, **54**:549–564.

Lund, J. P. and P. G. Dellow (1971). The influence of interactive stimuli on rhythmical masticatory movements in rabbits. *Arch. Oral Biol.*, **16**:215–223.

Lund, J. P. and Y. Lamarre (1973). The importance of positive feedback from periodontal pressoreceptors during voluntary isometric contraction of jaw closing muscles in man. *J. Biol. Buccale.*, **1**:345–351.

Lund, J. P. and Y. Lamarre (1974). Activity of neurons in the lower precentral cortex during voluntary and rhythmical jaw movements in the monkey. *Exp. Brain Res.*, **19**:282–299.

Lund, J. P. and B. Matthews (1979). Responses of muscle joint afferents recorded from the Gasserian ganglion of rabbits. *J. Physiol.*, **293**:38–39.

Lund, J. P. and B. Matthews (1981). Responses of temporomandibular joint afferents recorded in the Gasserian ganglion of the rabbit to passive movements of the mandible. In *Oral-Facial Sensory and Motor Functions*, Kawamura, Y., ed. Quintessence, Tokyo, pp. 153–160.

Lund, J. P. and K. A. Olsson (1983). The importance of reflexes and their control during jaw movement. *Trends Neurosci.*, **6**:458–463.

Lund, J. P. and S. Rossignol (1980). La mastication comme modèle d'étude du contrôle de la motricité. *Union Medicale du Canada.*, **6**:1–6.

Lund, J. P. and S. Rossignol (1981). Modulation of the amplitude of the digastric jaw opening reflex during the masticatory cycle. *Neurosci.*, **6**:95–98.

Lund, J. P., K. Appenteng, and J. J. Seguin (1982). Analogies and common features in the speech and masticatory control systems. In *Speech Motor Control*, Lubker, J. and A. Persson, eds. Pergamon Press, Oxford, pp. 231–245.

Lund, J. P., T. Drew, and S. Rossignol (1984). A study of jaw reflexes of the awake cat during mastication and locomotion. *Brain Behav. Evol.*, **25**:146–156.

Lund, J. P., S. Enomoto, H. Hayashi, K. Hiraba, M. Kotoh, Y. Nakamura, Y. Sahara, and M. Tairo (1983). Phase-linked variations in the amplitude of the digastric nerve jaw-opening reflex response during fictive mastication in the rabbit. *Can J. Physiol. Pharmacol.*, **61**:1122–1128.

Lund, J. P., F. J. R. Richmond, C. Touloumis, Y. Patry, and Y. Lamarre (1978). The distribution of golgi tendon organs and muscle spindles in masseter and temporalis muscles of the cat. *Neurosci.*, **3**:259–270.

Lund, J. P., S. Rossignol, and T. Murakami (1981). Interactions between the jaw opening reflex and mastication. *Can. J. Physiol. Pharmacol.*, **59**:683–690.

Lund, J. P., A. M. Smith, B. J. Sessle, and T. Murakami (1979). Activity of trigeminal alpha- and gamma-motoneurons and muscle afferents during performance of a biting task. *J. Neurophysiol.*, **42**:710–725.

Martensson, A. (1963). Reflex responses and recurrent discharges evoked by stimulation of laryngeal nerves. *Arch. Physiol. Scan.*, **57**:248–269.

Matsukawa, K., H. Kamei, K. Minoda, and M. Udo (1982). Interlimb coordination in cat locomotion investigated with perturbation, I. Behavioral and electromyographic study on symmetric limbs of decerebrate and awake walking cats, *Exp. Brain Res.*, **46**:425–437.

Matsunami, K. and K. Kubota (1972). Muscle afferents of trigeminal mesencephalic tract nucleus and mastication in chronic monkeys. *Jpn. J. Physiol.*, **22**:545–555.

McCloskey, D. I. (1978). Kinesthetic sensibility. *Physiol. Rev.*, **58**:763–820.

McIntyre, A. K., U. Proske, and D. J. Tracey (1978). Afferent fibres from muscle receptors in the posterior nerve of the cat's knee joint. *Exp. Brain Res.*, **33**:415–424.

Miller, S. and F. G. A. van der Meché (1976). Coordinated stepping of all four limbs in the high spinal cat. *Brain Res.*, **109**:395–398.

Miller, S., J. B. Ruit, and F. G. A. van der Meché (1977). Reversal of sign of long spinal reflexes dependent on the phase of the step cycle in the high decerebrate cat. *Brain Res.*, **128**:447–459.

Mott, F. W. and C. S. Sherrington (1895). Experiments upon the influence of sensory nerves upon movement and nutrition of the limbs. Preliminary communication. *Proc. R. Soc., London*, **57**:481–489.

Murphy, P. R., R. B. Stein, and J. Taylor (1984). Phasic and tonic modulation of impulse rates in gamma motoneurons during locomotion in premammillary cats. *J. Neurophysiol.*, **52**:228–243.

Nakamura, Y., Y. Kubo, S. Nozaki, and M. Takatori (1976). Cortically induced masticatory rhythm and its modification by tonic peripheral inputs in immobilized cats. *Bull. Tokyo Med. Dent. Univ.*, **23**:101–107.

Nashner, L. M. (1980). Balance adjustments of humans perturbed while walking. *J. Neurophysiol.*, **44**:650–664.

Nashner, L. M., M. Woollacott, and G. Tuma (1979). Organization of rapid responses to postural and locomotor-like perturbations of standing man. *Exp. Brain Res.*, **36**:463–476.

Ness, A. R. (1954). The mechanoreceptors of the rabbit incisor. *J. Physiol.*, **126**:475–493.

O'Donovan, M. J., M. J. Pinter, R. P. Dum, and R. E. Burke (1982). Actions of FDL and FHL muscles in intact cats: Functional dissociation between anatomical synergists. *J. Neurophysiol.*, **47**:1126–1143.

Olsson, K., K. Sasamoto, and J. P. Lund (1986). Modulation of transmission in rostral trigeminal sensory nuclei during chewing. *J. Neurophysiol.*, **55**:56–75.

Orlovsky, G. N. (1972). Activity of rubrospinal neurons during locomotion. *Brain Res.*, **46**:99–112.

Orlovsky, G. N. and A. G. Feldman (1972). Role of afferent activity in the generation of stepping movements. *Neurophysiol.*, **4**:304–310.

Pack, A. I. (1981). Sensory inputs to the medulla. *Ann. Rev. Physiol.*, **43**:73–90.

Paintal, A. S. (1969). Mechanism of stimulation of type J pulmonary receptors. *J. Physiol.*, **203**:511–532.

Paintal, A. S. (1973). Vagal sensory receptors and their reflex effects. *Physiol. Rev.*, **53**:159–227.

Paintal, A. S. (1977). The nature and effects of sensory inputs into the respiratory centers. *Fed. Proc.*, **36**:2428–2432.

Pearson, K. G. and J. Duysens (1976). Function of segmental reflexes in the control of stepping in cockroaches and cats. In *Neural Control of Locomotion*, Herman, R. M., S. Grillner, P. S. G. Stein, and D. G. Stuart, eds. Plenum Press, New York, pp. 519–537.

Perret, C. (1976). Neural control of locomotion in the decorticate cat. In *Neural Control of Locomotion*. Herman, R. M., S. Grillner, P. S. G. Stein, and D. G. Stuart, eds. Plenum Press, New York, pp. 587–615.

Perret, C. (1983). Centrally generated pattern of motoneuron activity during locomotion in the cat. In *Neural Origin of Rhythmic Movements*, Roberts, A. and B. Roberts, eds. Cambridge Univ. Press, London, pp. 405–422.

Perret, C. and A. Berthoz (1973). Evidence of static and dynamic fusimotor actions on the spindle response to sinusoidal stretch during locomotor activity in the cat. *Exp. Brain Res.*, **18**:178–188.

Perret, C. and J.-M. Cabelguen (1975). A new classification of flexor and extensor muscles revealed by study of the central locomotor program in the deafferentated cat. *Exp. Brain Res.*, **23**: Supplementum 160.

Perret, C. and J-M. Cabelguen (1980). Main characteristics of the hindlimb locomotor cycle in the decorticate cat with special reference to bifunctional muscles. *Brain Res.*, **187**:333–352.

Petrillo, G. A., L. Glass, and T. Trippenbach (1983). Phase locking of the respiratory rhythm in cats to a mechanical ventilator. *Can. J. Physiol. Pharmacol.*, **61**:599–607.

Prochazka, A. (1980). Muscle spindle activity during walking and during free fall. In *Spinal and Supraspinal Mechanisms of Voluntary Motor Control and Locomotion*, Desmedt, J. E., ed. Karger, New York, pp. 282–293.

Prochazka, A., K. H. Sontag, and P. Wand (1978). Motor reactions to perturbations of gait: proprioceptive and somesthetic involvement, *Neurosci. Lett.*, **7**:35–39.

Prochazka, A., J. A. Stephens, and P. Wand (1979). Muscle spindle discharge in normal and obstructed movements. *J. Physiol.*, **287**:57–66.

Prochazka, A., R. A. Westerman, and S. P. Ziccone (1976). Discharges of single hindlimb afferents in the freely moving cat. *J. Neurophysiol.*, **39**:1090–1104.

Prochazka, A., R. A. Westerman, and S. P. Ziccone (1977). Ia Afferent activity during a variety of voluntary movements in the cat. *J. Physiol.*, **268**:423–448.

Purves, M. J. (1979). What do we breathe for? In *Central Nervous Control Mechanisms in Breathing*, Euler, C. von and H. Lagercrantz, eds. Pergamon Press, New York, pp. 7–12.

Ranson, S. W. (1929). The parasympathetic control of muscle tonus. *Arch. Neurol. Psychiat.*, **22**:265–281.

Rasmussen,S. A., G. E. Goslow, Jr., and P. Hannon (1986). Kinematics of locomotion in cats with partially deafferented spinal cords: the spared-root preparation. *Neurosci. Lett.*, **65**:183–188.

Romfh, J. H., N. F. Capra, and G. B. Gatipon (1979). Trigeminal nerve and temporomandibular joint of the cat: a horseradish peroxidase study. *Exp. Neurol.*, **65**:99–106.

Rossignol, S. and T. Drew (1985). Interactions of segmental and suprasegmental inputs with the spinal pattern generator of locomotion. In *Feedback and Motor Control*, Barnes, W. J. P. and M. H. Gladden, eds. Croom Helm Ltd., London, pp. 355–377.

Rossignol, S. and T. Drew (1986). Phasic modulation of reflexes during rhythmic activity. In *Neurobiology of Vertebrate Locomotion*, Grillner, S., H. Forssberg, P. S. G. Stein, and D. Stuart, eds. Macmillan, London, pp. 517–534.

Rossignol, S., H. Barbeau, and C. Julien (1986). Locomotion of the adult chronic spinal cat and its modification by monoaminergic agonists and antagonists. In *Development and Plasticity of the Mammalian Spinal Cord.*, vol. III, Goldberger, M. E., A. Gorio and M. Murray, eds. Fidia Research Series, Liviana Press, Padova, pp. 323–345.

Rossignol, S., L. Gauthier, and C. Julien (1981a). Stimulus response relations during locomotion. *Can. J. Physiol. Pharmacol.*, **59**:667–674.

Rossignol, S., L. Gauthier, C. Julien, and J. P. Lund (1981b). State dependent responses during locomotion. In *Muscle Receptors and Movement*, Taylor, A. and A. Prochazka, eds. Macmillan, New York, pp. 389–402.

Rossignol, S., J. P. Lund, T. Drew, and R. Dubuc (1985). Genèse et adaptation des mouvements rythmiques. *L'Union Médicale du Canada.*, **114**:27–32.

Saltiel, P., J.-P. Gossard, T. Drew, and S. Rossignol (1986). Forelimb cutaneous reflexes during fictive locomotion in decorticate cats. *Soc. Neurosci. Abstr.*, **12**:879.

Sant'Ambrogio, G. (1982). Information arising from the tracheobronchial tree of mammals. *Physiol. Rev.*, **62**:532–569.

Sant'Ambrogio, G., O. P. Mathew, J. T. Fisher, and F. B. Sant'Ambrogio (1983). Laryngeal receptors responding to transmural pressure, airflow, and local muscle activity. *Resp. Physiol.*, **54**:317–330.

Sant'Ambrogio, G., J. E. Remmers, W. J. De Groot, G. Callas, and J. P. Mortola (1978). Localization of rapidly adapting receptors in the trachea and main stem bronchus of the dog. *Resp. Physiol.*, **33**:359–366.

Scarpelli, E. M., F. J. P. Real, and A. M. Rudolph (1965). Tracheal motion during eupnea. *J. Appl. Physiol.*, **20**:473–479.

Schomburg, E. D. and H. B. Behrends (1978a). The possibility of phase-dependent monosynaptic and polysynaptic Ia excitation to homonymous motoneurons during fictive locomotion. *Brain Res.*, **143**:533–537.

Schomburg, E. D. and H. B. Behrends (1978b). Phasic control of the transmission in the excitatory and inhibitory reflex pathways from cutaneous afferents to motoneurons during fictive locomotion in cats. *Neurosci. Lett.*, **8**:277–282.

Sears, T. A. (1964). Efferent discharges in alpha and fusimotor fibres of intercostal nerves of the cat. *J. Physiol.*, **174**:295–315.

Severin, F. V. (1970). The role of the gamma motor system in the activation of the extensor alpha motor neurones during controlled locomotion. *Biophysics USSR*, **15**:1138–1145.

Severin, F. V., G. N. Orlovsky, and M. L. Shik (1967). Work of the muscle receptors during controlled locomotion. *Biophysics USSR*, **12**:575–586.

Shefchyk, S. J., R. B. Stein, and L. M. Jordan (1984). Synaptic transmission from muscle afferents during fictive locomotion in the mesencephalic cat. *J. Neurophysiol.*, **51**:986–997.

Sherrington, C. S. (1910). Flexion reflex of the limb, crossed extension-reflex and reflex stepping and standing. *J. Physiol.*, **40**:28–121.

Shik, M. L., G. N. Orlovsky, and F. V. Severin (1966). Organization of locomotor synergism. *Biophysics USSR*, **11**:879–886.

Shimamura, M., I. Kogure, and T. Fuwa (1984). Role of joint afferents in relation to the initiation of forelimb stepping in thalamic cats. *Brain Res.*, **297**:225–234.

Siebens, A. A. and F. Puletti (1961). Afferent units in dorsal roots of cat driven by respiration. *Science*, **133**:1418–1419.

Sjostrom, A. and P. Zangger (1975). Alpha-gamma linkage in the spinal generator for locomotion in the cat. *Acta Physiol. Scand.*, **94**:130–132.

Sjostrom, A. and P. Zangger (1976). Muscle spindle control during locomotor movements generated by the deafferented spinal cord. *Acta Physiol. Scand.*, **97**:281–291.

Skoglund, S. (1956). Anatomical and physiological studies of knee joint innervation in the cat. *Acta. Physiol. Scand.*, **36**(Suppl 124):1–101.

Sprong, W. L. (1929). A study of reflexes in the deafferented leg of the cat and their relation to tonus. *Bull. John Hopkins Hosp.*, **45**:371–395.

Sumi, T. (1963). The segmental reflex relations of cutaneous afferent inflow to thoracic respiratory motoneurons. *J. Neurophysiol.*, **26**:478–493.

Székely, G., G. Czéh, and G. Y. Vörös (1969). The activity pattern of limb muscles in freely moving normal and de-afferented newts. *Exp. Brain Res.*, **9**:53–62.

Taub, E. (1976). Motor behavior following deafferentation in the developing and motorically mature monkey. In *Neural Control of Locomotion*, Herman, R. M., S. Grillner, P. S. G. Stein, and D. G. Stuart, eds. Plenum Press, New York, pp. 675–705.

Taylor, A. and K. Appenteng (1981). Distinctive modes of static and dynamic fusimotor drive in jaw muscles. In *Muscle Receptors and Movement*, Taylor A. and A. Prochazka, eds. Macmillan, New York, pp. 179–192.

Taylor, A., K. Appenteng, and T. Morimoto (1981). Proprioceptive input from the jaw muscles and its influence on lapping, chewing and posture. *Can. J. Physiol. Pharmacol.*, **59**:636–644.

Taylor, A. and F. W. J. Cody (1974). Jaw muscle spindle activity in the cat during normal movements of eating and drinking. *Brain Res.*, **71**:523–530.

Taylor, J., R. B. Stein, and P. R. Murphy (1985). Impulse rates and sensitivity to stretch of soleus muscle spindle afferent fibres during locomotion in premammillary cats. *J. Neurophysiol.*, **53**:341–360.

Teasdall, R. D. and G. W. Stavraky (1955). Tonic adaptions in deafferented limbs of the cat. *Can. J. Bioch. Physiol.*, **33**:139–155.

Viala, D. and P. Buser (1969a). The effects of L-dopa and 5-HTP on rhythmic efferent discharges in hindlimb nerves in the rabbit. *Brain Res.*, **12**:437–443.

Viala, D. and P. Buser (1971). Modalités d'obtention de rythmes locomoteurs chez le lapin spinal par traitements pharmacologiques (Dopa, 5-HTP, D-Amphétamine). *Brain Res.*, **35**:151–165.

Viala, D. and C. Vidal (1978). Evidence for distinct spinal locomotion generators supplying respectively fore- and hindlimbs in the rabbit. *Brain Res.*, **155**:182–186.

Viala, G. and P. Buser (1969b). Activités locomotrices rhythmiques stéréotypées chez le lapin sous anesthésie légère, étude de leurs caractéristiques générales. *Exp. Brain Res.*, **8**:346–363.

Viala, G. and P. Buser (1974). Inhibition des activités spinales a caractére locomoteur par une modalité particulière de stimulation somatique chez le lapin. *Exp. Brain Res.*, **21**:275–284.

Viala, G., D. Orsal, and P. Buser (1978). Cutaneous fiber groups involved in the inhibition of fictive locomotion in the rabbit. *Exp. Brain Res.*, **33**:257–267.

Vidal, C., D. Viala, and P. Buser (1979). Central locomotor programming in the rabbit. *Brain Res.*, **168**:57–73.

Wand, P., A. Prochazka, and K. H. Sontag (1980). Neuromuscular responses to gait perturbations in freely moving cats. *Exp. Brain Res.*, **38**:109–114.

Wetzel, M. C., A. E. Atwater, J. V. Wait, and D. G. Stuart (1976). Kinematics of locomotion by cats with a single hindlimb deafferentated. *J. Neurophysiol.*, **39**:667–678.

Widdicombe, J. G. (1954). Receptors in the trachea and bronchi of the cat. *J. Physiol.*, **123**:71–104.

Wiesendanger, M. (1964). Rigidity produced by deafferentation. *Acta Physiol. Scand.*, **62**:160–168.

Willigen, J. D. van and J. Weijs-Boot (1984). Phasic and rhythmic responses of the oral musculature to mechanical stimulation of the rat palate. *Arch. Oral. Biol.*, **29**:7–11.

Wyman, R. J. (1977). Neural generation of the breathing rhythm. *Ann. Rev. Physiol.*, **39**:417–448.

Zangger, P. (1978). Fictive locomotion in curarized high spinal cats elicited by 4-aminopyridine and Dopa. *Experimentia (Basel).*, **34**:904.

Zomlefer, M. R., J. Provencher, G. Blanchette, and S. Rossignol (1984). Electromyographic study of lumbar back muscles during locomotion in acute high decerebrate and in low spinal cats. *Brain Res.*, **290**:249–260.

Chapter Eight

CHEMICAL MODULATION OF CENTRAL PATTERN GENERATORS

RONALD M. HARRIS-WARRICK

Section of Neurobiology and Behavior
Cornell University
Ithaca, New York

1 EXPERIMENTAL PHASES IN CENTRAL PATTERN GENERATOR RESEARCH

The study of Central Pattern Generator (CPG) circuits has gone through several experimental phases. Early investigations were aimed at demonstrating that CPGs exist, that is, that simple rhythmic motor acts can be generated entirely within the central nervous system in the absence of sensory feedback. It is now generally agreed that most simple rhythmic behaviors are centrally generated in both invertebrates and vertebrates (Delcomyn, 1980; Grillner, 1981, 1985; Pinsker and Ayers, 1983). The second phase continues today with attempts to understand the neuronal organization of CPGs. The goal of this work is to provide a mechanistic explanation for the existence and detailed form of a rhythmic motor pattern. This has three major components: (1) identifying the component neurons of the CPG; (2) mapping the synaptic connectivity within the circuit; and (3) elucidating the intrinsic membrane properties of the component neurons. This goal has approached completion in only a few simpler invertebrate circuits (Roberts and Roberts, 1983, Selverston and Moulins,

1985). However, it is already clear that "understanding" a CPG is much more difficult than was originally thought and requires an understanding of all three components listed above as well as their interactions (Selverston, 1980; Grillner, 1985; Getting, this volume).

A new phase in the analysis of CPG function is aimed at understanding how outside influences can activate or modulate a CPG's motor pattern. Extrinsic inputs to the CPG are being sought that can activate or inactivate the motor pattern. However, it is now clear that, in addition to these activating inputs, there are many inputs to a CPG that play important "instructive" roles in the shaping of the final motor pattern. According to this approach, the CPG must be thought of, in a dynamic sense, as a loose organization of neurons which can interact with each other in many possible ways to generate a family of related behaviors. The functional CPG at any moment is "sculpted" by activity of extrinsic modulatory inputs from the anatomically defined network to assure that it is generating the most appropriate behavior for the situation. The output of the CPG thus depends not only on the intrinsic characteristics of its neurons and circuitry, but also on extrinsic inputs from other neuronal centers as well as sensory feedback and hormonal influences. These modulatory inputs are not properly members of the CPG itself, as they are neither necessary nor sufficient to generate a stereotyped motor output. However, the actual motor program at any moment results from a complex interaction of CPG components with these modulatory inputs.

1.1 Pharmacological Strategy for Study of CPG Modulation

How can we go about studying the mechanisms of CPG modulation? One method is to identify neurons or discrete tracts that provide modulatory input to the CPG, and to analyze the effects of their selective stimulation on the CPG (Kupfermann and Weiss, 1981; Nagy and Dickinson, 1983; McClellan and Grillner, 1984; Nusbaum and Kristan, 1986). However, in complex systems with a significant degree of redundancy, these neurons or tracts may be difficult to detect or to stimulate selectively, and a single neuron may not by itself produce a detectable change in CPG activity. An alternative approach, which I will discuss in this chapter, is to screen for endogenous chemical substances that modulate the CPG when bath-applied or iontophoresed. The mechanisms by which these compounds affect the CPG can then be analyzed. Furthermore, the morphology and ultrastructure of the neurons that use these compounds to affect the CPG can be studied with immunocytochemical and histochemical procedures. Although there are potential pitfalls with this method (including the loss of physical and temporal specificity of input to appropriate target sites), a good deal has been learned with the pharmacological approach to CPG modulation.

A large number of neuroactive compounds have been described, and

✓

Table 1. Chemical Initation of Movement

Movement	Species	Compound	Level of Analysis[a]	References
Walking	Cat	L-dopa	M, C	Grillner and Shik, 1973; Grillner and Zangger, 1974; Grillner, 1981; Omeniuk and Jordan, 1982
Crawling	*Aplysia*	Serotonin	M	Mackey and Carew, 1983
Walking	Locust	Octopamine	M, C	Sombati and Hoyle, 1984a,b
Flight	Locust	Octopamine	M, C	Sombati and Hoyle, 1984 a,b
Hopping	Rabbit	L-dopa	M	Viala and Buser, 1969, 1971
		5-HTP	M	
Swimming	Lamprey	NMDA, amino acids	M, C, I	Grillner et al., this vol. Sigvardt et al., 1985
Swimming	*Xenopus* embryo	NMDA, Kainate, amino acids	M, C, I	Roberts et al., 1983 Dale and Roberts, 1984
Swimming	Leech	Serotonin	M, C, I	Willard, 1981; Kristan and Weeks, 1983; Nusbaum, 1986; Nusbaum and Kristan, 1986
Swimmeret beating	Crayfish	Proctolin	M	Bradbury and Mulloney, 1982
Feeding	*Helisoma*	Serotonin	M, C	Granzow and Kater, 1977
Feeding	*Limax*	Dopamine	M	Wieland and Gelperin, 1983
Egg-laying	*Aplysia*	Bag cell peptides	M, C, I	Mayeri et al., 1979a,b
Egg-laying	*Caenorhabditis*	Serotonin	B, M	Horvitz et al., 1982
Eclosion	*Manduca*	Eclosion hormone	B, M	Truman and Weeks, 1983
Wandering	*Manduca*	Steroid hormones	B, M	Dominick and Truman, 1986

[a]Level of analysis: B, behavioral observations of animal activity; M, motor patterns monitored extracellularly from motor nerves; C, intracellular recordings from neurons in the motor pathway (cellular targets may or may not be identified); I, ionic mechanisms of chemical action on target cells studied.

one might expect that the roles of different types of compounds in CPG modulation will be different. Although there is a continuum of actions of different substances on the nervous system (Dismukes, 1979), neuroactive compounds are usually classified into three categories, based primarily on their time course of action. *Neurotransmitters* have fast actions in the msec time range, and their actions rarely outlast the presence of the compound. They are useful for rapid activation or adjustment of rhythmic movements such as locomotion, where moment-to-moment adjustment is essential. *Neuromodulators,* such as peptides and biogenic amines, act over seconds to minutes, and their actions usually outlast the presence of the com-

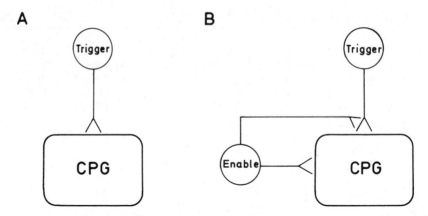

FIGURE 1. Model of triggering and enabling functions during activation of a CPG. (A) The CPG is activated by input from a trigger circuit, which may be specific or may be any excitatory input. By itself, this gives little flexibility in the activation process. (B) The enabling circuit modifies the effectiveness of the triggering input by modulating the amount of transmitter release from the trigger terminals or altering the responsiveness of the CPG neurons to the synaptic drive. This enabling function may be essential for the CPG to be activated.

pound. With their slower time courses, they are probably important in the slow modulation of ongoing motor programs. They could also bias a quiescent CPG to reduce the threshold for initiation of motor output, and thus act as initiators of longer-lasting or more tonically active motor programs. *Neurohormones,* including polypeptides and steroids, have very slow actions over hours or days. They could initiate prolonged motor programs that are only used under specific behavioral conditions. In addition, neurohormones may act over very long times in the formation and enabling of CPG networks during development or sexual maturation (Pfaff, 1983). It is important to recognize that any single substance can have a number of different physiological effects in several of these categories, depending on the type of receptor it encounters.

2   CHEMICAL ACTIVATION OF CPGs

How is rhythmic behavior initiated in a quiescent animal? This problem has been studied in a number of different systems, with differing levels of analysis (Table 1). The scientific rationale for studies of transmitters that activate CPGs has often been pragmatic instead of theoretical: if a compound reproducibly turns on a CPG, then that CPG can be studied more readily in an isolated preparation. Compounds that elicit rhythmic motor patterns in a highly dissected preparation must always be viewed with caution as to their normal role *in vivo*. While some of these agents may normally act as *triggers* to turn on CPG activity, others appear to have a more general role as *gain-setters* or *enablers* to prepare the CPG for activation by other neuronal inputs (Figure 1). I shall first describe a few systems in which these differences have been studied. Then I will discuss these concepts in more detail.

2.1   Amino Acid Activation of Locomotion in Lower Vertebrates

Poon (1980) and Cohen and Wallén (1980) showed that excitatory amino acids such as D-glutamate evoke rhythmic swimming movements in a semi-intact preparation or isolated spinal cord of the lamprey, *Ichthyomyzon unicuspis*. This motor pattern (Figure 2A) is very similar to that seen *in vivo* (Wallén and Williams, 1982, 1984). Grillner et al. (1981; Brodin et al., 1985) suggested that bath-applied amino acids interact primarily with N-methy-D-aspartate (NMDA)- and kainate-preferring receptors, which may use glutamate or aspartate as endogenous ligands (Watkins, 1981). This work has raised the possibility that the swim CPG is normally activated by an NMDA or kainate receptor-mediated mechanism. Supporting this, NMDA antagonists reduce low-intensity swimming in a semi-intact preparation elicited by stimulation of the brain stem or the tail fin (Grillner et al., 1981; McClellan and Grillner, 1984; Brodin and Grillner, 1985). However, strong swimming is only depressed by combined NMDA-kainate antagonists (Brodin and Grillner, 1985). Other mechanisms for activating the CPG also exist, as complete antagonism of NMDA and kainate receptors did not abolish swimming.

Similar experiments have been done in *Xenopus* embryos using a semi-intact preparation with exposed spinal cord (Roberts et al., 1983, 1985; Dale and Roberts, 1983, 1984). Activation of both NMDA- and kainate-preferring amino acid receptors can elicit swimming in this preparation (Figure 2B). A split-bath preparation was used to see whether amino acids are normally involved in activation of the swim CPG. The caudal half of the cord was exposed to amino acid antagonists, while the rostral half was bathed with normal saline. Transient dimming of the light can activate brief bouts of swimming in the semi-intact preparation; in the split-bath experiment, the rostral half of the cord generated normal swimming activity but the caudal half of the spinal cord (with amino acid antagonists) was inactive. These experiments suggest that a natural stimulus (a shadow) can elicit swimming by release of amino acids in the spinal cord. However, it is not possible to tell whether the amino acids are acting directly on the CPG or indirectly via activation of unidentified interneurons.

The cellular mechanisms for amino acid activation of these CPGs are only beginning to be studied (Grillner, this volume). In the lamprey, amino acids depolarize and excite many identified neurons (Rovainen, 1979; Buchanan and Cohen, 1982). Recently, Sigvardt, et al. (1985) studied the effects of NMDA on interneurons in the presence of tetrodotoxin (TTX). About one third of the neurons continued to show slow wave membrane

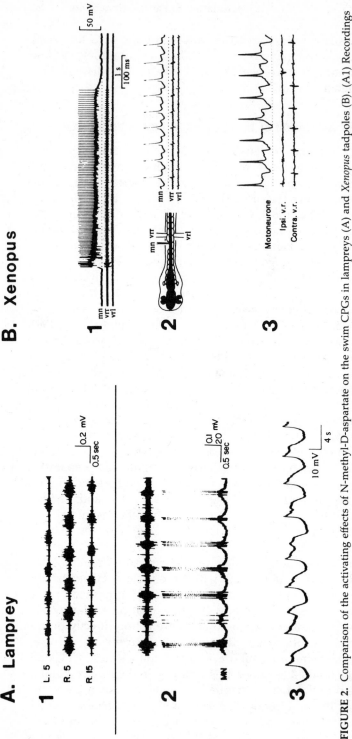

FIGURE 2. Comparison of the activating effects of N-methyl-D-aspartate on the swim CPGs in lampreys (A) and *Xenopus* tadpoles (B). (A1) Recordings from the isolated spinal cord of *Ichthyomyzon unicuspis*. The top three traces are extracellular recordings from a left (L) and two right (R.5, R.15) ventral root. (A2) Recording from a ventral root and intracellular recording from a swim motoneuron sending a process out that root. The motoneuron shows rhythmic oscillations in resting potential, with action potentials generated during the depolarized phase. (A1) and (A2) (Buchanan and Cohen, unpublished). (A3) Recording from a spinal interneuron in the presence of NMDA and 2×10^{-6}M TTX to block all action potentials in the preparation. The resting potential undergoes slow endogenous oscillations in resting potential (from Grillner et al., 1983). (B1) Activity of swim motoneurons during fictive locomotion in the tadpole elicited by a brief dimming of the illumination. The motoneuron (top trace, intracellular recording) undergoes a tonic depolarization and fires action potentials. (B2) high-speed trace of motoneuron activity, showing the regular cycle of motoneuron activity. Extracellular recordings from left (vrl) and right (vrr) ventral roots show strict alternation in spike activity. (B1 and B2) (from Roberts et al., 1983). (B3) Intracellular recording from a swim motoneuron during an NMDA-activated swim episode, with the same activity as the naturally induced swim cycle (from Dale and Roberts, 1983).

potential oscillations in the absence of action potentials (Fig. 2A$_3$), suggesting that these cells might be endogenously rhythmic during NMDA administration. Supporting this hypothesis, the frequency of oscillation could be varied by DC current injection (Wallén and Grillner, 1985). However, the possible contribution of non-spiking interactions to these potentials was not rigorously excluded. Some cells also exhibited bistable membrane properties similar to the plateau potentials that have been described in crustacean neurons (Russell and Hartline, 1978, 1981). These properties might be important in the activation of the spinal CPG for locomotion. The ionic mechanisms of NMDA have not been fully elucidated in the lamprey. In cultured embryonic mouse neurons, NMDA induces a change in the I/V relationship from a nearly linear one to one showing a pronounced N-shaped region of "negative conductance" (McDonald et al., 1982), which is typical of neurons exhibiting bistable behavior or endogenous bursting (Gola, 1976). This appears to arise from the activation of a voltage-insensitive inward current that is blocked in a voltage-sensitive manner by extracellular magnesium (Nowak et al., 1984). A similar mechanism appears to occur in the lamprey, since removal of magnesium causes oscillations to cease, with the cell highly depolarized. In addition, repolarization at the end of a burst requires calcium entry, possibly resulting in activation of calcium-activated potassium conductances (Grillner and Wallén, 1985).

In contrast, Roberts and co-workers have not observed endogenous membrane potential oscillations in *Xenopus* tadpole spinal neurons during NMDA-induced or naturally induced swimming episodes (Roberts et al., 1983, 1985; Dale and Roberts, 1984; Figure 2B). Instead, NMDA induces a prolonged depolarization by a conductance increase mechanism, during which phasic synaptic excitation and inhibition are observed. Based on these results, Roberts et al. (1983, 1985) suggested that network properties are primarily responsible for the organization and timing of the swimming motor program in the tadpole.

2.2 Amine-Induced Locomotion in Mammals

Jankowska et al. (1967) and Grillner (1969) showed that intravenous (IV) injection of the catecholamine precursor L-dopa can initiate stepping movements in spinal cats. When combined with treadmill stimulation, L-dopa-injected spinal cats walk with a fairly normal EMG pattern (Budakova, 1973; Forssberg and Grillner, 1973; Grillner, 1975). Rhythmic activity can be seen even after complete transection of all dorsal roots (Grillner and Zangger, 1979), showing that sensory feedback is unnecessary for amine-induced locomotion.

Injection of L-dopa or the serotonin precursor, 5-hydroxytryptophan (5-HTP), can elicit rhythmic alternating motor discharge in the flexor and extensor nerves of the hind legs in a curarized spinal rabbit (Viala and

Buser, 1969, 1971). A selective enhancement of flexor activity by 5-HTP and of extensor activity by L-dopa was observed, suggesting that serotonin and catecholamines may act as modulators of the flexor and extensor phases of the movement to provide a variety of forms of hop in the rabbit.

Although L-dopa can activate the CPG for locomotion in the cat and rabbit, the functional implications of this result are not clear. Several questions remain unanswered. First, what neurotransmitter pathways are activated by L-dopa? Norepinephrine is clearly implicated, as it is synthesized from L-dopa in the spinal cord. Supporting this conclusion, IV injection of the alpha-adrenergic agonist clonidine (Forssberg and Grillner, 1973) or intrathecal injection of norepinephrine in acute spinal cats (Omeniuk and Jordan, 1982; Jordan, 1983) can activate the spinal generator for locomotion. However, L-dopa also induces the release of dopamine and serotonin in the central nervous system (Ng et al., 1970; Comissiong and Sedgwick, 1979; Commissiong, 1981). Dopamine had only weak activating effects on locomotion when intrathecally injected into spinal cats (Omeniuk and Jordan, 1982). In the lamprey, L-dopa also initiates fictive locomotion, but pharmacological analysis suggests that it acts directly on excitatory amino acid receptors (Poon, 1980). Intrathecal glutamate can also induce rhythmic locomotor movements in spinal cats (Omeniuk and Jordan, 1982). Thus, the actions of L-dopa could be pharmacologically complex and may involve more than one transmitter pathway.

Second, are amines essential triggers for normal activation of the spinal CPG for locomotion? Noradrenergic neurons that send processes into the spinal cord (Westlund et al., 1982) are located within 200 μm of the mesencephalic locomotor region (MLR), where electrical stimulation can elicit locomotion in mesencephalic cats (Shik et al., 1966, 1967; Steeves et al., 1975, 1980). This led Grillner and Shik (1973) to propose that the descending noradrenergic coeruleospinal system could be a command system for the initiation of locomotion. However, pharmacological depletion of norepinephrine and serotonin in this region did not abolish MLR-evoked locomotion, and the catecholamine antagonist phenoxybenzamine did not block MLR-evoked locomotion (Steeves et al., 1980). These results suggest that monoamines are not essential for MLR-evoked locomotion, and that other transmitter systems are also involved in the activation of locomotion. Grillner (1981) has provided an insightful critique of the possible role of norepinephrine in the initiation of locomotion in the cat. He asserts that while it is true that large doses of NE can initiate locomotion, it is unlikely that such high concentrations are achieved under normal conditions. In addition, the noradrenergic system in the CNS has an extremely diffuse, widespread distribution, with single neurons projecting over large fractions of the brain (Moore and Bloom, 1979). It seems unlikely that such a system would play a role as a selective trigger for activating locomotion. An alternative explanation is that NE normally acts to prepare the CPG for activation by other inputs or to modulate ongoing movement (Barbeau and

Rossignol, 1982). In other systems, norepinephrine can raise the sensitivity of neurons to simultaneous synaptic inputs by a conductance decrease mechanism (Moore and Bloom, 1979). If this mechanism occurred in the spinal CPG, it could enable the CPG to be activated by other synaptic inputs that would not be adequate in the absence of aminergic modulation.

Third, what are the cellular mechanisms for L-dopa activation of the CPG for locomotion? A number of spinal neurons become active during L-dopa infusion, including interneurons discharging during all phases of the cycle (Jankowska et al., 1967), gamma motoneurons (Commissiong, 1981), and alpha motoneurons, but the direct actions of L-dopa on these cells are largely unknown. The only neurons that have been studied in detail are the alpha motoneurons. Recent work suggests that norepinephrine can produce a slow depolarization (Neuman, 1985) and a long-lasting facilitation by lowering the apparent threshold for action potential generation during glutamate iontophoresis (White and Neuman, 1980, 1983; Kuypers, 1982). These actions persist in the presence of high-magnesium saline or TTX, suggesting direct effects on the motoneurons (Neuman, 1985). In the facial nucleus, serotonin and norepinephrine facilitate glutamate excitation of motoneurons, accompanied by a slow depolarization and a modest decrease in membrane conductance (VanderMaelen and Aghajanian, 1980; Aghajanian, 1981). A similar mechanism could occur in the spinal cord. Further analysis of aminergic effects on the spinal CPG for locomotion must await unambiguous identification of the CPG components.

2.3 Serotonin and the Initiation of Locomotion in the Leech

The role of serotonin in the initiation of swimming in the leech has been examined by Kristan and colleagues (Kristan and Weeks, 1983). Each segmental ganglion contains 7 to 9 serotonergic neurons, including the large paired Retzius cells (Lent and Frazer, 1977). There appear to be two independent mechanisms whereby serotonergic neurons can initiate swimming in the leech. First, the Retzius cells appear to release serotonin as a neurohormone into the circulation (Willard, 1981). Elevated serotonin levels in the blood are correlated with enhanced probability of swimming, although with a significant delay after injection. Stimulation of the Retzius cells and addition of serotonin can elicit a swimming motor pattern in the isolated nerve cord (Willard, 1981). The Retzius cells do not synapse upon any of the identified swim-related interneurons. Thus, it appears that hormonal release of serotonin by the Retzius cells is adequate under certain conditions to release swimming activity, although with a prolonged delay.

In addition to this slow hormonal (and probably supportive) mechanism, stimulation of two pairs of serotonergic neurons, called cells 21 and 61, activates the swimming rhythm in vitro within a second of the onset of stimulation (Nusbaum and Kristan, 1986; Nusbaum, 1986). Cell 61 has been studied in some detail. This cell receives excitatory mechanosensory input as well as excitation from an identified swim initiator interneuron (cell 204). It fires rhythmically in bursts during swimming episodes and strongly excites a number of swim-related neurons, including an identified component of the swim CPG (neuron 208) and several swim motoneurons. However, it appears to only weakly excite the swim initiation cell 204 (Nusbaum, 1986). Cell 61 apparently excites the CPG neuron 208 by a conductance decrease of voltage-sensitive channels permeable to potassium or chloride. However, pressure-ejection of serotonin into the neuropil can have varied effects on cell 208, including both inhibition and a strong depolarization. Thus, serotonin may have multiple effects on this CPG neuron, and these effects may be spatially segregated. These results demonstrate that cells 21 and 61 have direct synaptic input to the swim CPG and probably use serotonin as a transmitter rather than as a hormone to affect swimming.

Does serotonin play an essential role in the initiation of swimming in the leech? To address this question, Glover and Kramer (1982) selectively ablated serotonergic neurons in embryonic leeches with 5,7-dihydroxytryptamine (5,7-DHT). When tested behaviorally, the 5,7-DHT-treated juveniles displayed a number of motor abnormalities and were unable to swim normally. However, when serotonin was injected into the coelom or animals were immersed in water containing 10^{-5}M serotonin, normal swimming appeared within 10 minutes, and other motor abnormalities disappeared. This effect was reversed upon removal of serotonin. These results suggest that serotonin-containing neurons are essential at some step in the initiation of swimming. However, Brodfuehrer and Friesen (1986a) have detected an interneuron (Tr2) in the subesophageal ganglion which can elicit swimming by a pathway that appears to be independent of the known serotonergic neurons and swim initiator neurons described above. It is not known whether this pathway is functional in 5,7-DHT-treated animals.

While serotonin and serotonergic neurons can initiate swimming in vitro, it is not clear that the amine plays this role in vivo. An alternative explanation is similar to that proposed for norepinephrine in cat locomotion: serotonin may play an essential enabling role to allow the CPG to be activated by another transmitter (Fig. 1). Serotonin could thus be a component of a "state-setting system," associated with readiness to swim (Brodfuehrer and Friesen, 1986b; Nusbaum, 1986). Lent and co-workers have also suggested that serotonin levels are modulated by the state of hunger in the leech, and that its activation of swimming may be part of a larger pattern of activation of feeding behaviors (Lent, 1985; Lent and Dickinsen, 1985).

2.4 Neurohormonal Activation of Complex Behavioral Acts

A number of hormones can elicit complex behavioral acts with prolonged time courses. In the developing tobacco hornworm, *Manduca sexta*, eclosion hormone triggers a complex set of motor patterns leading to ecdysis, a series of rhythmic peristaltic movements of the abdomen which free the pupa from the old cuticle (Truman and Weeks, 1983). Rhythmic movement starts about 1.5–2 hours after entry of the hormone into the blood. Such a time scale suggests that the CPGs for these movements are not directly triggered by the hormone. Instead, the hormone coordinates a number of steps that lead to activation of the CPGs. These steps could include functional formation of the CPG from preexisting network components.

In *Aplysia*, the two bag-cell clusters in the abdominal ganglion release several peptides that elicit a coordinated complex of behaviors associated with egg-laying (Scheller et al., 1984; Mayeri et al., 1979a,b). These behaviors include cessation of locomotion (Mackey and Carew, 1983), increase in heart rate and respiratory rate, egg-laying, head-waving and mucous secretion to attach the egg mass to a solid support. The peptides act as local neurotransmitters and as locally diffusing hormones within the abdominal ganglion, affecting different identified neurons by several excitatory and inhibitory mechanisms (Mayeri et al., 1985; Sigvardt et al., 1986). In addition, egg-laying hormone (ELH) acts as a circulating neurohormone to enhance contraction of the muscles in the reproductive duct. All these peptides appear to be cleavage products from a single high molecular weight protein precursor in the bag cells (Scheller et al., 1983). Thus, coexpression of these peptides results in the generation of a family of behaviors with a common goal (Scheller and Axel, 1984).

3 COMPARATIVE ANALYSIS OF CHEMICAL ACTIVATION OF CPGs

An analysis of the results obtained in these and other systems (Table I) leads to several general comments on the roles of identified transmitters and modulators as initiators of CPG activity.

1. *A compound can experimentally activate a motor pattern by either direct or indirect mechanisms.* First, it could directly excite neurons within the CPG circuit. To demonstrate this, at least some of the neurons comprising the CPG must be identified, and this has not yet been accomplished in any vertebrate system. Direct transmitter effects on CPG components have been demonstrated in several invertebrate CPGs (Nusbaum, 1986; Granzow and Kater, 1977). However, this does not assure a trigger function for these compounds (see below). Conversely, a compound could act indirectly to excite the elements of a "command system" (Kupfermann and Weiss, 1978) that normally activates the CPG. Since the ability of these compounds to activate the CPG would obviously vary with the excitability and efficacy of the command system, it may be misleading to consider them as "activators" of a CPG.

In many of the cases I have described, a compound directly excites motoneurons in addition to apparent effects at higher levels of the nervous system; such a multi-tiered activation of behavior may be a general mechanism. This multi-tiered action could enhance the movement by increasing the output at every level of neuronal organization.

2. *It is difficult to determine whether a compound normally plays a role to trigger activity of a CPG.* Since an animal can initiate locomotion very rapidly in a critical situation, pathways must exist that directly and rapidly trigger activity in CPG circuits. However, it has been difficult to identify the compounds that are used for this triggering role. Several approaches can be used. First, pharmacological antagonists of the compound can be tested for their ability to block a naturally induced activation of the CPG (Steeves et al., 1980; Dale and Roberts, 1983; Wieland and Gelperin, 1983; McClellan and Grillner, 1984; Brodin and Grillner, 1985). The specificity of the antagonist must be carefully examined to be sure that it functions as expected in each organism. In addition, if several independent mechanisms exist to activate a CPG, this test may yield false negative results. Also, as described below, if a compound plays an important role in preparing the CPG for activity but not in directly triggering it, pharmacological antagonism might disable the circuit. A second approach is to eliminate the neurons or terminals using the transmitter and see whether the motor pattern can still be activated (Steeves et al., 1980; Glover and Kramer, 1982). This approach really asks a different question: is the compound *essential* for CPG activation? Clearly it will fail when several pathways exist to activate a CPG. Care must be taken that the loss of these neurons has no other effects on the behavior in question. Again, this method cannot discriminate between compounds that trigger CPG activity and those that enable CPGs to be activated. A third approach is to identify the transmitters used by neurons that are active at appropriate times and which, when stimulated, elicit activity in the CPG. This method is most feasible in invertebrates, where the repeatable identification of neurons is relatively straightforward. It carries the potential problem that many neurons release more than one transmitter (Chan-Palay and Palay, 1984), and the entire package may be necessary to evoke the whole behavior. A particularly clear example of this is the bag cells in *Aplysia*, which release multiple peptides to elicit a complex of behaviors related to egg-laying; any one peptide only activates a portion of the entire behavioral pattern.

3. *A compound that activates a CPG in vitro may normally play an enabling or gain-setting role instead of a triggering role.* The search for compounds that trigger CPG activity also runs into problems of the definition of a trigger. Many neuromodulators change the responsiveness of a neuron to other synaptic inputs without themselves directly activating or inactivating the neuron (see below). These compounds could raise or lower the threshold for activation of a CPG by other neuronal inputs such as sensory feedback, descending commands, etc. Some CPGs might normally be activated by this enabling mechanism alone. The specificity for activation would then

lie in the preparatory modulation rather than in the actual triggering event. On the other hand, other CPGs may *require* a gain-setting change in addition to a direct triggering event for activation; that is, modulators may *gate* the ability of the normal triggering stimuli to activate the CPG. Such enabling inputs would be necessary but not sufficient to elicit CPG output (Figure 1).

4. *There is probably more than one mechanism for activating any CPG.* In several systems, transmitters have been identified that are sufficient but not necessary to elicit a motor pattern (Steeves et al., 1980; Brodin et al., 1984a,b). This suggests that additional activation mechanisms exist for these patterns. For many CPGs, both rapid "trigger" activation mechanisms and slower "modulatory" activation mechanisms would be useful for different behavioral circumstances.

5. *A number of different cellular mechanisms could be used to activate a CPG.* Since few CPGs are understood in any detail, little evidence is available to address that point. However, a number of possibilities can be described as reasonable mechanisms.

(a) *Generalized excitation.* For rapid activation of a CPG, standard excitation by a conductance increase mechanism could raise the activity of CPG components above threshold to start rhythmic activity within the CPG (Roberts et al., 1983).

(b) *Release from inhibition.* A CPG could be prevented from expressing its rhythmic motor output by tonic inhibition which decreases the excitability of the system below the level required to cycle. If this inhibitory input ceases, CPG output could begin. In a related mechanism, the CPG may cycle but the motor program would not be expressed due to tonic inhibition of the relevant motoneurons. Disinhibition or excitation of the motoneurons could allow the expression of CPG output.

(c) *Conductance decrease leading to cell activation.* A long-lasting conductance decrease mechanism increases the responsiveness of a neuron to other simultaneous synaptic inputs. By increasing the membrane resistance and thus decreasing the loss of synaptic current, EPSP's and IPSP's have greater amplitude at their initial sites, passively propagate over greater distances, and have longer time courses (Graubard and Calvin, 1979; Rall, 1981). These mechanisms enhance spatial and temporal summation of synaptic events and may result in spike initiation where previously the same inputs had yielded only subthreshold responses. This mechanism is clearly important in the modulation of CPG activity (see below). However, it acts slowly and, as described above, depends on other synaptic inputs to be the actual triggers. Thus, conductance decrease mechanisms seem inappropriate as rapid triggers, but are excellent for enabling roles or to maintain tonically active CPGs.

(d) *Activation of endogenous bursting in CPG neurons.* Most of the rhythmic CPGs that have been analyzed contain neurons with endogenous bursting pacemaker properties (Getting, this volume). Endogenous bursting in "conditional bursters" can be activated or inactivated by applied neuro-modulators (Ifshin et al., 1975; Drummond et al., 1980; Anderson and Barker, 1981; Marder and Eisen, 1984b; Flamm and Harris-Warrick, 1984, 1986b; Harris-Warrick and Flamm, 1986b) or stimulation of modulatory neurons (Nagy and Dickinson, 1983). These modulatory inputs probably act by enhancing the synthesis of second messengers such as cAMP, which has been shown to induce bursting in some silent cells (Connor, 1985; Flamm and Harris-Warrick, 1987). Clearly, generation of burst conductances in an essential CPG neuron could activate the CPG and at the same time provide temporal cues for the regulation of cycle period and intensity.

(e) *Modulation of other intrinsic nonlinear membrane properties of CPG neurons.* Other complex membrane properties such as postinhibitory rebound, plateau potentials, delayed excitation, and alterations in threshold are critically important to normal CPG activity (Getting, this volume). The membrane conductances that underly these properties can be regulated by neuromodulators (Russell and Hartline, 1978, 1981; Pellmar, 1981; Miller and Selverston, 1982), and their activation could turn on the CPG.

4   MODULATION OF ONGOING CPG ACTIVITY

All animals can adapt simple rhythmic motor programs to meet the changing demands of the environment. For example, a person can walk with a variety of gaits, quickly or slowly, and forward or backward. While each variation could in theory be produced by a different neuronal circuit, it is simpler to suppose that a single CPG is continuously modulated to produce all the variants on a common theme. Modifications of CPG activity by descending inputs and sensory feedback are reviewed in this volume (see Rossignol et al., and Grillner et al., this volume). Here, I wish to discuss the role of neuromodulators in the long-term modification of CPG-evoked motor patterns. By studying how these compounds act on a CPG and its associated motor pathway, we can further our knowledge of the organization of motor function, and approach an understanding of the cellular and molecular bases of behavioral plasticity.

A number of preparations have been studied in which identified transmitters or modulators change CPG activity (Table II). In many of these cases, the cellular targets of the transmitter have not yet been identified, and these will not be discussed further. I have chosen several systems to describe in some detail, as they illustrate important principles of CPG modulation which are discussed in the next section.

4.1   Serotonergic Modulation of Vertebrate Locomotion

Serotonin is present in small neurons and processes in the spinal cord of the lamprey, *Ichthyomyzon unicuspis* and *Petromyzon marinus* (Honma, 1970;

Table 2. Chemical Modulation of Movement

Movement	Species	Compound	Level of Analysis[a]	References
Swimming	Lamprey	Serotonin	M	Harris-Warrick and Cohen, 1985
Walking	Cat	Norepinephrine	B	Barbeau and Rossignol, 1982
		Serotonin	B	Barbeau and Rossignol, 1982
		Dopamine	B	Barbeau and Rossignol, 1982
Flight	*Manduca*	Octopamine	B, M	Kinnamon et al., 1984
Ventilation	Cat	ACh	B	Brimblecombe, 1977
		Serotonin	B	Armijo et al., 1979
		GABA	B	Yamada et al., 1981
		Glycine	B	Holtman et al., 1982
		Taurine	B	Holtman et al., 1983a
		CCK	B	Gillis et al., 1983
		Bombesin	B	Holtman et al., 1983b
	Rabbit	Substance P	B	Yamamoto et al., 1981
		TRH	B	
	Rat	Dopamine	B	Lundberg et al., 1979, 1982
		Serotonin	B	Mueller et al., 1980
		TRH	B	Hedner et al., 1981
	Corydalus	Serotonin	M	Bellah et al., 1984
Crawling	*Aplysia*	Bag cell peptides	M	Mackey and Carew, 1983
Posture	Lobster	Serotonin	M, C	Livingstone et al., 1980
		Octopamine	M, C	Harris-Warrick and Kravitz, 1984; Harris-Warrick, 1985
	Crayfish	Serotonin	B, M	Livingstone et al., 1980
		Octopamine	B, M	
	Crab	Serotonin	B, M	Bevengut and Clarac, 1982
		Octopamine	B, M	
Heartbeat	Crustacea	Serotonin	M, C, I	Cooke, 1966; Cooke and Hartline, 1975: Lemos and Berlind, 1981
		Dopamine	M, C, I	Miller et al., 1984; Cooke and Sullivan, 1982
		Octopamine	M, C	Florey and Rathmeyer, 1978 Benson, 1984
		Proctolin	M, C, I	Miller and Sullivan, 1981 Sullivan and Miller, 1984
	Limulus	Octopamine	M, C	Augustine et al., 1982
		Dopamine	M, C	Watson and Augustine, 1982
		Norepinephrine	M, C	Watson et al., 1985
		Serotonin	M, C	
		Proctolin	M, C	

Table 2. (Cont.)

Movement	Species	Compound	Level of Analysis[a]	References
	Leech	FMRFamide	M	Kuhlman et al., 1985
Scaphogna- thite beating	Crab	Serotonin	M	Berlind, 1977
Feeding	*Aplysia*	Serotonin	M, C, I	Kupfermann et al., 1979, 1981
				Kupfermann and Weiss, 1982
		SCP$_B$	M	Lloyd et al., 1984; Weiss et al., 1978
	Lymnaea	Serotonin	M, C	Benjamin, 1983; McCrohan and Benjamin, 1980; Benjamin et al., 1981
	Pleurobranchaea	Serotonin	M, C	Gillette and Davis, 1977
	Tritonia	Serotonin	M, C	Bulloch and Dorsett, 1979
	Helisoma	Dopamine	M, C	Trimble and Barker, 1984
Pyloric stomach rhythm	Lobster	Ach	M, C, I	Marder and Paupardin- Tritsch, 1978; Nagy and Dickinson, 1983; Dickinson and Nagy, 1983; Nagy et al., 1984, 1985
		Dopamine	M, C, I	Raper, 1979; Anderson and Barker, 1981; Marder and Eisen, 1984b; Flamm and Harris-Warrick, 1984, 1986ab; Harris-Warrick and Flamm, 1986
		Serotonin	M, C, I	Beltz et al., 1984; Flamm and Harris-Warrick, 1984, 1986a,b; Harris-Warrick and Flamm, 1986
		Octopamine	M, C, I	Flamm and Harris-Warrick, 1984, 1986a,b; Harris- Warrick and Flamm, 1986
		Histamine	M, C, I	Claiborne and Selverston, 1984
		Proctolin	M, C	Hooper and Marder, 1984; Marder et al., 1986
		FMRFamide	M, C	Hooper and Marder, 1984
Gastric stomach rhythm	Lobster	Octopamine	M, C	Wadepuhl and Selverston, 1984
		Proctolin	M, C	Marder et al., 1986; Marder and Hooper, 1985

[a]Level of analysis: B = behavioral; M = motor pattern; C = cellular; I = ionic mechanisms. See Table 1 for details.

Baumgarten, 1972; Ochi et al., 1979; Harris-Warrick et al., 1985; Van Dongen et al., 1985). Harris-Warrick and Cohen (1985) showed that serotonin can modulate fictive locomotion in the isolated lamprey spinal cord. At the segmental level, serotonin caused a dose-dependent reduction in the frequency and an increase in the intensity of rhythmic ventral root burst discharges. In addition, serotonin affected the intersegmental phase delay. This arose at least in part from a gradient of serotonin's effects on the segmental oscillators down the cord, with caudal segments more affected than rostral segments. Serotonin appears to affect primarily the locomotor CPG; when the CPG is not cycling (in the absence of D-glutamate), serotonin has no detectable effects. However, myotomal motoneurons also appear to be directly affected: part of the increased spike frequency during a burst of action potentials in serotonin appears to arise from a decreased duration of the spike afterhyperpolarization. Serotonin may thus act on motoneurons by blocking a potassium conductance (Van Dongen et al., 1986). Ayers and colleagues (1983) have proposed that the CPG for swimming in the lamprey spinal cord actually generates a family of related movements, including swimming, crawling, and burrowing. We have suggested that serotonin may be one of the neuromodulators that sculpt this CPG to produce a variety of related movements (Harris-Warrick and Cohen, 1985).

4.2   Amine Modulation of Posture in the Lobster

Injections of serotonin or octopamine into the hemolymph of freely moving lobsters (*Homarus americanus*) induce opposing static postures: serotonin causes a tonic flexion of all extremities, while octopamine causes a tonic extension (Livingstone et al., 1980; Harris-Warrick et al., 1980; Harris-Warrick and Kravitz, 1984). These amines affect the postural motor system at a number of different levels (Fig. 3). First, they act as circulating neurohormones and affect the postural exoskeletal muscles, where they have both pre- and postsynaptic effects (Battelle and Kravitz, 1978; Kravitz et al., 1980, 1981). On the opener muscle in the walking leg, both serotonin and octopamine directly induce a long-lasting contracture and allow the production of calcium-dependent action potentials by increasing a voltage-dependent calcium current (Glusman et al., 1980; Kravitz et al., 1981). Serotonin also enhances the release of both excitatory and inhibitory transmitters from motoneuron terminals (Glusman and Kravitz, 1982). Each amine has different effects on different muscles in the lobster, but it always has symmetrical effects on a functionally opposing flexor-extensor pair (Harris-Warrick and Kravitz, 1984). Thus, the peripheral actions of amines do not specify postural flexion or extension. Instead, they act to adjust the amplitude of muscle response for a given neural command.

The postures observed in vivo arise from amine actions within central ganglia to alter the pattern of postural motoneuron activity (Livingstone et al., 1980; Harris-Warrick and Kravitz, 1984). Similar results have been reported in the crayfish, *Procambarus* (Livingstone et al., 1980) and in the

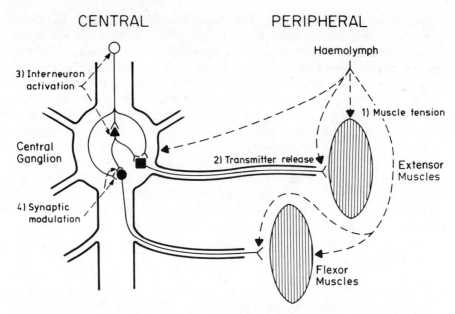

FIGURE 3. Targets of amine modulation in the postural motor system in the lobster. Serotonin and octopamine act as circulating hormones to modulate muscle tension (1) and release of transmitter from motoneuron terminals (2). Both amines are also found within cells and processes in the central ganglia, where they modulate the activity of postural interneurons (3) and regulate the efficacy of their synapses onto postural motoneurons (4).

crab, *Carcinus* (Bevengut and Clarac, 1982). The amines alter this motor pattern at least in part by increasing or decreasing the activity of premotor interneurons that drive the postural motoneurons (Harris-Warrick and Kravitz, 1984).

In addition to changing the level of activity of postural interneurons, octopamine and serotonin modulate the efficacy of their synapses onto postural motoneurons (Harris-Warrick, 1985). An extended family of interneurons called "command fibers" (Evoy and Kennedy, 1967) or "command elements" (Kupfermann and Weiss, 1979) controls posture in the crustacean abdomen (Jellies and Larimer, 1983; Larimer et al., 1985). These cells synapse both monosynaptically and polysynaptically onto postural motoneurons (Thompson and Page, 1981, 1982; Miall and Larimer, 1982; Harris-Warrick, 1985). The postural motor pattern induced by an extension command element is dramatically enhanced by octopamine and reduced by serotonin. This results at least in part from corresponding increases and decreases in the amplitude of the final epsp onto postural motoneurons (Harris-Warrick, 1985). Thus, the strength of the motor pattern generated by the central postural control circuits can be modified by modulating the motoneuron response to a given synaptic input.

In summary, octopamine and serotonin act in a highly coordinated fashion at multiple levels from CNS to muscle to affect the motor system for tonic posture in the lobster (Figure 3). Beltz and Kravitz (1984) have shown that the same neuron can release serotonin both centrally within neural ganglia and peripherally into the hemolymph. Thus, the transmitter and hormonal actions of serotonin might be temporally coupled to provide a coherent multi-level modulation of posture.

4.3 Serotonergic Modulation of Feeding Motor Programs in Molluscs

The neuronal circuitry underlying the initiation and control of feeding has been extensively studied in a variety of molluscs (for review, see Benjamin, 1983). A pair of large serotonergic cells, called the metacerebral cells (MCCs) plays an important modulatory role in feeding. Activity of these cells is correlated with behavioral arousal for feeding (Kupfermann and Weiss, 1982). Stimulation of an MCC in quiescent, semi-intact preparations can sometimes elicit feeding (Granzow and Kater, 1977, Croll et al., 1985), but it always modulates ongoing feeding motor programs, increasing the burst strength and frequency. The targets of MCC synapses and bath-applied serotonin include neuronal structures for feeding at every possible level (Fig. 4). These include: (1) monosynaptic excitation of cells that ap-

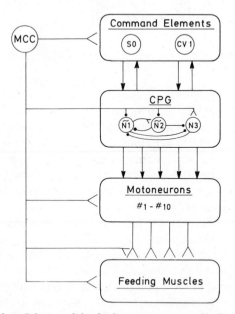

FIGURE 4. Targets of modulation of the feeding motor system by the serotonergic metacerebral cell (MCC) in molluscs. The MCC affects every level of this system, with monosynaptic inputs to command elements, CPG neurons, motoneurons, motoneuron terminals and feeding muscles. The activity is highly coordinated to enhance feeding behavior at every level. This figure shows combined data from *Lymnaea* and *Aplysia*. Adapted from Benjamin, 1983 and Elliot and Benjamin, 1985.

pear to be members of the command system for initiation of feeding behavior (Benjamin, 1983); (2) monosynaptic excitation or polysynaptic inhibition of putative members of the feeding CPG (McCrohan and Benjamin, 1980b; Benjamin et al., 1981; Benjamin, 1983); (3) modulatory excitation of many of the feeding motoneurons, where a train of MCC pulses induces a prolonged depolarization that reduces the threshold for activation (Kupfermann and Weiss, 1981); and (4) direct modulation of the feeding musculature (Kupfermann and Weiss, 1981). In the accessory radula closer muscle (ARC), MCC stimulation has little effect alone, but it enhances the nerve-evoked muscle contraction. Part of this effect results from an enhancement of transmitter release from the motoneuron terminals. However, the greatest effect appears to be directly on the muscles and may involve cAMP-dependent phosphorylation of myofibrillar proteins (Kupfermann and Weiss, 1981; Weiss et al., 1979). As with crustacean postural muscles, serotonin can have different effects on different feeding muscles (Ram et al., 1981).

These experiments show the strikingly broad effects of the serotonergic MCC within the feeding circuit. Serotonin acts at every level of the pathway, from the decision-making cells to the muscle fibers. Other modulators also effect feeding at different levels, including a small cardioactive peptide (SCP$_B$) which mimics serotonin's effects on the ARC muscle (Lloyd et al., 1984). Thus, parallel peptidergic and serotonergic pathways can mediate the peripheral aspects of feeding arousal.

4.4   Modulation of the Pyloric Rhythm in the Lobster Stomatogastric Ganglion

The stomatogastric ganglion of *Panulirus interruptus* consists of about 30 neurons and contains the CPGs for two rhythmic stomach movements, the gastric rhythm and the pyloric rhythm (Selverston et al., 1976, 1983; Miller and Selverston, 1985). The pyloric rhythm CPG generates a rhythmic pumping and filtering movement in the pyloric region of the stomach. It has been analyzed very thoroughly, and is the best understood CPG at the present time. It contains 14 neurons in six major classes (Fig. 5). The synaptic connectivity and transmitters used in the pyloric CPG have been elucidated (Miller and Selverston, 1982a,b; Eisen and Marder, 1982; Fig. 5), and many of the intrinsic properties of its neurons are known. The mechanistic basis for the rhythmic bursting motor pattern has been qualitatively described (Miller and Selverston, 1982b; Selverston et al., 1983). The existence of the pattern is based upon the intrinsic bursting properties of many of the neurons, in combination with the pattern of mutually inhibitory synapses within the network. The actual phase relations depend on the pattern of synaptic connectivity as well as intrinsic properties of the neurons such as plateau potentials (Russell and Hartline, 1978, 1981), bursting pacemaker potentials (Miller and Selverston, 1982a), post-inhibitory re-

A. Pyloric circuit

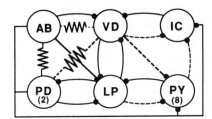

B. Combined

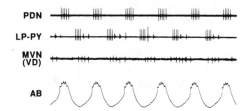

C. Sucrose block

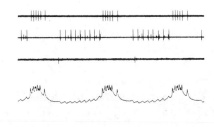

D. Dopamine

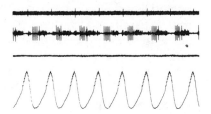

E. Octopamine

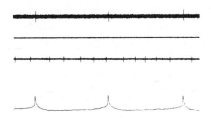

F. Serotonin

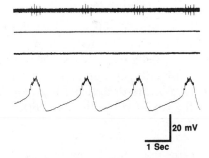

20 mV

1 Sec

FIGURE 5. Motor patterns generated by the pyloric circuit of the lobster stomatogastric ganglion. (A) Schematic diagram of the pyloric circuit. The synaptic connections are either electrical (resistor symbols) or chemical inhibitory (filled circles). Some of the synaptic connections are functionally weaker (dashed lines), while others are stronger (solid lines). (B) Typical activity of the pyloric circuit with intact modulatory input from the commissural and esophageal ganglia. The top three traces are extracellular records from motor nerves carrying axons of the indicated motoneurons. The AB is the only cell in the circuit that is not a motoneuron: intracellular recordings of its activity are shown in the bottom trace. (C) Reduced activity in the isolated stomatogastric ganglion when modulatory inputs from the commissural and esophageal ganglia are blocked with a sucrose pool on the stomatogastric nerve. Many cells become silent, and others fire tonically at low frequencies. (D,E,F) Activity of an isolated stomatogastric ganglion with bath-applied dopamine, octopamine and serotonin. From Harris-Warrick and Flamm, 1986a.

bound and differences in relative synaptic strengths (Selverston et al., 1976; Miller and Selverston, 1982b). The AB interneuron appears to be the most important neuron for timing of the cycle; it is electrically coupled to the two PD neurons and has very strong inhibitory synapses onto all the other neurons.

Although the pyloric circuit can generate a basal rhythm in the absence of any other synaptic input, it is normally under modulatory control from other ganglia (Selverston et al., 1976; Marder, 1984). If input from the commissural and esophageal ganglia is left intact, the rhythm is highly active and all the neurons fire in bursts (Russell, 1979). However, upon isolation of the ganglion, the rhythm slows down and occasionally stops; many of the neurons are silent (Fig. 5). This is due to the inactivation of plateau potential and bursting pacemaker potential capabilities in the pyloric neurons (Russell and Hartline, 1978, 1981; Miller and Selverston, 1982a,b). Since these intrinsic membrane properties are under modulatory control, many of the pyloric neurons have been termed "conditional bursters" (Miller and Selverston, 1982a,b). A number of neurotransmitters and neuromodulators are present in the stomatogastric nerve (STN) which provides the sole input to the STG from other ganglia (Table 2). Many of these compounds can modify the form of the pyloric rhythm (Fig. 5). Thus, the small 14-neuron circuit can be modulated to produce a very large variety of motor patterns (Marder, 1984).

4.5   Amine Modulation of the Pyloric Rhythm

Our data on the effects of dopamine, octopamine and serotonin on the pyloric rhythm are shown in Figures 6–8 (Harris-Warrick and Flamm, 1984; Beltz et al., 1984; Flamm and Harris-Warrick, 1986a,b). In these experiments, modulatory input from the other ganglia was blocked to attain a basal, non-modulated state of the STG. The natural neuromodulators of the circuit could then be added back one at a time, and their effects measured.

Each amine enhanced activity in the pyloric circuit, but the motor patterns in each case were unique both in their neuronal composition (which cells were active) as well as in the activity of the component neurons (Figs. 5 and 6). Each amine activated some neurons while inhibiting others. The quality of the amine effects on different cells in the circuit was also different. Marder and colleagues have shown that the peptides Proctolin and FMRFamide (Hooper and Marder, 1984; Marder et al., 1986) and red pigment concentrating hormone (Nusbaum and Marder, 1986), as well as the muscarinic agonist pilocarpine (Nagy and Dickinson, 1983; Marder, 1985) can all elicit further unique patterns from the pyloric CPG. These data show that a single anatomically defined neuronal network can be modulated to generate a number of functionally different circuits (Fig. 8). Each functional circuit is produced by the interactions of a subset of the CPG

Intact Circuit

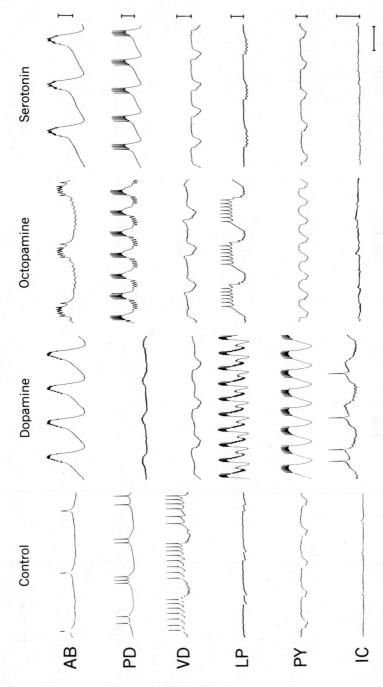

FIGURE 6. Effects of dopamine, octopamine, and serotonin on the six cell classes in the pyloric CPG. Intracellular records from different cells are from different experiments. Each amine elicits a unique constellation of effects on the pyloric neurons, resulting in different motor patterns. Adapted from Flamm and Harris-Warrick, 1985a. Time marker: 1 second. Voltage markers: 10mV.

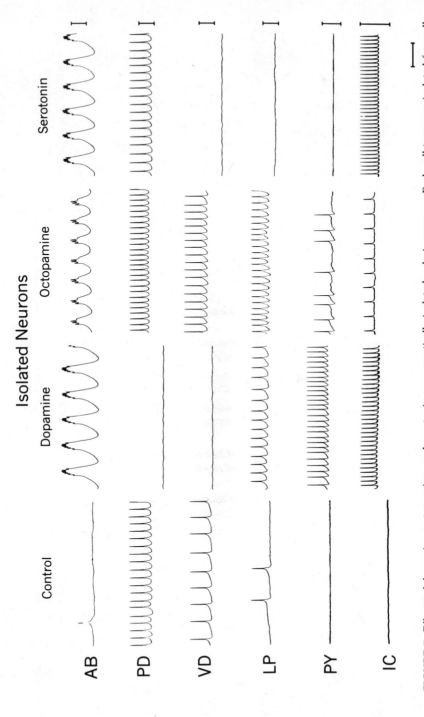

Isolated Neurons

Control Dopamine Octopamine Serotonin

AB

PD

VD

LP

PY

IC

FIGURE 7. Effects of dopamine, octopamine, and serotonin on synaptically isolated pyloric neurons. Each cell type was isolated from all known synaptic inputs as described in the text. Dopamine and octopamine have direct excitatory or inhibitory effects on every cell type in the pyloric CPG, while serotonin affects four of the six classes. The AB neuron is induced to burst endogenously with amines; other neurons fire tonically or are inhibited. From Harris-Warrick and Flamm, 1986a. Time marker: 1 second. Voltage markers: 10 mV.

TARGETS   ACTIVE CIRCUIT

Control

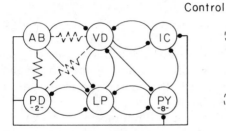

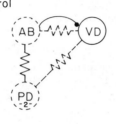

10^{-4}M Dopamine

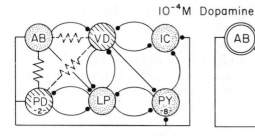

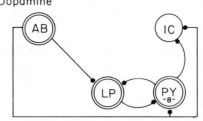

10^{-4} M Octopamine

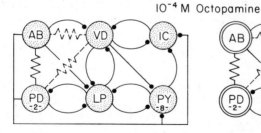

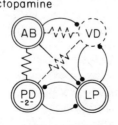

10^{-5}M Serotonin

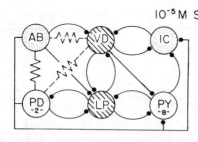

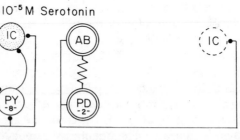

FIGURE 8. Summary of the direct neuronal targets of dopamine, octopamine and serotonin in the pyloric CPG (left), and the active circuits that result from each amine (right). Stippled cells are excited by the amine, stripped cells are inhibited and clear cells are not affected. Spike activity in the active circuit is given by the circle type, with double circle as strong activity, single circle as moderate activity, dashed circle as weak activity and no circle as inactive. From Flamm and Harris-Warrick, 1986b.

network's neurons, and each generates a unique motor pattern (Marder, 1984).

In addition, we have observed concentration-dependent differences in the stable motor patterns generated by dopamine and octopamine (Flamm and Harris-Warrick, 1986b). This suggests that alterations in the rate or intensity of activity of neurons releasing these amines can result in qualitatively different motor patterns. Biochemical, immunocytochemical, and physiological experiments also suggest that while dopamine and octopamine are released from nerve terminals in the STG, serotonin normally acts as a circulating hormone to affect the pyloric rhythm in *Panulirus* (Beltz et al, 1984). The STG, because it is located within the anterior ophthalmic artery, has access to blood-borne hormones. Serotonin is active at concentrations found in the hemolymph (10^{-9}M: Livingstone et al., 1980; Cooke and Sullivan, 1982) and is not biochemically or immunocytochemically detectable in the stomatogastric nervous system of *Panulirus interruptus* (Beltz et al., 1984).

4.6   Cellular Targets of Amine Action in the Pyloric CPG

In order to understand how a neuromodulator shapes a CPG circuit, it is essential to determine which neurons in the circuit are direct targets of modulatory input. The pyloric CPG offers a unique opportunity to answer this question, because it is possible to isolate any given cell from all detectable synaptic input in situ and determine its direct responses to a modulator. Three steps are taken to synaptically isolate a pyloric neuron (Flamm and Harris-Warrick, 1984, 1986b): (1) eliminate input from other ganglia with a sucrose/TTX block on the input STN; (2) use lucifer yellow photoinactivation (Selverston and Miller, 1980; Miller and Selverston, 1979, 1982a,b) to kill stomatogastric neurons that synapse on the cell; in this system, electrically coupled cells are *not* dye-coupled (Miller and Selverston, 1982a,b); and (3) inhibit other stomatogastric synaptic inputs with pharmacological blockade of the pyloric transmitters (Marder, 1974, 1976; Lingle, 1981; Marder and Eisen, 1984a). These procedures leave the neuron intact with normal dendritic arborization and receptors, but with no detectable synaptic input (Fig. 7, control). Neuromodulators can then be added and direct effects on the isolated neuron determined in the absence of confounding synaptic inputs. Figure 7 shows the effects of dopamine, octopamine, and serotonin on each of the six classes of synaptically isolated pyloric neurons. The qualitative targets of amine action and the resulting modified neuronal circuits are summarized in Figure 8.

Several conclusions can be drawn from these results. First, each amine has a unique constellation of effects on the neurons in the pyloric circuit (Fig. 7). This underlies the unique variants of the pyloric motor pattern generated in the synaptically intact circuit. (Figs. 6 and 8). Second, each amine affects almost every cell in the circuit. There is no single "target neuron" for an amine; rather, the entire population of neurons in the circuit is usually affected by each amine. Third, each amine can have multiple physiological effects on different cells within this small circuit. For example, dopamine elicits endogenous bursting pacemaker potentials in the AB cell, tonic firing in the LP, PY and IC cells, and tonic inhibition of the PD and VD neurons. Note that the AB and PD neurons, which are electrically coupled and usually fire synchronously, are oppositely affected by dopamine (Eisen and Marder, 1984). Octopamine and serotonin also have multiple effects on pyloric neurons. This diversity of modulator action on different neurons within the circuit allows for a greatly increased variety of motor patterns when compared to a system where each modulator has only one mechanism of action or only acts on one or a few neurons in the circuit.

4.7 Modulation of Intrinsic Properties of Pyloric Neurons

In addition to determining which neurons are active or inactive, a neuromodulator can change the motor pattern produced by a CPG by modifying the intrinsic properties of the component neurons. In the lobster *Jasus lalandii*, stimulation of the cholinergic anterior pyloric modulator (APM cell), or bath application of muscarinic agonists, can induce plateau potential capabilities in quiescent pyloric neurons (Dickinson and Nagy, 1983). During this time, a brief depolarization will elicit a prolonged depolarized plateau with high frequency spiking. The ionic mechanisms underlying plateau potential induction have not been fully elucidated, but may include a reduction of a tonic TEA-sensitive potassium conductance. This depolarizes the cell and unmasks a voltage-sensitive calcium conductance that underlies the sustained depolarization during the plateau potential (Nagy et al., 1984, 1985). Other conductance changes are also likely to be involved.

The AB neuron in *Panulirus interruptus* is a conditional burster. When synaptically isolated, it is silent, but a number of inputs and neuromodulators can induce rhythmic bursting, with a large bursting pacemaker potential (BPP) underlying each burst (Flamm and Harris-Warrick, 1986b; Marder and Eisen, 1984b; Marder et al., 1986). We have compared the ionic dependences of BPPs induced by dopamine, serotonin, and octopamine (Harris-Warrick and Flamm, 1986b). The BPP frequency, amplitude and shape are different for each of the three amines (Fig. 9). Experiments using ion substitution and pharmacological blockade have shown that there are quantitative differences in the contributions of sodium, calcium, and potassium currents in the BPPs induced by the three amines (Fig. 9). For example, BPPs initiated by serotonin or octopamine are rapidly eliminated by tetrodotoxin or low-sodium saline, but dopamine-induced BPPs are not. In contrast dopamine-induced BPPs are eliminated by reductions in extracellular calcium to 25% of normal, while serotonin- and octopamine-

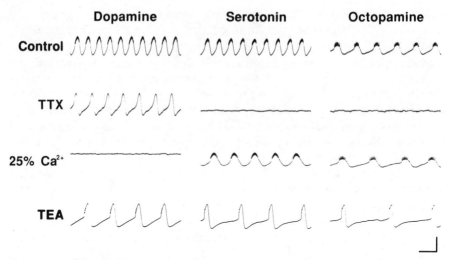

FIGURE 9. Effects of dopamine, serotonin and octopamine on synaptically isolated AB neurons under different conditions. *Control:* with normal saline, all three amines induce rhythmic bursting pacemaker potentials (BPPs) with different amplitudes, frequencies and shapes. *TTX:* in the presence of 10^{-7}M TTX, dopamine still generates large BPPs, but serotonin- and octopamine-induced BPPs are abolished. Identical results are seen with low-sodium saline (Harris-Warrick and Flamm, 1986b). *25% Ca²⁺:* with reduced calcium, dopamine-induced BPPs are abolished, and the cell remains depolarized near the peak of the BPP. Serotonin- and octopamine-induced BPPs are modified but not abolished. *TEA:* addition of TEA nearly eliminates the difference in BPP amplitudes induced by the three amines. Voltage marker: 20mV, except 10mV for TTX. Time marker: 1 second, except 2.5 second for TTX (Note: amplitude and frequency of dopamine-induced BPPs were not altered by TTX: this figure is from a different experiment than the control above. From Harris-Warrick and Flamm, 1986b.)

induced BPPs are not. These results and others show that this single neuron can be modulated to burst by a variety of different ionic mechanisms; bursting does not depend on a particular, carefully balanced combination of conductance changes. These different bursting mechanisms in the AB neuron have important biological consequences for the pyloric rhythm, resulting in changes in cycle frequency and phase relations between pyloric neurons (Harris-Warrick and Flamm, 1986b).

4.8   Modulation of Synaptic Efficacy in the Pyloric CPG

In addition to changing the activity of isolated neurons in a CPG, neuromodulators can also alter the strength of synaptic interactions within the circuit, thus functionally altering the "wiring diagram" of the circuit. In *Jasus lalandii*, stimulation of the APM neuron induces a dramatic reorganization of the pyloric rhythm, including changes in the cycle frequency, the amplitudes of slow wave depolarizations of many of the neurons, and the phase relationships between neurons (Nagy and Dickinson, 1983;

Dickinson and Nagy, 1983). Many of these changes are due to the enabling of plateau potential capabilities in the pyloric neurons, as described above. APM stimulation affects many synaptic interactions within the circuit: some inhibitory synapses are functionally strengthened, while others are weakened. APM activation of plateau potentials in the postsynaptic cells can explain part of these effects: a cell firing from a plateau potential will actively resist weak inhibitory inputs while allowing a full repolarizing response to strong inhibitory inputs which can terminate the plateau potential (Dickinson and Nagy, 1983). In addition, transmitter release may also be altered by APM stimulation. These alterations in synaptic efficacy and plateau potential capability can explain the observed changes in the phase relations between pyloric neurons during APM stimulation.

In *Panulirus interruptus*, phase relationships between pyloric neurons are altered by dopamine, and this results in part from opposing effects of dopamine on the electrically coupled AB and PD neurons (Fig. 7; Marder and Eisen, 1984b). These cells usually fire synchronously and synapse on the same follower cells but release different transmitters. AB uses glutamate to elicit a rapid ipsp, while PD releases acetylcholine to elicit a much slower, more prolonged ipsp. The compound ipsp observed in the follower cells thus has a rapid onset (from the AB) and a slow recovery (from the PD) (Eisen and Marder, 1982, 1984). In dopamine, the AB is excited but the PD is inhibited (Eisen and Marder, 1984b; Flamm and Harris-Warrick, 1984, 1986a,b). As a consequence, the new compound ipsp reflects mainly AB activity and is shortened in time course. This allows the follower cells such as the LP to recover more quickly and begin to burst at an earlier phase in the cycle. We have also obtained preliminary evidence that octopamine, and perhaps serotonin as well, can modulate the strength of synapses between identified pyloric neurons (Johnson and Harris-Warrick, unpublished).

4.9 Reconstruction of Modified Pyloric Rhythm from Amine Effects on Single Cells in the Circuit

These results point out the difficulty of determining exactly how a neuromodulator generates a new motor pattern from a CPG. The final pattern represents a complex interaction between the direct effects of the modulator on (1) the activity of each of the CPG neurons, (2) the intrinsic properies of those neurons, and (3) the synaptic connectivity of the system, which itself can be modulated (Selverston, 1980). For example, octopamine directly excites all six classes of pyloric neurons (Figs. 7 and 8; Flamm and Harris-Warrick, 1986a,b). However, in the synaptically intact circuit, only three classes of neurons (AB, PD and LP) are highly active; the others are very weakly active or silent (Figs. 6 and 8). This apparent discrepancy can only be understood within the full context of the circuit. The AB and LP neurons are quantitatively more strongly excited by octopamine than the other neurons. These cells together synaptically inhibit all the other neurons throughout the cycle except the PD, which is electrically coupled to the AB. Thus, even though the other neurons are excited by octopamine, the synaptic connectivity of the circuit prevents the manifestation of that excitation (Flamm and Harris-Warrick, 1985b). This result shows clearly that the effects of neuromodulators must be interpreted within the constraints of the circuit in order to understand the motor patterns that result from modulation.

5   COMPARATIVE ANALYSIS OF MODULATION OF CPGs

Any attempt to draw definitive conclusions about the mechanisms for modulation of CPG circuits is hampered by the small number of systems that have been carefully analyzed (Table 2). The major obstacle has been the difficulty in defining the CPG components so that the targets of modulation can be unambiguously studied. This has only been accomplished in a few invertebrate systems. The following conclusions obtained in a few simpler systems should thus be considered as testable hypotheses for more complex systems. I will first list some principles concerning neuromodulation of motor systems in general. Then I will describe some principles for neuromodulation of CPG circuits in particular.

5.1   Neuromodulation of Motor Patterns

1. *One CPG can generate a large variety of motor patterns, and different neuromodulators generate unique variants on the basic pattern.* An animal must be able to modulate simple motor patterns in order to adapt its behavior to the changing demands of the environment. The CPG is a prime target for modulation to allow this behavioral plasticity to occur. With the pyloric rhythm of the stomatogastric ganglion, every aspect of the circuit can be modulated, including the active components of the circuit, the intrinsic properties of the active neurons, and the synaptic connectivity in the circuit. A large number of neuromodulators can act to produce variants on the basic motor theme elicited by one CPG. In systems where an appreciable number of modulators have been identified, each one has a unique constellation of effects on the motor pattern. For example, in the STG, acetylcholine, dopamine, octopamine, serotonin, histamine, proctolin, and FMRFamide all produce different variants of the pyloric rhythm (Table II).

2. *Any single neuromodulator will affect the motor pattern at many levels in the motor system.* In several invertebrate systems, a single neuromodulator has been shown to act on the pattern-initiating components, the CPG neurons, the motoneurons, and the peripheral muscles (Figs. 3, 4, and Table 2). This probably also occurs in vertebrates, where modulatory effects in

the brain and spinal cord may interact to produce a modified motor output. In addition, monoamines and peptides modulate transmission at the vertebrate neuromuscular junction (Bergman et al., 1981; Johnston et al., 1983); the possible temporal integration of hormonal and central effects of these compounds in vertebrates has not been studied.

3. *Modulation occurs in interactions between unit oscillators.* Stein (1978) and Grillner (1981, 1985) have discussed the existence of multiple independent oscillator circuits, called "unit burst generators" or "local control centers", that control separate parts of a movement and interact to generate complex rhythmic movements such as locomotion in a quadruped. For example, Grillner (1981) has suggested that, for a horse to switch gait from a trot (with alternation of forelimbs) to a gallop (with synchrony of forelimbs), it need merely change the strength and net sign of coupling between the unit burst generators for the limbs. This alteration in synaptic interactions could be accomplished by modulatory inputs. In the lamprey spinal cord, Cohen and Harris-Warrick (1984) showed that the glycine antagonist, strychnine, can modify fictive swimming to switch the motor output between left and right sides of a single segment from strict alternation to strict synchrony. We proposed that this synchronous strychnine-induced bursting resulted from a blockade of crossed inhibition between the unit burst generators that control rhythmic output from each ventral root. This allowed weaker crossed excitatory synapses to be unmasked. Endogenous transmitters or modulators could have similar actions to alter the relative coordination between different oscillators and thus change the gait of a complex rhythmic motor output (Cohen *et al.*, 1982). For example, serotonin modulates intersegmental coordination in the lamprey spinal cord, although the mechanisms are not fully understood (Harris-Warrick and Cohen, 1985). Kopell, and Rand et al. (this volume) present further discussions of such systems of coupled oscillators.

4. *Neuromodulators can gain access to motor systems by a variety of routes.* A neuromodulator can be released from nerve terminals and act locally as a neurotransmitter. At other sites, a compound may be released locally from nerve terminals but diffuse over a wide area to affect many nearby neurons as a "paracrine hormone" (Jan et al., 1983). Finally, a compound can act globally as a circulating hormone (Kravitz et al., 1980). Any single compound can affect a motor system by several of these routes simultaneously (Benjamin, 1983; Beltz and Kravitz, 1984).

5.2   Mechanisms for Neuromodulation of CPG Circuits

1. *A full understanding of the effects of a neuromodulator on a CPG requires a thorough knowledge of the intrinsic properties of the CPG.* It is clear that a modulatory act must be analyzed within the context of the circuit to determine its functional significance for a motor pattern (Flamm and Harris-Warrick, 1986a,b). In addition, the *state* of the CPG can be altered by other inputs,

with attendant changes in the intrinsic properties of the circuit. The behavioral consequences of a modulator's activity may be very different when this occurs (see below).

2. *A neuromodulator can have a number of different physiological effects on the component neurons in a CPG.* Even with the limited data available, it is clear that a neuromodulator does not have a single mechanism of action within a given circuit. This is especially obvious in the stomatogastric ganglion, where dopamine and serotonin each have at least three different effects on pyloric neurons in this 14-neuron circuit. The simplest interpretation of these data is that different cells have different receptors or biochemical responses to the amine, and different ionic conductances are expressed. However, it is also possible that an amine has only one mechanism of action, but different neurons have different responses to this mechanism. For example, an amine might enhance the calcium conductance in two cells: one cell may respond with calcium-dependent endogenous bursting while the other cell may hyperpolarize due to enhancement of a calcium-activated potassium conductance. In any case, the functional consequences of a neuromodulator's actions on the different cells within a single CPG circuit can be very different. The elucidation of a neuromodulator's effect on one neuron in a CPG gives *no* information about its effects on other neurons in the circuit.

3. *Neuromodulators can redefine the active CPG circuit by a selective excitation and inhibition of the component neurons.* By changing the cells that are active, a neuromodulator can sculpt a new circuit from the anatomically defined network (Fig. 8). Each of the functional circuits sculpted by a different modulator can be thought of as an efficient CPG that controls a specific and stable motor pattern. Thus, the anatomically defined CPG network can be thought of as the basic framework from which active subcircuits can be chosen by the appropriate mixture of neuromodulators.

4. *Neuromodulators can alter the basic motor pattern by changing the intrinsic properties of neurons in a CPG circuit.* Properties such as endogenous bursting (Fig. 9) and plateau potentials (Nagy and Dickinson, 1983) are clearly under modulatory control. This is not limited to invertebrates. The peptide TRH can induce endogenous bursting in neurons of the guinea pig nucleus tractus solitarius (Dekin et al., 1985). Hounsgaard et al. (1984; Hounsgaard and Kiehn, 1985) have shown that the serotonin precursor, 5-hydroxytryptophan, can induce calcium-dependent bistable plateau potential properties in cat and turtle spinal motoneurons. NMDA can induce bursting and plateau potentials in lamprey spinal interneurons and motoneurons (Sigvardt et al., 1985; Grillner and Wallen, 1985). Similar effects are seen in other preparations. These changes in the intrinsic activity of CPG neurons have dramatic effects on motor patterns, including changes in phase relationships and in the frequency and intensity of motor output.

5. *Neuromodulators can change the "wiring diagram" in a CPG by altering the efficacy of specific synapses within the circuit.* This is a well-known action of

neuromodulators, and it is no surprise that it is important in the shaping of motor patterns. Changes in synaptic strength can result from a number of different physiological mechanisms, including alteration of transmitter release, variation in the specific responsiveness of the post-synaptic cell to the transmitter, and generalized changes in the membrane resistance of the pre- or post-synaptic cell (Kupfermann, 1979; Shain and Carpenter, 1981). The coupling coefficients of electrical synapses within a circuit can also be modulated (Spira and Bennett, 1980; Piccolino et al., 1984). Thus, neuromodulators can change the quantitative wiring diagram in a CPG circuit, and this can lead to changes in relative phasing of neuronal activity.

6. *Multiple ionic and biochemical mechanisms underly these circuit changes.* The actions of neuromodulators on isolated neurons, neuromuscular junctions, and other simplified systems have been recently reviewed (Kupfermann, 1979; Dismukes, 1980; Hartzell, 1981; Pellmar, 1981). Neuromodulators can act by a number of different mechanisms to modify the activity and excitabilty of neurons. These mechanisms are of obvious importance in modifying the output of a highly interacting circuit such as a CPG. For example, a neuromodulator could act by a standard conductance increase mechanism but of prolonged duration. By altering the resting membrane potential, a simple conductance increase could not only change the cell's excitability but also enable or disable the expression of voltage-sensitive conductances that determine the intrinsic firing properties of the neuron. Another common neuromodulator mechanism involves a decrease in the resting membrane conductance. As described earlier, this will enhance a cell's responsiveness to all synaptic input (excitatory and inhibitory alike) and thus its integrative capabilities. Conductance decrease mechanisms have been called "enabling" or "bias-adjusting" systems (Moore and Bloom, 1979) to reflect these general activating features. Third, neuromodulators can directly increase or decrease the density of voltage-sensitive conductances. This can affect the expression of a number of intrinsic properties of CPG neurons as well as synaptic transmission within the circuit.

A number of biochemical mechanisms not directly involving ionic conductances could also modulate the activity of CPG neurons. First, alteration in the activity of the electrogenic Na^+, $K^+ - ATPase$ (which maintains ionic gradients across the neuronal membrane) could cause long-term changes in membrane potential. The prolonged hyperpolarization of muscle by catecholamines appears to use this mechanism (Phillis and Wu, 1982). Second, modulation of intracellular ion buffering mechanisms can affect neurotransmission. For example, if the sequestration of calcium at the nerve terminal is modulated, transmitter release would be affected for prolonged periods (Glusman and Kravitz, 1982). The second messenger inositol trisphosphate, generated by the hydrolysis of phosphatidylinositol, appears to act by liberating calcium from intracellular stores (Berridge and Irvine, 1984). Third, the post-synaptic cell's responsiveness to a transmitter can be directly modulated. For example, benzodiazepines enhance the responsiveness to GABA in a number of vertebrate tissues by a direct interaction with the GABA receptor-ionophore complex (Choi et al., 1981; Olsen, 1981; Tallman et al., 1980), and it is likely that an endogenous ligand has a similar role (Costa et al., 1983). Finally, general changes in metabolic activity could affect the level of activity in rhythmically active neurons (Connor et al., 1976; Connor, 1985).

7. *Neuromodulators acting in concert may give different results than the sum of their effects alone.* We have very little information on the frequency, intensity, or complexity of modulatory input to a CPG. However, it is very likely that a large number of modulatory inputs are simultaneously active, resulting in a mixture of effects on the CPG. By changing the mixture of many modulatory inputs, variations in motor pattern can be evoked that are both more subtle and more complex than we can observe experimentally by adding one neuromodulator at a time. Given the prolonged and voltage-dependent mechanisms of action of neuromodulators, the results of changing mixtures of modulators will be difficult to predict. Changes in the working membrane potential range could affect the expression of voltage-sensitive conductances which, themselves, could be activated or inactivated by modulators. Combinations of conductance increase and decrease mechanisms may give qualitatively different results depending on the exact quantitative levels of each change. In addition, many neurons have now been shown to release two or more transmitters, and the co-release of a biogenic amine and a peptide is especially common (Hokfelt et al., 1980; Chan-Palay and Palay, 1984). The effects of these multiple-transmitter neurons could also be complex and activity-dependent.

CONCLUSION

The Central Pattern Generator concept has been of immense value in focussing our attention on the organization of central neuronal circuits that generate simple rhythmic movements. It is now clear, however, that the concept of a CPG as a fixed or static circuit must be discarded. Modulatory inputs to these circuits can alter every aspect of their function, including the neuronal composition of the active circuit, the synaptic wiring diagram connecting the cells, and the intrinsic properties of the cells. This extensive "sculpting" of the CPG circuit results in the formation of many alternative functional circuits, each capable of generating its own motor pattern. As a result, a very large number of unique variants on the basic motor pattern can be generated from a single anatomically defined network. The anatomical network alone does not specify the behavior that will result from its activation; rather, it represents a library of possible interactions from which behaviors are built. Modulatory inputs to the circuit, therefore, play an "instructive" role in determining the final motor pattern. These inputs cannot be regarded as members of the CPG circuit, as they are not necessary for the generation of a rhythmic motor pattern. However, they must be included in any study of the movements an animal actually makes in its constant adaptations to its environment.

ACKNOWLEDGMENTS

I thank Dr. Avis Cohen for valuable discussions and critical reading of earlier drafts of this paper; R. Hoy, P. Katz and R. Flamm for reading the manuscript; B. Seely for preparing the manuscript; and M. Howland for help in preparing the figures. Supported in part by NIH research grant NS17323 and HATCH grant NYC191410.

REFERENCES

Aghajanian, G. K. (1981). The modulatory role of serotonin at multiple receptors in brain. In *Serotonin Neurotransmission and Behavior*, B. L. Jacobs and A. Gelperin, eds. MIT Press, Cambridge, MA, pp. 156–185.

Anderson, W. W. and D. L. Barker (1981). Synaptic mechanisms that generate network oscillations in the absence of discrete postsynaptic potentials. *J. Exp. Zool.*, **216**:187–191.

Armijo, A., A. Mediavilla, and J. Florez. (1979). Inhibition of the activity of the respiratory and vasomotor centers by centrally administered 5-hydroxytryptamine in cats. *Rev. Esp. Fisiol.*, **35**:219–228.

Augustine, G. J., R. Fetterer, and W. H. Watson (1982). Amine modulation of the neurogenic *Limulus* heart. *J. Neurobiol.*, **13**:61–74.

Ayers, J., G. A. Carpenter, S. Currie, and J. Kinch (1983). Which behavior does the lamprey central motor program mediate? *Science*, **221**:1312–1315.

Barbeau, H. and S. Rossignol (1982). Modulation of the locomotor pattern by noradrenergic, serotonergic, and dopaminergic agonists in the adult chronic spinal cat. *Neurosci. Abst.*, **8**:163.

Battelle, B-A. and E. A. Kravitz (1978). Targets of octopamine action in the lobster. Cyclic nucleotide changes and physiological effects in hemolymph, heart and exoskeletal muscle. *J. Pharm. Exp. Ther.*, **205**:438–448.

Baumgarten, H. G. (1972). Biogenic amines in the cyclostome and lower vertebrate brain. *Prog. Histochem. Cytochem.*, **4**:1–90.

Bellah, K. L., G. K. Fitch, and A. E. Kammer (1984). Central action of octopamine on ventilation frequency in *Corydalus cornutus*. *J. Exp. Zool.*, **231**:289–292.

Beltz, B. and E. A. Kravitz (1984). Morphological analyses of identified serotonin-proctolin containing neurons in the lobster. *Neurosci. Abst.*, **10**:152.

Beltz, B. S., J. S. Eisen, R. Flamm, R. M. Harris-Warrick, S. Hooper, and E. Marder (1984). Serotonergic innervation and modulation of the stomatogastric ganglion of three decapod crustaceans (*Homarus americanus*, *Cancer irroratus*, and *Panulirus interruptus*). *J. Exp. Biol.*, **109**:35–54.

Benjamin, P. R. (1983). Gastropod feeding: behavioural and neural analysis of a complex multicomponent system. In *Symp. Soc. Exp. Biol.*, **27**:*Neural Origin of Rhythmic Movements*, pp. 159–194.

Benjamin, P. R., C. R. McCrohan, and R. M. Rose (1981). Higher order interneurons which initiate and modulate feeding in the pond snail, *Lymnaea stagnalis*. In *Neurobiology of Invertebrates, Mechanisms of Integration*, J. Salanki, ed., Oxford, Pergamon Press, pp. 171–200.

Benson, J. A. (1984). Octopamine alters rhythmic activity in the isolated cardiac ganglion of the crab, *Portunus sanguinolentus*. *Neurosci. Lett.*, **44**:59–64.

Bergman, H., S. Glusman, R. M. Harris-Warrick, E. A. Kravitz, I. Nussinovitch, and R. Rahimimoff (1981). Noradrenaline augments tetanic potentiation of transmitter release by a calcium dependent process. *Brain Res.*, **214**:200–204.

Berlind, A. (1977). Neurohumoral and reflex control of scaphognathite beating in the crab *Carcinus maenas*. *J. Comp. Physiol.*, **116**:77–90.

Berridge, M. J. and R. F. Irvine (1984). Inositol trisphosphate, a novel second messenger in cellular signal transduction. *Nature*, **312**:315–321.

Bevengut, M. and F. Clarac (1982). Contrôle de la posture du Crabe *Carcinus maenas* par des amines biogènes. *C.R. Acad. Sc. Paris. Serie. III*, **295**:23–28.

Bradbury, A. G. and B. Mulloney (1982). Proctolin activates and octopamine inhibits swimmeret beating. *Neurosci. Abst.*, **8**:736.

Brimblecombe, R. W. (1977). Drugs acting on central cholinergic mechanisms and affecting respiration. *Pharmacol. Ther. Pt. B Gen. Syst. Pharmacol.*, **3**:65–74.

Brodfuehrer, P. D. and W. O. Friesen (1986a). Initiation of swimming activity by trigger neurons in the leech subesophageal ganglion. I. Output connections of Tr1 and Tr2. *J. Comp. Physiol.*, **159**:489–502 .

Brodfuehrer, P. D. and W. O. Friesen (1986b). Initiation of swimming activity by trigger neurons in the leech subesophageal ganglion. II. Role of segmental swim-initiating interneurons. *J. Comp. Physiol.*, **159**: 503–510.

Brodin, L., S. Grillner, and C. M. Rovainen (1985). NMDA, kainate and quisqualate receptors and the generation of fictive locomotion in the lamprey spinal cord. *Brain Res.*, **325**:302–306.

Brodin, L. and S. Grillner (1985). The role of putative excitatory amino acid neurotransmitters in the initiation of locomotion in the lamprey spinal cord. I. The effects of excitatory amino acid antagonists. *Brain Res.*, **360**:139–148.

Buchanan, J. T. and A. H. Cohen (1982). Activities of identified interneurons, motoneurons, and muscle fibers during fictive swimming in the lamprey and effects of reticulospinal and dorsal cell stimulation. *J. Neurophysiol.*, **47**:948–960.

Budakova, N. N. (1973). Stepping movements in the spinal cat due to L-dopa administration. *Fiziol. Zh. SSSR*, **59**:1190–1198.

Bulloch, A. G. M. and D. A. Dorsett (1979). The integration of the patterned output of buccal motoneurones during feeding in *Tritonia hombergi*. *J. Exp. Biol.*, **79**:23–40.

Chan-Palay, V. and S. L. Palay, eds. (1984). *Coexistence of Neuroactive Substances in Neurons*, Wiley, New York.

Choi, D. W., D. H. Farb, and G. D. Fischbach (1981). Chlordiazepoxide selectively potentiates GABA conductance of spinal cord and sensory neurons in cell culture. *J. Neurophysiol.*, **45**:621–631.

Claiborne, B. J. and A. I. Selverston (1984). Histamine as a neurotransmitter in the stomatogastric nervous system of the spiny lobster. *J. Neurosci.*, **4**:708–721.

Cohen, A. H. and P. Wallén (1980). The neuronal correlates of locomotion in fish: 'fictive swimming' induced in an *in vitro* preparation of the lamprey spinal cord. *Exp. Brain Res.*, **41**:11–18.

Cohen, A. H. and R. M. Harris-Warrick (1984). Strychnine eliminates alternating motor output during fictive locomotion in the lamprey. *Brain Res.*, **293**:164–167.

Cohen, A. H., P. J. Holmes, and R. H. Rand (1982). The nature of the coupling between segmental oscillators of the lamprey spinal generator for locomotion: a mathematical model. *J. Math. Biol.*, **13**:345–369.

Commissiong, J. W. and E. M. Sedgwick (1979). A pharmacological study of the adrenergic mechanisms involved in the stretch reflex of the decerebrate rat. *Br. J. Pharmacol.*, **50**:365–374.

Commissiong, J. W. (1981). Spinal monoaminergic systems: an aspect of somatic motor function. *Fed. Proc.*, **40**:2771–2777.

Connor, J. A. (1985). Neural pacemakers and rhythmicity. *Ann. Rev. Physiol.*, **47**:17–28.

Connor, J. A., D. L. Krevlen, and C. L. Prosser (1976). Relation between oxidative metabolism and slow rhythmic potentials. *Proc. Natl. Acad. Sci.* **73**:4329–4243.

Cooke, I. M. (1966). The sites of action of pericardial organ extract and 5-hydroxytryptamine in the decapod crustacean heart. *Am. Zool.*, **6**:107–121.

Cooke, I. M. and D. K. Hartline (1975). Neurohormonal alteration of integrative properties of the cardiac ganglion of the lobster, *Homarus americanus. J. Exp. Biol.*, **63**:33–52.

Cooke, I. M. and R. E. Sullivan (1982). Hormones and secretion. In *The Biology of Crustacea: Vol. 3: Neurobiology: Structure and Function*, H. L. Atwood and D. C. Sandeman, eds. Academic Press, New York, pp. 206–291.

Costa, E., G. Corda, B. Epstein, C. Forchetti, and A. Guidotti (1983). GABA-benzodiazepine interactions. In *The Benzodiazines: From Molecular Biology to Clinical Practice*, E. Costa, ed. Raven Press, New York, pp. 117–136.

Croll, R. P., M. P. Kovac, W. J. Davis, and E. M. Matera (1985). Neural mechanisms of motor program switching in the mollusc *Pleurobranchaea*. III. Role of the paracerebral neurons and other identified brain neurons. *J. Neurosci.*, **5**:64–71.

Dale, N. and A. Roberts (1983). Excitatory amino acid receptors in the *Xenopus* embryo spinal cord and their role in the activation of swimming. *J. Physiol.*, *(Lond.)* **348**:527–543.

Dekin, M. S., G. B. Richerson, and P. A. Getting (1985). Thyrotropin-releasing hormone induces rhythmic bursting in neurons of the nucleus tractus solitarius. *Science*, **229**:67–69.

Delcomyn, F. (1980). Neural basis of rhythmic behavior in animals. *Science*, **210**:492–498.

Dickinson, P. S. and F. Nagy (1983). Control of a central pattern generator by an identified modulatory interneuron in *Crustacea*. II. Induction and modification of plateau properties in pyloric neurones. *J. Exp. Biol.*, **105**:59–82.

Dismukes, R. K. (1979). New concepts of molecular communication among neurons. *Behav. Brain Sci.*, **2**:409–448.

Dominick, O. S. and J. W. Truman (1986). The physiology of wandering behavior in *Manduca sexta*. IV. Hormonal induction of wandering behavior from the isolated nervous system. *J. Exp. Biol.*, **121**:133–151.

Drummond, A. H., J. A. Benson, and I. B. Levitan (1980). Serotonin-induced hyperpolarization of an identified *Aplysia* neuron is mediated by cyclic AMP. *Proc. Natl. Acad. Sci.*, **77**:5013–5017.

Eisen, J. S. and E. Marder. (1982). Mechanisms underlying pattern generation in lobster stomatogastric ganglion as determined by selective inactivation of identified neurons. III. Synaptic interactions of electrically coupled pyloric neurons. *J. Neurophysiol.*, **48**:1392–1415.

Eisen, J. S. and E. Marder (1984). A mechanism for the production of phase shifts in a pattern generator. *J. Neurophysiol.* **51**:1375–1393.

Elliot, C. J. H. and P. R. Benjamin (1985). Interactions of pattern-generating interneurons controlling feeding in *Lymnaea stagnalis*. *J. Neurophysiol.*, **54**:1396–1411.

Evoy, W. H. and D. Kennedy (1967). The central nervous organization underlying control of antagonistic muscles in the crayfish. I. Types of command fibers. *J. Exp. Zool.*, **165**:223–238.

Flamm, R. E. and R. M. Harris-Warrick (1984). Neuronal targets of dopamine, octopamine and serotonin in the pyloric central pattern generator of the stomatogastric ganglion in the lobster, *Panulirus interruptus*. *Neurosci., Abst.* **10**:149.

Flamm, R. E. and R. M. Harris-Warrick (1986a). Aminergic modulation in lobster stomatogastric ganglion. I. Effects on motor pattern and activity of neurons within the pyloric circuit. *J. Neurophysiol.*, **55**:847–865.

Flamm, R. E. and R. M. Harris-Warrick (1986b). Aminergic modulation in lobster stomatogastric ganglion. II. Target neurons of dopamine, octopamine and serotonin within the pyloric circuit. *J. Neurophysiol.*, **55**:866–881.

Flamm, R. E. and R. M. Harris-Warrick (1987). Pharmacologically induced changes in intracellular cAMP levels produce changes in physiological activity in pyloric CPG neurons from *Panulirus interruptus*. *J. Neurophysiol.* (In press).

Florey, E. and M. Rathmeyer (1978). The effects of octopamine and other amines on the heart and on neuromuscular transmission in decapod crustaceans: further evidence for a role as a neurohormone. *Comp. Biochem. Physiol.*, **61C**:229–237.

Forssberg, H. and S. Grillner (1973). The locomotion of the acute spinal cat injected with clonidine i.v. *Brain Res.*, **50**:184–186.

Getting, P. A. (this volume).

Gillette, R. and W. J. Davis (1977). The role of the metacerebral giant neuron in the feeding behavior of *Pleurobranchaea*. *J. Comp. Physiol.*, **116**:129–159.

Gillis, R. A., J. A. Quest, F. D. Pagani, J. Dias Souza, A. M. T. DaSilva, R. T. Jenson, T. Q. Garvey, and P. Hamosh (1983). Activation of CNS cholecystokinin receptors stimulates respiration in the cat. *J. Pharm. Exp. Ther.*, **224**:408–414.

Glover, J. C. and A. P. Kramer (1982). Serotonin analog selectively ablates identified neurons in the leech embryo. *Science*, **216**:317–319.

Glusman, S., J. W. Moore and E. A. Kravitz (1980). The modulatory action of serotonin at lobster neuromuscular junctions. *Neurosci. Abst.*, **6**:702.

Glusman, S. and E. A. Kravitz (1982). The action of serotonin on excitatory nerve terminals in lobster nerve-muscle preparations. *J. Physiol. Lond.*, **325**:223–241.

Gola, M. (1976). Electrical properties of bursting pacemaker neurons. In *Neurobiology of Invertebrates*, J. Salanki, ed. Akademiai Kiado, Budapest, pp. 381–421.

Granzow, B. and S. B. Kater (1977). Identified higher-order neurons controlling the feeding motor program of *Helisoma*. *Neurosci.*, **2**:1049–1063.

Graubard, K. and W. H. Calvin (1979). Presynaptic dendrites: Implications of spikeless synaptic transmission and dendritic geometry. *The Neurosciences: Fourth Study Program*, pp. 317–331.

Grillner, S. (1969). Supraspinal and segmental control of static and dynamic gamma-motoneurones in the cat. *Acta Physiol. Scand. Suppl.*, **327**:1–34.

Grillner, S. (1975). Locomotion in vertebrates: Central mechanisms and reflex interactions. *Physiol. Rev.*, **55**:247–304.

Grillner, S. (1981). Control of locomotion in bipeds, tetrapods and fish. In *Handbook of Physiology, Section 1: The Nervous System*, vol. II, Part 2, V. B. Brooks, ed., Amer. Physiol. Soc., Bethesda, pp. 1179–1236.

Grillner, S. (1985). Neurobiological bases of rhythmic motor acts in vertebrates. *Science*, **228**:143–148.

Grillner, S., J. T. Buchanan, P. Wallén, and L. Brodin. (this volume).

Grillner, S. and M. L. Shik (1973) On the descending control of the lumbosacral spinal cord from the "mesencephalic locomotor region." *Acta Physiol. Scand.*, **87**:320–333.

Grillner, S., P. Wallén, A. McClellan, K. Sigvardt, T. Williams, and J. Feldman (1983). The neural generation of locomotion in the lamprey: an incomplete account. *Symp. Soc. Exp. Biol.*, **37**:285–304.

Grillner, S. and P. Wallén (1985). The ionic mechanisms underlying N-methyl-D-aspartate receptor-induced, tetrodotoxin-resistant membrane potential oscillations in lamprey neurons active during locomotion. *Neurosci. Lett.*, **60**:289–294.

Grillner, S. and P. Zangger (1979). On the central pattern generation of locomotion in the low spinal cat. *Exp. Brain Res.*, **34**:241–262.

Grillner, S., A. McClellan, K. Sigvardt, P. Wallén, and M. Wilén (1981). Activation of NMDA-receptors elicits 'fictive locomotion' in lamprey spinal cord in vitro. *Acta Physiol. Scand.*, **113**:549–551.

Harris-Warrick, R. M. (1985). Amine modulation of extension command element-evoked motor activity in the lobster abdomen. *J. Comp. Physiol. A.*, **156**:875–884.

Harris-Warrick, R. M. and A. H. Cohen (1985) Serotonin modulates the central pattern generator for locomotion in the isolated lamprey spinal cord. *J. Exp. Biol.*, **116**:27–46.

Harris-Warrick, R. M. and R. E. Flamm (1984). Aminergic modulation of the pyloric rhythm in the stomatogastric ganglion of *Panulirus interruptus*. *Neurosci. Abst.*, **10**:149.

Harris-Warrick, R. M. and R. E. Flamm (1986a). Chemical modulation of a small central pattern generator circuit. *Trends in Neurosci.*, **9**:432–437.

Harris-Warrick, R. M. and R. E. Flamm (1986b). Multiple mechanisms of bursting in a conditional bursting neuron. *J. Neurosci.* **7**:2113–2128.

Harris-Warrick, R. M. and E. A. Kravitz (1984). Cellular mechanisms for modulation of posture by octopamine and serotonin in the lobster. *J. Neurosci.*, **4**:1976–1993.

Harris-Warrick, R. M., M. S. Livingstone, and E. A. Kravitz. (1980). Central effects of octopamine and serotonin on postural motor systems in the lobster. *Neurosci. Abst.*, **6**:27.

Harris-Warrick, R. M., J. C. McPhee, and J. A. Filler (1985). Distribution of serotonergic neurons and processes in the lamprey spinal cord. *Neurosci.*, **14**:1127–1140.

Hartzell, H. C. (1981). Mechanisms of slow postsynaptic potentials. *Nature,* **291**:539–544.

Hedner, J., T. Hedner, J. Jonason, and D. B. A. Lundberg (1981). Central respiratory stimulant effect by thyrotropin releasing hormone in the rat. *Neurosci. Lett.,* **25**:317–320.

Hedner, J., T. Hedner, J. Jonason, and D. B. A. Lundberg (1982). Evidence for a dopamine interaction with the central respiratory control system in the rat. *Eur. J. Pharmacol.,* **81**:603–615.

Hokfelt, T., O. Johansson, A. Ljungdahl, J. M. Lundberg, and M. Schultzberg (1980). Peptidergic neurones. *Nature,* **284**:515–521.

Holtman, J. R., A. Buller, P. Hamosh, A. M. T. DaSilva, and R. A. Gillis (1982). Respiratory depression produced by glycine injected into the cisterna magna of cats. *Neuropharmacol.,* **21**:1223–1225.

Holtman, J. R., A. A. Buller, A. M. T. DaSilva, P. Hamosh and R. A. Gillis (1983a). Respiratory depression produced by centrally administered taurine in the cat. *Life Sci.,* **32**:2313–2320.

Holtman, J. R., R. T. Jensen, A. Buller, P. Hamosh, A. M. T. DaSilva, and R. A. Gillis (1983b). Central respiratory stimulant effect of bombesin in the cat. *Eur. J. Pharm.,* **90**:449–451.

Honma, S. (1970). Presence of monoaminergic neurons in the spinal cord and intestine of the lamprey, *Lampetra japonica. Arch. Histol. Jpn.,* **32**:383–393.

Hooper, S. L. and E. Marder (1984). Modulation of a central pattern generator by two neuropeptides, proctolin and FMRFamide. *Brain Res.,* **305**:186–191.

Horvitz, H. R., M. Chalfie, C. Trent, J. E. Sulston, and P. D. Evans (1982). Serotonin and octopamine in the nematode *Caenorhabditis elegans. Science,* **216**:1012–1014.

Hounsgaard, J., H. Hultborn, B. Jespersen, and O. Kiehn. (1984). Intrinsic membrane properties causing bistable behavior of α-motoneurones. *Exp. Brain Res.,* **55**:391–394.

Hounsgaard, J. and O. Kiehn (1985). Ca^{++} dependent bistability induced by serotonin in spinal motoneurons. *Exp. Brain Res.,* **57**:422–425.

Ifshin, M. S., H. Gainer, and J. L. Barker (1975). Peptide factor extracted from molluscan ganglia that modulates bursting pacemaker activity. *Nature,* **254**:72–74.

Jan, Y. N., C. W. Bowers, D. Branton, L. Evans, and L. Y. Jan. (1983). Peptides in neuronal function-studies using frog autonomic ganglia. *Cold Spring Harbor Symp. Quant. Biol.*, **48**:363–374.

Jankowska, E., M. G. M. Jukes, S. Lund, and A. Lundberg (1967). The effect of L-dopa on the spinal cord. 5. Reciprocal organization of pathways transmitting excitatory action to alpha motoneurones of flexors and extensors. *Acta Physiol. Scand.*, **70**:369–388.

Jellies, J. and J. L. Larimer (1983). Synaptic interactions between flexion-producing interneurons in crayfish. *Neurosci. Abst.*, **9**:382.

Johnston, M. F., E. A. Kravitz, H. Meiri, and R. Rahamimoff (1983). Adrenocorticotropic hormone causes long-lasting potentiation of transmitter release from frog motor nerve terminals. *Science*, **220**:1071–1072.

Jordan, L. M. (1983). Factors determining motoneuron rhythmicity during fictive locomotion. *Symp. Soc. Exp. Biol.* **37**:423–444.

Kinnamon, S. C., L. W. Klaassen, A. E. Kammer, and D. Claassen (1984). Octopamine and chlordimeform enhance sensory responsiveness and production of the flight motor pattern in developing and adult moths. *J. Neurobiol.*, **15**:283–293.

Kravitz, E. A., S. Glusman, R. M. Harris-Warrick, M. S. Livingstone, T. Schwarz and M. F. Goy (1980). Amines and a peptide as neurohormones in lobsters. *J. Exp. Biol.* **89**:159–175.

Kravitz, E. A., S. Glusman, M. Livingstone, and R. M. Harris-Warrick (1981). Serotonin and octopamine in the lobster nervous system: mechanisms of action at neuromuscular junctions and preliminary behavioral studies. In *Serotonin Neurotransmission and Behavior*, B. L. Jacobs and A. Gelperin, eds. MIT Press, Cambridge, MA, pp. 188–210.

Kristan, W. B. and J. C. Weeks (1983). Neurons controlling the initiation, generation and modulation of leech swimming. *Symp. Soc. Exp. Biol.*, **37**:243–260.

Kuhlman, J. R., C. Li, and R. L. Calabrese (1985). FMRFamide-like substances in the leech: bioactivity on the heartbeat system. *J. Neurosci.*, **5**:2310–2317.

Kupfermann, I. (1979). Modulatory actions of neurotransmitters. *Ann. Rev. Neurosci.*, **2**:447–465.

Kupfermann, I., J. L. Cohen, D. E. Mandelbaum, M. Schonberg, A. J. Susswein, and K. R. Weiss. (1979). Functional role of serotonergic neuromodulation in *Aplysia*. *Fed. Proc.*, **38**:2095–2102.

Kupfermann, I. and K. R. Weiss (1978). The command neuron concept. *Behav. Brain Sci.*, **1**:3–39.

Kupfermann, I. and K. R. Weiss (1981). The role of serotonin in arousal of feeding behavior in *Aplysia*. In *Serotonin Neurotransmission and Behavior*, B. L. Jacobs and A. Gelperin, eds. MIT Press, Cambridge, MA, pp. 255–287.

Kupfermann, I. and K. R. Weiss (1982). Activity of an identified serotonergic neuron in freely moving *Aplysia* correlates with behavioral arousal. *Brain Res.*, **241**:334–337.

Kuypers, H. G. J. M. (1982). A new look at the organization of the motor system. *Descending pathways to the spinal cord, Progress in Brain Research*, 57: 381–403.

Larimer, J. L., J. Jellies, and D. Moore (1986). The crayfish position on command neurons. *Beh. Brain Sci.* (in press).

Lemos, J. R. and A. Berlind (1981). Cyclic adenosine monophosphate mediation of peptide neurohormone effects on the lobster cardiac ganglion. *J. Exp. Biol.,* **90**:307–326.

Lent, C. M. (1985). Serotonergic modulation of the feeding behavior of the medicinal leech. *Brain Res. Bull.,* **14**:643–655.

Lent, C. M. and B. M. Frazer (1977). Connectivity of the monoamine-containing neurons in central nervous system of leech. *Nature (London),* **266**:844–847.

Lent, C. M. and M. H. Dickinson (1985). Serotonin integrates the feeding behavior of the medicinal leech. *J. Comp. Physiol.* (in press).

Lingle, C. J. (1980) Sensitivity of decapod foregut muscles to acetylcholine and glutamate. *J. Comp. Physiol,* **138**:187–199.

Livingstone, M. S., R. M. Harris-Warrick, and E. A. Kravitz (1980). Serotonin and octopamine produce opposite postures in lobsters. *Science,* **208**:76–79.

Lloyd, P. E., I. Kupfermann, and K. R. Weiss (1984). Evidence for parallel actions of a molluscan neuropeptide and serotonin in mediating arousal in *Aplysia. Proc. Natl. Acad. Sci.* **81**:2934–2937.

Lundberg, D. B. A., G. R. Breese, and R. A. Mueller (1979). Dopaminergic interaction with the respiratory control system in the rat. *Eur. J. Pharmacol.* **54**:153–159.

Mackey, S. and T. J. Carew (1983). Locomotion in *Aplysia:* triggering by serotonin and modulation by bag cell extract. *J. Neurosci.,* **3**:1469–1477.

Marder, E. (1974). Acetylcholine as an excitatory neuromuscular transmitter in the stomatogastric system of the lobster. *Nature,* **251**:730–731.

Marder, E. (1976). Cholinergic motor neurones in the stomatogastric system of the lobster. *J. Physiol.,* **257**:63–86.

Marder, E. (1984). Mechanisms underlying neurotransmitter modulation of a neuronal circuit. *Trends Neurosci.,* **7**:48–53.

Marder, E. and J. S. Eisen (1984a). Transmitter identification of pyloric neurons: Electrically coupled neurons use different transmitters. *J. Neurophysiol.,* **51**:1345–1361.

Marder, E. and J. S. Eisen (1984b). Electrically coupled pacemaker neurons respond differently to the same physiological inputs and neurotransmitters. *J. Neurophysiol.,* **51**:1362–1374.

Marder, E. and S. L. Hooper (1985). Neurotransmitter modulation of the stomatogastric ganglion of decapod crustaceans. In A. I. Selverston, ed., *Model Neural Networks and Behavior,* Plenum Press, New York, pp. 319–337.

Marder, E., S. L. Hooper, and K. Siwicki (1986). Modulatory action and distribution of the neuropeptide Proctolin in the crustacean stomatogastric nervous system. *J. Comp. Neurol.,* **243**:454–467.

Marder, E. and D. Paupardin-Tritsch (1978). The pharmacological properties of some crustacean neuronal acetylcholine, GABA and L-glutamate responses. *J. Physiol.,* **280**:213–236.

Mayeri, E., P. Brownell, W. D. Branton, and S. B. Simon (1979a). Multiple, prolonged actions of neuroendocrine bag cells on neurons in *Aplysia.* I. Effects on bursting pacemaker neurons. *J. Neurophysiol.,* **42**:1165–1184.

Mayeri, E., P. Brownell, W. D. Branton, and S. B. Simon (1979b). Multiple, prolonged actions of neuroendocrine bag cells on neurons in *Aplysia.* II. Effects on beating pacemaker and silent neurons. *J. Neurophysiol.,* **42**:1185–1197.

Mayeri, E., B. S. Rothman, P. H. Brownell, W. D. Branton, and L. Padgett (1985). Nonsynaptic characteristics of neurotransmission mediated by egg-laying hormone in the abdominal ganglion of *Aplysia*. *J. Neurosci.*, **5**:2060–2077.

McClellan, A. D. and S. Grillner (1984). Activation of 'fictive swimming' by electrical microstimulation of brainstem locomotor regions in an in vitro preparation of the lamprey central nervous system. *Brain Res.*, **300**:357–361.

McCrohan, C. R. and P. R. Benjamin (1980). Synaptic relationships of the cerebral giant cells with motoneurons in the feeding system of *Lymnaea stagnalis*. *J. Exp. Biol.*, **85**:169–186.

McDonald, J. F., A. V. Porietis, and J. M. Wojtowic (1982). Aspartic acid induces a region of negative slope conductance in the current-voltage relationship of cultured spinal cord neurons. *Brain Res.*, **237**:248–253.

Miall, R. C. and J. L. Larimer (1982). Interneurons involved in abdominal posture in crayfish: structure, function and command fiber responses. *J. Comp. Physiol.* **148**:159–173.

Miller, J. P. and A. I. Selverston (1979). Rapid killing of single neurons by irradiation of intracellularly injected dye. *Science*, **206**:702–704.

Miller, J. P. and A. I. Selverston (1982a). Mechanisms underlying pattern generation in lobster stomatogastric ganglion as determined by selective inactivation of identified neurons. II. Oscillatory properties of pyloric neurons. *J. Neurophysiol.*, **48**:1378–1391.

Miller, J. P. and A. I. Selverston (1982b). Mechanisms underlying pattern generation in lobster stomatogastric ganglion as determined by selective inactivation of identified neurons. IV. Network properties of pyloric system. *J. Neurophysiol.*, **48**:1416–1432.

Miller, J. P. and A. I. Selverston (1985). Neural mechanisms for the production of the lobster pyloric motor pattern. In *Model Neural Networks and Behavior*, A. I. Selverston, ed. Plenum Press, New York, pp. 49–68.

Miller, M. W. and R. E. Sullivan (1981). Some effects of proctolin on the cardiac ganglion of the Maine lobster, *Homarus americanus*. *J. Neurobiol.*, **12**:629–639.

Miller, M. W., J. A. Benson, and A. Berlind (1984). Excitatory effects of dopamine on the cardiac ganglion of the crabs *Portunus sanguinolentus* and *Podophthalmus vigil*. *J. Exp. Biol.*, **108**:97–118.

Moore, R. Y. and F. E. Bloom, (1979). Central catecholamine neuron systems: anatomy and physiology of the norepinephrine and epinephrine systems. *Ann. Rev. Neurosci.*, **2**:113–168.

Mueller, R. A., D. Lundberg, and G. R. Breese (1980). Evidence that respiratory depression by serotonin agonists may be exerted in the central nervous system. *Pharmacol. Biochem. Behav.*, **13**:247–255.

Nagy, F., J. A. Benson and M. Moulins (1984). Cholinergic activation of burst generating oscillations mediated by opening of calcium channels in lobster pyloric neurons. *Neurosci. Abst.*, **10**:148.

Nagy, F., J. A. Benson, and M. Moulins (1985). Cholinergic inputs reduce a steady outward K^+ current allowing activation of a Ca^{2+} conductance which underlies the burst-generating oscillations in lobster pyloric neurons. *Neurosci. Abst.*, **11**:1022.

Nagy, F. and P. S. Dickinson (1983). Control of a central pattern generator by an identified modulatory interneurone in *Crustacea*. I. Modulation of the pyloric motor output. *J. Exp. Biol.*, **105**:33–58.

Neuman, R. S. (1985). Action of serotonin and norepinephrine on spinal motoneurons following blockage of synaptic transmission. *Can. J. Physiol. Pharmacol.*, **63**:735–738.

Ng, K. Y., T. N. Chase, R. W. Colburn, and I. J. Kopin (1970). L-dopa-induced release of cerebral monoamines. *Science*, **170**:76–79.

Nowak, L., P. Bregestovski, P. Ascher, A. Herbet, and A. Prochiantz (1984). Magnesium gates glutamate-activated channels in mouse central neurones. *Nature*, **307**:462–465.

Nusbaum, M. P. and W. B. Kristan (1986). Swim initiation in the leech by serotonin-containing interneurones, cells 21 and 61. *J. Exp. Biol.*, **122**:277–302.

Nusbaum, M. P. (1986). Synaptic basis of swim initiation in the Leech. III. Synaptic effects of serotonin-containing interneurones (cells 21 and 61) on swim CPG neurones (cells 18 and 208). *J. Exp. Biol.*, **122**:303–321.

Nusbaum, M. P. and E. Marder. Novel neuronal role for crustacean red pigment concentrating hormone. *Nature*, (submitted).

Ochi, J., T. Yamamoto, and Y. Hosoya (1979). Comparative study of the monoamine neuron system in the spinal cord of the lamprey and hagfish. *Arch. Histol. Jap.*, **42**:327–336.

Olsen, R. W. (1981). GABA-benzodiazepine-barbiturate receptor interactions. *J. Neurochem.*, **37**:1–13.

Omeniuk, D. J. and L. M. Jordan (1982). Locomotion induced by intrathecal drug administration in spinal cats. *Neurosci. Abst.*, **8**:165.

Pfaff, D. W. (1983). Impact of estrogens on hypothalamic nerve cells: ultrastructural, chemical and electric effects. *Rec. Prog. Hormone Res.*, **39**:127–179.

Pellmar, T. C. (1981). Transmitter control of voltage-dependent currents. *Life Sci.* **28**:2199–2205.

Phillis, J. W. and P. H. Wu (1981). (Na$^+$, K$^+$)ATPase and adrenoceptors. In *Adrenoceptors and Catecholamine Action*, G. Kunos, ed. Wiley, New York, pp. 273–296.

Piccolino, M., J. Neyton and H. M. Gerschenfeld (1984). Decrease of gap junction permeability induced by dopamine and cyclic adenosine 3′, 5′-monophosphate. *J. Neurosci.*, **4**:2477–2488.

Pinsker, H. M. and J. L. Ayers (1983). Neuronal Oscillators. In *The Clinical Neurosciences*, Vol. 5: *Neurobiology*, R. N. Rosenberg, ed. Churchill Livingstone, New York, pp. 203–266.

Poon, M. (1980). Induction of swimming in lamprey by L-DOPA and amino acids. *J. Comp. Physiol.*, **136**:337–344.

Rall, W. (1981). Funtional aspects of neuronal geometry. In *Neurones Without Impulses*, A. Roberts and B. M. H. Bush, eds. Cambridge Univ. Press, Cambridge, MA, pp. 223–254.

Ram, J. L., U. A. Shukla, G. S. Ajimal (1981). Serotonin has both excitatory and inhibitory modulatory effects on feeding muscles in *Aplysia*. *J. Neurobiol.*, **12** 613–621.

Raper, J. A. (1979). Nonimpulse-mediated synaptic transmission during the generation of a cyclic motor program. *Science*, **205**:304–306.

Roberts, A., N. Dale, W. H. Evoy, and S. R. Saffe (1985). Synaptic potentials in motoneurons during fictive swimming in spinal *Xenopus* embryos. *J. Neurophysiol.*, **54**:1–10.

Roberts, A. and B. L. Roberts, eds. (1983). *Neural Origin of Rhythmic Movements*, *Symp. Soc. Exp. Biol.*, **37**, Cambridge Univ. Press, Cambridge, MA, 503 pp.

Roberts, A., S. R. Soffe, J. D. W. Clarke, and N. Dale. (1983). Initiation and control of swimming in amphibian embryos. *Symp. Soc. Exp. Biol.*, **37**:261–284.

Rossignol, S., J. P. Lund, and T. Drew (this volume).

Rovainen, C. M. (1979) Neurobiology of lampreys. *Physiol. Rev.*, **59**:1007–1077.

Russell, D. F. (1979). CNS control of pattern generators in the lobster stomatogastric ganglion. *Brain Res.*, **177**:598–602.

Russell, D. F. and D. K. Hartline (1978). Bursting neural networks: A reexamination. *Science*, **200**:453–456.

Russell, D. F. and D. K. Hartline (1981). Slow active potentials and bursting motor patterns in pyloric network of the lobster, *Panulirus interruptus. J. Neurophysiol.*, **48**:914–937.

Scheller, R. H. and R. Axel (1984). How genes control an innate behavior. *Sci. Am.*, **250**:54–62.

Scheller, R. H., J. F. Jackson, L. B. McAllister, B. S. Rothman, E. Mayeri, and R. Axel (1983). A single gene encodes multiple neuropeptides mediating a stereotyped behavior. *Cell*, **32**:7–22.

Scheller, R. H., R-R. Kaldany, T. Kriener, A. C. Mahon, J. R. Nambu, M. Schaefer, and R. Taasig (1984). Neuropeptides: mediators of behavior in *Aplysia*. *Science*, **225**:1300–1308.

Selverston, A. I., D. G. King, D. F. Russell, and J. P. Miller, (1976). The stomatogastric nervous system: Structure and function of a small neural network. *Prog. Neurobiol.*, **7**:215–290.

Selverston, A. I. (1980). Are central pattern generators understandable? *Behav. Brain Sci.*, **3**:535–571.

Selverston, A. I. and J. P. Miller (1980). Mechanisms underlying pattern generation in lobster stomatogastric ganglion as determined by selective inactivation of identified neurons. I. Pyloric system. *J. Neurophysiol.*, **44**:1102–1121.

Selverston, A. I. and J. P. Miller (1982). Application of a cell inactivation technique to the study of a small neural network. *Trends Neurosci.*, **5**:120–123.

Selverston, A. I., J. P. Miller and M. Wadepuhl (1983). Cooperative mechanisms for the production of rhythmic movements. *Symp. Scc. Exp. Biol.*, **37**:55–88.

Selverston, A. I. and M. Moulins (1985). Oscillatory neural networks. *Ann. Rev. Physiol.*, **47**:29–48.

Shain, W. and D. O. Carpenter (1981). Mechanisms of synaptic modulation. *Int. Rev. Neurobiol.*, **22**:205–250.

Shik, M. L., F. V. Severin, and G. N. Orlovsky, (1966). Control of walking and running by means of electrical stimulation of the midbrain. *Biofizika*, **11**:659–666.

Shik, M. L., F. V. Severin, and G. N. Orlovsky, (1967). Structures of the brain stem responsible for evoked locomotion. *Fiziol. Zh. SSSR*, **12**:660–668.

Sigvardt, K. A., S. Grillner, P. Wallén, and P. A. M. van Dongen, (1985). Activation of NMDA receptors elicits fictive locomotion and bistable membrane properties in the lamprey spinal cord. *Brain Res.*, **336**:390–395.

Sigvardt, K. A., B. S. Rothman, R. O. Brown, and E. Mayeri (1986). The bag cells of *Aplysia* as a multitransmitter system: identifcation of alpha-bag cell peptide as a second neurotransmitter. *J. Neurosci.*, **6**:803–813.

Sombati, S. and G. Hoyle (1984a). Central nervous sensitization and dishabituation of reflex action in an insect by the neuromodulator octopamine. *J. Neurobiol.*, **15**:455–480.

Sombati, S. and G. Hoyle (1984b). Generation of specific behaviors in a locust by local release into neuropil of the natural neuromodulator octopamine. *J. Neurobiol.*, **15**:481–506.

Spira, M. E. and M. V. L. Bennett (1980). Synaptic control of electrotonic coupling between neurons. *Brain Res.*, **37**:294–300.

Steeves, J. D., L. M. Jordan, and N. Lake (1975). The close proximity of catecholamine-containing cells to the 'mesencephalic locomotor region'. *Brain Res.*, **100**: 663–670.

Steeves, J. D., B. J. Schmidt, B. J. Skovgaard, and L. M. Jordan (1980). The effect of noradrenaline and 5-hydroxytryptamine depletion on locomotion in the cat. *Brain Res.*, **185**:349–362.

Stein, P. S. G. (1978). Motor systems, with specific reference to the control of locomotion. *Ann. Rev. Neurosci.*, **1**:61–82.

Sullivan, R. E. and M. W. Miller, (1984). Dual effects of protolin on the rhythmic burst activity of the cardiac ganglion. *J. Neurobiol.*, **15**:173–196.

Tallman, J. F., S. M. Paul, P. Skolnik, and D. W. Gallager (1980). Receptors for the age of anxiety: pharmacology of the benzodiazepines. *Science*, **207**:274–281.

Thompson, C. S. and C. H. Page (1981). Interneuronal control of postural motoneurons in the lobster abdomen. *J. Neurobiol.*, **12**:87–91.

Thompson, C. S. and C. H. Page (1982). Command fiber activation of superficial flexor motoneurons in the lobster abdomen. *J. Comp. Physiol.*, **148**:515–527.

Trimble, D. L. and D. L. Barker (1984). Activation by dopamine of patterned motor output from the buccal ganglia of *Helisoma trivolvis*. *J. Neurobiol.*, **15**:37–48.

Truman, J. W. and J. C. Weeks (1983). Hormonal control of the development and release of rhythmic ecdysis behaviours in insects. *Symp. Soc. Exp. Biol.*, **37**: 223–242.

VanderMaelen, C. P. and G. K. Aghajanian (1980). Intracellular studies showing modulation of facial motoneurone excitability by serotonin. *Nature*, **287**: 346–347.

Van Dongen, P. A., T. Hokfelt, S. Grillner, A. A. Verhofstad, H. W. Steinbusch, A. C. Cuello, and L. Terenius (1985). Immunohistochemical demonstration of some putative neurotransmitters in the lamprey spinal cord and spinal ganglion: 5-hydroxytryptamine-, tachykinin-, and neuropeptide Y-immuno-reactive neurons and fibers. *J. Comp. Neurol.*, **234**:501–522.

Van Dongen, P. A. M., S. Grillner, and T. Hokfelt, (1986). *Brain Research* (In press).

Viala, D. and P. Buser (1969). The effects of L-dopa and 5-HTP on rhythmic efferent discharges in hind-limb nerves in the rabbit. *Brain Res.*, **12**:437–443.

Viala, D. and P. Buser (1971). Modalités d'obtention de rhythmes locomoteurs chez le lapin spinal par traitements pharmacologiques (L-dopa, 5-HTP, D-Amphetamine). *Brain Res.*, **35**:151–165.

Wadepuhl, M. and A. I. Selverston (1984). Octopamine induces slow pacemaker potentials. *Neurosci. Abst.*, **10**:148.

Wallén, P. and S. Grillner (1985). The effects of current passage on N-methyl-D-aspartate-induced, tetrodotoxin-resistant membrane potential oscillations in lamprey neurons active during locomotion. *Neurosci. Lett.*, **56**:87–93.

Wallén, P. and T. Williams (1984). Fictive locomotion in the lamprey spinal cord in vitro compared with swimming in the intact and spinal animal. *J. Physiol.*, **347**:225–239.

Watkins, J. C. and R. H. Evans (1981). Excitatory amino acid transmitters. *Ann. Rev. Pharmacol. Toxicol.*, **21**:165–204.

Watson, W. H. and G. J. Augustine (1982). Peptide and amine modulation of the *Limulus* heart: a simple neural network and its target tissue. *Peptides*, **3**:485–492.

Watson, W. H., T. Hoshi, J. Colburne, G. J. Augustine, (1985). Neurohormonal modulation of the *Limulus* heart: actions on neuromuscular transmission and cardiac muscle. *J. exp. Biol.*, **118**:71–84.

Wieland, S. J. and A. Gelperin (1983). Dopamine elicits feeding motor program in *Limax maximus*. *J. Neurosci.*, **3**:1735–1745.

Weiss, K. R., J. L. Cohen, and I. Kupfermann (1978). Modulatory control of buccal musculature by a serotonergic neuron (metacerebral cell) in *Aplysia*. *J. Neurophysiol.*, **41**:181–203.

Weiss, K. R., D. E. Mandelbaum, M. Schonberg, and I. Kupfermann (1979). Modulation of buccal muscle contractility by serotonergic metacerebral cells in *Aplysia:* evidence for a role of cycle adenosine monophosphate. *J. Neurophysiol*, **42**:791–803.

Westlund, K. N., R. M. Bowker, M. G. Ziegler, and J. D. Coulter (1982). Descending noradrenergic projections and their spinal terminations. In: *Descending Pathways to the Spinal Cord*, H. G. J. M. Kuypers and G. F. Martin, eds. *Progress in Brain Research*, **57**:219–238.

White, S. R. and R. S. Neuman (1980). Facilitation of spinal motoneurone excitability by 5-hydroxytryptamine and noradrenaline. *Brain Res.*, **188**:119–127.

White, S. R. and R. S. Neuman (1983). Pharmacological antagonism of facititatory but not inhibitory effects of serotonin and norepinephrine on excitability of spinal motoneurons. *Neuropharmacol.*, **22**:489–494.

Willard, A. L. (1981). Effects of serotonin on the generation of the motor pattern for swimming by the medicinal leech. *J. Neurosci.*, **1**:936–944.

Yamada, K. A., P. Hamosh, and R. A. Gillis (1981). Respiratory depression produced by activation of GABA receptors in hindbrain of cat. *J. Appl. Physiol*, **51**:1278–1286.

Yamamoto, Y., H. Lagercrantz, and C. VonEuler (1981). Effects of Substance P and TRH on ventilation and pattern of breathing in newborn rabbits. *Acta Physiol. Scand.*, **113**:541–543.

Chapter Nine

SYSTEMS OF COUPLED OSCILLATORS AS MODELS OF CENTRAL PATTERN GENERATORS

RICHARD H. RAND
AVIS H. COHEN
PHILIP J. HOLMES

Department of Theoretical and Applied Mechanics
Section of Neurobiology and Behavior
Cornell University
Ithaca, New York

1 INTRODUCTION

In the development of the mathematical framework that follows, we are motivated by three major goals. The first is to construct models which will allow us to test assertions regarding the structure and function of the intersegmental coordinating system of the lamprey central pattern generator (CPG) for locomotion (Cohen and Wallén, 1980; see Grillner et al., Chapt. 1, for the description of the motor pattern). In the process, we hope, secondly, to formulate some general concepts which might be useful in understanding other biological systems of coupled oscillators. Finally, we will formulate a method for analysis of CPGs. In view of these considerations, we have allowed the lamprey experimental data to guide our thinking while at the same time emphasizing those aspects of the dynamical behavior of the models which should be shared by a rather general class of systems. In some instances we sacrifice considerable physiological and anatomical detail in order to obtain tractability of the equations or generality of the model. While a general theory is still far from complete, in this chapter we offer some basic results we have obtained. During the course of the discussion, we point out the relevant relations to the lamprey as well as draw analogies with other CPGs to which the model might be applied. In her chapter, Kopell further develops these ideas. She also develops the mathematics which is required for the changes and provides additional examples of the usefulness of the models.

The mathematics used both in our chapter and in that of Kopell requires some knowledge of advanced calculus, linear algebra, and differential equations. It is not expected to be easily accessible to mathematically inexperienced readers. However, we will attempt to relate the ideas to biological systems represented elsewhere in the book in hopes of motivating the biologist to seek an applied mathematician with whom to collaborate. Generally, we have tried to separate the biological and mathematical components of the discussion. The mathematical treatments will begin with a description of the biological significance of the assumptions and will end with conclusions again placed in a biological context. Unfortunately, some jargon is unavoidable, and some terms must be used which are impossible to define adequately in a few words. However, these can often be finessed

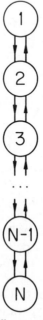

FIGURE 1. A system of N oscillators with nearest neighbor interactions.

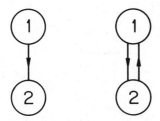

17   **FIGURE 2.** One-way coupling versus two-way coupling.

by the reader and the general meaning can still be derived. We encourage this approach. *Feel free to note the assumptions, skip the mathematics, and read ahead to see if the conclusions look compelling.* Those who want more mathematical background in dynamical systems, the area of mathematics relevant to the models, can turn to a series by Abraham and Shaw (1983) called *Dynamics—the Geometry of Behavior.* These books are profusely illustrated, entertaining, and assume only basic calculus.

By a system of coupled oscillators we shall mean a number of individual oscillating units, each of which is able to oscillate stably on its own when uncoupled from the others, but all of which can affect each other's behavior due to coupling. The effect of one oscillator on another may be direct, as in the case of two neighboring oscillators in a system with nearest neighbor interactions (see Fig. 1), or it may be indirect, as in the case of two distantly separated oscillators in the same system. Note that the interaction between two oscillators may be one-way, as in studies of biological clocks forced by the daily solar cycle (in which case the sun is seen as an oscillator which forces the biological system, but is unaffected itself by the interaction), or the interaction may involve two-way coupling, in which case both oscillators influence each other's behavior (Fig. 2). This formulation is similar to that proposed for the vertebrate locomotor CPG by Grillner (1981) and by Cohen and Wallén (1980).

2 BIOLOGICAL OSCILLATORS

By a biological oscillator we shall mean a biological system which may be modeled by a *structurally stable* dynamical system which exhibits a unique and *asymptotically stable limit cycle.* Structural stability means that the system continues to behave in a qualitatively consistent fashion, *no matter how it is changed,* assuming only that the changes are sufficiently small. Such mathematical changes (called "perturbations") could represent physical changes made by the experimenter, such as dissection of the organism to study the system more easily. Alternatively, they could be due to sensory input arising naturally or artificially, or they could be due to input from

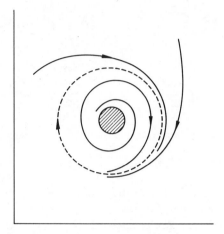

FIGURE 3. Limit cycle oscillator in a two dimensional state space. Shaded region shows quiescent states which do not lie in the basin of attraction of the limit cycle (the dashed trajectory).

other oscillators to which the oscillator in question is coupled. In any case, we assume that the individual unit can oscillate both when it is alone (uncoupled) as well as when it is in the system. That is, we assume that it exhibits stable periodic behavior (called a "limit cycle") which represents the long-time behavior of almost every motion of the system, independent of its initial state. The "basin of attraction" of a limit cycle is all those initial conditions which lead the system to eventually approach that limit cycle. We note that there may be some initial conditions such as extreme temperature and anoxia from which the system cannot attain stable behavior because the conditions do not lie in the basin of attraction of the limit cycle, but we shall ignore the possibility that the oscillator reaches such states (Fig. 3). In other models of excitable membranes the possibility of conditional oscillation or bistable membrane behavior (i.e., either oscillatory or quiescent, depending upon initial conditions or parameters), may be important, but we do not consider such models here. See Harris-Warrick (Chap. 8) and Kopell (Chap. 10) for further discussion of these concepts.

We make no assumptions about the nature of the "state space" which contains the dynamics of the individual oscillator. The state space should be thought of as a space with axes taken as relevant quantities, possibly measurable, such as ionic concentrations, membrane potentials, ionic currents, displacements, velocities, and so on. Thus, a point in the state space represents a particular set of values for the variables being measured (i.e., a "state") and a path parametrized by time in the state space represents the evolving states of the system. We do not claim that the state variables represent any particular specified quantities, although in a specific example one may apply the general theory to a definite state space. In practice, such a model is highly general, requiring knowledge only of the phenomenologically observed oscillations of the system. The mechanisms giving rise to the oscillations need not be understood. Such a model makes no attempt to model the structure of the oscillator itself and will not be useful for studying the origin of the oscillation, but is quite useful for studying the collective behavior of a system of oscillators whose underlying neuronal structure is unknown.

We now consider the mathematical representation of a single uncoupled biological oscillator. We shall distinguish between the following two effects for motions which start inside the basin of attraction of the stable limit cycle: first, there is the fairly rapid attraction onto the limit cycle, and, second, there is the oscillatory motion around the limit cycle. The first effect possibly corresponds to start-up, for example, as the elements of the oscillators are excited above threshold. This phase is transient and, in many biological systems, disappears after one or two cycles (Pavlidis, 1973, Winfree, 1980). In view of the transient nature of this effect, and in order to obtain a simpler mathematical model, we shall neglect the transient approach to the limit cycle and shall, rather, assume that the oscillator is on its steady state limit cycle at all times. This permits us to specify the state of a single oscillator by a single variable $\theta(t)$, where $\theta(t)$ represents the position of the oscillator *around* its limit cycle at time t, i.e., $\theta(t)$ is the *phase* of the limit cycle (see Fig. 4). Thus the phase of the oscillator is a single variable which realistically reflects the behavior of the most important variables which underlie the oscillation. While this is a dramatic simplification, it seems to be legitimate biologically. We shall rescale θ so that it goes from 0 to 2π radians (= 360 degrees) over one cycle, and we shall parametrize θ so that it flows uniformly around the limit cycle. That is, θ is proportional to the fraction of the period which has elapsed. In applying this model to experimental situations, we will ignore the fine structure of the cycle and look only at some well defined event such as the onset of the

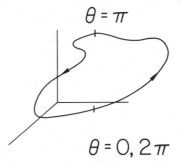

FIGURE 4. The state of a limit cycle oscillator in an n-dimensional state space is represented by the single variable $\theta(t)$, its phase, chosen to run from 0 to 2π around one cycle, and computed mod 2π.

burst. The comparable point will be used in all cycles to delineate $\theta = 0$. This yields the following simple differential equation characterizing a single oscillator:

$$\frac{d\theta}{dt} = \omega \tag{1}$$

where ω is the frequency of the oscillator and $2\pi/\omega$ its period. The solution of this equation is:

$$\theta(t) = \omega t + \theta(0) \tag{2}$$

where $\theta(0)$ is the initial value (at time $t = 0$) of θ.

Although this equation predicts that (t) is an ever increasing function of t, we shall interpret θ to always lie between 0 and 2π. Since motion around the limit cycle is topologically circular, we do not distinguish between one oscillation and the next, but rather start measuring θ anew each time θ crosses 2π. This is accomplished mathematically by using modular arithmetic: Given a value of θ, we add or subtract multiples of 2π to it until the result lies in the interval $0 \le \theta < 2\pi$. In this case eq. (2) is written:

$$\theta(t) = \omega t + \theta(0) \ (\text{mod } 2\pi) \tag{2}$$

Geometrically this means that θ is pictured as a point moving on a topological circle rather than on a straight line.

Note that in terms of a state variable $x(t)$ (an axis of the state space), the motion of the oscillator around its limit cycle is given by its projection onto the x-axis. The model offers no prediction as to the wave shape of the resulting periodic function, except that its period must be $2\pi/\omega$ (see Fig. 5). This apparently serious shortcoming of the model is the price we pay for tractability of the ensuing equations. Mathematically speaking, we cannot distinguish between almost sinusoidal (weak) limit cycles and relaxation oscillations (cf. Kopell, Chapt. 10). In short, we have eliminated all references to wave shape except for the phase $\theta(t)$. To account for the observed ventral root output of the lamprey cord, one imagines that a threshold effect causes the spiking process to occur only for a definite range of values of the phase $\theta(t)$, see Figure 5.

For several applications where the oscillator is known purely phenomenologically, this treatment is particularly suitable, in spite of its limitations. In such systems the only measurable variable may be the presence or absence of nerve or muscle activity, or membrane polarization of passively driven output elements, the details of the internal variables being essentially unknown. Thus, one could model the CPG for mastication beginning with the assumption that the CPG is composed of a group of coupled oscillators, each of which controls the activity of one muscle or

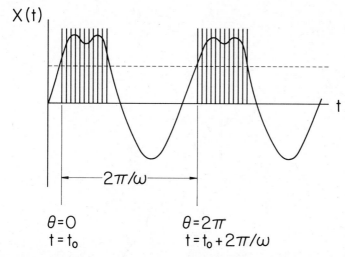

$X(t)$

$2\pi/\omega$

$\theta = 0$
$t = t_0$

$\theta = 2\pi$
$t = t_0 + 2\pi/\omega$

FIGURE 5. Relationship between $\theta(t)$ and $x(t)$ in a limit cycle oscillator which spikes when $x(t)$ is larger than some threshold value (shown dashed).

group of synergistic muscles. In such a model, one could simply use the onset of muscle activity in the various muscle groups to denote $\theta = 0$ for each oscillator. Similarly, in cat locomotion one could make the same set of assumptions with $\theta = 0$ as the onset of activity in the limb muscles. This approach permits us to test assertions regarding the coordinating system while knowing little about the oscillator *per se,* and is in contrast to work in which fairly detailed models of specific physiological processes are developed (e.g., Rinzel, to appear; Chay and Rinzel, to appear).

3 COUPLED OSCILLATORS

Since one of our goals is to develop a method rather than a specific model, we have chosen to use the simplest formulations for our equations. We constructed the oscillators of our models to be non-linear and stable but easily dealt with analytically. Particular assumptions can be added or changed to make them more like a given system or to test a specific hypothesis regarding some component of the system. Such a change will alter the behavior of the system in ways that must be determined for each case. The coupling we have chosen is also characterized by its simplicity, rather than its reality. Again, it can be changed in each case as information is obtained, and again, the behavior of the system in each case must be redetermined. As the discussion progresses we will compare the assumptions used here to those of Kopell. We will also point out the effect the differences have on the conclusions we derive. Essentially, Kopell has gen-

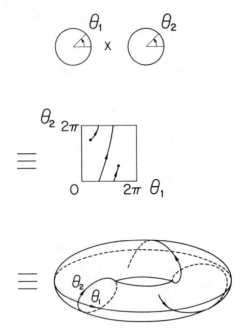

FIGURE 6. Two oscillators are viewed as living on a torus instead of on their individual circles.

eralized the basic formulation set forth in Cohen et. al. (1982) and summarized here. She has also included refinements which make the model conform more to the biology. Some people may find it helpful to start with our formulation which, although unrealistically simplified, is designed to be a skeleton upon which assumptions can be hung and within which changes can be made. Further discussion of the differences between the two approaches will be presented as relevant now and in Kopell's chapter (Chapt. 10).

Let us consider a system of N coupled biological oscillators, each modeled in the manner just described. Corresponding to the ith oscillator (where i is an integer between 1 and N) there will be a phase $\theta_i(t)$ which describes its state at time t. Each phase θ_i will be viewed as living on a circle, $0 \le \theta_i < 2\pi$. Hence the entire system of N oscillators will live on N such circles. Rather than think in terms of N circles, we will use the usual mathematical convention of "multiplying" these together to give an N dimensional torus T^N. (For example, in the case of $N = 2$ oscillators, we may picture the relationship between the two circles and the 2 dimensional torus T^2 via the intermediate step of identifying the sides of a square in the $\theta_1 - \theta_2$ plane. See Fig. 6.) Thus a vector $\bar{\theta} = (\theta_1, \theta_2, \ldots, \theta_i, \ldots, \theta_N)$ specifies a point on T^N; the N components of the vector tells us where we are relative to each independent circular coordinate.

Here we assume that the limit cycles which characterize the dynamics of the individual oscillators continue to exist after the oscillators are coupled together. Although the shape of the individual limit cycles may change as the nature of the coupling changes, our scheme for parametrizing the θ_i's to run from 0 to 2π around a cycle always permits us to refer to the same N-torus T^N to describe the motion of the system. Our assumption of the structural stability of the individual oscillators implies that, for sufficiently weak coupling relative to the individual oscillator's transient dynamics, the system of coupled oscillators will continue to oscillate stably.

We may obtain a mathematical representation of the system of N oscillators by including coupling terms in eq. (1) written for the ith oscillator:

$$\frac{d\theta_i}{dt} = \omega_i + h_i\,(\theta_1, \theta_2, \ldots, \theta_N) \tag{3}$$

in which ω_i is the (uncoupled) frequency of the ith oscillator, and the function h_i represents the direct effects of coupling by other oscillators on the ith oscillator. The frequencies ω_i of the individual oscillators may or may not be equal. In the lamprey, for example, the frequencies of the oscillators in a given cord have been found to be equal in some cases, but generally are not (Fig. 7; Cohen, 1984). There will be more detailed discussion of the effect of the ω_i parameters in later sections of this paper.

If the oscillator is more complex, some more complicated function could be added to this equation. For example, if one were modeling the interaction between the cerebellum and the locomotor CPG of cats, one would first note that the cells of the dorsal spinocerebellar tract (DSCT) were not themselves oscillatory but are rhythmically driven by input from the CPG (cf. Gelfand et al., this volume). To model such a neuron one might choose a function $f(\theta)$ with zeroes (points θ^* at which $f(\theta^*) = 0$) so that the equation for the cell $\theta_k' = f(\theta_k)$ sits at a constant phase when isolated. Addition of couplings $h_k\,(\theta_1, \ldots, \theta_N)$ can then set it in oscillatory motion at the same frequency as the CPG. Such a cell also receives influences from other neurons in the brain and sensory inputs ascending from the limbs and so its equation should include a term which incorporates the influences from these other structures.

Since in our basic model the ith oscillator is described by reference only to its phase θ_i, the coupling function h_i also depends only on the θ_i's (and not, for example, on the size of the limit cycle, or any other characteristics of its wave shape.) The coupling function h_i we must choose to be 2π-periodic in each of its arguments, in order that the "flow" (3) be uniquely defined on the torus T^N. That is, the rate of change of θ_i is to depend only upon the position of each of the N oscillators in their cycles, and not upon how many cycles have already passed (cf. the modular arithmetic discussion above.)

We further assume that the coupling may be separated into contribu-

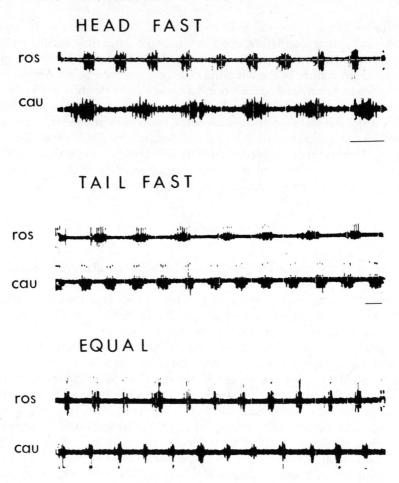

FIGURE 7. Ventral root bursting of separated rostral and caudal pieces of isolated lamprey spinal cords. Prior to cutting, the cords all generated well-coordinated traveling waves when stimulated with D-glutamate. The cords, all treated alike, were cut through at their mid-segments, kept under the same conditions and recordings continued. These traces were photographed after the drug was removed and reapplied to allow damaged fibers to quiet down.

tions due to the interaction between any two pairs of oscillators. In each part of the equation one oscillator is presynaptic and the other postsynaptic. Mathematically this means that we may write the coupling function h_i as the sum of a series of N terms:

$$h_i(\theta_1, \theta_2, \ldots, \theta_N) = \sum_{j=1}^{N} h_{ij}(\theta_i, \theta_j) \qquad (4)$$

where the function h_{ij} represents the effect of the jth oscillator on the ith oscillator (and hence depends only on θ_i and θ_j). The jth oscillator is, therefore, presynaptic to the ith oscillator in (4), and h is assumed to be 2π-periodic in its arguments.

How shall we specify the coupling functions h_{ij}? To begin with, we will require that h_{ij} be zero when both oscillators are at the same points in their cycles, i.e., when θ_i equals θ_j. This assumption will, as we shall see, permit two identical coupled oscillators to oscillate in phase with each other, as intuition requires. (See Kopell, Chapt. 10, for an alternative form of coupling she terms "synaptic coupling.") Mathematically, this can be accomplished by requiring that h_{ij} depend only on the difference between θ_i and θ_j:

$$h_{ij}(\theta_i, \theta_j) = h_{ij}(\theta_j - \theta_i) \tag{5}$$

such that $h_{ij}(0) = 0$. Such coupling is called diffusive coupling. In Kopell's formulation, h_{ij} also depends on $(\theta_j - \theta_i)$ but need not be zero when $\theta_j - \theta_i = 0$. (Cf. Kopell for further discussion of the significance of this assumption.) Now since the function h_{ij} must be 2π-periodic, we can develop it in a Fourier series of sines and cosines. Taking just the first terms of the Fourier series, we obtain:

$$h_{ij}(\theta_i, \theta_j) = a \sin(\theta_j - \theta_i) + b [1 - \cos(\theta_j - \theta_i)] \tag{6}$$

where a and b are coupling coefficients. We shall take $b = 0$ in what follows (after Cohen et al., 1982), thus making h the pure sine function, but we note that Ermentrout and Kopell (1984) have discussed the effects of including the cosine terms. The latter play an important role in some situations especially with respect to the resultant frequency of the system and to the uniformity of the phase lags in a chain of many oscillators. A coupling function of the form (6) was derived by an independent approach (a perturbation method) in the case of two weakly coupled van der Pol oscillators (Rand & Holmes, 1980), and in more general situations by Neu (1979, 1980).

Substituting (4) – (6) into (3) we obtain:

$$\frac{d\theta_i}{dt} = \omega_i + \sum_{j=1}^{N} a_{ij} \sin(\theta_j - \theta_i) \tag{7}$$

where a_{ij} is the coupling coefficient representing the influence of oscillator j on oscillator i. a_{ij} is assumed to be independent of the oscillator, undoubtedly an incorrect assumption. However, superficial attempts to change this have not yielded anything very interesting to date, but more needs to be done to explore fully this level of complexity. Note that *positive* values of a_{ij}

tend to advance the phase of θ_i, if θ_j leads θ_i by a small amount, and hence are called *excitatory*. Similarly, *negative a_{ij}* are called *inhibitory* (cf. Kopell, Chapt. 10 in which the terms "desynchronizing" and "synchronizing" are used instead).

These differential equations (7) are nonlinear and no exact general solution can be expected to be found for arbitrary parameter values. Nevertheless, it is possible to learn much about the behavior of these equations by (1) looking for exact special solutions and (2) numerically integrating them on a digital computer.

In the rest of this chapter, we shall consider various special cases of eqs. (7) and associated applications, as well as extensions of the model to more complicated coupling functions.

4   TWO COUPLED OSCILLATORS

Many biological systems can be modeled as consisting of two coupled oscillators. For example, the CPGs for each limb of a quadruped can be modeled as a chain of several oscillators (cf. Grillner, 1981; Cohen, Chapt. 5). However in dealing with the coordination between the two limbs of a single girdle, they can more conveniently be viewed as a pair of coupled oscillators where the oscillators for the various muscle groups are lumped together and taken as a single limb oscillator. Moreover, the following simple systems serve as a good introduction to help understand the behaviors exhibited by larger collections of oscillators. In the case of two oscillators, eqs. (7) become:

$$\frac{d\theta_1}{dt} = \omega_1 + a_{12} \sin(\theta_2 - \theta_1) \tag{8a}$$

$$\frac{d\theta_2}{dt} = \omega_2 + a_{21} \sin(\theta_1 - \theta_2) \tag{8b}$$

It is convenient to define a quantity

$$\varphi(t) = \theta_1(t) - \theta_2(t) \tag{9}$$

which represents the phase lag of oscillator 2 relative to oscillator 1. Like θ_1 and θ_2, φ lives on a circle. The phase lag φ satisfies a relatively simple differential equation which is obtained by subtracting (8b) from (8a), giving:

$$\frac{d\varphi}{dt} = (\omega_1 - \omega_2) - (a_{12} + a_{21}) \sin \varphi \tag{10}$$

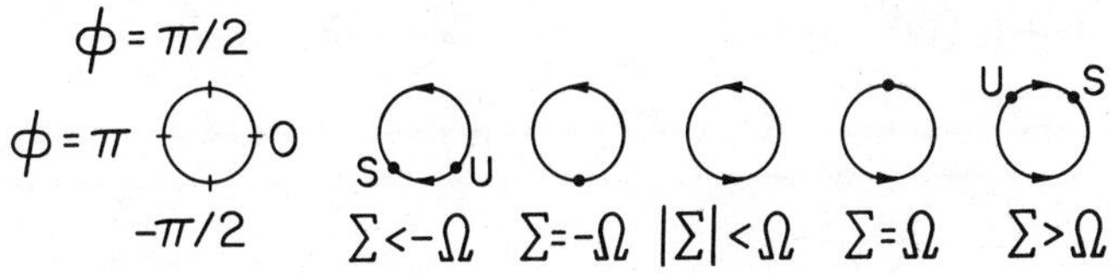

FIGURE 8. Bifurcation of equilibrium states of eq. (10) (representing phase-locked motions). In this sequence of flows on the φ circle, we assume that $\omega_1 > \omega_2$ (and set $\Omega = \omega_1 - \omega_2 > 0$). We let $\Sigma = a_{12} + a_{21}$ vary from $-\infty$ to $+\infty$. The positions of the equilibria are given by dots, the location of which are found from eq. (11). As indicated by the directions of the arrows, the stable equilibria are marked S, and the unstable U. For $0 < \Omega < \Sigma$ (excitatory coupling), the stable equilibrium point satisfies $0 < \varphi < \pi/2$ and oscillator 1 (the faster of the two) leads oscillator 2. For $\Sigma < -\Omega < 0$ (inhibitory coupling), on other hand, the stable equilibrium satisfies $-\pi < \varphi < -\pi/2$ and the slower oscillator (oscillator 2) leads.

This single differential equation can be solved exactly (see Cohen et al., 1982). It is sufficient for us here, however, to look for special solutions, called 1:1 phase-locked motions, in which the phase lag $\varphi(t)$ is a constant over time. These motions are represented by the equilibria of (10), and may be obtained by equating the right-hand side of (10) to zero:

$$\varphi = \arcsin \frac{\omega_1 - \omega_2}{a_{12} + a_{21}} \tag{11}$$

Eq. (11) has either 0, 1, or 2 solutions, depending upon whether the key quantity, the ratio of frequency difference to coupling.

$$\left| \frac{\omega_1 - \omega_2}{a_{12} + a_{21}} \right| \tag{12}$$

is greater than, equal to, or less than unity. (Since the sine function always has absolute value less than or equal to unity, there will be no solutions if (12) is greater than 1. Note that this result depends on the form assumed for the coupling function h (eqs. (6), (7).) If a different function h were chosen, a similar analysis would be required and the results may or may not support phase-locked motions (see Fig. 8). In the case that no such phase-locked solutions occur, the system is said to drift. The same qualitative bifurcation into drift will hold for any bounded 2π periodic function, although more than one stable solution might exist in the locked region.

In words, this result states that phase (and frequency) locking will occur if the difference between the frequencies of the two oscillators is sufficiently small, compared to the net coupling between them. For two given oscillators (with their frequencies ω_1 and ω_2 fixed), the coupling may be increased until a critical value is reached at which point the system goes from drift to phase-locked motion. As we will see later, in the transitions

A. FICTIVE SWIMMING: D-glutamate

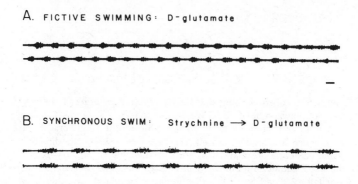

B. SYNCHRONOUS SWIM: Strychnine ⟶ D-glutamate

FIGURE 9. Strychnine-induced synchronous bursting. The recordings are from the left and right roots of a single segment. Top traces: before strychnine with D-glutamate alone. Lower traces: after strychnine was applied to cord, removed and D-glutamate readded. (Adapted from Cohen & Harris-Warrick, 1984. See reference for details). Time bar = 1 second.

there may be what has been termed "relative coordination" (von Holst, 1939, transl. 1973), as has been observed in fish by von Holst (1939, transl. 1973) and in lamprey by Cohen (Cohen et al., 1982; Cohen, 1984). From eq. (11) it follows that once locking has occurred, if the net coupling is positive (excitatory), then the faster oscillator will lead by a phase angle between 0 and 90 degrees, while if the net coupling is negative (inhibitory), then the slower oscillator will lead by a phase angle between 90 and 180 degrees. These last conclusions follow from consideration of the stability of the phase-locked states, and can be seen from the direction of the arrows generating the flow on the φ circle in Figure 8. It is interesting to observe that in a simple, two-oscillator system, this could afford a mechanism for reversing the direction of motion, say, from forwards to backwards, simply by changing the relative frequencies of the oscillators.

As an example of an application of this model to a biological problem in which the two oscillators have similar frequencies, we consider an experiment by Cohen and Harris-Warrick (1984) involving the treatment of the isolated lamprey spinal cord with strychnine. Briefly, we postulate that each segment, or small group of segments of the cord contains two oscillators which normally burst about 180 degrees (π radians) out-of-phase. In the in vitro preparation, this is called "fictive swimming" (cf. Grillner et al., Chapt. 1 and Cohen, Chapt. 5). After pre-treatment with strychnine, the two sides are observed to oscillate approximately in phase, with roughly synchronous bursting (Fig. 9). Although the details of the effect of strychnine are not completely known, it is known that in the lamprey spinal cord strychnine blocks inhibitory glycinergic synapses (Homma and Rovainen, 1978).

In order to explain this behavior with the foregoing model, we assume that the left and right sides of the cord can be "lumped" into two oscillators with approximately the same uncoupled frequencies ($\omega_1 \approx \omega_2$). The oscillators along the entire cord almost certainly do not have the same frequencies but the two within each segment almost certainly do have very close frequencies. Thus, $\omega_1 - \omega_2 \approx 0$. Since the normal functioning of the cord displays phase-locked alternation with $\varphi = \pi$, we assume that the net coupling is initially inhibitory ($a_{12} + a_{21} < 0$). The addition of strychnine is then modeled as removing the inhibitory coupling, leaving a net excitatory coupling ($a_{12} + a_{21} > 0$). This moves the dynamical state from the initial state out-of-phase equilibrium $\varphi \approx \pi$ to a new in-phase equilibrium given by $\varphi \approx 0$. Moreover, the model predicts that as the strychnine gradually takes effect, the net coupling must pass through zero (since it goes from net negative to net positive). For some range of coupling values around zero (depending on the frequency difference $\omega_1 - \omega_2$) no phase-locked states exist (cf. eq. (11)), and the model predicts a temporary period of drift. The model system, although it must drift for a time, can move continuously through the transition from alternation to synchrony. However, in the experimental system, the situation is more complex. The cord is unable to pass into and out of the period of drift. Adding strychnine directly to a fictively swimming preparation causes the cord to burst unstably and, finally, tonically, with all evidence of oscillation gone. The only method of application that produces stable bursting is to remove the glutamate from the bath, perfuse the cord with strychnine for some time, and immediately add the glutamate after removing the strychnine (which remains bound to the receptors for well over half an hour). The supposition is that this difference between the model and the cord will be reflected in the imbedding of the two oscillators in their respective multidimensional phase spaces, an aspect which our simple phase model cannot address and which we have so far ignored.

This simple formulation of the model can also be applied to experiments by Young et al. (1980) on the *scaphognathite* of the lobster, *Homarus americanus*, and by Kammer on several species of Lepidoptera (1968). In the experiments of Young et al., picrotoxin, which blocks inhibitory synapses, was able to induce changes in the ventilatory motor output pattern very similar to those predicted in the discussion above. The bursting was transformed by picrotoxin from an out-of-phase mode, through a long period of instability and drift, to a stable in-phase mode (Fig. 10). Kammer recorded motor activity during the change from warm-up to flight in several species of moths. She obtained a variety of "shivering" patterns, but a relatively common observation was that muscles would fairly rapidly switch from the synchrony of shivering to the alternation needed for flight. This would suggest a mechanism similar to that proposed above, but with the switch being from excitatory to inhibitory coupling. Kammer proposed a model qualitatively similar to ours in order to explain her findings.

The transition from trot to gallop in tetrapods may also have some of

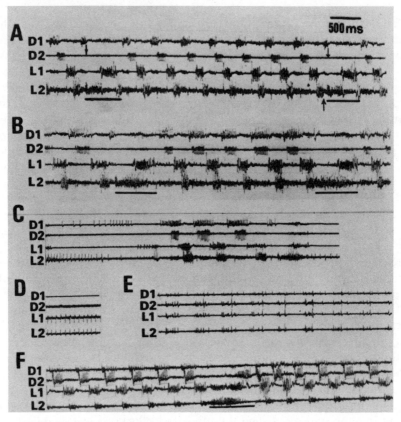

FIGURE 10. Effect of picrotoxin (ptx) on phasing of the scaphognathite muscles during rhythmic activity. (A) Activity before ptx treatment. Bursts underscored are reversals, arrows indicate changes in pattern associated with the reversal. Notice the minimum overlap between D1 and D2. (B) Activity 6 minutes after treatment with the ptx. Notice the phasing has changed with D1 and D2 now overlapping considerably. L and D groups still alternate (C) Activity 9 minutes after treatment. Brief periods of rhythmic pumping interrupt periods of long, overlapping though still weakly reciprocating bursts of increasing length. By 10 minutes no rhythmic activity was seen. (D) BY 15 minutes L1 started firing and the two L group muscles showed tonic, synchronous activity for about 15 minutes. (E) By 65 minutes tonic synchronous spikes and bursts appeared in all groups. (F) By 90 minutes normal rhythmic activity returned. (Adapted from Young et al., 1980. See reference for more details.)

the model's features. In cats, each limb continues to oscillate normally as the animal changes from trot to other fast gaits, such as canter and gallop. However, English has noted (1979) that the limbs pass through highly variable phase relations as they change from the slower alternating to the faster non-alternating gaits. One interpretation for the variability is that drift occurs between limb oscillators as the coupling between the limbs changes from inhibitory to excitatory coupling.

As a different type of example of the two-oscillator model, we consider the experiments of Cohen concerning the surgical lesioning of the isolated lamprey cord. Briefly, the experiment consists of making a specific lesion in the cord and observing the changes in dynamics of bursting. It is found that the groups of segments rostral and caudal to the lesion remain internally phase-locked, but the two groups can be seen to drift with respect to one another. The extent and nature of the drift is dependent on the kind of lesion. The drift state can be characterized by plotting "period" of oscillation (i.e., time between consecutive appearances of the same phase in the cycle, in this case the onset of the bursting) as a function of time (see Fig. 11).

This situation has been modeled (Cohen et al., 1982) by taking the rostral and caudal groups of segments on either side of the lesion as individual oscillators. We assume, in accord with the more common experimental observation, that the frequencies of the oscillators differ (Cohen, 1984). In order to compare the model with the experiment, we graph the behavior of the model oscillators as described above. The period of time between consecutive zero phases is plotted against time for both oscillator 1 and oscillator 2 (see Fig. 12). Note that in the extreme case of one-way descending coupling, where the lesion has destroyed all the ascending coupling, the forcing oscillator is perfectly stable while the forced oscillator shows great instability. Comparison of Figures 11 and 12 led to the conjecture that, in the experimental cord, the spared medial tracts contain fibers which primarily descend from head to tail. Similar types of evidence suggest that the lateral tracts contain both descending and ascending fibers (Cohen, 1986; Rovainen, 1985). More experimental work is needed to confirm these conjectures, but they remain as working hypotheses.

It is important to note that with h, the coupling, as the sine function, the frequency of the pair of coupled oscillators will be intermediate between the frequencies of the uncoupled pair. However, with couplings other than the sine function, the frequency of the coupled system will still depend on ω_1, ω_2 and h, but it need not be intermediate between ω_1 and ω_2 (cf. Kopell, Chapt. 10).

5   CHAIN OF N OSCILLATORS WITH NEAREST NEIGHBOR COUPLING

We return now to consideration of eqs. (7) in the general case of N coupled oscillators. We start by considering a chain of N oscillators with nearest neighbor coupling (Fig. 1), a configuration which is certainly oversimplified, but which is useful in beginning to model the lamprey CPG (Cohen et al., 1982). It also applies to waves in the mammalian intestine (Ermentrout and Kopell, 1984), and stomatal oscillations in the leaves of green plants (Rand et al., 1982). In this case, eqs. (7) become:

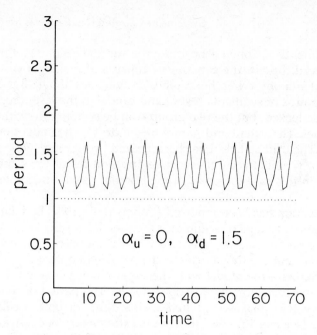

FIGURE 11. Upper figure. Graph of period versus time for two model oscillators. The dotted line is the "rostral" and the solid, the "caudal". We assume the ascending coupling (α_u) has been lesioned leaving only the descending ocupling (α_d) reduced but still present. When uncoupled period of "rostral" is 1 and "caudal" is 1.5. (From Cohen et al., 1982.)

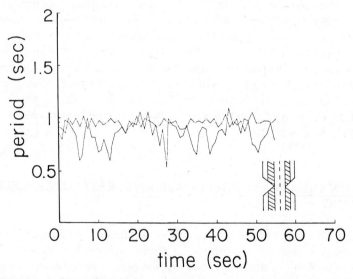

FIGURE 12. Lower figure. Period of successive bursts versus time for two ventral roots of a lesioned lamprey spinal cord (see insert) Rostral root is dotted, caudal is solid. Caudal is considerably more variable than rostral with pattern of variability similar to that of theoretical oscillators in Fig. 11. (From Cohen et al., 1982.)

$$\frac{d\theta_1}{dt} = \omega_1 + a\,\sin(\theta_2 - \theta_1)$$

$$\frac{d\theta_i}{dt} = \omega_i + a\,\sin(\theta_{i+1} - \theta_i) + a\,\sin(\theta_{i-1} - \theta_i) \tag{13}$$

$$\frac{d\theta_N}{dt} = \omega_N + a\,\sin(\theta_{N-1} - \theta_N)$$

where $i = 1,2, \ldots ,N$ and where we have assumed for convenience that all the coupling constants are equal, $a_{ij} = a$.

Following the treatment of the two oscillator case, we set $\varphi_i = \theta_i - \theta_{i+1}$ for $i = 1,2, \ldots ,N-1$, cf. eq. (9). From eqs. (13) we obtain the following $N - 1$ eqs. on the ϕ_i, which we write in matrix form:

$$\frac{d\bar{\varphi}}{dt} = \bar{\Omega} + \bar{A}\bar{S} \tag{14}$$

where

$$\bar{\varphi} = \begin{bmatrix} \varphi_1 \\ \ldots \\ \varphi_{N-1} \end{bmatrix}, \quad \bar{S} = \begin{bmatrix} \sin \varphi_1 \\ \ldots \\ \sin \varphi_{N-1} \end{bmatrix}, \quad \bar{\Omega} = \begin{bmatrix} \omega_1 - \omega_2 \\ \ldots \\ \omega_{N-1} - \omega_N \end{bmatrix}$$

are $N-1$ vectors and where

$$\bar{A} = a \begin{bmatrix} -2 & 1 & & \\ 1 & -2 & 1 & \\ & 1 & -2 & 1 \\ & & 1 & -2 \end{bmatrix}$$

is a tri-diagonal $N-1 \times N-1$ matrix representing the coupling constants between all N oscillators.

As in the two oscillator case, we investigate the existence of 1:1 phase locked motions by requiring the φ_i to be constants in (14), giving $d\bar{\varphi}/dt = \bar{0}$ and:

$$\bar{S} = -\bar{A}^{-1}\bar{\Omega} \tag{15}$$

No solution of (15) exists if any of the components of $\bar{A}^{-1}\bar{\Omega}$ are larger than unity in absolute value (since each of the components of S are sines).

Now it turns out (Cohen et al., 1982) that the matrix $\bar{A}$, although arbitrarily large, is tractable, since it can be inverted in closed form. For example, in the case of $N = 6$ oscillators, $\bar{A}$ is a 5×5 matrix with inverse:

$$\bar{A}^{-1} = -\frac{1}{6a}\begin{bmatrix} 5\ 4\ 3\ 2\ 1 \\ 4\ 8\ 6\ 4\ 2 \\ 3\ 6\ 9\ 6\ 3 \\ 2\ 4\ 6\ 8\ 4 \\ 1\ 2\ 3\ 4\ 5 \end{bmatrix} \tag{16}$$

Thus, we can compute the phase lag vector $\bar{\varphi}$ in closed form.

As an example, suppose that the difference in frequencies, ω_i along the chain is a constant, i.e., $\omega_1 - \omega_2 = \omega_2 - \omega_3 = \ldots = e$. Then

$$\bar{\Omega} = e\begin{bmatrix} 1 \\ 1 \\ \cdots \\ 1 \end{bmatrix} \tag{17}$$

and in the case of $N = 6$ oscillators, eq. (15) becomes (using (16)):

$$\begin{bmatrix} \sin\varphi_1 \\ \sin\varphi_2 \\ \sin\varphi_3 \\ \sin\varphi_4 \\ \sin\varphi_5 \end{bmatrix} = \frac{e}{2a}\begin{bmatrix} 5 \\ 8 \\ 9 \\ 8 \\ 5 \end{bmatrix} \tag{18}$$

Note that the condition on φ_3 is the hardest to satisfy, and phase-locked solutions exist only if

$$\left\|\frac{e}{a}\right\| \leq \frac{2}{9} \tag{19}$$

For general N, it can be shown that eq. (19) generalizes to $|e/a| \leq 8/N^2$ (N even), or $|e/a| \leq 8/(N^2-1)$ (N odd), and that the resulting motion is frequency-locked at the average frequency of the uncoupled oscillators. For $N = 2$ this gives $|e/a| \leq 2$, which is just expression (12) equated to unity. When $e = 0$, the chain oscillates in unison with $\varphi = 0$, that is, there is no traveling wave.

Returning to the example of $N=6$ oscillators, Fig. 13 shows the predicted phase lags for $e/a = 0.01$ and 0.22. Since each of the φ_i's is positive, the faster oscillators lead the slower ones in each pair of neighbors (assuming e and a are positive), the greatest phase difference occurring at the middle of the chain, between oscillators 3 and 4. It should be noted that the experimentally measured phase difference between nearby oscillators in the midbody region and at the ends of the cord is actually always quite small. Moreover, no differences in phase lags have so far been observed along the cord, but a small difference could be difficult to measure reliably.

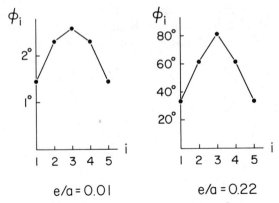

FIGURE 13. Plot of φ_i for a system of 6 oscillators with $\bar{\Omega} = (e, e, e, \ldots, e)$.

Alternatively, this discrepancy could be an indication that the ratio of the frequency difference to coupling constant e/a is quite small or that the assumptions of sine coupling and strictly nearest neighbor coupling are inappropriate for the lamprey (cf. Kopell for h, not the sine function).

In the case that eq. (19) is not satisfied, the system of $N = 6$ oscillators is not 1:1 phase-locked. Ermentrout and Kopell, (1984) have studied what happens to a chain of N oscillators with nearest neighbor coupling when the parameters are tuned to just outside the point of phase-locking. Their results, interpreted in terms of the $N = 6$ example, show that if e/a is just slightly larger than 2/9, oscillators 1, 2, and 3 tend to oscillate as one unit; oscillators 4, 5, and 6 oscillate as another unit; but the two groups drift with respect to one another. Ermentrout and Kopell (1984) have followed earlier authors and called this phenomenon "frequency plateaus," and have identified it with the normal functioning of mammalian intestines. In some situations, several plateaus can appear in a long chain of oscillators. In the formulation of Kopell and Ermentrout (cf. Kopell, chapt. 10) N oscillators, with nearest neighbor coupling, can produce a traveling wave with uniform phase lags along the cord. They assume $e = 0$, i.e., that there are little or no frequency differences among the oscillators and that the coupling is "synaptic" ($h(0) \neq 0$). They can address frequency differences of a significant magnitude if they add multiple neighbor interactions (see Kopell, Chapt. 10).

6 DOUBLE CHAIN MODEL

There is considerable, albeit indirect, evidence that the lamprey CPG is actually composed of a double chain of oscillators (Cohen and Harris-Warrick, 1984; Cohen and Wallén, 1980; Grillner et al., Chapt. 1). This fact is proven unequivocally in the *Xenopus* tadpole, since each half of a sub-divided cord can continue to burst (Kahn and Roberts, 1982). To account for this evidence, in the following equation we extend the previous single chain model to a double chain. By doing this we can also begin to demonstrate how the approach presented in this chapter could be applied to a variety of situations. This extension, for example, brings us closer to the realm of more complex CPGs, such as the mammalian locomotor CPG. In such complex CPGs the brachial and lumbar enlargements control their respective joints and limbs with their respective sets of flexors and extensors (Viala and Vidal, 1979); each limb generator in turn is coupled to each other limb generator. As is reflected in the range of gaits limbed animals display (Gambary an, 1974; Hildebrand, 1976), the potential for controlling the coordination under these conditions is enormous, as is the task of understanding them (cf. Cohen, Chapt. 5).

This model involves $2N$ oscillators with phases θ_i^R and θ_i^L for i from 1 to N (L = left, R = right) see Figure 14. The governing equations become:

$$\frac{d\theta_i^L}{dt} = \omega_i + a\,\sin(\theta_{i-1}^L - \theta_i^L) + a\,\sin(\theta_{i+1}^L - \theta_i^L) + k\,\sin(\theta_{i-1}^R - \theta_i^L) +$$
$$k\,\sin(\theta_{i+1}^R - \theta_i^L) + c\,\sin(\theta_i^R - \theta_i^L) \tag{20}$$

$$\frac{d\theta_i^R}{dt} = \omega_i + a\,\sin(\theta_{i-1}^R - \theta_i^R) + a\,\sin(\theta_{i+1}^R - \theta_i^R) +$$
$$k\,\sin(\theta_{i-1}^L - \theta_i^R) + k\,\sin(\theta_{i+1}^L - \theta_i^R) + c\,\sin(\theta_i^L - \theta_i^R) \tag{21}$$

where a, k, and c are coupling constants (see Fig. 14), and where we have assumed that θ_i^L and θ_i^R both have the same uncoupled frequencies ω_i. Note that when k and c are zero, eqs. (20), (21) each reduce to eq. (13) for the single chain model.

We now seek a phase-locked solution for "fictive swimming" by setting:

$$\theta_i^R(t) = \theta_i^L(t) + P, \qquad P = 0 \text{ or } \pi \tag{22}$$

Eq. (22) is based on the experimental observation that the left and right sides of the cord are normally 180 degrees out-of-phase, but, with the addition of strychnine, can be made to oscillate in-phase (cf. the foregoing discussion of the two oscillator model). We also take into account the well-known observation that the locomotor CPGs of mammals permit either alternating (trot) or a range of gaits in which the limbs are more or less in-phase (e.g., gallop, bound, hop) (Gambaryan, 1974). In this latter case we make no assumptions regarding the origin of the coupling. It could be propriospinal neurons, descending controlling neurons, or sensory inputs. Here, rather than fixing coupling and frequency parameter values and seeking a phase locked solution, we specify a desired solution and seek the parameter values which would yield it. This approach yields an

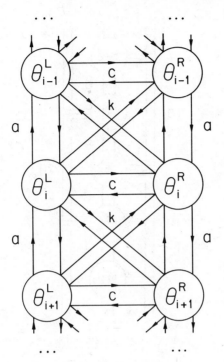

FIGURE 14. Double chain model.

exact solution to the governing equations, but it does not eliminate the possibility that other solutions may exist.

Substitution of (22) into (20), (21) gives:

$$\frac{d\theta_i^L}{dt} = \omega_i + (a \pm k)\left[\sin(\theta_{i-1}^L - \theta_i^L) + \sin(\theta_{i+1}^L - \theta_i^L)\right] \qquad (23)$$

where the upper sign corresponds to $P = 0$ and the lower sign corresponds to $P = \pi$, and where, due to (22), we obtain an identical equation on θ_i^R.

Note that the form of eq. (23) is identical to that of the single chain eq. (13), except that the coupling constant a has been replaced by $a \pm k$. (The reason that the single chain model has bearing on the double chain is because we have assumed the special solution (22) in which both sides of the double chain are phase locked together.) In the case that $a = 0$, $k < 0$, and $P = \pi$, the analysis of the single chain model shows that this system exhibits phase-locked motions. This allows us to draw the following important conclusion: The double chain model shows that the lamprey cord can exhibit normal fictive swimming (with left and right sides 180 degrees out-

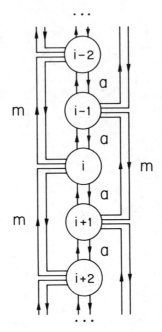

FIGURE 15. A chain of N oscillators with nearest and second nearest neighbor coupling.

of-phase) without excitatory coupling a, but rather with inhibitory coupling k from each oscillator to its upper and lower neighbors on the opposite side of the cord. This fact is particularly interesting in view of results obtained with strychnine. In the lamprey cord, strychnine pretreatment does not block intersegmental coordination, but it does degrade it and change it (Cohen, 1983). This implies that there are both glyceringic fibers (presumably inhibitory) and non-glyceringic fibers (presumably at least partly excitatory), which are components of the intersegmental coordinating system. The model results suggest that the inhibitory fibers may be crossed fibers while the excitatory are uncrossed (see also Rovainen, 1985).

7   CHAIN WITH NEAREST AND SECOND-NEAREST NEIGHBOR COUPLING

Next we shall extend the single chain model (13) to include both nearest and second-nearest neighbor coupling. The lamprey CPG has been shown to have both short and long coordinating fibers (Cohen, 1984). The long fibers can extend over ten or more segments. A model incorporating such a wide range of coordinating fiber lengths would be extremely difficult to deal with mathematically. Second-nearest neighbor coupling is expected to offer a generalization which, while still far from the actual situation, is a step closer to resembling the features of the cord which we can identify. Referring to Figure 15, the governing equations become:

$$\frac{d\theta_i}{dt} = \omega_i + a\,\sin(\theta_{i+1} - \theta_i)$$
$$+ a\,\sin(\theta_{i-1} - \theta_i) + \tag{24}$$
$$m\,\sin(\theta_{i+2} - \theta_i) + m\,\sin(\theta_{i-2} - \theta_i)$$

where a and m are coupling coefficients. Once again, defining $\varphi_i = \theta_i - \theta_{i+1}$, we obtain the following matrix equation on the φ_i, expressed in the notation of eq. (14):

$$\frac{d\bar{\varphi}}{dt} = \bar{\Omega} + \bar{A}\bar{S} + \bar{M}\bar{T} \tag{25}$$

where $\bar{\varphi}$, $\bar{\Omega}$, $\bar{A}$, $\bar{S}$ are as in eq. (14), and where $\bar{M}$ is an $N-1 \times N-2$ matrix of next to nearest neighbor coupling coefficients $\bar{T}$ is an $N-2$ vector given by:

$$M = m\begin{bmatrix} -1 & 1 & & & & \\ -1 & -1 & 1 & & & \\ 1 & -1 & -1 & 1 & & \\ & 1 & -1 & -1 & 1 & \\ & & \ddots & & & \\ & & & 1 & -1 & 1 \\ & & & & 1 & -1 \\ & & & & & -1 \end{bmatrix} , \; T = \begin{bmatrix} \sin(\varphi_1 + \varphi_2) \\ \sin(\varphi_2 + \varphi_3) \\ \dots \\ \sin(\varphi_{N-3} + \varphi_{N-2}) \\ \sin(\varphi_{N-2} + \varphi_{N-1}) \end{bmatrix}$$

Note that when $m = 0$ eq. (25) reduces to eq. (14) for the chain with nearest neighbor coupling.

We investigated eq. (25) using numerical integration on a digital computer. We chose the parameter values $\bar{\Omega} = \bar{0}$, i.e., $\omega_1 = \omega_2 = \dots \omega_N$ (identical uncoupled oscillators), and $a = 1$, $m = -1$. This models the case in which the nearest neighbor coupling is excitatory, while the second-nearest neighbor coupling is inhibitory. Before discussing the results, we note that in the case $\bar{\Omega} = \bar{0}$, $a = 1$ and $m = 0$ (oscillators with identical frequencies and nearest neighbor coupling only), eq. (14) predicts that the system will be phase-locked with zero phase lag between any two oscillators (cf. eq. (18) with $e = 0$), i.e., there will be only synchronous bursting with no traveling wave.

The addition of inhibitory nearest neighbor coupling produces the results displayed in Figure 16, which is now drastically different. Eq. (25) was numerically integrated until a steady state was reached. The initial

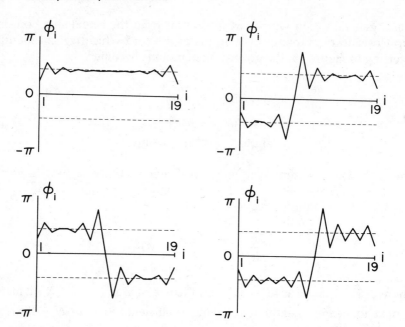

FIGURE 16. Results of numerical integration to a steady state for the system of Fig. 15, eq. (25), for $a = 1$, $m = -1$, $\omega_1 = \omega_2 = \ldots = \omega_{20}$ in the case of $N = 20$ identical oscillators.

conditions were randomly chosen for the four displayed runs (the coupling and frequency parameters were identical). The great diversity in results means that each of the displayed phase-locked solutions is only locally asymptotically stable, and that the actual state achieved by the system is strongly dependent on the choice of initial conditions. No biological system can afford to operate in this fashion.

Thus, a system of identical oscillators with excitatory nearest neighbor coupling can be destabilized (in the sense of creating an unstable steady state) by adding enough inhibitory second-nearest neighbor coupling. How much inhibitory second-nearest neighbor coupling can be added without destabilizing the zero phase difference state? In order to obtain an analytical answer to this question, we have considered the continuum model in the Appendix.

8   2:1 PHASE-LOCKING

In some cases, after a lamprey cord has been lesioned, the segments above and below the lesion can be phase-locked but with the frequency of those segments on one side of the lesion twice the frequency of those on the other (Fig. 17). Stable 2:1 bursting is rare; it does not occur following any particular lesion or under conditions we can precisely specify. However, a pattern of two-burst cycles for each movement cycle can be obtained by imposing movement on the caudal end of the cord which is too far outside the preferred frequency of the segmental oscillators (Grillner et al., 1981). 2:1 stepping patterns have also been observed upon occasion in high-spinal turtles (Stein, 1978) and decerebrate chickens (Jacobson and Holly-day, 1982). More stable 2:1 stepping patterns can be induced in decerebrate (Kulagin and Shik, 1970) or chronic spinal kittens (Forssberg, 1980), by placing each of the hind limbs on a separate treadmill belt moving at different speeds. All these examples are cases in which the normal pattern generated by the system of coupled oscillators is a stable 1:1 phase locked motion. Unfortunately, in none of the cases is it known whether the 2:1 pattern arises because of a change in the underlying oscillator frequency or in the coupling. In the sensory induced 2:1 patterns, the sensory input could be serving either to alter the coupling or to change the drive on the oscillators. Similarly, in the other examples, the two components cannot be separated adequately. We discuss here one possible model in which changes in the coupling and/or frequency differences can give rise to transitions from 1:1 to 2:1 activity in such systems (Keith and Rand, 1984).

In order to permit the model based on eqs. (3), (4) to exhibit 2:1 phase locking, we may extend the coupling to include terms of the form $h_{ij}(\theta_i, \theta_j) = h_{ij}(\theta_i - 2\theta_j)$. Specifically, we consider a system of the form:

$$\frac{d\theta_1}{dt} = \omega_1 + a \sin(\theta_2 - \theta_1) + p \sin(2\theta_2 - \theta_1) \tag{26a}$$

$$\frac{d\theta_2}{dt} = \omega_2 + a \sin(\theta_1 - \theta_2) + p \sin(\theta_1 - 2\theta_2) \tag{26b}$$

When $p = 0$ we recover the system (8) described earlier which has been shown to exhibit 1:1 phase-locked motions if the absolute value of $(\omega_1 - \omega_2)/2a$ is less than unity (cf. eq. (11)).

When $a = 0$, it may be shown that (26) can exhibit 2:1 phase-locking by letting $\psi(t) = \theta_1(t) - 2\theta_2(t)$. Then subtracting twice (26b) from (26a) gives:

$$\frac{d\psi}{dt} = (\omega_1 - 2\omega_2) - 3p \sin \psi \tag{27}$$

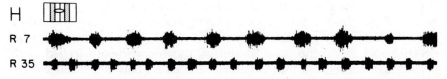

FIGURE 17. 2:1 activity following a medial lesion in a lamprey spinal cord.

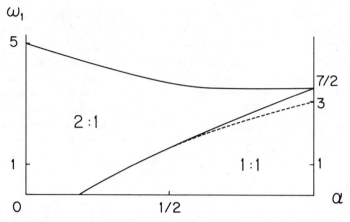

FIGURE 18. Regions of 1:1 and 2:1 phase entrainment for eqs. (34) with $p = 1 - a$ and $\omega_2 = 1$. From Keith and Rand, 1984.

2:1 phase-locked solutions correspond to equilibria of (27), since if $d\psi/dt$ is identically zero, then $d\theta_1/dt$ is twice $d\theta_2/dt$. Thus (27) exhibits 2:1 locking whenever the absolute value of $(\omega_1 - 2\omega_2)/3p$ is less than unity.

When neither a nor p are zero, eqs. (26) are more difficult to treat. Using numerical integration as well as various analytical methods, it has been shown (Keith and Rand, 1984) that as one sweeps across a parameter space defined by setting $p = 1 - a$ and $\omega_2 = 1$, there is a wide range of values for which the system (26) is 1:1 or 2:1 phase-entrained (Fig. 18).

Here we must distinguish between 1:1 *phase-locking*, in which the two phases are linearly related, i.e., $\theta_2(t) \equiv \theta_1(t)$ plus a constant, and 1:1 *phase-entrainment*, in which θ_2 completes one cycle in the same time that θ_1 does, but not necessarily by maintaining a constant phase difference. The distinction between phase-locking and phase-entrainment can be illustrated by reference to the phase torus in Figure 19.

Now let us consider the results displayed in Figure 18. The 1:1 phase-entrained region includes the points $\omega_1 < 3$, $a = 1$ (for which 1:1 locking occurs), while the 2:1 region includes the points $\omega_1 < 5$, $a = 0$ (for which 2:1 locking occurs). Both regions extend far from their respective locked states, however, showing that it is possible to obtain 2:1 entrainment under a broad range of conditions. These even include an uncoupled frequency ratio of 1:1. In the neighborhood of $a = 1$, the 2:1 region grows out of a 2:1 drift state at $\omega_1 = 7/2$, $a = 1$, into a wedge-shaped region.

Of mathematical interest is the nature of the bifurcation which occurs as one crosses from 1:1 to 2:1 phase entrainment. It has been shown numerically that many $p{:}q$ phase-entrained motions occur, where p/q lies between 1 and 2. On the basis of general dynamical theory (called circle maps), it is conjectured that in fact all rational p/q between 1 and 2 occur for small open sets of parameter values between the 1:1 and 2:1 regions.

The biological significance of this work lies in the relationship between the parameter variation and the kind of phase-entrainment that the system sees. Unfortunately for the analysis of the CPGs, until more is known about the underlying mechanisms governing CPGs and their coordinating systems, the models will be helpful only in so far as they delineate the possibilities. These are many, but the modeling will be unable to differentiate between the options since it is possible to induce 2:1 entrainment in this system by changing either the coupling between the oscillators or their uncoupled frequencies.

9 CONCLUSIONS

Although we have made only modest progress towards the goal of obtaining a general theory of coupled oscillators, we have, nevertheless, provided the biological researcher with a model of coupled oscillators which may be adapted to a wide variety of applications. The model has been shown to be able to account for phase and frequency-locking in a system of N oscillators, and it offers predictions as to which parameters are important in achieving such steady states. By extending the model to include such details as double chains, second-nearest neighbor coupling, and 2:1 entrainment, we are able to further assess the importance of these parameters in particular applications. We look forward to the continued development of this approach, as we feel that the dynamics which it supports is very rich and largely uninvestigated at the present time.

ACKNOWLEDGMENTS

The authors would like to thank Nancy Kopell for several extremely useful discussions and critical comments on the manuscript. The work reported here was partially funded by the following grants, NIH: NS16803 and NSF: CME84-02069.

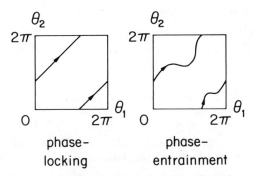

FIGURE 19. Distinction between 1:1 phase-locking and 1:1 phase-entrainment.

APPENDIX: CONTINUUM MODEL

In any real biological system, N, the number of oscillators, will always be finite. Nevertheless, we have found it useful to pass to the continuum limit by letting N approach infinity mathematically. A syncytium of neurons, or a group of neurons tightly coupled electrically, which were all endogenous oscillators would come close to this, but would still not precisely reflect the image. The continuum limit replaces the system of ordinary differential equations (ODEs) on $\varphi_i(t)$ (for example, eq. (13) or (25)), by a single partial differential equation (PDE) on $\varphi(x,t)$. That is, the continuous variable x now tags which oscillator we are interested in, whereas in the finite N case, the index i did this job. The point of this computation is that the single partial differential equation (PDE) may be easier to deal with mathematically than the system of N ordinary differential equations (ODEs).

Note that we view the continuum limit as an approximation to the more appropriate N oscillator case. This is quite the opposite of the situation in classical continuum mechanics, in which one uses finite differences to replace a PDE (considered an exact model) by a system of N ODEs (considered an approximation).

We will work with eq. (24), which includes eq. (13) as a special case. Let be the distance between two neighboring oscillators. Then as $\to 0$, the differences approach derivatives as follows:

$$\frac{\theta_{i+1} - \theta_i}{} \to \left.\frac{\partial\theta}{\partial x}\right|_i \quad \text{and} \quad \frac{\theta_{i+2} - \theta_i}{2} \to \left.\frac{\partial\theta}{\partial x}\right|_i \tag{A1}$$

so that eq. (24) becomes

$$\frac{\partial\theta}{\partial t} = \omega(x) + a\frac{\partial}{\partial x}\sin\left[\frac{\partial\theta}{\partial x}\right] + 2\,m\frac{\partial}{\partial x}\sin\left[2\frac{\partial\theta}{\partial x}\right] \tag{A2}$$

Now differentiate ($A2$) and multiply by to get:

$$\frac{\partial\varphi}{\partial t} = \Omega(x) + a^*\frac{\partial^2}{\partial x^2}\sin\varphi + 2\,m^*\frac{\partial^2}{\partial x^2}\sin 2\varphi \tag{A3}$$

where $\varphi(x,t) = (\partial\theta/\partial x)$, $\Omega(x) = (\partial\omega/\partial x)$, $a^* = a^2$, $m^* = m^2$.

We are interested in steady state (phase-locked) solutions to (A3) subject to some reasonable boundary conditions, say $\varphi = 0$ at $x = 0$ and L, where L is the length of the cord. We begin by considering nearest neighbor coupling only, and we set $m^* = 0$, giving the continuum version of eq. (15):

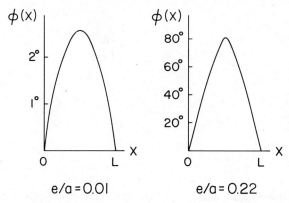

e/a = 0.01   e/a = 0.22

FIGURE A1. Phase difference ω(x) from continuum model with nearest neighbor coupling only, eq. (A5). In order to compare with the discrete case of N = 6 oscillators, Fig. 13, we use L/l = N and $a^* = al^2$ to obtain $eL^2/a^* = N^2e/a = 36e/a$. Since e/a = 0.01 and 0.22 in Fig. 13, we use eL^2/a^* = 0.36 and 7.92 here.

$$\sin \varphi = -\frac{1}{a^*} \iint \Omega(x)\, dx\, dx + c_1 x + c_2 \qquad (A4)$$

where c_1 and c_2 are constants of integration. In order to extend the comparison, we assume that there is a constant gradient of frequencies down the system, i.e., $\Omega(x) = e$. This gives, using the boundary conditions $\varphi = 0$ at $x = 0$ and L.

$$\sin \varphi = \frac{e}{2a^*} x\, (L - x) \qquad (A5)$$

which is the continuum version of eq. (18), cf. Figures 13 and A1.

Now we consider the case of a continuum of identical oscillators $(\Omega(x) = 0)$ with second-nearest neighbor coupling added to the foregoing case. Eq. (A3) gives, in the steady state:

$$a^* \sin \varphi + 2m^* \sin 2\varphi = c_1 x + c_2 \qquad (A6)$$

Applying the boundary conditions $\varphi = 0$ at $x = 0$ and L, we obtain $c_1 = c_2 = 0$ and

$$(a^* + 4\, m^* \cos \varphi)\, \sin \varphi = 0 \qquad (A7)$$

which has the roots

$$\varphi = 0,\ \pi,\ \arccos\left[-\frac{a^*}{4m^*} \right] \qquad (A8)$$

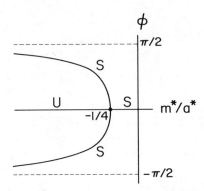

FIGURE A2. Constant phase difference φ from continuum model with nearest and second-nearest neighbor coupling, eq. (A8). The zero phase difference state is unstable for $m^*/a^* \leq \frac{1}{4}$ (U = unstable, S = stable).

These roots are displayed in Figure A2. Numerical integration of eq. (A3) for $m^*/a^* < -1/4$, $\Omega(x) = 0$, and the foregoing boundary conditions, shows that it exhibits a steady state solution which is piecewise constant in x, the solution taking on one of the values $\arccos(-a^*/4m^*)$ on each subinterval. The actual form of the piecewise constant steady state is found to be extremely sensitive to the initial conditions. In order to compare the continuum model with the finite N case of Figure 16, we set the two coupling coefficients to have equal strength, but with opposite signs, so that $m^*/a^* = -1$, and obtain the roots $\varphi = \arccos(1/4) = \pm 1.318$ radians, in approximate agreement with Figure 16.

A question was raised at the end of the section on the chain with nearest and second-nearest neighbor coupling, regarding the minimum value of inhibitory second-nearest neighbor coupling required to destablilize the zero phase difference solution of a system of N identical oscillators. We note that if the absolute value of m^*/a^* is less than 1/4, then the only roots of (A8) are $\varphi = 0$ and π. Thus the PDE suggests that the answer to the ODE question is that we require $m/a < -1/4$ to destabilize $\varphi = 0$, a result that is confirmed by numerical integration of the ODEs (25).

Before leaving the continuum model, we note that Kopell (Chapt. 10) has shown that the even function coupling terms in eq. (6) (i.e., the terms $b\,[1 - \cos(\theta_j - \theta_i)]$), play a more important role in the continuum model than do the odd terms $a \sin(\theta_j - \theta_i)$ which we have focused on in this chapter. Specifically, when the terms

$$b\,[1 - \cos(\theta_{i+1} - \theta_i)] + b\,[1 - \cos(\theta_{i-1} - \theta_i)] \qquad (A9)$$

are appended to eq. (24), and the limiting processes of eqs. (A1)–(A3) are applied, there results an additional term in eq. (A3) of the form:

$$- 2\,b^* \frac{\partial}{\partial x} \cos \varphi \qquad\qquad (A10)$$

where $b^* = bl$. In order to compare the relative importance of the even versus odd terms in eq. (6), we take $m^* = 0$ in (A3), i.e., we include only nearest neighbor coupling. Then the coefficient b^* is proportional to the small quantity l, while the coefficient a^* in (A3) is proportional to the square of l, and hence a^* is expected to be much smaller than b^* (assuming a and b are of the same order of magnitude). However, the a^* term involves a second derivative while the b^* term involves a first derivative. The net effect is to produce a *singular perturbation problem* (in the limit in which a^* is much smaller than b^*). The effect of the small second derivative terms is to produce localized boundary layers at the ends of the chain (Bender and Orszag, 1978).

REFERENCES

Abraham, R. H. and C. D. Shaw (1983). *Dynamics—The Geometry of Behavior.* Aerial Press, Santa Cruz, CA.

Bender, C. M. and S. A. Orszag (1978). *Advanced Mathematical Methods for Scientists and Engineers,* McGraw-Hill, New York.

Chay, T. R. and J. Rinzel Bursting. Beating and chaos in an excitable membrane model. *Biopys. J.* (to appear).

Cohen, A. H. (1983). Strychnine induces "fictive galloping" in the isolated spinal cord of the lamprey. *Soc. for Neurosci. Abst.,* **221**:4.

Cohen, A. H. (1984). The structure of the intersegmental coordinating system of the lamprey CPG for locomotion. *Soc. Neurosci. Abst.,* **218**:3.

Cohen, A. H. and R. M. Harris-Warrick (1984). Strychnine eliminates alternating motor output during fictive locomotion in the lamprey. *Brain Res.,* **293**:164–167.

Cohen, A. H., P. J. Holmes, and R. H. Rand (1982). The nature of the coupling between segmental oscillators of the lamprey spinal generator for locomotion: A mathematical model. *J. Math Biol.* **13**:345–369.

Cohen, A. H. and P. Wallén (1980). The neuronal correlate of locomotion in fish. "Fictive swimming" induced in an in vitro preparation of the lamprey spinal cord. *Exp. Brain Res.,* **41**:11–18.

English, A. W. and P. R. Leonard (1982). Interlimb coordination during stepping in the cat: In-phase stepping and gait transitions. *Brain Res.,* **245**:353–364.

Ermentrout, G. B. and N. Kopell (1984). Frequency Plateaus in a Chain of Weakly Coupled Oscillators, I. *SIAM J. Math. Anal.,* **15**:215–237.

Forssberg, H., S. Grillner, J. Halbertsma, and S. Rossignol (1980). The locomotion of the low spinal cat. 2: Interlimb coordination. *Acta Physiol. Scand.,* **108**:283–295.

Gambaryan, P. P. (1974). *How Mammals Run.* Halsted Press, New York.

Grillner, S. (1981). Control of locomotion in bipeds, tetrapods, and fish. In: *Handbook of Physiology*. Section 1: The Nervous System, Vol. II, Part 2. Ed. V. B. Brooks, Amer. Physiol. Soc., Bethesda, MD 1179–1236.

Grillner, S., A. McClellan, and C. Perret (1981). Entrainment of the spinal pattern generators for swimming by mechanosensitive elements in the lamprey spinal cord in vitro. *Brain Res.*, **217**:380–386.

Hildebrand, M. (1976). Analysis of tetrapod gaits: General considerations and symmetrical gaits. In *Neural Control of Locomotion*, Herman, R. H., Grillner, S., Stein, P., and Stuart, D., eds. Plenum Press, New York, pp. 203–236.

Holst, E. von (1973). *The Behavioral Physiology of Animals and Man: The Collected Papers of Erick von Holst*, vol. 1. University of Miami Press, Coral Gables.

Homma, S. and C. M. Rovainen (1978). Conductance increases produced by glycine and aminobutyric acid in lamprey interneurons. *J. Physiol. (Lond.)*, **279**:231–252.

Jacobson, R. D. and M. Hollyday (1982). Electrically evoked walking and fictive locomotion in the chick. *J. Neurophysiol.*, **48**:257–270.

Jones, A. and B. Smith (1973). Regulation of function. *J. Neurophysiol.* **27**:229–289.

Kahn, J. A. and A. Roberts (1982). Experiments on the central pattern generator for swimming in embryos of the amphibian *Xenopus laevis*, *Phil. Trans. Roy. Soc. London, Ser. B*, **296**:229–243.

Kammer, A. E. (1968). Motor patterns during flight and warm-up in Lepidoptera, *J. Exp. Biol.* **48**:89–109.

Keith, W. L. and R. H. Rand (1984). 1:1 and 2:1 phase entrainment in a system of two coupled limit cycle oscillators, *J. Math Biology,* **20**:133–152.

Kulagin, A. S. and M. L. Shik (1970). Interaction of symmetrical limbs during controlled locomotion *Biofizika*, **15**:164–170 (Engl. transl. 171–178).

Mehler, W. R. (1960). More nonsense. In *The Book*, D. Purpura and Y. Yahr, eds. Press, New York, pp. 101–110.

Neu, J. C. (1979). Coupled chemical oscillators, *SIAM J. Appl. Math*, **37**:307–315.

Neu, J. C. (1980). Large populations of coupled chemical oscillators, *SIAM J. Appl. Math.*, **38**:189–208.

Pavlidis, T. (1973). *Biological Oscillators: Their Mathematical Analysis*, Academic Press, New York.

Rand, R. H. and P. J. Holmes (1980). Bifurcation of periodic motions in two weakly coupled van der Pol oscillators *Int. J. Nonlinear Mechanics*, **15**:387–399.

Rand, R. H., D. W. Storti, S. K. Upadhyaya, and J. R. Cooke (1982). Dynamics of coupled stomatal oscillators, *J. Math. Biology,* **15**:131–149.

Rinzel, J., Bursting oscillations in an excitable membrane model. In *Proc. 8th Dundee Conf. on the Theory of Ordinary and Partial Differential Equations*, B. D. Sleeman, R. J. Jarvis, and D. S. Jones, eds. Springer Verlag, to appear.

Rovainen, C. M. (1985). Effects of propriospinal interneurons on fictive swimming in lamprey. *J. Neurophysiol.*, **54**:959–977.

Stein, P. S. G. (1978). Swimming movements elicited by electrical stimulation of the turtle spinal cord: the high spinal preparation. *J. Comp. Physiol.*, **124**:203–210.

Viala, D. and C. Vidal (1978). Evidence for distinct spinal locomotion generators supplying respectively fore- and hind-limbs in the rabbit. *Brain Res.*, **155**:182–186.

Winfree, A. T. (1980). *The Geometry of Biological Time.* Springer-Verlag, New York.

Young, R. E., J. L. Wilkens, and C. Dodd (1980). Pharmacological dissection of a neural pattern generator. *J. Comp. Physiol.*, **139**:1–10.

Chapter Ten

TOWARD A THEORY OF MODELLING CENTRAL PATTERN GENERATORS

NANCY KOPELL

Department of Mathematics
Boston University
Boston, Massachusetts

1 INTRODUCTION

Central pattern generators (CPGs) are believed to involve collections of oscillators, often large in number. The oscillators are usually not understood in detail, and the coupling among them and between them and controlling elements is even less specified. Indeed, if a given oscillatory system consists of many interacting parts, this information will probably never be available, or it may vary in detail from one individual to another within a species.

In such a situation, one might ask if mathematical modelling is premature, or even impossible (Selverston, 1980). This may be true for some questions, but for those involving the behavior of the entire system, the situation is quite hopeful. Indeed, much of the behavior of oscillators, when forced or coupled to other systems, is relatively insensitive to the detailed description of the oscillators or the coupling. The main aim of this chapter is to discuss such behavior, and relate it to CPGs. A more am-

bitious aim is to point toward a mathematical theory of collections of oscillators and "almost oscillators" designed to interpret available and
potentially available data. This theory is qualitative, deducing qualitative
but detailed—and not necessarily intuitively clear—conclusions from robust qualitative hypotheses.

This approach is related to that of Cohen et al. (1982) and Rand et al.
(Chapt. 9). The latter, however, choose particular simple models which
display certain behavior, and which are easy to analyze completely. By
contrast, we shall be more concerned with large classes of models, within
which one may expect to find behavior such as entrainment. The goal is to
sort out those phenomena that are expectable on general mathematical
grounds from those due to extra biological structure, which then require
further investigation. (See e.g., Section 2.2.)

In this theory, it will make no difference whether the neural unit is a
single cell with a biochemical oscillation or a network of cells, none or only
some of which oscillates endogenously. Rather, from phenomenological
properties of the oscillator units, we predict the behavior of those units
when they are forced or coupled to other units. Note that what is considered a "unit" depends on the problem considered. If the problem involves
a change of gait, the unit could be an entire limb. If, however, the question
concerns the roles of different cells of a pacemaker (e.g., the AB and PD
cells of the lobster pyloric pacemaker (Eisen and Marder, 1984), then the
units must be the individual cells.

The chapter is structured so that its main conclusions can be accessible
to those who do not wish to follow all the mathematical reasoning. The
mathematical points have been isolated into some subsections; their applications to particular examples are done in other subsections whose main
point is scientific, rather than mathematical. The reader is invited to
browse first through Section 6 and Section 4.3, which present examples of
biological phenomena that are clarified by the methods developed here.
Sections 3.1.3 and 3.1.4 describe some of the differences between the approach used here and that used by Rand et al. in Chapter 9. Sections labelled "Example: . . . ." illustrate how the math can be used.

Section 1 orients the reader to the kinds of mathematical hypotheses
being made in the chapter, and the reasons for the choices. Sections 2, 3,
and 4 develop, with examples from the CPG literature, a mathematical
theory that is applicable in some situations in which the more usual phase
response curve (PRC) analysis is inappropriate or awkward. This theory,
which is only a primitive beginning, is by no means universally applicable;
but even at this stage, it expands considerably the available arsenal of
mathematical tools for thinking about CPG phenomena. The more technical parts of Section 2, and applications of those parts, are discussed in a
sequence of Appendices (A1–A4). Section 5 hints at a more general theory
that could include non-oscillating elements as well. Section 6 discusses the
philosophy of modelling that is implicit in the chapter. The conclusions of

the mathematics become progressively less intuitively clear in successive sections. The full strength of the "APD theory" is used in the section on linear arrays of oscillators, which relies on relatively deep mathematics. Nevertheless, the case study (section 4.3) that this is intended to illuminate can be read without (most of) the mathematics.

1.1 Equations with Limit Cycles

The systems we describe have variables that change continuously in time, with the rate of change dependent on the state of the system, so they can be modelled by ordinary differential equations

$$\dot{X} = F(X). \tag{1.1}$$

Here t is time and X is a vector whose components may represent any variables (mechanical, electrical, chemical). For CPGs, the variables need not be localized in the spinal cord or even the nervous system, but may include quantities partially determined by descending control or by afferent feedback. (See Sections 3.2.2 and 3.2.3 for examples in which such considerations are included.) Thus, the theory is compatible with the spirit advocated by some (Grillner, 1975; Rossignol et al, Chapt. 7), in which there is no longer a complete dichotomy between *central* pattern generators and reflex chains, and the purely spinal rhythmic activity can be investigated in its larger context.

Most of the systems will also have the property that the variables oscillate regularly in time. Then (1.1) is required to have a periodic solution. The systems must also be stable under perturbation of initial conditions and of parameters as are biological systems. (See Hirsch and Smale, 1974, for further discussion of stability.) Linear systems do not have this stability property. If a linear equation has a periodic solution, a change in initial condition can change the amplitude of the periodic solution. More importantly, a small change in parameters can eliminate all periodic solutions. Because of this instability, we shall discuss only nonlinear equations. We shall be interested in equations which have a "stable limit-cycle solution," that is, a periodic solution with the property that all solutions with nearby initial conditions tend, as t increases, toward the limit cycle (Hirsch and Smale, 1974). Not all nonlinear equations with periodic solutions have limit cycles; many oscillators from nonlinear mechanics, such as the equation of the undamped pendulum, do not.

One important feature shared by limit cycle oscillators is that coordinates can be chosen in a region around the limit cycle so as to greatly simplify the analysis. The most important coordinate is "phase," or angular change around the limit cycle; the others measure distance to the limit cycle. The coordinates can be assigned so that, on the limit cycle, the phase changes uniformly in time; off the limit cycle, two points are assigned the same phase if, as time increases, the distance between the trajectories (i.e., solutions) through those points decreases exponentially. A curve of points having the same phase is sometimes called an "isochron" (Winfree, 1980; Guckenheimer, 1975).

1.2   A Digression on Limits and Computability

The word "limit" will be used often and requires some explanation (it does *not* mean the same as the "limit" of "limit cycle"). The motivation is similar to that of studying the most primitive kind of biological structure: catch some phenomenon as it emerges, before other complicating, and possibly irrelevant, factors intrude. By "limits" or "limiting cases," we shall mean that some quantity is infinitely large or infinitely small; this leads to a simplification of the description, which may allow the use of analytic tools not otherwise available. Even more importantly, the analysis can then usually be extended to apply when such a quantity is merely "small enough," or "large enough." Indeed, investigation of limiting cases often provides a reliable guide to intuition quite far from the limits, where the detailed analysis is considerably more difficult.

In the case of nonlinear oscillators, there are many such limits one could study, and different limits may be relevant in different situations. One case familiar to biologists is the limit in which the decay of a perturbation from the limit cycle is instantaneous, i.e., the transient time is "infinitely small". Such a limiting case is essentially assumed in the calculation of phase response curves (PRCs), which measure the eventual change in phase of an oscillator due to an instantaneous pulse perturbation. PRCs tend to work well provided the decay is "fast enough"; in practice, this means the transient is no longer noticeable after one cycle. PRCs will be discussed in section 2.1. and Appendix 1.

Another familiar and important case close to a limit is that of "relaxation oscillators." For such classes of oscillators, parts of the limit cycle are almost instantaneous. One famous example is the van der Pol oscillator. Oscillations with at least two distinct time scales in the limit cycle are common among biological oscillators (Berridge and Rapp, 1979), making the relaxation limit an important one. Oscillations close to the relaxation limit have a very useful property: since part of the cycle is extremely fast, the period of the oscillation is determined by the slower segments. It is easy to change the frequency of such an oscillator by alterations in the equations which extend or shorten the slow segment. Because of this, for such oscillators, increasing amplitude is usually associated with decreasing frequency. Some models of biological oscillators, such as the "integrate and fire" model (Glass and Mackey, 1979), are relaxation oscillators in the limit.

In some situations involving a kind of limit, the behavior of a complicated set of equations can be understood from a simpler set obtained by averaging the effects of the coupling over each cycle of the oscillator. When such averaging is valid, the coupling in the resulting equations turns out to depend only on the difference of the phases of the oscillators, not on the phases themselves. At first glance, it is counter-intuitive to use such equations in a physiological setting, since coupling signals among cells often occur during only part of the cycle of the signalling cell, and a signal may create a reaction only if the reacting cell is in an appropriate part of its own cycle. Nevertheless, the phaselocking behavior of the full system may, under some circumstances, be completely determined by the averaged system, which is far easier to analyze (see 2.1 for a definition of phaselocking). That is, even though the signals come at varied times in the cycle, and their effects are not dependent only on phase differences, the locking behavior can be predicted by analyzing the averaged effects of the coupling signals.

One such circumstance is when the coupling among the oscillators is "weak enough." As in the other cases of limits discussed above, the mathematical statements can often be *proved* only close to the limit (i.e., very small coupling). However, the conclusions can be expected to hold quite far from the limit. Indeed, recent numerical simulations by G. B. Ermentrout (pers. comm.) show that the locking behavior of a pair of coupled oscillators, each of which emits a coupling signal at only one point in a cycle, is surprisingly close to that of the averaged equations, even for moderately strong coupling.

Whenever a description involving limits is used, the question arises as to how far from the limit the description is valid. How instantaneous must a transient be to use PRC analysis? How weak is "weak coupling"? This question is indeed a serious one, and it has no complete answers. For particular equations it can be answered, but the point of the theory is to get answers in the absence of such complete knowledge. One can make reasonable guesses: "weak coupling" will not suffice to induce phaselocking in oscillators whose frequencies are 100% apart. However, if the differences are 20% to 30% apart, phaselocking is observed, and it takes more than one cycle to reach the steady oscillation from some initial conditions, then the techniques are probably applicable. An important point to recognize is that this question is as serious for PRC analysis as it is for "weak coupling."

There are other settings, involving strong coupling, in which it may be valid to use averaging. One, presently under investigation, is when each of the interacting oscillators has many components which emit coupling signals at different times in the cycle, as in leech (Friesen et al., 1978). Another setting, discussed in Section 4.3.4, involves strong coupling made up of many weak ties.

We shall refer to the equations obtained by averaging as the *averaged phase difference* (APD) equations, and the body of conclusions that can be drawn from them as "APD theory." This choice of simplification is in the tradition of the ideas of von Holst (1939); the study of systems of oscillators is reduced to an investigation of the interactions of their phases, as in von Holst's "magnetic effects." However, these interactions are not obvious without the mathematics, and the theory to be presented provides a grounding for some of his (and later) observations, as well as conclusions that can guide further observations.

2.   FORCED OSCILLATORS

The simplest interaction between two oscillators is that of one oscillator forced by another. Many of the early references in the biological literature to the mathematics of forced oscillators concern the implications of PRC data for periodic forcing. In section 2.1, we look at the strengths and weaknesses of that approach and propose an alternative applicable to CPGs in some circumstances when PRCs are not appropriate to use.

2.1   APD Theory for Forced Oscillators

Two oscillators that are coupled, either one way (i.e., forced) or mutually, are said to be 1:1 phaselocked if they oscillate at the same frequency, with a fixed phase difference between them. It has been much noted (Winfree, 1980; Perkel et al., 1964; Pittendrigh and Minis, 1964) that information about such phaselocking can be derived from PRC data. In particular, the theory addresses the question of whether, if a perturbing pulse is given periodically, the forced oscillator will have a periodic response of the same period. A brief review of PRC theory is given in Appendix 1.

This is a good theory when the transients decay quickly and the perturbations are impulses. Such hypotheses hold well for some circadian rhythms, with the perturbations given by light pulses, or for a very strong membrane oscillator perturbed by an action potential. However, there are many instances relevant to CPGs in which this formalism is inappropriate. For example, if the connection between the forced and forcing oscillators is via interneurons which operate in a continuous and graded way (Pearson and Fourtner, 1975), and/or the transients do not damp within one cycle (Stein, 1976), the situation is not well described by PRCs. Moreover, for some spiking cells, even when hyperpolarized, neurotransmitter release can be graded and sensitively dependent on membrane potential, (Marder and Eisen, 1984; Graubard et al., 1983); hence, even if the interneurons are spiking, their effect on the forced cells may not be impulse-like. Similarly, if the connections between two oscillator units are complex, and the output signals are at different times in the cycle (Friesen et al., 1978), the total effect of one unit on another may be closer to being continuous than impulse-like.

We develop here another formalism better suited to describing such interactions. This formalism, unlike PRCs, will also enable us to handle pairs of oscillators coupled mutually, as well as large collections of coupled oscillators. As in the PRC theory, something must be assumed in order to make the mathematics tractable; we shall assume that we are in a range where averaging methods are valid, for example, the situation of "weak" coupling. As described above, in practice this covers quite a range of effective coupling strengths.

The general equation for a forced oscillator is

$$\dot{X} = F(X) + g(t) \tag{2.1}$$

where (1.1) has a limit cycle with period σ, and $g(t)$ has period τ. If the limit cycle of (1.1) is fairly strongly attracting, and $g(t)$ is not extremely large, then it is possible to reduce the study of (2.1) to the study of how the phase of (1.1) is perturbed by the forcing (Chow and Hale, 1982). (This does not require very weak forcing, and for given equations (1.1), the phrase "not extremely large" can be made precise. However, that is quite technical.) The effect of the forcing is then averaged over a cycle of the forcing function to get the APD equations. These averaged equations have the form

$$\dot{\theta} = \omega + H(\theta_0 - \theta) \tag{2.2a}$$
$$\dot{\theta}_0 = \omega_0 \tag{2.2b}$$

where θ and θ_0 are the phases of the forced and forcing oscillators, and $\omega = 1/\sigma$, $\omega_0 = 1/\tau$. H is a scalar (i.e., real-valued) function that is periodic (with period one); if equation (1.1) is known explicitly, then H can also be computed explicitly. For example, if (1.1) is given by a commonly used simple nonlinear model (Kopell and Howard, 1973), and $g(t)$ is the limit cycle of this equation, then H has the form $H(\phi) = A \sin 2\pi\phi + B \cos 2\pi\phi$ (see Ermentrout and Kopell, 1984). In general, H depends on (1.1) in a region around the limit cycle, not just on the limit cycle; indeed, the phase-locking behavior of (2.1) can be changed by altering F without changing the limit cycle solution, i.e., the phaselocking behavior depends on the transients as well as the limit cycle and, in particular, is affected by the shape of the isochrons (St. Vincent, 1987). Also, unlike a PRC curve, H depends on the frequency of the forcing as well as on the forced oscillator.

Equations (2.2) are not equivalent to the full ones (2.1); however, in some circumstances, such as weak enough coupling (Guckenheimer and Holmes, 1983), it can be proved that conclusions derived from (2.2) about phaselocking also hold for (2.1). Even if the forcing is not weak, if the oscillation is forced by a single pulse per cycle, and the PRC is the usual "type 1" (Winfree, 1980), the conclusions from APD analysis are similar to those from PRC analysis for 1:1 locking, though APD theory predicts *stable* locking in a larger range. The validity of APD theory for other kinds of strong forcing is under investigation.

The function H plays the same role in the APD theory that PRCs play in the above theory of periodically forced oscillators. That is, experiments can be done which *directly* give the information about H needed to make conclusions about phaselocking, independent of (probably unobtainable) information about the complete equations (1.1) and the forcing.

The use of APD theory to handle the same questions as PRC theory is illustrated in Appendix 2, and the ideas are applied there to observations about spinal dogfish. It is not easy to measure H directly. There is, however, a related function called a Poincaré map that is as easy to measure as a PRC, and which contains the essential information. This is discussed in Appendix 3, along with an application to the crayfish swimmeret system. Appendix 4 is devoted to the more subtle phenomenon of relative coordination from the point of view of APD theory and an application to some results of Perkel et al. (1964).

If the forcing is weak, APD theory can also be used to deduce the behavior of the amplitude and wave form of the oscillation. In this case, the phase equations are independent of the amplitude, so it is possible to solve for their behavior alone, as we have done. By contrast, the amplitude is "slaved" to the phase, i.e., the solution for the phase $\theta(t)$ determines the entire solution $X(t)$ to (2.1) (Neu, 1979; Rand and Holmes, 1980). In particular, if the forcing frequency is considerably higher or lower than the natural frequency, the amplitude will be modulated at the forcing frequency, but the details of the modulation will vary with the system. APD methods can sometimes also be used to get information about amplitudes when the forcing is large (Aronson et al., 1987).

2.2 Example (Dogfish): Mathematics and Physiological Mechanisms

We focus here on the findings of Grillner and Wallén on mechanical forcing of fictive swimming in dogfish, in particular, data concerning incomplete entrainment. (See Grillner and Wallén, 1982, Figs. 8A–C.) Our goal will be to assess the implications of the findings for physiological mechanisms. The forcing was done by moving the tail of the dogfish at various frequencies and amplitudes.

For weak forcing (14° of movement) at forcing frequencies somewhat less than one-third of the natural (rest) frequency, the ventral root activity is modulated by, but not phaselocked to, the slow sinusoidal forcing. The data suggest drift, as expected for parameter values near the interval of 3:1 locking. (See Appendix 4). For larger forcing, (Figs. 8B and 8C of Grillner and Wallén, 1982), APD theory is probably not relevant, but the behavior for quite large forcing (60°) is consistent with known behavior of nonlinear oscillators (see Section 2.3); the intermediate forcing case has been less investigated.

Two plausible physiological mechanisms are suggested by the authors to explain these data. They involve action on the segmental pattern generator as a functional unit or, alternatively, on just a part of the CPG network such as some premotor interneurons. The authors tentatively favor the second, on the grounds that the incomplete entrainment for weak forcing could be interpreted as competing interactions between the directly entrained part of the CPG network and the rest of the network. Similarly, they suggest that the reduction in amplitude at very high frequency and larger amplitude forcing may indicate that only part of the network is entrained.

As seen in Appendix 4, however, the incomplete modulation of the amplitude and entrainment of the phases is consistent with the theory of a single weakly forced oscillator. APD theory cannot in general address larger forcing, but there are simple examples in which the amplitude of the response decreases as the forcing frequency becomes further from the natural frequency (Aronson, et al., 1987). (To get 1:1 locking, this requires larger and larger forcing.) Thus, the mathematics cannot prove, but is consistent with, the hypothesis that the sensory input acts directly on the segmental oscillators. One need not posit that the effects of the weaker input are via entrainment of some subset of the CPG.

2.3 More Complicated Behavior of Forced Oscillators

The results obtained by studying limiting cases tend to be qualitatively correct even at some distance from the limits involved, but sufficiently far from the limiting cases, other phenomena can occur. If the forcing is large, there may be 1:1 locking for very large differences between the rates of the unforced oscillator and the forcing term (Hoppensteadt and Keener, 1982; St. Vincent, 1987; Levi, 1981) as was seen by Grillner and Wallén with forcing frequencies 3 or 6 times the natural frequency. There may even be new types of behavior. For example, an oscillator such as the van der Pol oscillator can have multiple stable periodic responses and very complex aperiodic solutions for the same forcing term (Cartwright and Littlewood, 1945; Levi, 1981). This "chaotic" behavior appears to be associated with medium strong forcing, as opposed to "weak" or "very strong." Even when there is such complicated behavior, analysis in terms of phase can still be useful. (Guevara and Glass, 1982; Levi, 1981).

3. PAIRS OF COUPLED OSCILLATORS

PRC theory predicts the response of one oscillator to another, provided that there is no other disturbing influence. Two coupled oscillators, however, perturb each other in ways undetermined until the dynamics is worked out. This makes PRC theory an awkward way to handle mutually coupled oscillators. By contrast, APD theory is easily extendable to a pair of coupled oscillators, and even to large collections of them (see Section 4.) We first discuss the important case of *two* coupled oscillators, which has some special properties not shared by greater numbers of coupled oscillators. (See also Ermentrout, 1981; Rand and Holmes, 1980; Neu, 1979.)

3.1   1:1 Phaselocking

3.1.1   The APD Equations

The general equations of a pair of coupled oscillators is

$$\dot{X}_1 = F_1(X_1) + G_1(X_1, X_2)$$
$$\dot{X}_2 = F_2(X_2) + G_2(X_2, X_1).$$
(3.1)

Here, X_1 and X_2 are vectors of variables of any dimensions (not necessarily the same). We assume, as usual, that $\dot{X}_i = F_i(X_i)$ has a limit cycle oscillation for $i = 1, 2$. As in the case of a single forced oscillator, if the coupling is not extremely strong, the high dimensional set of equations (3.1) can be reduced to equations describing the interactions of two phases θ_1 and θ_2. After those equations are averaged, the resulting equations have the form

$$\dot{\theta}_1 = \omega_1 + H_1(\theta_2 - \theta_1)$$
(3.2a)

$$\dot{\theta}_2 = \omega_2 + H_2(\theta_1 - \theta_2)$$
(3.2b)

(Ermentrout and Rinzel, 1984). ω_1 and ω_2 are the natural frequencies of the two oscillators. The functions H_1 and H_2 can be determined mathematically as before, and again are periodic with period 1. As before, the averaged equations are not equivalent to the full equations (3.1), but in some circumstances contain all the relevant information about phaselocking. One such circumstance is again that of weak coupling. In that case, the H_i can be computed separately: H_1 is found by forcing the oscillator X_1 with the limit cycle of X_2, and similarly for H_2. It is currently being investigated under what circumstances (3.2) may by used when the coupling is not weak (see Section 1.2).

As will be seen below, the analysis of (3.2) is far easier than that of two oscillators coupled by PRCs. One reason is that the PRC formulation gives the phase just before a pulse in terms of the phase before the previous pulse, the delay function and the time between pulses. However, unless the delay function $\Delta(\sigma\theta)$ is "small"—in which case the PRC theory is a special case of APD theory—the timing of a pulse from either oscillator is not known a priori. By contrast, because the APD equations are derived by averaging over a cycle, in APD theory, the analysis doesn't require a priori information about the time at which a particular phase is reached.

3.1.2 Analysis and Implications

We shall first look for 1:1 phaselocking. The mathematics is very similar to the special case of forced oscillators in which G_2, and hence H_2, is identically zero. However, there are some interesting new observations that can be read off the analysis. As in Appendix 2, we let $\phi = \theta_2 - \theta_1$ be the phase difference. The full equations can display phaselocking even if $\theta_2 - \theta_1$ is not constant; however, in the averaged equations, which can be an accurate predictor of phaselocking, 1:1 locking is equivalent to having a constant phase difference. The equation for ϕ is

$$\dot{\phi} = [\delta + H_2(-\phi) - H_1(\phi)] \tag{3.3}$$

where $\omega_2 - \omega_1 = \delta \geq 0$. There is a solution in which the two oscillators have the same frequency, with constant phase difference ϕ, if

$$0 = \delta + H_2(-\phi) - H_1(\phi) \tag{3.4}$$

can be solved for ϕ. This solution is stable if

$$\frac{d}{d\phi}[H_2(-\phi) - H_1(\phi)] < 0. \tag{3.5}$$

To see what this implies, consider the special case of two identical oscillators coupled the same in both directions. (This is called *isotropic* coupling.) Thus $F_1 = F_2$ and $G_1 = G_2$, so $H_1 = H_2 = H$. In that case, (3.4) can be simplified by decomposing H into its odd and even parts $H(\phi) = He(\phi) + Ho(\phi)$. (An even function $He(\phi)$ such as $\cos 2\pi\phi$ satisfies $He(-\phi) = He(\phi)$; an odd function such as $\sin 2\pi\phi$ satisfies $Ho(-\phi) = -Ho(\phi)$. Any function can be so decomposed.) Using this decomposition, (3.4) and (3.5) become

$$0 = -2Ho(\phi) \tag{3.6}$$

$$Ho'(\phi) > 0. \tag{3.7}$$

For any Ho periodic and odd, $\phi = 0$ (inphase) and $\phi = 1/2$ (antiphase) are solutions to (3.6); if these are the only two, then one is stable and one is unstable. (For complicated F, (3.6) may also be satisfied by other ϕ.) From (3.6), (3.7), we see that Ho alone determines at what phase the oscillators stably phaselock. However, the *frequency* at which the oscillators run when coupled depends on the function He as well as Ho. Indeed, from (3.2a), if the oscillators run stably inphase ($\phi = 0$, $Ho'(0) > 0$), then the frequency is

$$\dot{\theta}_1 = \omega + H(0) = \omega + He(0) \tag{3.8}$$

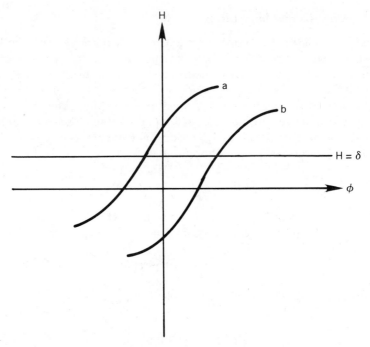

FIGURE 1. Plot of h vs. ϕ for two different functions H. If $H'(\phi) > 0$ near $\phi = 0$ and $H(0) > 0$ then, for $\sigma = 0$, the solution to (2.5) is < 0; if $H(0) < 0$, the solution is > 0. Thus, the sign of $H(0)$ determines whether there is a phase lag or lead. For either function, the solution to (2.5) is an increasing function of σ, so a larger difference in frequency between the forced and forcing oscillators leads to a later response for the forced oscillator.

where $\omega = \omega_1 = \omega_2$, and $He(0) = H(0)$ since $Ho(0) = 0$. (Every odd function vanishes at 0.) Thus, depending on the sign of $He(0)$, the frequency of the coupled system may be higher or lower than that of the uncoupled oscillators. The fact that the frequency of the coupled system is not necessarily the same as the uncoupled frequency depends on the coupling being more general than the "diffusive" coupling assumed by Cohen et al. (1982; Rand et al., Chapt. 9; see Section 3.1.3). Two similar oscillators can drive each other to go faster, yet still maintain synchrony at a finite frequency. *A change in coupling alone, without change in the oscillators, can change the frequency by changing He.*

The APD theory makes predictions about how two mutually and weakly coupled equal oscillators behave if the output of a related unilaterally forced system is known. Specifically, suppose that in a unilaterally forced system given by (2.2) with $\omega = \omega_0$, the forced oscillator lags (i.e., $\phi > 0$ in (A2.2) with $\delta = 0$). Suppose that $H'(\phi) > 0$ in an interval that includes the solution to (A2.2) and $\phi = 0$. $H'(\phi) > 0$ implies that the graph of $H(\phi)$ increases from left to right, so that if $H(\phi) = 0$ (i.e., ϕ solves (A2.2), with $\delta = 0$) for $\phi > 0$, then $H(0) < 0$. (see Fig. 1). As seen above, $H'(0) > 0$ implies that, for two mutually coupled oscillators, the inphase solution is stable. Also $H(0) < 0$ implies that this solution has a frequency below that of the natural frequencies. *This shows that, if in the forced system, the forced oscillator lags, then the mutually coupled system slows down. Conversely, if the forced oscillator leads, then the pair speeds up when mutually coupled.*

A similar analysis shows that if the oscillators are not equal, the frequency of the mutually coupled pair need not lie between the two natural frequencies. If it does, this frequency need not be the average, the highest or the lowest of the natural frequencies. The details for any given system must be worked out, but the general theory points out the diversity of the possible behavior.

3.1.3 Diffusive Versus Synaptic Coupling

We pause to make explicit a distinction we have been using implicitly, and which will be a key idea in analyzing large collections of oscillators. The distinction is between coupling that is *diffusive*, as used in Cohen et al., (1982) and in Rand et al., (Chapter 9), and coupling that is "synaptic." By diffusive coupling we mean coupling in which the functions G_i of (3.1) satisfy $G_i = 0$ whenever $X_1 = X_2$, i.e., the oscillators do not affect one another if their state variables are all equal. This coupling term is an appropriate mathematical description of chemical (or electrical) diffusion across a permeable boundary or electrotonic coupling of nerve cells. It is not appropriate for coupling via chemical synapses, in which the effect of one oscillator on another need not vanish when the oscillators are in the same state. For "synaptic" coupling, to be defined below, there is interaction even for synchronous oscillators. We define this coupling in terms of the averaged interactions.

In the averaged equations, for *any* G_i, the functions H_1 and H_2 depend on only the differences of the phases (Ermentrout and Rinzel, 1984). If the G_i are of the special diffusive type, then the H_i have the extra property that $H_i(0) = 0$. By synaptic coupling we shall mean that $H_i(0) \neq 0$, i.e., the averaged interaction does not vanish for synchronous oscillators. A diffusively coupled system of two equal oscillators has an oscillatory solution whose frequency is the common natural one; for synaptic coupling, we have seen that this is not necessarily true. For another important implication of this distinction, see section 4.2.2. Note that our use of the word "synaptic" includes ordinary chemical synaptic coupling between two cells, but is also applicable to coupling between larger groups of neurons, and includes coupling between cells that is partly due to synapses and partly electrotonic. (See Kawato and Suzuki (1980), a model which uses coupling that is "synaptic" in the above sense.)

3.1.4   Excitation, Inhibition, and APD Theory

A fundamental distinction often made when the oscillators involve changes in transmembrane potential is between excitatory (depolarizing) and inhibitory (hyperpolarizing) coupling. Excitatory forcing is generally thought to be synchronizing, and inhibitory connections are implicated in producing antiphase behavior of coupled oscillators (see Grillner, 1981, for some references). In APD theory, there is also an important distinction when $H_1 = H_2$ between $H'(\phi) > 0$ and $H'(\phi) < 0$ for ϕ near zero. This sign determines if the synchronous solution ($\phi = 0$) is stable; if not, the system might be stable in antiphase.

Theoretically, it is not clear a priori that all models with excitatory coupling between equal oscillators should lead to stable inphase solutions ($H'(0) > 0$), and all models with inhibitory connections should lead to stable antiphase solutions ($H'(0) < 0$, but $H'(.5) > 0$). (This is implicitly assumed in Rand et al., (Chapt. 9) when they label coupling functions $H(\phi)$ satisfying $H'(0) > 0$ as "excitatory.") However, G. B. Ermentrout (pers. comm.) has shown that for simple models of weak enough excitatory and inhibitory connections, excitatory coupling *does* lead to stable inphase solutions and inhibitory connections to stable antiphase behavior. It remains to do the mathematical work of understanding how general is this principle. It should be noted that even for models involving excitatory coupling, $H(0)$ can take either sign. This implies that two oscillators, coupled in an excitatory way, can slow down from their natural frequencies when coupled. It may be that physiological oscillators have extra properties so that they always speed up with excitatory input, but this is not well understood.

Although the two distinctions may turn out to be equivalent when they are both applicable, the classification of interactions as excitatory or inhibitory is much more limited than the classification by stability properties of the connections (i.e., connections which lead to inphase or antiphase behavior for a pair of equal coupled oscillators.) An oscillator cell or network may receive both inhibitory and excitatory pulses (e.g., Getting, 1983); also, the cells need not interact only via pulses. Furthermore, even a single pulse may not be easily classifiable as excitatory or inhibitory (e.g., if a transmitter has a more complex effect on the postsynaptic cell than the production of an IPSP or EPSP). Finally, a network with crossed inhibitory connections can be equivalent to a simpler one with excitatory interactions (Rand et al., Chapt. 9). What is critical is the net coordinating effect of all the interactions. Thus we suggest that the distinction between "synchronizing connections" (i.e., $H'(0) > 0$) and "desynchronizing connections" (i.e., $H'(0) < 0$) may be more fundamental than the one between excitatory and inhibitory connections. The use of the word "desynchronizing" for $H'(0) < 0$ is motivated partly by models involving large collections of oscillators in which the phases of the oscillators appear to disperse as widely as possible (Winfree, 1967). For two oscillators, "as widely as possible" is antiphase.

3.2 j:k Phaselocking in Coupled Oscillators

3.2.1 Generalities

As in the case of forced oscillators, two mutually (and weakly) coupled oscillators (not necessarily equally coupled) can be expected to phaselock if the ratio ω_1/ω_2 of their natural (uncoupled) frequencies is a rational number j/k with j, k small (such as 2 or 1/2). As before, this implies that for the coupled oscillators, the pair then stays phaselocked even if the natural frequencies are varied somewhat. This follows as in Appendix 4 from the theory of circle maps. For details of how the circle map (again called a Poincaré map) is defined from (3.1) or (3.2), see Guckenheimer and Holmes (1983). Some examples of $j:k$ phaselocking in mutually coupled biological oscillators are given below; for others, see Stein (1976).

3.2.2 Example: "Phasic Forcing" and Split Belt Experiments

There are many biological examples of 2:1 locking of rhythms (for some examples in circadian rhythms, see Winfree, 1980). In the context of CPGs, one of the more interesting examples concerns split belt experiments in cat locomotion (Kulagin and Shik, 1970). Kulagin and Shik investigated the effects of placing the contralateral limbs on treadmills going at different speeds. They found that at nearby treadmill speeds, the preparation compensated (by changes in the duration of the stance phase) for the treadmill differences, and the limbs moved at the same frequency. For sufficiently large differences in treadmill speed, (i.e., one speed four to six times the other) the limbs moved at different frequencies, one twice that of the other.

To understand the relation between this effect and the above mathematics, we make another distinction, between *temporal* forcing and *phasic* forcing. By temporal forcing, we mean periodic influences on the system which depend explicitly on time, and which may be independent of the state of the system. (The effects of these influences, of course, are not independent of the state at which they are received.) Such temporal forcing is described by equation (2.1), with $g(t)$ the forcing. By contrast, phasic forcing means an influence that is exerted when the system is in a particular state, independent of what time that state (i.e., set of phases) is reached. An example of this is a swing that is pushed whenever it is at its lowest point. If a system (1.1) is phasically forced, the new mathematical description is not (2.1) but a time independent system of the same dimension as (1.1), i.e., (2.1) with $g(t)$ replaced by $g(X)$.

The effect of the treadmill is mathematically akin to pushing a swing; it provides phasic forcing (during the phases corresponding to the stance state). Thus, if we consider each limb to be governed by an oscillator (Grillner, 1975), the effect of the treadmill on the limb is to change the oscillator. Since the frequency of nonlinear oscillators can change under changes of parameters, with different treadmill speeds for the contralateral limbs, the pair of coupled oscillators have different intrinsic speeds. ("Intrinsic" here refers to the system of *oscillator plus phasic forcing*, without interlimb coupling.) By the theory of phaselocking, one expects intervals in the parameter space (the parameter is the ratio of treadmill speeds) for which there is 1:1 or 2:1 locking. Also expected is an in-between, less stable, region corresponding to rotation numbers between 1 and 1/2 (see Appendix 4). This is also observed (Kulagin and Shik, 1970). The fact that it takes such a large ratio of treadmill speeds to get 2:1 locking suggests that it takes a large amount of phasic forcing to double the intrinsic limb frequency (i.e., the limb frequency is not extremely sensitive to changes in parameters). This strong phasic forcing does not rule out the use of APD theory, provided, for example, that the contralateral limbs are not strongly coupled.

The afferent feedback is treated in this conceptualization as having its primary effect on the oscillators, and only at most a minor effect on the coupling. If this is false, one needs a more complicated model (see Rand et al., Chapter 9, for one mathematical possibility).

3.2.3   Example: Tonic Forcing and Locking in Turtle Limbs

Another preparation showing 2:1 locking is the high spinal preparation of the turtle, *Pseudemys scipta elegans* (Stein, 1978). This effect is sometimes elicited by tonic electrical stimulation applied to the dorsolateral funiculus (DLF). In most preparations in which swimming movements could be elicited, Stein found 1:1 coordination between the fore and hind limbs contralateral to the stimulation. However, by appropriate placement of the electrode in the DLF, he could sometimes (in the same preparation) also get 2:1 locking (two cycles of the forelimb for each of the hindlimb). This is understandable in terms of the above theory once it is clear that the relevant system that defines the limb oscillator must include the tonic stimulation from supraspinal structures. Like phasic forcing, tonic excitation can effect the frequency of a nonlinear oscillator by changing the equations. Under normal swimming conditions, this tonic excitation is such that the natural intrinsic frequencies of the fore and hind limb are sufficiently close to achieve 1:1 locking. With abnormally distributed excitation, the uncoupled frequencies of the fore and hind limbs might be much further apart. To confirm this requires a preparation in which one could measure the frequency of each limb in the absence of mutual interference.

3.3   More Complicated Behavior of Coupled Oscillators

Mutually coupled oscillators whose coupling is not very weak or very strong can have the complex behavior discussed in Section 2.3 for the special case of forced oscillators. In addition, they can sometimes exhibit the extinguishing of all rhythm. That is, if two limit cycle oscillations having sufficiently different frequencies are coupled in some range of intermediate strengths of forcing, the coupled systems can display a stable rest point (Bar-Eli, 1984, Aronson et al., 1987). This appears to be related to the decrease in response amplitude that can be seen when one oscillator is forced by another of much higher frequency. Even identical oscillators, when coupled in a way that cannot be averaged, may stop oscillating (Ermentrout and Kopell, 1987); indeed, this is an important motivation for the study of averaged systems, as in APD theory.

4   LINEAR ARRAYS OF OSCILLATORS

We now go to interactions of larger populations of oscillators, arranged in a chain, where the power of the APD formalism is more evident. We shall deal with phenomena that have not been treated with other methods, and find results that are not necessarily intuitive without the mathematics. At the end of this section we apply the results to swimming of fish and development of locomotion. (See also Grasman and Jansen, 1979; Neu, 1980; Winfree 1967.)

4.1   General Assumptions

As in the rest of this chapter, we seek conclusions that are robust consequences of very general hypotheses. Thus, we shall make no assumptions about the oscillators other than requiring that they be limit cycle oscillators, and that all the oscillators be similar though not necessarily identical, in dynamics. For the coupling, we assume that only nearest neighbors have a direct effect on a given oscillator, and that this effect is not too strong. The equations are general enough to provide a flexible framework within which to consider the effects of gradients in frequency, pacemakers, synaptic coupling, differences in strength and timing of rostral vs. caudal coupling, and such experimental interventions as split bath experiments and lesions. Many of the conclusions will be laid out in a future paper, and here we merely give some idea of the framework and a few conclusions. Generalizations of these ideas involving multiple neighbor connections are discussed in Section 4.3.4.

For $N + 1$ oscillators, the full equations are

$$\dot{X}_k = F_k(X_k) + [G_k^+(X_k, X_{k+1}) + G_k^-(X_k, X_{k-1})].$$
$$k = 1, \dots, N+1$$
(4.1)

Here X_k is a vector with any number of variables,

$$\dot{X}_k = F_k(X_k)$$
(4.2)

has a stable limit cycle, and the F_k are all approximately the same. The functions G_k^+ and G_k^- represent respectively the backward and forward effects on oscillator k of its nearest neighbors. G_k^+ and G_k^- are allowed to be different, but not too large. The oscillators at the ends of the chain have only one nearest neighbor, so the corresponding term in (4.1) must be set equal to zero. That is,

$$G_{N+1}^+(X_{N+1}, X_{N+2}) \equiv 0 \equiv G_1^-(X_1, X_0). \tag{4.3}$$

4.1.1 APD Phase Equations

As in the case of two coupled oscillators, one can derive a set of averaged equations for the phase differences. If $\theta_1, \ldots, \theta_{N+1}$ are the phases of the $N+1$ oscillators, and $\phi_k = \theta_{k+1} - \theta_k$ are the phase differences then, after averaging, the ϕ's satisfy equations which depend only on the other phase differences and not on the phases themselves. These equations have the special form

$$\dot{\phi}_k = [\delta_k + H_{k+1}^+(\phi_{k+1}) - H_k^+(\phi_k) + H_{k+1}^-(-\phi_k) - H_k^-(-\phi_{k-1})]. \tag{4.4}$$

Here δ_k is the frequency difference between the $(k+1)$st and kth oscillators, i.e., $\delta_k = \omega_{k+1} - \omega_k$, where ω_k is the frequency of the limit cycle of (4.2). $H_k^\pm$ can be explicitly computed from the F_k and $G_k^\pm$, and are periodic with period 1. From (4.3) we get

$$H_{N+1}^+(\phi_{N+1}) = 0 = H_1^-(-\phi_0) \tag{4.5}$$

As before, at least in the case of weak coupling, the phaselocking behavior of the full equations (4.1) is the same as that of Equations (4.4). Note that equations of the form (4.4) include those used by Rand et al. (Chapt. 9). For a derivation of (4.4), see Ermentrout and Kopell (1984).

4.2 Ensemble Properties

In general, the functions F_k and $G_k^\pm$ are not known in detail. Hence, we continue to connect properties of the solutions to (4.4) to properties of $H_k^\pm$ and the Δ_k's that are more measurable. A crucial concern for CPGs is the generation of appropriate and stable phase relationships among the oscillators. For a phase difference equation such as (4.4), phase relationships fixed in time correspond to critical points or time-independent solutions ($\dot{\phi}_k = 0$, all k). Thus, the mathematical problem is to understand how the properties of $H_k^\pm$ and the δ_k's affect the existence and stability of critical points of (4.4), and the spatial pattern of lags and leads corresponding to the stable critical points. We consider for simplicity the case in which coupling is constant along the cord, i.e., H^+ and H^- are independent of k.

As we will see below, synaptic coupling has essential consequences for the properties of the resulting solutions. For a pair of equal coupled oscillators, we have seen that the *synaptic coupling hypothesis* $H^\pm(0) \neq 0$ implies that the frequency of such a pair of oscillators need not be the same as the uncoupled frequency. The locked solution, however, may be synchronous ($\phi = 0$). For three or more oscillators, the effects of synaptic coupling become even more important. For example, when there are at least three equal oscillators in a chain, and $H^\pm(0) \neq 0$, then the homogeneous in-phase configuration ($\phi_k = 0$, all k) is not a time independent solution to (4.4), (4.5). Instead, the synaptic coupling produces travelling waves of electrical activity. The mechanism may be thought of as a generalization to bidirectional coupling of the kind of analysis used by P. Stein (1976) in describing the metachronal waves in the crayfish swimmeret system.

In Cohen et al. (1982) and Rand et al. (Chapt. 9), a model using diffusive coupling is discussed in which the natural frequencies of the uncoupled oscillators display a rostral to caudal gradient. We shall reexamine the effects of such a gradient in the context of equations (4.4), or equivalently (4.1), in order to make two points. First, if there is a gradient in the natural frequency of the uncoupled oscillators (rostral higher) and $H^+ = H^- = H$, there is always a travelling wave down the chain of oscillators; this is true independent of the choice of $H^\pm$. (In Cohen et al., 1982, and Rand et al., Chapt. 9, $H^\pm(\phi) = \sin 2\pi\phi$.) Secondly, the detailed properties of the wave do depend on some (measurable) properties of $H^\pm$. In general, although the phase lag between any two oscillators is constant over time, it varies down the chain; thus, for the model of Cohen et al., the waves do not have lags independent of position. In Section 4.2.2 we shall discuss mathematical situations which do produce travelling waves with constant speed as in dogfish (Grillner, 1974; Grillner and Kashin, 1976).

4.2.1 *An Associated Partial Differential Equation and an Implication*

The analysis of (4.4) is considerably more difficult than that in Rand et al. (Chapt. 9). Indeed, the advantage of their choice of $H^\pm(\phi) = \sin 2\pi\phi$ is precisely that it allows the explicit calculation of solutions. However, as we shall see, more general (and realistic) coupling functions have some quite different mathematical properties.

Except for very special choices of $H^\pm$, it is difficult to find any of the critical points of (4.4), (4.5). However, if the number of oscillators is sufficiently large, then the time independent behavior of (4.4), (4.5) can be read off from an associated continuum equation. (N need not be very large: in numerical studies, $N = 20$ yielded results very close to those for N extremely large. See Kopell and Ermentrout, 1986a, which also contains rigorous but unfortunately long proofs. A condensed version of the ideas may be found in Kopell, 1986. The more mathematical readers should note that the equation below is derived from different assumptions than, and is not equivalent to, the continuum equation in Rand et al.)

The associated equation has the form

$$0 = -\beta + 2[f(\phi)]_x + \frac{1}{N}[g(\phi)]_{xx}$$

$$H^-(-\phi) = 0 \text{ at } x = 0;$$
$$H^+(\phi) = 0 \quad \text{at } x = 1; \qquad 0 \le x \le 1 \tag{4.6}$$

Here f and g can be computed from H^+ and H^-; if $H^+ = H^-$, then $f = He$ and $g = Ho$. $\delta_k = -\beta/N$; for ease of exposition, we are assuming that δ_k is independent of k, which means that, if there is a gradient in natural frequencies (i.e., $\delta_k \ne 0$), then the gradient is linear. For $\beta > 0$, the frequency is higher at the end where the counting begins, which we identify with the rostral end. A solution $\phi(x)$ to (4.6) corresponds approximately to a critical point $(\phi_1, \phi_2, \ldots, \phi_N)$ of (4.4), (4.5), with ϕ_k approximately equal to $\phi(k/[N + 1])$. We illustrate the solution to (4.6) in Figure 2, for the functions $H^{\pm} = A \sin 2\pi\phi + B \cos 2\pi\phi$, A, B, β, > 0. The solution to (4.4), (4.5), with that H and β, is approximately obtained by making the continuous curve $\phi(x)$ into a dotted curve, i.e., plotting only the points ϕ_k at each $x = k/[N + 1]$.

It is much easier to solve (4.6) than (4.4), (4.5) and from the solutions we can read off many implications. The first concerns travelling waves in the presence of frequency gradients. If $\beta > 0$ and H^+, H^- are nearly the same, the solution $\phi(x)$ satisfies $\phi(x) < 0$ over almost all of the interval, except in a so-called "shock layer," which gets very thin for N large. (See Kopell and Ermentrout, 1986a, for the technical hypotheses. If $H^+ \ne H^-$, both boundary conditions may be on the same side of $\phi = 0$, so there need be no reversal at all.) Recall that ϕ_k represents the phase difference between two successive oscillators, so $\phi_k < 0$ means that the higher numbered oscillator lags behind its lower numbered neighbor. Thus, if there is a frequency gradient in the natural frequencies, with the higher frequency at the rostral end, then there are always travelling waves going rostral to caudal. Furthermore, the size of the phase lags give information about the speed of the wave; the speed at a point along the wave is inversely proportional to the absolute value of ϕ_k. Thus, in Figure 2, the wave speed increases rostral to caudal (at least away from the boundary layer); in the mirror image graph (which is the solution if $B < 0$) it decreases rostral to caudal. In either case, *as long as there is a frequency gradient, the wave speed is never constant. Thus, for those instances of fish swimming* (e.g., in the dogfish; see Grillner, 1974; Grillner and Kashin, 1976) *in which the phase lag is uniform down the cord and thus the wave speed is constant, the existence of a frequency gradient cannot be the primary mechanism for producing the waves.* Also note: when there is a frequency gradient, e.g., rostral to caudal, the phase lags can either increase in size or decrease in size along the cord, depending here on the sign of B; thus, this property could differ among different species. The details of the phase lags also depend on anisotropy in the cou-

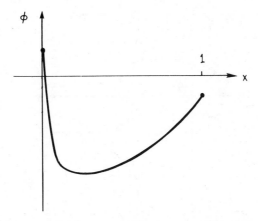

FIGURE 2. The solution to the continuum problem (4.6) for $H^{\pm} = A \sin 2\pi\phi + B \cos 2\pi\phi$, $A, B > 0$, when there is a gradient in natural frequencies (decreasing rostral to caudal). The chain of discrete oscillators has phase differences which approximately fit on this curve, with the x − axis replaced by the k − axis. Since $\phi < 0$ (except very near $x = 0$), the solution corresponds to a rostral to caudal travelling wave. Since ϕ is not independent of k, the wave speed is not constant. In this picture, the wave speed decreases as x (and hence k) increases, except for a small number of oscillators near $k = 0$.

pling and the changes in size and timing of the coupling signals along the cord; this requires analysis of more general equations than (4.6), and will be discussed in a later publication.

4.2.2   Constant Speed Waves and Synaptic Coupling

We now discuss mechanisms that *can* stably produce constant speed waves. These mechanisms do not rely importantly on frequency differences; rather, the "cause" of the waves is the synaptic drive, as in the work of P. Stein (1974), which uses one-way coupling. However, some of the observed phenomena, e.g., in dogfish (Grillner, 1974), are incompatible with one-way coupling.

The important point is that, when the coupling is synaptic, the synchronous configuration ($\phi_k = 0$ for all k, or no phase delays) is not a solution to equation (4.6), and so some phase lags must form. Unless there is some frequency gradient, or anisotropy in the coupling, there is nothing to bias the waves in one direction or another; indeed, the waves then go in both directions, either outward from, or inward to, the center. Figure 3A illustrates the solution for $H^{\pm} = A \sin 2\pi\phi + B \cos 2\pi\phi$, $B > 0$; as before, the picture for the case $H^{\pm}(0) < 0$ (i.e., $B < 0$) is the mirror image. In Figure 3A, $\phi(x)$ is positive and almost constant in the caudal half. This corresponds to a travelling wave moving outward at constant speed from the center. (For the mirror image picture, the solution corresponds to a pair of waves moving inward toward the center.)

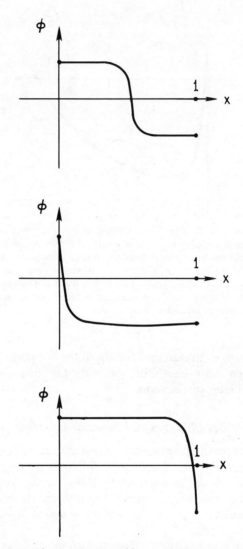

FIGURE 3. The solution to the continuum problem, with $H^{\pm} = A \sin 2\pi\phi + B \cos 2\pi\phi$, A, $B > 0$, when (A) There is no frequency gradient and no anisotrophy in the coupling. Waves travel outward in both directions from the midpoint of the chain of oscillators. (B) There is (i) a tiny frequency gradient (rostral frequency higher) or ii) no frequency gradient, but the backward coupling is stronger than the forward. Waves travel at a constant speed in the caudal direction. (C) There is no frequency gradient and the forward coupling is stronger than the backward. waves travel at constant speed in the rostral direction.

When the coupling is synaptic, the position of the shock layer is very sensitive to changes in both coupling and frequency parameters (cf. Fig. 3B for a tiny $\beta > 0$). This means that if there is a large number of oscillators, the shock layer can be moved anywhere from the middle to the rostral end by a very small rostral to caudal frequency gradient. Even without a frequency gradient, the system can be biased by making the strength or timing of the coupling signals different in the rostral and caudal directions. For example, if H^- is just a multiple of H^+, then for the case $H^{\pm}(0) > 0$, stronger backward coupling leads to solutions as in Figure 3B, corresponding to a wave going rostral to caudal; stronger forward coupling leads to solutions as in Figure 3C, corresponding to a wave going caudal to rostral. To get a solution with the leading segment near the rostral end, the model requires slightly stronger backward coupling. (If instead we have $H^{\pm}(0) < 0$, stronger *forward* coupling has this effect.) With anistropy, there can even be waves in the appropriate rostral to caudal direction in the presence of a small adverse frequency gradient (i.e., frequency higher caudally). P. Stein has noticed this for one-way coupling (Stein, 1974); also see Davis and Kennedy (1972); Pearce and Friesen (1985a,b); and Section 4.3 below.

In general, the model provides a framework for analyzing the possibly competing effects of frequency differences and non-isotropic coupling. The model can also be extended to deal with coupling that depends on position within the chain. It is not within the scope of this chapter to give a full analysis of the implications. However, it can be said that the position of the leading segment is determined by a balance between the anisotropy and the frequency differences. Thus, as mentioned above, even with isotropic coupling, the leading segment can be moved to one end or the other by a small bias in natural frequencies. If there are substantial differences in natural frequency, one would expect the leading segment to be close to the high frequency end.

4.3   A Case Study: Swimming in Fish

4.3.1   Some Phenomena

We now apply the theory described above to swimming of fish; much of the data comes from experiments in intact and spinal dogfish (Grillner, 1974; Grillner and Kashin, 1976), though similar results have been found in other species. Measurements of EMG or ventral root recordings from segments along the body show periodic bursts of activity all at the same frequency (Grillner, 1974; Grillner and Wallén, 1982). The two muscles or ventral roots of a single segment are usually 180° out of phase. There is a phase difference between the bursts of activity of one segment and that of its rostral or caudal neighbor. This phase difference is thought to be independent of position along the body of the fish and is constant over changes in swimming speed (Grillner and Kashin, 1976). In spinal swimming, the leading segment need not be at the head of the fish; it can be somewhere in the most rostral third and appears to be sensitive to small changes even during a given experiment (Grillner, 1974). From the leading segment, there are phase lags in both directions, so waves of activity pass both caudal and rostral from the leading segment at constant speed. Under appropriate conditions, the fish can swim backwards, with the wave passing caudal to rostral (Grillner, 1974). Portions of the cord, isolated from the rest, can fictively swim forwards or backwards (Grillner, 1974).

4.3.2   Nonmathematical Assumptions

The application of the above theory to these phenomena in dogfish requires some nonmathematical assumptions. One is that, under the conditions of excitation appropriate to stereotypic swimming, there is some neural network within each segment, driving the motoneurons, that is capable of endogenous oscillation, independent of the other segments. Since fictive swimming has not yet been elicited in dogfish with less than eight segments (Grillner, 1974), this is a serious assumption. (The mathematics is a correct description even if each oscillator spans more or less than one segment; it must be modified if the oscillators are not distinct, i.e., share components.) Another assumption is that the *direct* electrical and chemical connections among the segmental oscillators are only between nearest neighbors. The latter assumption is probably anatomically wrong. However, the results do not appear to depend crucially on this; in Section 4.3.4, we discuss multiple neighbor connections. (Also see Rand et al. (Chapt. 9) for a discussion of synchronizing interactions from contralateral inhibition. One generalization of nearest neighbor coupling which does qualitatively change the results has short-range excitation and long-range inhibition (Cohen et al. 1982; Rand et al., Chapt. 9).)

4.3.3   The Dogfish CPG as Seen Through APD Theory

The dogfish CPG is modelled here as a chain of weakly coupled oscillators (see Section 4.3.4 for conclusions about non-weak coupling). To understand the phenomena described earlier, only one of the two parallel chains need be considered, since the paired oscillators operate in antiphase. (To understand experiments which change that antiphase relationship (Rand et al., Chapt. 9), both chains must be explicitly considered.) The first conclusion of the analysis is that, if the strength of the coupling does not strongly depend on the position of the segment, then to get a wave moving along the cord with uniform phase lags, i.e., at a constant speed, there must be no gradient in natural frequencies (or, at most, a small one), and the oscillators must be coupled "synaptically" (see 3.1.3). If the oscillators are coupled by multiple neighbor connections, gradients may not have so severe an impact on the wave speed (see Section 4.3.4).

A revealing fact about the dogfish CPG is that the leading segment need not be the most rostral. From the analysis, we see that there *are* solutions to the APD equations which, like the spinal swimming in dogfish, have waves progressing in both directions. However, according to APD theory, this can happen only if the forward and backward coupling are almost equal in strength. In that case, the leading segment would indeed be very sensitive to changes in parameters, the sensitivity increasing with the number of oscillators (there are over 65 segments in dogfish—Grillner, 1974). This sensitivity implies a simple mechanism for allowing a reversal of wave direction: a small bias in the coupling due to synapses activated preferentially in rostral to caudal fibers or caudal to rostral fibers can shift the leading segment to one end or the other. (A small bias in the natural frequencies can have the same effect.) So can shifts in timing of the signals going rostral or caudal, as in recent simulations of Pearce and Friesen (pers. comm.).

The effect of a bias in coupling depends on the sign of the coupling functions $H^\pm(0)$ (if H^+ and H^- differ only in magnitude). In order that there be a solution to (4.4), (4.5) with waves travelling outward from some segment, as in dogfish, $H^\pm$ must satisfy $H^\pm(0) > 0$. For this choice of sign, to get waves moving rostrally, the coupling must be increased in the caudal direction. Thus, the model suggests that backward swimming can be provoked by an increase in coupling strength in the rostral to caudal fibers. As discussed in Section 4.2.2, this could also be accomplished by a temporary caudal bias in natural frequency.

The constancy of phase lags over wide ranges of frequency (Grillner and Kashin, 1976) is easily handled within the framework of this model. Suppose that the frequency of the system is changed by an increase in excitation which increases the frequency of each oscillator without affecting the coupling, i.e., the functions $H^\pm$ remain the same. Then the phase lag ϕ between successive segments, which is determined by (4.4), also remains the same. If ϕ is unchanged but the cycle period decreases, then the intersegmental time delays decrease and, as observed, there is an increase in the propagation speed down the spinal cord, which is proportional to the swimming velocity in an intact fish (Grillner and Kashin, 1976). The solution to (4.4) is unchanged by altering the number of oscillators; hence the model predicts the same phase lag per segment independent of the number of segments in an isolated piece of cord (provided the latter is not too small.) We note that the model does not require the existence of specially located "pacemakers," which would be an awkward assumption for isolated portions of the cord.

4.3.4 Multiple Neighbor Coupling

The coupling among the segmental oscillators extends considerably beyond nearest neighbor segments. In the lamprey, it is known that some coordination remains when as many as ten segments are blocked (Cohen, 1986). Some hypothesized interneurons thought to be important in intersegmental coordination have processes which extend five to ten segments in the caudal direction and a few in the rostral (Rovainen, 1985; Grillner et al., Chapt. 1). In the leech, in which a single segment is known to be capable of oscillation (Weeks, 1981), similar multiple coupling has been found (Pearce and Friesen, 1985a,b).

The mathematical model described in Sections 4.1 and 4.2 can be generalized to include such multiple connections. Investigations of such generalized systems are not yet as advanced as for nearest neighbor systems, but preliminary numerical and analytical investigations suggest that the conclusions discussed in the previous section on dogfish swimming continue to hold when there are multiple neighbor connections.

In addition, the multiple coupling helps to account for some phenomena in the isolated lamprey cord that are incompatible with weak nearest neighbor coupling. One such observation is that when a lamprey cord is cut into two or three pieces, the phaselocked frequencies of the groups can be quite different (Cohen, 1987). Similarly, by dividing the bath into compartments, and changing the chemical concentrations in the different parts of the bath, it is possible to make parts of the cord have a natural frequency considerably larger than another part of the cord; yet phaselocking is preserved between the parts, with phase differences that remain very small (Rovainen, pers. comm.). If the coupling were to be both weak and nearest neighbor, phaselocking would break down, and/or there would be large phase differences between nearby segments.

Preliminary investigations by Kopell and Ermentrout suggest that these phenomena can be understood from multiple neighbor coupling, each link of which may be weak, but whose total strength is not small. Phaselocking is then possible with large frequency differences. The resulting phase lags appear to be both small and relatively independent of frequency differences. This is an important property that could help in explaining the relatively strong regulation of phase lags in the presence of possibly noisy local frequencies. It also helps to explain how constant speed waves can exist in the lamprey cord in the apparent presence of significant differences in natural frequencies (see Section 4.3.3). Related work using multiple coupling has recently been done by Pearce and Friesen (pers. comm.).

4.3.5   A Variation: The CPG of Electric Fish

The fin movements of *Eigenmannia* and *Gymnarchus* (cf. Cohen, Chapt. 5) can also be understood from the above mathematics. Of particular interest are the rapid movements of the leading segment and the variation in the number of wavelengths within the fin. For synaptic coupling, the former can be accomplished by small, uniform changes in the relative strengths of the forward and backward coupling. If these changes are substantial, they can affect the observed wavelength. The mathematics shows that changes in leading segment and wavelength can also be accomplished by changing the gradient of frequencies along the cord. It could also possibly be done by a moving "pacemaker" with a sufficiently large frequency difference from the rest of the cord. The different mechanisms (or combinations of them) give rise to different detailed predictions, but the current data is not sufficient to distinguish them.

4.3.6 Developmental Implications

The C-coils of early embryonic muscle involve simultaneous contractions of the myotomal muscles on one side of the embryo (see Cohen, Chapt. 5). Such activity, in which the phase lag between oscillators is zero, is expected if the coupling among the neural or muscular cells is electrotonic (a special case of "diffusive" coupling; see Section 3.1.3). Furshpan and Potter (1968) report electric coupling in early embryos of various species. In chicks, these appear to exist before synaptogenesis (Trelstad et al., 1966). By contrast, as shown above, synchronizing synaptic coupling, e.g., by excitatory synapses, gives rise to travelling waves (see Section 3.1.4 for the meaning of "synchronizing"). The mathematics suggests that the later development of the capacity to produce travelling waves is a consequence of the development of appropriate ipsilateral synapses. If the simultaneous firing of cells aids in the formation and strengthening of synapses between them, the early synchronous form of organization may be a necessary precursor to the later state.

After the development of undulatory swimming, fish are still capable of undergoing simultaneous contractions (with no phase lags) on one side of the body, as in escape swimming. This is consistent with the above, if, e.g., there is a fast conduction system like the Mauthner axon to simultaneously excite all the oscillators along the cord.

5   ALMOST OSCILLATORS

Pattern generating networks make use of elements which are more general than those discussed above; they can include units that do not oscillate, but have special properties that make them susceptible to oscillation if they are coupled to endogenous oscillators, or if some parameters are changed (cf. Harris-Warrick, Chapt. 8). The mathematics of systems on the border of oscillation is more difficult and considerably less developed than that of limit cycle oscillators (for references to one such body of work, see Rinzel, 1981). In Section 5, we discuss two ways in which a system can be "on the verge of oscillation" and some ways in which these systems can interact with oscillators.

5.1   Damped Oscillations

One way in which a system can be on the edge of oscillation is if it is a slightly damped oscillator. The amplitude of such a system decreases to zero unless the system is repeatedly excited; when perturbed, the phase changes periodically. Physiological examples include cardiac cells (Tsien et al., 1979). Slightly damped oscillators, perturbed by some phasic forcing (see Section 3.2.2), can easily become a stable oscillator. Sensory inputs can act via reflex pathways to perturb and force the system periodically (Andersson et al., 1981; Rossignol et al. Chapt. 7). This mechanism could provide appropriate phasic forcing at different points in the locomotion cycle; as T. McMahon points out (McMahon, 1984, Chapter 7), this, plus damped oscillations, can yield a stable oscillator. Thus, with sensory feedback, there can be oscillations for physiological parameter ranges in which the CPG does not spontaneously oscillate. Lightly damped oscillators can also be considered to be a kind of tuning mechanism: when coupled to oscillators of a nearby frequency, they can respond by oscillating at the forcing frequency.

5.2   Excitable Systems

Another example of an almost oscillator is called an excitable system or a "one shot oscillator." Without stimulation, such a system remains in stable equilibrium; however, a small threshold change in initial conditions away from a stable equilibrium point leads to a much larger excursion of the solution before the system returns to rest. A classic example is, of course, a nerve membrane capable of producing an action potential.

In general, a small change in the parameters of an excitable system can lead it to become oscillatory. For example, depolarizing current applied to a nerve axon leads to periodic firing. The mathematics of this is described in Rinzel (1981). We emphasize that the notion of excitable system has a general mathematical meaning which can be applied to larger units such as networks of cells.

An excitable system can become oscillatory through lightly damped oscillations, as above. Another way is illustrated in the phase-plane pictures in Figures 4A, B. As noted by Rinzel and Ermentrout, the system in these pictures corresponds to a mechanism for excitability that occurs in what has been called "class I axons" (Connor et al., 1977). The horizontal axis is membrane potential (V); the vertical axis (n) is an "activator" for gates allowing the ionic flow of potassium (see Ermentrout and Kopell, 1986; Kopell and Ermentrout, 1986b, for further discussion). In Figure 4A, the system has a stable rest point and a threshold. It also has an unstable saddle-type point, whose two departing trajectories both enter the stable rest point and, hence, form a circle containing the saddle and stable rest points. As a parameter is changed, the stable rest point and the saddle coalesce and disappear, and the circle changes into a limit cycle (see Figure 4B). In this case, the original (excitable) system has no intrinsic frequency (unlike the damped oscillations discussed above). Just past the change-over value of the parameter, the period of the oscillation is arbitrarily large.

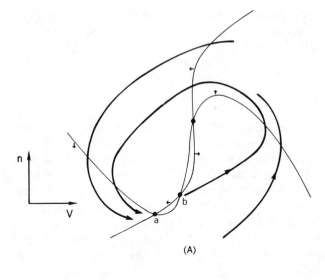

(A)

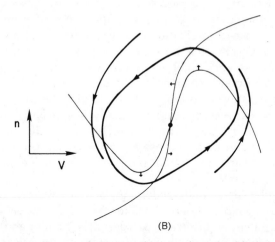

(B)

FIGURE 4. Phase plane diagrams for systems that come from simplifications of the Hodgkin-Huxley equations. The axes are V (voltage) and n (a recovery variable). The light curves represent "nullclines", i.e. the points satisfying $\dot{V} = 0$ or $\dot{n} = 0$. The dark curves are solutions to the differential equation. (A) There is a stable rest point (a) and a threshold (b). (B) There is a stable limit cycle.

If the system is given a perturbation which allows it to oscillate temporarily, then, as the system decays to stability, the periods increase while the amplitude remains almost constant. The oscillations in *Tritonia* swim network (Getting, 1983) behave like this.

5.2.1 Parabolic Bursting

To give an idea of how qualitative theory can be useful in understanding coupled systems of oscillators and excitable units, we now discuss one particular result. As in the rest of the chapter, the result concerns very general equations (see Kopell and Ermentrout, 1986b, for the equations). The equations describe two coupled systems. One system, with variables called $x(t)$, is assumed to be near the border between excitability and oscillation, as in Figure 4. It is coupled to another system, with variables $y(t)$, which oscillates slowly even if $x(t)$ is held fixed. Here, "slow" means that the period is long compared with the time scale of the excursion of the excitable system.

The conclusion is that the coupled system has a complicated periodic solution in which $x(t)$ undergoes some number k of cycles for each slow period in $y(t)$; for different parameters, there are different numbers of oscillations in x for each oscillation in y (Ermentrout and Kopell, 1986). If the x-system represents the transmembrane potential and the voltage-controlled activators and inhibitors of a nerve cell, then one oscillation in the x-system corresponds to an action potential, and the function $x(t)$ corresponds to a bursting solution. If, furthermore, the influence of the y-oscillator on the excitable system is qualitatively sinusoidal in shape, then the bursting is "parabolic" (Strumwasser, 1967); i.e., the interspike intervals first decrease and then increase again. By contrast, if the slow waveform is an increasing triangular ramp, the interspike intervals keep decreasing within a burst.

As an example, such an interaction may hold between two types of cells thought to be the main part of the CPG for the pyloric system of the lobster stomatogastric ganglion (Eisen and Marder, 1984; Marder and Eisen, 1984). The AB cell oscillates endogenously, often without spikes, and with a frequency of the order of a second. In the intact network in which the AB and PD cells are coupled electrically to one another, the PD cells burst parabolically exactly when the wave form of the AB cell is qualitatively sinusoidal (cf. Fig. 2 of Marder and Eisen, 1984, to Fig. 1 of Eisen and Marder, 1984).

The formalism discussed above holds generally whenever an excitable unit (as in Figs. 4A,B) is coupled to a slow oscillation. Thus, this mechanism may hold in situations in which there is a subcellular (Tsien, et al., 1979), or metabolic, oscillation in a cell, coupled to membrane properties through a metabolically sensitive sodium-potassium pump, or calcium-dependent conductance. Such oscillations have been experimentally verified in smooth muscle (Connor, 1979; Ohba et al., 1977), and damped oscillations are found in cardiac Purkinje cells (Tsien et al., 1979). The parabolic nature of the bursting in the *Aplysia* neuron R15 (for which the underlying slow oscillation is qualitatively sinusoidal) suggests such a mechanism for R15. This is argued in Kopell and Ermentrout (1986b). See Adams (1985), Plant and Kim (1976), and Rinzel and Lee (1986) for other points of view.

The above discussion can be compared to "threshold" models for bursting (Junge and Stephens, 1973), which postulate that action potentials appear whenever the potential of the slow oscillation is sufficiently high (depolarized), *and* that the local frequency of the spikes varies with the level of depolarization. By contrast, the above analysis provides a very general mathematical mechanism which automatically produces the latter conclusion, in the absence of detailed knowledge of ionic currents. Of course, to apply these ideas in any particular case, it would be necessary to check the general hypotheses. With a few more qualitative assumptions usually made about nerve models (Rinzel, 1981; Carpenter, 1979), one can conclude much about the fine structure of the burst, e.g., the qualitative behavior of the undershoots (Kopell and Ermentrout, 1986b).

6 A PHILOSOPHY OF MODELLING

The theory toward which the work presented here is pointing is not just about weak coupling, or even, more generally, about situations in which averaging is valid. Rather, the ideal is to develop a body of mathematics that can help decide, with minimal a priori guessing, which differences do indeed make a difference. Thus, the method is to work with robust classes of equations and, within these, to attempt to sort out which conclusions are essentially universal and which depend on further structure. For example, in the case study modelling dogfish swimming, one always finds waves with uniform phase lags if the coupling is "synaptic," but there are simultaneous waves in both directions only if the forward and backward coupling are closely balanced. Similarly, it is very general for two coupled oscillators to phaselock, but the frequency at which they will lock depends on the oscillators, and can be higher than, or lower than, both of the interacting oscillators.

As will be apparent to the reader of this book, there are many different reasons for modelling, and many points of view about what constitutes the successes and pitfalls of this art. It is well understood that a model can be "too simple." Particular examples are used to gain intuition, to make otherwise difficult calculations, to focus attention on phenomena that are more easily seen in simple situations. If predictions made from such descriptions turn out to be wrong in some details, one can always modify, and make the description more complex.

This process of successive modification does not, however, address a more subtle pitfall, that of inappropriate specificity. A model is something more than a catalogue of facts, some of which are in flux; it is part of an attempt to create a coherent context for those facts. To that end, an initial description or model is used to generate predictions which, if substantiated, lend weight to the description. Some phenomena, though, are so robust that they are independent of many special choices that may be made as part of the description. Hence, it is misleading to explain such phenomena in terms of detailed properties that are not necessarily essential. For example, membrane properties are surely important in the question of whether a given neuron is capable of being an oscillator (i.e., a burster); however, the question of whether two such neurons will oscillate in synchrony or in antiphase or neither can often be decided by knowing only that each neuron *does* burst, and some phenomenological properties of the burst and the coupling. That is, the level of detail needed to account for a particular phenomenon depends on the phenomenon. In working with a "realistic," i.e., detailed model, one can lose sight of why it is working, and whether it would continue to work if some ad hoc part of the description is modified. By contrast, the approach taken here is to try to seek out general and verifiable hypotheses which give the essential reason for the behavior in question.

The work exposed above is the outline of only a small part of a CPG theory, dealing mainly with CNS components that are oscillatory. To fill the many gaps of this outline will require the close collaboration of mathematicians and neurobiologists.

APPENDIX 1: REVIEW OF PRC THEORY

Let Δ denote the delay in phase (after transients have died) due to a pulse perturbation at some time t (measured from an arbitrary starting point in the cycle). It is convenient to write Δ in terms of phase θ rather than time t, with phase changing between 0 and 1. Thus $\theta = t/\sigma$, where σ is the period of the forced oscillator and, since $t = \sigma\theta$, we write $\Delta = \Delta(\sigma\theta)$; Δ is a periodic function of θ with period 1, and a periodic function of the time variable t with period σ. We adhere to the convention that $\Delta > 0$ implies a phase delay. If a perturbing pulse is given periodically, with period τ, one can ask if the forced oscillation will have a periodic response with period τ. If so, will the response be stable under changes in the initial condition, and how will the phase of the output be changed by the periodic inputs? For a fixed perturbing pulse (whose transient effects decay "sufficiently fast"), these questions can be answered from analyzing $\Delta(\sigma\theta)$. It is shown in Perkel et al. (1964) that there is a periodic response with a delay of θ_1 provided that the equation

$$\Delta(\sigma\theta_1) = \frac{1}{\sigma}(\tau - \sigma) \tag{A1.1}$$

can be solved for θ_1. The response is stable if $\Delta'(\sigma\theta_1)$ lies between 0 and 2. For more details, see, e.g., Perkel et al. (1964).

APPENDIX 2:   THE USE OF APD THEORY AND AN APPLICATION TO SPINAL DOGFISH

To understand how to use APD theory, we begin by asking the same questions of (2.2) that could be handled by PRC theory: for ω_0, ω, and H, does (2.2) have a stable phaselocked solution, and with what phase delay or advance? If the oscillators are to be phaselocked, we require a solution to (2.2) in which $\theta_0 - \theta$ is constant in time. Letting $\phi = \theta_0 - \theta$, and subtracting (2.2b) from (2.2a), we get

$$\dot{\phi} = [\delta - H(\phi)] \tag{A2.1}$$

where $\delta = \omega_0 - \omega$. We are looking for a solution to (A2.1) with $\dot{\phi} = 0$ [i.e., a critical point of (A2.1)]. Any such critical point solves

$$\delta - H(\phi) = 0. \tag{A2.2}$$

The critical point for (A2.1) is stable (and so then is the rhythmic behavior described by the periodic solution to (2.2) if $H'(\phi) > 0$.

A2.1   Implications of APD Theory (Applied to Spinal Dogfish)

Much qualitative information is implied by (A2.2). For example, if the forced and forcing oscillations have the same frequency ($\delta = 0$), and $H'(\phi) > 0$ in an interval around $\phi = 0$ including the solution to (A2.2), then the sign of $H(0)$ determines whether the forced oscillator will lead or lag ($H(0) < 0$ implies the solution ϕ to (A2.2) satisfies $\phi > 0$, so the forced oscillator lags by ϕ; see Fig. 1). Similarly, if $H'(\phi) < 0$ in a region around $\phi = 0$, any stable critical point must be far from $\phi = 0$, and so the lag or lead must be outside that region.

If the oscillators are not the same, (A2.2) relates the size of the lag to the amount of the frequency difference. For example, consider the experiments of Grillner and Wallén (1982), who imposed sinusoidal mechanical movements on the tail region of curarized spinal dogfish during fictive locomotion. They found that at forcing rates near the natural ("resting") rate, the higher the forcing frequency of the mechanical motion, the later within the cycle was the bursting response in the ventral root; this was true for a wide range of amplitudes. Where the forced and forcing rhythms are not alike, the choices of phase to be labelled $\theta = 0$, $\theta_0 = 0$ are made independently, so "$\phi = 0$" is not a special point. Nevertheless, the model makes predictions about the *change* in phase differences as a parameter (such as $\omega_0 - \omega$) is varied. As an example, suppose that ϕ_0 is a stable solution to (A2.2) with $\delta = 0$ (forcing frequency equals rest frequency). Since $H'(\phi)$ must be positive near any ϕ_0 which is a *stable* solution, equation (A2.2) says that an increase in δ near $\delta = 0$ leads to a larger phase difference, i.e., a fixed phase in the responding oscillation will occur later for higher forcing frequencies, as was observed (see Fig. 1). Similarly, a decrease in δ leads to a smaller phase difference. With no specific knowledge of H, this can be deduced from stability, which is necessary if locking can be observed at all. This implies that the results are general properties of forced oscillators and do not depend on the details of the mechanism involved.

Other consequences predicted by APD theory are the 1:1 entrainment observed by Grillner and Wallén within some interval of forcing frequencies, and the fact that this interval gets larger as the amplitude of the mechanical forcing is increased. The latter follows from the theory because increased forcing "stretches" the range of the function H. For instance, multiplying g in equation (2.1) by a number larger than 1 does the same for H in (2.2). This increases the interval of δ's for which (A2.2) can be solved. The amplitude of the mechanical forcing is presumed to be correlated with the strength of forcing that it provides. For low amplitude forcing of much higher or much lower frequency, 1:1 entrainment is impossible, but APD theory predicts other kinds of entrainment which, in fact, correspond to the observed data (see Appendix 4). For large forcing amplitudes, the APD theory is probably not relevant, since large amplitude forcing corresponds to "strong" coupling, as discussed in Section 2.3.

APPENDIX 3: POINCARÉ MAPS AND AN APPLICATION TO THE CRAYFISH SWIMMERET SYSTEM

A3.1 Poincaré Maps and the Measurement of H

When averaging is valid, the periodic function H contains all the information necessary to decide if a forced oscillator will phaselock. However, it is not easy to measure H directly. There is, though, a related function, central to the theory of nonlinear oscillators, that is as easy to measure as a PRC. This is the so-called Poincaré map (Guckenheimer and Holmes, 1983).

To understand Poincaré maps, it is useful to first discuss a special case that is very close to the phase transition curve (PTC). The PTC maps a phase just before a pulse into the new phase right after the pulse (assuming instant decay of transients). If Δ is the delay function, the PTC is

$$\theta \rightarrow [\theta - \Delta(\sigma\theta)] \bmod 1. \qquad (A3.1)$$

("mod 1" means integer multiples are ignored; only the fractional part is kept. See Figure 5 for the graphs of a PRC and its associated PTC.) If an

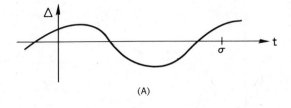

(A)

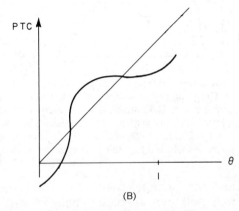

(B)

FIGURE 5. (A) Schematic PRC or delay curve: delay Δ in phase due to a pulse vs. time t at which the pulse is given. This graph is periodic with period σ. (B) Associated PTC; the horizontal axis is phase before a pulse and the vertical one is phase after a pulse. The intersection of the graph with the 45 degree line corresponds to the zeros of the curve in Figure 5(a).

oscillator is periodically forced by pulses, the Poincaré map P takes a phase θ measured at one point in the forcing cycle (e.g., just before a pulse is given) to the phase achieved at the next similar point (i.e., just before the next pulse is given). The formula for P is obtained by adding to (A3.1) the phase change due to normal movement of the oscillator between pulses:

$$P(\theta) = [\theta - \Delta(\sigma\theta) + \frac{1}{\sigma}\tau] \bmod 1 \qquad (A3.2)$$

(see Fig. 6 for the graph).

For a general forced oscillator, the Poincaré map P takes a phase θ at one point in the forcing cycle to the phase achieved one full forcing cycle later. Unlike a PRC, which encodes only the response to a single pulse, the Poincaré map, like H, depends on the period of the forcing (see Fig. 6). 1:1 phaselocking corresponds to a "fixed point" of P, i.e., a value $\hat{\theta}$ for which $P(\hat{\theta}) = \hat{\theta}$; that is, if the response is periodic with the same period as the forcing, there must be some phase $\hat{\theta}$ of the forced oscillator that returns to

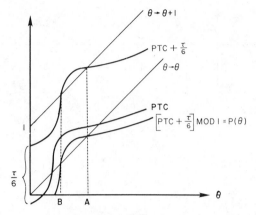

FIGURE 6. A Poincaré map computed from a PTC. The upper curve is the graph of the PTC translated upward by τ/σ; The graph of $P(\theta)$ is obtained by shifting downward by 1 the portion of this graph that rises above $\theta = 1$. The horizontal axis in each case is the phase at the start of the cycle. For the graph of $P(\theta)$, the vertical axis represents phase after one cycle of the forcing oscillator. If $\tau = \sigma$, the graphs of $P(\theta)$ and the PTC coincide. The points A and B are the fixed points of P, i.e., phases which return to themselves after each cycle of the forcing.

itself after one cycle of the forcing oscillator (see Fig. 6; the points labelled A and B are fixed points). If there are natural points $\theta = 0$ and $\theta_0 = 0$ from which to measure the beginnings of the cycle for each of the oscillators, (e.g., the onset of bursting in some cell), then this $\hat{\theta}$ measures the phase lag ($\hat{\theta} > 0$) or lead ($\hat{\theta} < 0$) of the forcing oscillator to the forced one with respect to these natural starting points. In PRC theory, the phaselocked solution is stable if $\Delta'(\sigma\theta_1)$ lies between 0 and 2 (see equation A1.1). The analogue for the Poincaré map is that $|P'(\hat{\theta})| < 1$. Point A of Figure 6 is stable; point B is not.

The measurement of P is analogous to that of a PRC: starting from a given phase, the oscillator is forced for one cycle of the forcing oscillator, and the new phase is determined (see below for an experimentally measured Poincaré map). To use this information about P, it is necessary to connect P with H, in particular to relate the phase $\hat{\theta}$ to the phase difference ϕ that obtains when there is phaselocking. Recall that $\phi = \theta_0 - \theta$. In the averaged equations, when there is phaselocking, ϕ does not change with time, and so can be measured at any fixed time t. At $t = 0$, we have $\theta_0 = 0$ and $\theta = \hat{\theta}$; thus, $\phi = -\hat{\theta}$. It can be shown that the two notions of stability discussed above, i.e., $|P'(\hat{\theta})| < 1$ and $H'(\phi) > 0$, are equivalent. If $\phi > 0$, the forcing oscillator leads the forced one; if $\phi < 0$, the forcing oscillator lags. This discussion connects P and H only near fixed points of P. However, this is the only part of P that is related to 1:1 locking.

A3.2   Example: Crayfish Swimmerets

As an application of these ideas, consider the crayfish swimmeret system studied by P. Stein (1971). In the swimmeret system, there is a wave of activity which moves progressively rostral, i.e., recordings from the motor nerves of successively more rostral swimmeret ganglia have fixed phase delays relative to more caudal ganglia. Stein shows that the connections between neighboring ganglia are much stronger in the caudal to rostral direction than in the other, though there is some influence in the other direction (Stein, 1971). He measures a "first PRC" for a single swimmeret oscillator and uses the formalism of PRC theory to conclude that the wave of electrical activity is a predictable consequence.

As Stein points out, this formalism is not really applicable because the transients take several cycles to adequately die out. Also, the signals from one ganglion to another are of long duration; thus an ad hoc argument is invoked to separate (conceptually) the signal into pieces having different effects, with no time between the pieces for the transients to die out. Nevertheless, if the coupling is not inappropriately strong, or the coupling signals are sufficiently dispersed throughout the cycle to justify averaging, APD theory says that his conclusion is correct: his measurements do imply the existence of the metachronal waves.

To see this, we assume (as he does) that the swimmeret oscillators are essentially equivalent, and that there are no rostral to caudal connections. Then any neighboring pair of oscillators can be considered to be a forced oscillator system. The forced and forcing oscillators are equal with the forcing oscillator the more caudal one. In Stein (1976), the correct data for a Poincaré map is measured, but it is plotted there, in Figure 4, in the way usually associated with PRCs. If the data is replotted as explained above, then it can be seen that there is a $\hat{\theta}$ near 1 (which is equivalent, mod 1, to a negative phase $\hat{\theta}$ near 0) such that $P(\hat{\theta}) = \hat{\theta}$ and $0 < P'(\hat{\theta}) < 1$. (Recall that Figures 5 and 6 show how to go from a PRC to a Poincaré map. In this application $\tau/\sigma = 1$, and so P has the same graph as the PTC. Figure 7 of this chapter replots the essential part of Figure 4 of Stein (1976) and the associated Poincaré map.) Since $\hat{\theta} < 0$, this implies that $\phi = - \hat{\theta} > 0$. (See A3.1 above.) Recall that ϕ is the phase of the forcing oscillator minus that of the forced one; thus $\phi > 0$ means that the caudal oscillator leads the rostral one, and the coordinating neurons do, indeed, generate a metachronal wave from caudal to rostral.

APPENDIX 4: ROTATION NUMBER AND RELATIVE COORDINATION

We have seen that APD theory gives conditions for stable 1:1 phaselocking which are equivalent to those given by PRC theory when the latter applies. For more subtle phenomena, the theories are not equivalent. However, there is a more general theory that encompasses both theories, which predicts considerably more than 1:1 locking, and which sheds light on phenomena that might otherwise seem mysterious or paradoxical (Perkel et al. 1964). It is an important theme of this chapter (see Section 6) that expla-

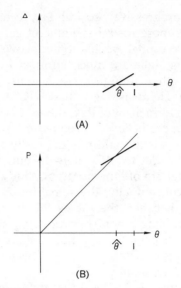

FIGURE 7. (A) A schematic graph of the relevant part of the measured "first PRC" of crayfish swimmerets, after Stein (1976). (B) The relevant part of the associated Poincaré map, derived from Figure 7a as in Figures 5 and 6, with $\sigma = \tau$. The fixed point $\hat{\theta}$ of P is the zero of the delay function Δ. Since $P'(\hat{\theta}) = 1 - \Delta'(\hat{\theta})$, if $\Delta'(\hat{\theta})$ is between 0 and 1, so is $P'(\hat{\theta})$. Hence, $\hat{\theta}$ corresponds to a stable phaselocked solution.

nations of phenomena should not be tied more closely than necessary to unknowable specifics, and we suggest that an understanding of the generality of some observed phenomena should, at the very least, lead to caution about accepting the validity of detailed models having such observations as conclusions. Another reason for including this material is that much of the modern mathematical literature on oscillators takes this theory as a starting point, and hence this material may be helpful to those readers who want access to that literature.

The general theory is that of circle maps (Guckenheimer and Holmes, 1983). We shall first briefly describe the theory and its conclusions, then connect this to PRC and APD theories and to neural experiments.

A4.1   Circle Maps, Rotation Number, and Periodic Solutions

The Poincaré map of a weakly forced oscillator (2.2), described in Appendix 3, can also be represented as a "circle map." That is, both the input and output quantities are angular variables that can be thought of as points on a circle. For such maps there is a theory whose predictions are directly relevant to phenomena of entrainment and locking.

For this section, it helps to think geometrically: instead of regarding the Poincaré map as a graph (as in Figure 6), think of it as an algorithm that moves each point (i.e., phase θ) to another position on the circle (e.g., for

$P(\theta)$ in Figure 6, the point $\theta = 0$ is moved clockwise, points A and B are left alone, and the points between B and A are moved counter-clockwise; see Figure 8). The central idea in the theory of circle maps is that of the *rotation number* $\rho(f)$ of a map f. $\rho(f)$ measures the fraction of a circle that each point is moved, on the average, by f. For example, if f rotates the circle counterclockwise through 90°, then $\rho(f) = 1/4$.

The formal definition of $\rho(f)$ is quite technical and can be found in Guckenheimer and Holmes (1983). For the purposes of this chapter, it suffices to know some of the facts about rotation number. First of all, the rotation number determines much of the qualitative behavior of f, especially the existence of periodic points. (f is said to have a periodic point θ of period k if, after k applications of the map f, the image of the point θ ends up again at θ. For example, if f rotates the circle through 90°, every point has period $k = 4$.) The theory of circle maps shows that f has at least one periodic point of period k exactly when $\rho(f)$ is a fraction whose denominator is k. Periodic points for the relevant circle maps correspond to absolute and relative coordination (or locking) of the oscillators, so knowledge about periodic points is of central importance.

For the examples we discuss below there is, not a single circle map, but a family of them. For example, the period τ of the forcing oscillator can be considered to be a parameter. For Poincaré maps that come from PTCs, the graphs of such a family are obtained from any one by raising or lowering the graph by $(1 - \tau/\sigma)$ as in Figure 6. The second fact about rotation number is that it varies continuously as parameters are changed. This implies that, as the rotation number passes from one number to another, it must hit all the rational numbers in between. The final important point about rotation numbers is that for "most" one-parameter families of circle maps,

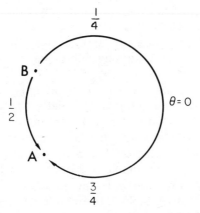

FIGURE 8. A geometrical picture of the Poincaré map $P(\theta)$ in Figure 6. The points A and B are the fixed points of P. Phases are attracted to point A and repelled from point B.

the rotation number is constant in some parameter interval around each rational number. That is, every time the rotation number passes a rational number, it "sticks," or gets locked in. (The size of the lock-in interval gets smaller and smaller as the denominator of the fraction increases.) Outside of these intervals, there is drift, or other behavior, rather than phaselocking (See below).

A4.2   PRC, APD, and Phaselocking

We now focus on the relevance of the above ideas for the PRC and APD theories. We start with APD theory, and write P_τ for the Poincaré map of an oscillator forced periodically with period τ. We concentrate on the case $\tau \leq \sigma$, i.e., the frequency of the forcing oscillator is at least as high as that of the forced. When the forcing is weak, $\rho(P_\tau)$ is close to τ/σ, so if $\tau = \sigma$, the rotation number is near 1. By the above theory, there is then usually an interval in τ around $\tau = \sigma$ for which the rotation number is still 1. This corresponds to 1:1 phaselocking, i.e., one response for each forcing cycle, even when the natural and forcing frequencies are somewhat different. See Appendix 3 for more detail available from measurable data.

If τ is approximately $\sigma/2$ (i.e., the forcing frequency is about twice as fast as the natural frequency), then the associated rotation number is about 1/2, so there is usually an interval of phaselocking for which there is one response of the forced oscillator for every two forcing cycles. In general, for each rational number $0 \leq j/k \leq 1$, there can be an interval of locking in which there are j responses for k forcing cycles. Such locking, for which the number of response cycles is not equal to the number of forcing cycles, has often been noticed (von Holst, 1973; Reid, 1969; Guttman et. al. 1980) in biological systems, and is sometimes called "relative coordination".

In PRC theory, the role of the one-parameter family is taken by $P_\tau(\theta)$, the right hand side of equation (A3.2). As τ is decreased from $\tau = \sigma$, the rotation number decreases from approximately 1, and there are intervals of phaselocking as above. In this theory, the delay function Δ need not be small. However, if Δ is sufficiently large, even the qualitative conclusions about locking may change, especially if the PRC changes from "type 1" to "type 0" (Winfree, 1980).

For j,k small, if the rotation number is j/k, there is likely to be an interval of locking. In between these intervals, the patterns are more complicated. One standard pattern is "drift," also known as "gliding coordination," which is seen for parameter values just outside an interval of locking. For example, near 1:1 locking, the oscillators appear to lock temporarily into a preferred phase relation, then move quickly relative to one another until they reach that preferred relation again; this is repeated (Ermentrout and Rinzel, 1984). A biological example can be found in Wendler (1966).

A4.3   Example: Inhibitory Pulsing and "Paradoxical" Regions

We now apply some of these ideas to some results of Perkel et al. (1964) on simulations of the effect of inhibitory periodic pulsing on the firing rate of neurons. They show that, even with inhibitory pulsing, for some ranges of forcing period, there is a stable periodic response at a fractional multiple of the forcing rate. This is also seen experimentally in the *Procambarus* thoracic stretch receptor (Perkel et al. 1964). Within those intervals, the frequency of the response goes up with the frequency of the forcing. This may seem paradoxical, since one might expect inhibitory forcing to lower the firing rate. However, the above theory says that, independent of the properties of the forcing, one obtains stable intervals in which the response rate is the same fractional multiple of the perturbation rate. The major difference between inhibitory and excitatory forcing is not the rate of the response, but the phase delay imposed by the forcing (see Section 3.1.4).

ACKNOWLEDGMENTS

I am happy to acknowledge many debts to A. Cohen, who suggested this project, did her best to educate me, and prodded me toward a readable output. I am also indebted to A.Beckoff, G. B. Ermentrout, S. Grillner, R. Pearce, C. Rovainen, P. S. G. Stein and S. Strogatz for very helpful comments and much appreciated encouragement, to the NSF and the AFOSR for partial support, and to the Guggenheim Foundation for the leisure to think.

REFERENCES

Adams, W. B. (1985). Slow depolarizing and hyperpolarizing currents which mediate bursting in Aplysia neuron R15. *J. Physiol.*, **360**:51–68.

Andersson, O. H., Forssberg, S. Grillner, and P. Wallén (1981). Peripheral feedback mechanisms acting on the central pattern generator for locomotion in fish and cat. *Can. J. Physiol. Pharmacol.*, **59**:713–726.

Aronson, D., G. B. Ermentrout, and N. Kopell (1987). Amplitude response of forced and coupled oscillators. Preprint.

Bar-Eli, K. (1984). On the coupling of chemical oscillators. *J. Phys. Chem.*, **88**:3616–3622.

Berridge, M. J. and P. E. Rapp (1979). A comparative survey of the function, mechanism and control of cellular oscillators. *J. Exp. Biol.*, **81**:217–279.

Blackshaw, S. E. and A. E. Warner (1976). Low resistance junctions between mesoderm cells during development of trunk muscles. *J. Physiol. (London)* **255**:209–230.

Carpenter, G. A. (1979). Bursting phenomena in excitable membranes. *SIAM J. Appl. Math.*, **36**:334–372.

Cartwright, M. L. and J. E. Littlewood (1945). On nonlinear differential equations of the second order, I. *J. Lond. Math. Soc.*, **20**:180–189.

Chow, S. N. and J. K. Hale (1982). *Methods of Bifurcation Theory*, Springer-Verlag, New York.

Cohen, A. H. (1987). Intersegmental coordinating system of the lamprey central pattern generator for locomotion. *J. Comp. Phys. A.*, **160**:181–193.

Cohen, A. H. (1986). Experimental and theoretical studies of the intersegmental coordinating system of the lamprey CPG. In *Neurobiology of Vertebrate Locomotion*, Grillner, P., Stein, R., Herman, eds., Stockholm Symp. Vol. 5, 371–382.

Cohen, A. H., P. J. Holmes, and R. H. Rand, (1982). The nature of the coupling between segmental oscillators of the lamprey spinal generator for locomotion: a mathematical model. *J. Math. Biol.*, **13**:345–369.

Connor, J. A., D. Walter, and R. McKown, (1977). Neural repetitive firing: modifications of the Hodgkin-Huxley axon suggested by experimental results from crustacean axons. *Biophys. J.*, **18**:81–102.

Connor, J. A. (1979). On exploring the basis for slow potential oscillations in the mammalian stomach and intestine. *J. Exp. Biol.*, **81**:153–173.

Davis, W. J. and D. Kennedy, (1972). Command neurons controlling swimmeret movements in the lobster, I. Types of effects on motoneurons. *J. Neurophys.*, **35**:1–12.

Eisen, J. S. and E. Marder, (1984). A mechanism for production of phase shifts in a pattern generator. *J. Neurophys.*, **51**:1375–1393.

Ermentrout, G. B. (1981). n:m phaselocking of weakly coupled oscillators. *J. Math. Biol.*, **12**:327–342.

Ermentrout, G. B. and N. Kopell (1984). Frequency plateaus in a chain of weakly coupled oscillators, I. *SIAM J. Math. Anal.*, **15**:215–237.

Ermentrout, G. B., and N. Kopell (1986). Parabolic bursting in an excitable system coupled with a slow oscillation. *SIAM J. Appl. Math.*, **46**:233–253.

Ermentrout, G. B. and N. Kopell (1987). Oscillator death in systems of coupled neural oscillators. Preprint.

Ermentrout, G. B. and J. Rinzel (1984). Beyond a pacemaker's entrainment limit: phase walk-through. *Am J. Phys.*, **246**:R102–R106.

Forssberg, H., S. Grillner, S. Rossignol, and P. Wallén (1976). Phasic control of reflexes during locomotion in vertebrates. In *Neural Control of Locomotion*, R. M. Herman, S. Grillner, P. S. G. Stein, and D. G. Stuart, eds. Plenum, New York, pp. 647–674.

Friesen, W. O., M. Poon, and G. Stent, (1978). Neuronal control of swimming in the medicinal leech, IV. Identification of a network of oscillatory interneurons. *J. Exp. Biol.*, **75**:25–43.

Furshpan, E. J. and D. D. Potter (1968). Low resistance junctions between cells in embryos and tissue culture, In *Current Topics in Developmental Biology, 3*, A. Moscona and A. Monroy, eds. Academic Press, New York, 95–127.

Getting, P. (1983). Mechanisms of pattern generation underlying swimming in *Tritonia*. II. Network reconstruction. *J. Neurophys.* **49**:1017–1035.

Glass, L. and M. C. Mackey (1979). A simple model for phase locking of biological oscillators. *J. Math. Biol.*, **7**:339–352.

Goldstein, S. S. and W. Rall (1974). Changes in action potential shape and velocity for changing core geometries. *Biophys. J.*, **14**:731–737.

Grasman, J. and M. J. W. Jansen (1979). Mutually synchronized relaxation oscillators as prototypes of oscillating systems in biology. *J. Math. Biol.*, **7**:171–197.

Graubard, K., J. A. Raper, and D. K. Hartline (1983). Graded synaptic transmission between identified spiking neurons. *J. Neurophysiol.*, **50**:508–521.

Grillner, S. (1974). On the generation of locomotion in the spinal dogfish. *Exp. Brain Res.*, **20**:459–470.

Grillner, S. (1975). Locomotion in vertebrates: central mechanisms and reflex interaction. *Physiol. Rev.*, **55**:247–304.

Grillner, S. (1981). Control of locomotion in bipeds, tetrapods and fish. In *Handbook of Physiology, Section 1: The Nervous System, Vol. II, Part 2.* V. B. Brooks, ed. Amer. Physiol. Soc., Bethesda, 1179–1236.

Grillner, S. and S. Kashin (1976). On the generation and performance of swimming in fish. In *Neural Control of Locomotion*, R. M. Herman, S. Grillner, P. S. G. Stein, and D. G. Stuart, eds. Plenum, New York, 181–202.

Grillner, S. and P. Wallén (1982). On peripheral control mechanisms acting on the central pattern generators for swimming in the dogfish. *J. Exp. Biol.*, **98**:1–22.

Guckenheimer, J. (1975). Isochrons and phaseless sets. *J. Math. Biol.*, **1**:259–273.

Guckenheimer, J. and P. Holmes (1983). *Nonlinear Oscillations, Dynamical Systems and Bifurcations of Vector Fields*, Springer, New York.

Guevara, M. R. and L. Glass (1982). Phase locking, period doubling bifurcations and chaos in a mathematical model of a periodically driven oscillator: a theory of entrainment of biological oscillators and the generation of cardiac dysrthymias. *J. Math. Biol.*, **14**:1–23.

Guttman, R., L. Feldman, and E. Jakobsson (1980). Frequency entrainment of squid axon membrane. *J. Memb. Biol.*, **56**:9–18.

Herman, M. R. (1977). Mesure de Lebesque et nombre de rotation, In *Lecture Notes in Math. 597, Geometry and Topology.* Springer, Berlin, pp. 271–293.

Hirsch, M. W. and S. Smale (1974). *Differential Equations, Dynamical Systems and Linear Algebra.* Academic Press, New York.

Holst, E. von (1939). Die relative Koordination als Phänomen und als Methode zentralnervösen Funktionanalyse. *Ergebn. Physiol.*, **42**:288–306.

Holst, E. von (1973). *The Behavioral Physiology of Animals and Man: The Collected Papers of E. von Holst*, Vol. 1, R. Martin, trans. Methuen, London.

Hoppensteadt, F. C. and J. P. Keener, (1982). Phase locking of biological clocks. *J. Math. Biol.*, **15**:339–349.

Junge, D. and C. L. Stephens, (1973). Cyclic variation of potassium conductance in a burst generating neuron in Aplysia. *J. Physiol.*, **235**:155–181.

Kawato, M. and R. Suzuki (1980). Two coupled neural oscillators as a model of the circadian pacemaker. *J. Theor. Biol.*, **86**:547–575.

Kopell, N. (1986). Coupled oscillators and locomotion by fish. In *Nonlinear Oscillators in Biology and Chemistry*, H. Othmer. ed. *Lectures in Biomath.*, **66**:160–174.

Kopell, N. and G. B. Ermentrout (1986a). Symmetry and phaselocking in chains of weakly coupled oscillators. *Comm. Pure Appl. Math.* **39**:623–660.

Kopell, N. and G. B. Ermentrout (1986b). Subcellular oscillations and bursting. *Math. Biosciences,* **78**:265–291.

Kopell, N. and L. N. Howard (1973). Plane wave solutions to reaction-diffusion equations. *Studies Appl. Math.,* **52**:291–328.

Kulagin, A. S. and M. L. Shik, (1970). Interaction of symmetrical limbs during controlled locomotion. *Biofizyka,* **15**:164–170.

Levi, M. (1981). *Qualitative Analysis of the Periodically Forced Relaxation Oscillations, Memoirs of the AMS,* 32, A.M.S. Providence, 1981.

Levinson, N. (1950). Small periodic perturbations of an autonomous system with a stable orbit. *Ann. Math.,* **52**:727–738.

Lin, C. C. and L. A. Segel, *Mathematics Applied to Deterministic Problems in the Natural Sciences.* Macmillan, New York.

MacMahon, T. A. (1984). *Muscle, Reflexes and Locomotion,* Princeton Univ. Press, Princeton.

Marder, E. and J. S. Eisen (1984). Electrically coupled pacemaker neurons respond differently to same physiological inputs and neurotransmitters. *J. Neurophysiol.,* **51**:1362–1374.

Neu, J. C. (1979). Coupled oscillators. *SIAM J. Appl. Math.,* **37**:307–315.

Neu, J. C. (1980). Large populations of coupled chemical oscillators. *SIAM J. Appl. Math.,* **38**:305–316.

Ohba, M., Y. Sakamoto, and T. Tomita (1977). Effects of sodium potassium and calcium ions on the slow wave in the circular muscle of the guinea-pig stomach. *J. Physiol.,* **267**:167–180.

Pearce, R. A. and W. O. Friesen (1985). Intersegmental coordination of the leech swimming rhythm: I. Intrinsic period gradient and coupling strength, *J. Neurophysiol.,* **54**:1444–1459; II. Comparison of long and short chains of ganglia, *J. Neurophysiol.,* **54**:1460–1472.

Pearson, K. G. and C. R. Fourtner, (1975). Nonspiking interneurons in the walking system of the cockroach. *J. Neurophysiol.,* **38**:33–51.

Perkel, D. H., J. H. Schulman, T. H. Bullock, G. P. Moore, and J. P. Segundo (1964). Pacemaker neurons: effects of regularly spaced synaptic input. *Science,* **145**:61–63.

Pittendrigh, C. S. and D. H. Minis (1964). The entrainment of circadian oscillations by light and their role as photoperiodic clocks. *Amer. Nat.,* **98**:261–294.

Plant, R. E. and M. Kim (1976). Mathematical description of a bursting pacemaker neuron by a modification of the Hodgkin-Huxley equations. *Biophys. J.,* **16**:227–244.

Rand, R. H. and P. J. Holmes (1980). Bifurcation of periodic motions in two weakly coupled van der Pol oscillators. *Int. J. Nonlinear Mech.,* **15**:387–399.

Reid, J. V. O. (1969). The cardiac pacemaker: effects of regularly spaced nervous input. *Amer. Heart J.,* **78**:58–64.

Rinzel, J. (1981). Models in Neurobiology. In *Nonlinear Phenomena in Physics and Biology,* R. H. Enns, B. L. Jones, R. M. Miura, and S. S. Rangnekar, eds. Plenum, New York, pp. 345–367.

Rinzel, J. and Y. S. Lee (1986). Dissection of a model for neuronal parabolic bursting. Preprint.

Rovainen, C. (1985). Effects of groups of propriospinal interneurons on fictive swimming in the isolated spinal cord of the lamprey. *J. Neurophysiol.*, **54**:959–977.

Selverston, A. I. (1980). Are central pattern generators understandable?, *Behavioral and Brain Sciences*, **3**:535–571.

St. Vincent, M. (1987). Entrainment of a limit cycle oscillator with shear by large amplitude forcing, *SIAM J. Appl. Math*, in press.

Stein, P. S. G. (1971). Intersegmental coordination of swimmeret motorneuron activity in crayfish. *J. Neurophysiol.*, **34**:310–318.

Stein, P. S. G. (1974). Neural control of interappendage phase during locomotion. *Am. Zool.*, **14**:1003–1016.

Stein, P. S. G. (1976). Mechanisms of interlimb phase control. In *Neural Control of Locomotion*, R. M. Herman, S. Grillner, P. S. G. Stein, D. G. Stuart, eds. Plenum, New York, pp. 456–487.

Stein, P. S. G. (1978). Swimming movements elicited by electrical stimulation of the turtle spinal cord: the high spinal preparation. *J. Comp. Physiol.*, **124**:203–210.

Strumwasser, F. (1967). Types of information stored in a single neuron. In *Invertebrate Nervous Systems*, C. A. G. Wiersma, ed. Univ. of Chicago Press, Chicago, pp. 291–319.

Trelstad, R. L., J. P. Revel, and E. D. Hay, (1966). Tight junctions between cells in the early chick embryo as visualized with the electron microscope. *J. Cell Biol.*, **31**:C6–C10.

Tsien, R. W., R. S. Kass, and R. Weingart (1979). Cellular and subcellular mechanisms of cardiac pacemaker oscillations. *J. Exp. Biol.*, **81**:205–215.

Wendler, G. (1966). The coordination of walking movements in arthropods. *Symp. Soc. Exp. Biol.*, **20**:229–249.

Winfree, A. T. (1967). Biological rhythms and the behavior of populations of coupled oscillators. *J. Theor. Biol.*, **16**:15–42.

Winfree, A. T. (1980). *The Geometry of Biological Time*. Springer, New York.

Weeks, J. C. (1981). Neuronal basis of leech swimming: separation of swim initiation, pattern selection, and intersegmental coordination by selective lesions. *J. Neurophysiol.*, **45**:698–723.

Chapter Eleven

THE ROLES OF SYNTHETIC MODELS IN THE STUDY OF CENTRAL PATTERN GENERATORS

BRIAN MULLONEY

Department of Zoology
University of California
Davis, California

DONALD H. PERKEL

Psychobiology Department
University of California
Irvine, California

1 INTRODUCTION

When we set out to understand how the central nervous system generates a motor pattern, we set out to understand the dynamic performance of a complex system with nonlinear parts. Static summaries of the synaptic organization of the pattern generating circuits, like those reviewed in earlier chapters, can only be the beginnning of our understanding. To proceed from these circuit diagrams to a grasp of the dynamic performance of the circuit, we must add a description of the important active responses of the component neurons, and some quantitative description of the properties of their synapses. These additions are not impossible; physiologists who work regularly with a pattern generating circuit often develop an ability to predict quantitatively the outcome of the different physiological perturbations and to explain in semiquantitative terms how the system works. Their abilities depend on a quantitative feel for the cellular properties of the neurons involved, and ideas about the sources of the circuit's performance. However, to test these ideas as formal hypotheses or to teach the explanation to critical colleagues who lack the same experience is difficult and sometimes impossible without incorporating these quantitative properties into the circuit diagram, in other words, without a quantitative model of the system.

Several different motives lead people to construct synthetic models. These models can state succinctly the results of some experiments, and at the same time illustrate the author's ideas about the meaning of these results. They can be used in the context of a working hypothesis to test the sufficiency of experimental data to account for the performance of the system. Synthetic models based on experimental data can, like input-output models, be used to predict and control the performance of the system they describe (e.g., Edelson, 1981), although practical applications of this type are rare in neurobiology. Synthetic models are also useful in testing the plausibility of a complex idea or hypothesis, particularly of an inherently quantitative idea that can only be evaluated by systematic and quantitative exploration of its consequences. Once a model has been explored and tested to the point where we can be confident that it describes well and predicts accurately the performance of the real nervous system, the model can be used to do thought experiments that are either technically infeasible in the real nervous system, or that explore novel combinations of parameters that describe non-existent variants of the nervous system. Such explorations are one way to discover whether the observed natural range of performance is an accident of the nervous system's evolutionary history, or is a reflection of severe natural selection.

This chapter attempts to introduce readers to synthetic models of neuronal dynamics, to illustrate them with selected examples, and to discuss critically the requirements of a successful model. We hope to encourage more neurobiologists to tackle the problems of understanding these dynamic systems, to show how quantitative models can help, and to give readers some guidance in making the critical decisions that determine the success of their own modeling efforts. The examples were chosen to illustrate alternative forms a model might take and to highlight the critical abstractions and simplifications that are needed for a successful model of any complex system. This chapter is divided into four sections that treat, first, the preludes to construction of a model and the various forms the model might take, and then review examples of models of single neurons and neuronal circuits.

TABLE 1. Examples of Neural Phenomena and the Levels of Analysis
Appropriate to Them

	Level	Phenomena
(Animals)	Behavior	Movements Perception
(Brains)	Systems of circuits	Motor patterns Modulation
(Motor and sensory nuclei & cortical columns)	Circuits of neurons	Dynamics of circuit
(Cells)	Neurons	Synaptic integration Active responses Connectivity
(Macromolecules)	Membranes, channels, and receptors	Voltage-gated and transmitter-gated currents

2 WHAT IS A SYNTHETIC MODEL?

Synthetic models are formal conceptual constructs made by abstracting
from our knowledge of a nervous system's organization and from the data
about its performance those factors that are most important. Synthetic
models differ from "black box models" that are based solely on the relations between input and output because they include a hypothesis about
how the nervous system achieves the observed performance. Successful
synthetic models have two characteristics: they duplicate and predict satisfactorily the performance of the nervous system, and they provide
insight into the mechanism of the system. Richard Levins (quoted in
Schoener, 1972) stated four desirable features of any model—generality,
precision, reality, and analytical tractability—and concluded that most
models achieve at best two. From the perspective of neurobiology, Levins
is an optimist.

Nervous systems are rather more complex than most systems that have
been modeled successfully. This complexity is apparent in the several levels at which we study them (Table 1), and the phenomena that we attempt
to understand. If a model is to succeed, it is critical to choose a level of
description appropriate to the phenomenon we want to understand. At
this level, the model needs accuracy and realistic detail. At lower levels,
the model needs thoughtful simplification and abstraction. Channel kinetics and Ca^{++} concentrations are not the stuff of models of the whole cortex. The need for simplification and abstraction comes in part from the
biological complexity of neurons and synaptic circuits, and in part from

the limited formalisms available to describe them.For example, real neurons have many voltage-sensitive and transmitter-gated currents that interact to control their membrane potentials (reviewed in Adams et al., 1980). In a heterogeneous collection of neurons, each kind will have its characteristic mix of currents (Smith, 1978; Partridge et al., 1979; Hume et al., 1982). Under the best of conditions, it is difficult to separate, measure and describe each of these currents, and in many interesting circuits it is all but impossible. If the neuron is not isopotential, the shape of a neuron will also affect the interactions of these currents. The available methods to take into account a neuron's shape can describe accurately the integration of synaptic and active currents in a neuron, but to use them complicates the description of each neuron in a circuit. These biological and conceptual problems, then, put a premium on insightful simplification of the system at the beginning of the modelling effort. We will see that the most successful efforts have either ignored most active responses or ignored the integrative structures of neurons in the circuit.

3   THE POSSIBLE FORMS OF A MODEL

Synthetic models of a given circuit can take different forms, and the form chosen to implement the model can determine its success or failure. The major alternatives are continuous mathematical models, discrete mathematical models, and analog models. The common approach to a description of a neuron or a circuit in mathematical terms is to write a differential equation that describes the currents that flow in each neuron or region of neurons as functions of equilibrium potentials, membrane resistances and capacitances, transmitter-gated changes in resistance, and resistive coupling to other parts of the circuit. The underlying notion is that Ohm's Law and Kirchhoff's Law apply to neurons too, and so can be used to describe quantitatively the flow of ions across the membrane and throughout each neuron (Rall, 1977). It is an important virtue of such models of ionic currents, synaptic integration, and passive properties that they follow naturally from a consideration of the physical properties of membranes and currents, and so can be interpreted in mechanistic terms. This is a powerful approach because the description—the model—is in a form that can be manipulated with the tools of linear algebra and numerical integration, which have been thoroughly developed for similar systems of equations by engineers, economists, and applied mathematicians (e.g., Churchhouse, 1981). A continuous mathematical model is the best form for quantitative analysis of the factors that underlie a circuit's dynamics because the tools of mathematics are well suited to such analyses. For individual neurons, or for small circuits with relatively simple properties, mathematical models can sometimes be analysed directly, and major properties of the system can be explored and explained directly from this analysis (e.g.,

Zucker, 1973). Plant, in a lucid paper written for biologists (1982), has illustrated how phase-plane analysis, singular perturbation theory and bifurcation theory can be used to understand the equations that describe the currents that cause bursts of impulses in some gastropod neurons. Analyses like Plant's could usefully be performed for small sets of synapsing neurons, and might lead to a better understanding of the motor patterns they produce.

Continuous models can treat both the dynamics of interactions between neurons and integration of currents within one neuron. For cases where the numbers of neurons are small and the circuit is known in some detail, two alternative schemes are in common use for constructing a continuous mathematical model of the passive, or linear, electrical structure of a neuron that includes information about the neuron's shape: equivalent-cylinder models and compartmental models. Both describe a neuron as a set of regions linked by cytoplasmic resistances. The equivalent cylinder scheme finds the dimensions of a membrane-bound cylinder of cytoplasm that has electrical properties equivalent to those of the neuron's different branches, and then solves the equations that describe this cylinder.* The model can, therefore, be as structurally simple as is appropriate for the questions being addressed, and a useful array of mathematical tools is available to solve these models as a problem in one-dimensional cable theory (Jack et al., 1975). Provided the original neuron's dimensions fall within a well-defined set of size relations, the spread of current in the entire branching structure can be analysed (Rall, 1977). Koch and Poggio (1985) have developed an algorithm that overcomes this limitation on the structures that can be analysed with this approach.

A compartmental model represents a neuron as a set of interconnected regions, each with a resistance and capacitance to ground, and connected to other regions by coupling resistances (Rall, 1977). Compartmental models are not restricted to particular size relations in the structures of a neuron's branches. Such models can accurately describe the integration of synaptic currents in a neuron when they are developed from measurements of the neuron's membrane resistance and measurements of the neuron's shape (Perkel and Mulloney, 1978 a,b; Perkel, Mulloney, and Budelli, 1981; Edwards and Mulloney, 1984; Johnston and Brown, 1983; Glantz and Viancour, 1983). The mathematical tools used to solve the equations of a compartmental model are different from those used for equivalent-cylinder models, but the two approaches yield the same answers when applied to the same problem (e.g., Perkel and Mulloney, 1978a). A com-

---

*The appendix of Rall (1981) is a remarkably detailed and explicit description of his procedure for constructing equivalent-cylinder models. This description merits careful study by anyone who wants to build structurally detailed models. It also could be a specification for an interactive computer program that would construct such models from parameters given by the user.

partmental model whose structure reflects the shape of the original neuron can, therefore, be used to analyze how that neuron integrated synaptic currents, and how currents that originated at well-defined anatomical loci interact in the dendritic structure of the neuron.

Discrete models simplify a neuron to a simple threshold device that exists in a few discrete states, e.g., firing or silent. The transition between states is then controlled by summing the states of other neurons connected to it (e.g., McCulloch and Pitts, 1943; Szekely, 1965; Thompson and Gibson, 1981a,b). These models also have a mathematical form, but do not include time as a continuous parameter. Rather, they impose a rigid, discontinuous structure on the time variable. The power of such models is that they formalize the synaptic organization of a neural circuit so that the consequences and probabilities of a state change in a neuron, from firing to silent, can be analysed in an orderly way. Discrete models force us to focus on the synaptic organization of a circuit, and to isolate the consequences of this organization.

Analog models are usually made of electronic components. The simplest such model—a parallel resistor and capacitor to ground used to simulate a neuron in a recording circuit—is familiar to most electrophysiologists. Analog models of the passive properties of neurons and circuits of neurons are useful tools, and have the singular virtue that most electrophysiologists can understand them by inspection. More elaborate models use batteries, transistors, and resistor networks to simulate active responses and synaptic integration (e.g., Lewis, 1968). The principal attribute of these models is that their parameters can be adjusted rapidly, and their performance— or output—can be examined with the same tools used to study the real nervous system. They can usually be comprehended and used by neurophysiologists without the need to employ unfamiliar or long-forgotten mathematical tools, and they are particularly useful in calibrating and testing experimental apparatus.

All these forms have inherent problems and limitations, consideration of which make clear the importance of the choice of form, and of the level of description and understanding desired.

3.1   Problems with Mathematical Models

Three problems must be tackled before any mathematical approach can be successful. The first is biological, and calls for insightful simplification; each parameter in each equation must be specified before the equations can be solved. An analysis of the equations, like that illustrated by Plant (1982), does not require this specification, but if one wants to know what the membrane potential will be in a particular neuron or branch or *bouton* at some future time, then the equations must be solved, and that means one must specify the parameters.Clearly, the initial advantage is to models with few parameters.

For continuous models, the necessary parameters include the membrane time constant, and the resistances or capacitances of each region. The membrane time constant is needed to calculate R_m, the specific membrane resitivity. In different biological membranes, R_m ranges from 10^{-3} to at least 10^3 kohm·cm² (e.g., Keynes and Martins-Ferreira, 1953; Bennett, 1971; Gorman and Mirolli, 1972), and we have no a priori guide to the appropriate choice of this parameter for any kind of neuron. The specification of R_m is too important to leave to guesswork, particularly since R_m can be measured. To do so, the voltage response to a step of current is analysed as the sum of a constant and a series of exponential functions (e.g., Rall, 1969; Brown et al., 1981; Edwards and Mulloney, 1984). This sum can be used to write an expression that accurately predicts all linear voltage responses of the neuron. The necessary exponential series can be recovered from the voltage response by peeling the exponentials off the log transform of the voltage response in time. Peeling is a recursive procedure for fitting a regression line to the straight portion of a semilog plot of voltage against time, subtracting the regression line from the data, and replotting the results until the last data points are well fitted by the last regression. Given biological data, the usual limit of this procedure is three peels, and so three regression lines. The intercepts and slopes of each regression line then become coefficients and time constants in the exponential series (Rall, 1969). Because the specific capacitance of the membrane, C_m, is 1.0 μF/cm² (Rall, 1977), and the time constant of the membrane, T_m, is the same as the longest time constant in the measured series of exponentials, we can calculate

$$R_m = \frac{\tau_m}{c_m} \tag{1}$$

if we assume the specific resistance of the membrane, R_m, is uniform. The series of exponentials that can be peeled from a neuron's passive voltage response also describes the properties of a multi-region RC network, a compartmental model, that closely approximates the responses of the neuron, and can be used to specify the values of each component of that network (Edwards and Mulloney, 1984). Two papers that treat, from the perspective of pharmacology, the problems of alternative interpretations of multiexponential series and errors in their measurement should be read and considered by anyone who uses these methods (DeStefano and Landaw, 1984; Landaw and DeStefano, 1984).

The second problem with continuous mathematical models is conceptual, and arises particulary when the equations don't have an explicit algebraic solution, but must be solved numerically. An algebraic solution to an equation, or set of equations, is a solution obtained by applying the rules of algebra and calculus to obtain a function that satisfies the relationship described by the equation. Not all differential equations have algebraic solutions (Uspensky, 1948), and insoluble equations often arise when membrane conductances or experimental or synaptic currents are concentration-dependent or vary in time. Nonetheless, numerical methods exist to use these "unsolvable" equations to calculate the time-courses of neuronal properties and the dynamics of circuits, once the parameters and initial conditions have been specified. These numerical methods are powerful, but they are not intuitive, and are not part of the intellectual armory of most biologists. Edelson (1981) stated the conceptual problem clearly: "The use of mathematics to obtain the behavior of a physical or chemical system from [a synthetic] model yields a description in which the variables are related to each other by functions that contain parameters characteristic of various components of the model. If this description can be obtained in analytic form, the dependence of the behavior on these parameters is transparent, and it is a simple matter to calculate the effect of changes in them, or to see the relative importance of parts of the model. When these solutions must be obtained by computer, however, this connection between input and output is lost, and the more complex the model becomes, the more difficult it is to deduce the parts of the mechanism responsible for certain features of the simulation, or to see how changes would affect this behavior." This problem limits us in two ways. For the one who makes the model, the insight and predictions that were the goal of the modeling effort come at the expense of repeated calculations with slightly varied parameters. When the original equations are stiff (see below), the time required for these calculations may be forbidding. Worse, once the insight and predictions are achieved, other colleagues unfamiliar with numerical methods of solution will inevitably maintain an unhealthy scepticism about the original statement of the problem, the choice of parameters and the relation of the model to reality.

The third problem is mathematical and arises when the circuit under study produces a motor pattern that has a period seconds long and the factors thought to regulate that period have time-constants that are much briefer, perhaps less than a millisecond. Systems of equations that describe slow processes governed by fast rate-constants are called stiff equations, and their numerical solution encounters interesting difficulties. Numerical integration can be as accurate as a biologist could wish, but the time necessary to solve a system of equations grows with the number of equations and the number of terms in each equation, as well as with the length of time one wishes to simulate. We are fortunate that a quarter of a century of effort has already gone into efficient methods for solving these beasts (e.g., Hamming, 1973; Forsythe, Malcolm, and Moler, 1977). Today, biologists have available well-developed packages of subroutines for the integration of stiff equations (e.g, Plant, 1979; Byrne, 1981) and are well-advised to use these packages, if they cannot avoid the basic problem.

3.2   Problems with Discrete Models

Because discrete models simplify each neuron to a two-state device, they are ill-suited to an analysis of the roles of continuous cellular phenomena, like accommodation or postinhibitory rebound or spatial integration, in the performance of the circuit. They are also inappropriate for the calculation of the time-courses of motor patterns or the time-courses of perturbations that the user might want to simulate, because time is not a continuous variable in these models. In the context of this review, these criticisms are tautologous, but they have occasionally been forgotten by enthusiasts for models of this form*.

3.3   Problems with Analog Models

All these difficulties recommend analog circuits as alternative forms for modeling neural circuits. Analog models also require specification of each parameter, but once this is done, construction can go quickly. Analog models of the active properties are difficult to design, construct and comprehend, but their components are familiar enough to electrophysiologists, and their output can be so like that of the nervous system that we can be lulled into accepting them uncritically as successful models of the system under study without testing their performance carefully. The most serious shortcoming of analog models is that, for most of them, it is difficult to measure the various parameters of the model during a simulation, or to set and to vary these parameters systematically. It is also difficult to calculate the standard deviations, confidence limits, and other statistics that give the reader some guidance to the robustness of the results. For this reason, the analog models now available are ill-suited to a quantitative exploration of a complex non-linear system.

4   EXAMPLES OF SYNTHETIC MODELS

This section presents and criticizes examples selected to illustrate both forms of models and the simplifications and abstractions that went into their construction. It includes not only models of locomotory systems but also of single neurons and of networks of receptors, selected because they illustrate particularly well the use of synthetic models to test hypotheses. The section begins with models that ignore the shapes of neurons, and then reviews more complex models that include shape as a factor governing synaptic integration.

---

*For example, Thompson and Gibson (1981a) dismiss as "secondary effects" all time-dependent neuronal features and phenomena, including the membrane's time constant and changes in excitability, and the time-courses of synaptic potentials.

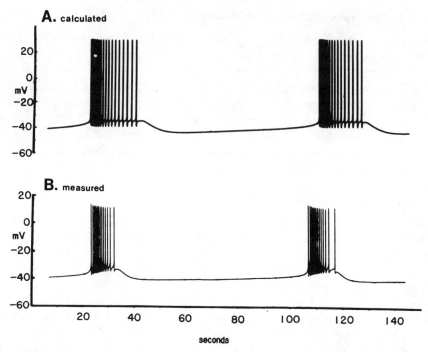

FIGURE 1. (A) Membrane potential waveform calculated from voltage clamp descriptions of seven ionic currents. (B) Membrane potential waveform recorded in *Tritonia* cell LP1 3 at 10° C. From Smith (1978).

4.1   Models That Ignore the Integrative Structures of Neurons

4.1.1   *Endogenous Bursters*

The endogenous bursts of impulses that occur in a few identified neurons in gastropods, crustaceans, and leeches have a broad appeal and fascination for neurophysiologists. After repeated earlier attempts to explain this property in terms of membrane currents or other cellular phenomena, two simultaneous independent efforts constructed similar successful explanations that the interplay of an inward Ca^{++} current and a Ca^{++}-gated K^+-current would lead to bursts of impulses (Smith, 1978; Plant, 1978). These two papers, then, addressed the same question but from different perspectives. They each succeeded in part because they simplified a bursting neuron to a system of membrane currents and a Ca^{++} concentration and chose to ignore the neurons' size and shape.

Smith set out to measure all the membrane currents he could find in a neuron that fired bursts of impulses. He found seven, measured them, and summed these currents to calculate the total membrane current:

$$I_M = C_s \, dV/dt + I_I + I_K + I_A + I_B + I_C + I_D + I_L \qquad (2)$$

He then calculated membrane potential as a function of time using this equation and supplementary equations that described the kinetics of each current, to see if potential oscillated in time. He also asked how closely such an oscillatory solution resembled the bursts of impulses that occur in the neuron itself. Thus, the model Smith constructed was a test both of the plausibility of the hypothesis—that bursts can arise because of the interactions of membrane currents—and of the adequacy of his experimental measurements to describe these currents. The ability of Smith's model to predict the behavior of these neurons is impressive (Fig. 1). This result supports the original hypothesis and increases our confidence that he identified and measured accurately the significant currents in these neu-

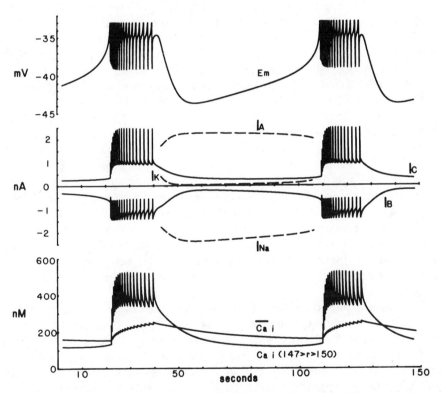

FIGURE 2. Time courses of selected variables calculated in reconstructing the burst cycle. Time axes in each panel are identical and simultaneous. Top panel shows same membrane potential waveform as Figure 1A. Expanded vertical scale truncates spikes but emphasizes subthreshold potential variations. Middle panel shows variations of individual ionic current components, identified by capital letters near each trace. For clarity, all traces except I_B and I_C have been suppressed during the firing burst (but see Fig. 3). I_D is not shown in this figure since it is within the trace width of zero a all times, except during action potentials. Bottom panel shows variations of intracellular calcium concentrations near the inner membrane surface and as a volume average throughout the cell, as indicated. From Smith (1978).

rons. There may be yet other factors that influence bursting here, but these currents suffice for a detailed explanation.

Smith's model, because it was written in a mathematical form that allowed him to explore the behavior of its variables in time, also yielded new insights into the quantitative interplay of these membrane currents during an action potential and during a burst of impulses (Figs. 2, 3). Two of them, I_B and I_C, interact with a long duration hysteresis that is the source of the burst period. I_B is an inward Ca^{++} current, and I_C is Ca^{++}-gated. These are quite small currents relative to those that occur during each impulse, but together they govern the periodicity of bursts of impulses in the neuron. These results point out the significance of the small components of membrane current in all neurons, components that can sculpt the neuron's dynamic properties.

Plant's (1978) hypothesis was based on insightful consideration of other workers' experimental data. He constructed two alternative models that described different hypotheses about how Ca^{++} interacts with the Ca^{++}-dependent K^+-channels. One model treated Ca^{++} concentration as the significant variable, the other model treated Ca^{++} binding as a function of the voltage field across the channel. His models, then, are examples of a test of the plausibility of a quantitative hypothesis. His results establish that these hypotheses are both plausible, but favor the Ca^{++}-concentration version. Further investigation of Smith's equation reveals a high degree of sensitivity to Ca^{++} parameters and confirms Plant's preference for the Ca^{++}-concentration alternative (Perkel, unpublished). Small changes in the time constants for removal of Ca^{++} from the outmost shell of cytoplasm produce marked changes in the structure of a burst and in the duration of the interburst interval. Like the related work of Chay and Rinzel (1985), these simulations imply that minor variations in the regulation of free Ca^{++} can drastically affect the rhythmic behavior of the neuron, and suggest an explanation for the marked temperature sensitivity characteristic of this bursting behavior (Smith and S. H. Thompson, personal communication).

Plant also explored the mathematical properties of the equations that described the hypothetical membrane currents, and of their solutions. He assigned values to each parameter in the equations, solved them numerically to demonstrate the periodic bursts of impulses and their responses to imposed currents, and then explored the ranges of parameters within which his models would generate stable bursts. Plant (1981) continued this analysis by considering how the consequences of different experimental manipulations of a bursting neuron, e.g., TTX poisoning, are predicted by his model. These continuous mathematical models, although they required numerical solutions, have led to a deeper understanding of the dynamics of endogenously bursting neurons. Plant's analysis of the stability of the periodic solution and of the bifurcations that occur is an excellent introduction for the biologist to these modes of thought. It also generates a deep interpretation of the real neuron's performance.

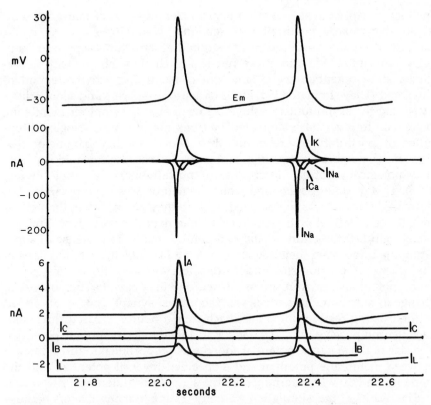

FIGURE 3. Time courses of ionic currents during reconstructed action potential firing. Time axes in each panel are identical and simultaneous. Values shown are from the same computing run as those in Fig. 3, but with the time scale expanded as indicated on the abscissa. The top panel shows the reconstructed membrane potential waveform; the lower two panels show membrane currents plotted with two different vertical scale factors to accommodate the differing magnitudes of the seven components. The behavior of ionic currents is essentially the same during each action potential of the burst, except for the changes in I_B and I_C evident in Fig. 2. From Smith (1978).

4.1.2 The Dynamics of Small Circuits

Here we review five cases that illustrate particular strategies of modeling neuronal circuits. The first two cases look at reciprocal inhibitory networks—one theoretical and one controversial. The third case analyzes networks of photoreceptors with complex membrane currents. The fourth considers a pattern-generating network with complex synapses. Finally, we look at discrete models and analog models of recurrent inhibition.

The notion that neurons organized by reciprocal inhibitory synapses would fire alternately goes back at least to Brown (1911). Attempts to analyze the plausibility of this idea and the consequences of various synaptic and cellular properties in such circuits have been made by many authors. Perkel and Mulloney (1974) simulated pairs of neurons with reciprocal inhibitory synapses to see what influence different kinds of neuronal excitability, particularly postinhibitory rebound, would have on the motor patterns the pairs produced. They ignored all structural aspects of neurons; each simulated neuron was merely a patch of membrane with a specified resting potential, membrane time-constant and activity-dependent threshold. They simulated two kinds of neurons—pacers and silent cells—by setting the asymptotic threshold below or above asymptotic membrane potential. To give these simulated neurons the phenomenological properties of postinhibitory rebound, they added another parameter that decreased membrane potential and also decreased threshold—a phenomenologically correct description of postinhibitory rebound (Perkel, 1976). This parameter increased when the neuron was hyperpolarized but decreased when it was depolarized, and decayed more slowly than either membrane potential or threshold when the neuron was at rest. This parameter, in fact the entire model of a neuron, made no pretense of simulating the underlying membrane currents and pumps that are the basis of the emergent phenomena under consideration—the fluctuating membrane potentials and thresholds of neurons in a circuit. The sources of change in membrane potentials were simulated synaptic potentials added to the existing resting potentials. Each time a neuron crossed threshold, each neuron postsynaptic to it had a PSP added to its membrane potential. The size of the synaptic potential added was proportional to the difference between membrane potential and a specified reversal potential, and the sign of each PSP was determined by the sign of this difference.

The results of this simulation were interesting to many readers because they showed not only that the circuit performed as predicted when pacers were used (Fig. 4A) or when excitatory synaptic drive was shared by both neurons—results that had been reported by earlier authors, e.g., Wilson and Waldron (1968)—but also that stable alternating bursts would be produced from pairs of silent neurons if they once were stimulated to fire, as long as the parameters that described rebound fell within a modestly broad range of values (Fig. 4B). Furthermore, the period and intensity of the bursts of impulses in these alternating neurons could be modulated by other synaptic input to the neurons. A final insight from these simulations was that the dominant factor that determined the period of the motor patterns that emerged during the simulations was the time-constant of the rebound parameter. In cellular terms, this means that the kinetics of the small currents that affect excitability—currents like those described by Smith, above—could set the period of motor patterns, and, therefore, must be attended to by physiologists attempting to understand how a neuronal circuit worked.

These insights were achieved from consideration of a restricted subset of a neuron's features; no membrane currents and no spatial integration of synaptic potentials were simulated as such. Therefore, the results of this simulation are, at most, a test of the plausibility of the original hypothe-

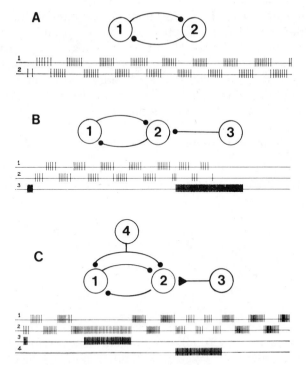

FIGURE 4. Impulse trains in pairs of reciprocally inhibitory neurons that exhibit postinhibitory rebound. In the circuit diagrams, a dark circle indicates an inhibitory synapse, the triangle indicates an excitatory synapse, and the numbers refer to the "neurons" whose activity is displayed on lines of impulse traces. (A) Pacemaker neurons; spontaneous development of stable pattern of alternating bursts; the pattern continues indefinitely. (B) Nonpacemaker neurons. The burst pattern is triggered by a brief barrage of small IPSPs to neuron 2; the pattern continues until stopped by a longer barrage of IPSPs diminishing in size, produced by the same axon. (C) Modification and resetting of pattern by sustained input. An excitatory barrage to one neuron interrupts the pattern, which resumes after excitation stops. Weak inhibition of both neurons decreases the number of spikes in each burst and increases the rate of alternation; the pattern is subsequently restored. Redrawn from Perkel & Mulloney (1974).

sis—that postinhibitory rebound could stabilize the firing of reciprocally inhibitory neurons into patterns of alternating bursts of impulses. Furthermore, no hypotheses about the underlying cellular mechanisms from which rebound emerges were included, so these simulations could not contribute to discussion of the basis of rebound. The simulation was truly synthetic, however, because it included a hypothesis about the consequences of cellular phenomena for a circuit of neurons, a hypothesis about the source of the motor pattern.

More recently, we have repeated this analysis, first by constructing circuits of neurons with time-dependent synaptic conductances, synaptic currents that were proportional to membrane potential and a phenomenologically accurate model of postinhibitory rebound (Mulloney et al., 1981), and then with voltage-sensitive membrane currents (Perkel, unpublished). Both new models described the physiological properties of neurons more accurately than did the original work, and both confirm the original insights and conclusions. The additional details affect the internal structures of individual bursts, but burst period was determined primarily by the time-course of postinhibitory rebound.

4.1.3   Reciprocal Inhibition of Flight Motor Neurons in Flies

The five motor neurons that innervate each dorsolongitudinal muscle of flies fire in a distinctive pattern. Each neuron fires one impulse at a time when the rest are silent; together they form a phase-constant pattern that is stable as spike-frequency changes. The order in which they fire is not immutable, but a few of the possible patterns are much more common than the others, and the physiological basis of these patterns has provoked an interesting and protracted controversy. The hypotheses that have been proposed describe two different kinds of synaptic organization among these motor neurons. Wilson (1966) and Wyman (1966) proposed that these neurons were reciprocally inhibitory; each neuron inhibited each of the others that innervated the muscle. Wilson explored the consequences of this idea using an early simulation program that summed synaptic potentials (an antecedent of Perkel, 1976), and demonstrated that reciprocal inhibition could generate phase-constant patterns in the face of frequency changes. Subsequent experimental work demonstrated that the neurons responded to antidromic stimulation as if they were themselves in a reciprocally inhibitory synaptic network (Mulloney, 1970), and these data have been confirmed repeatedly (Levine, 1973; Harcombe and Wyman, 1977). It was interesting, then, that Koenig and Ikeda (1980) proposed a different hypothesis about the organization of these neurons. They proposed that these motor neurons are electrically coupled, and that the electrical synapses are the source of the motor pattern. Well-formed alternative hypotheses like these are well-suited to exploration by modeling.

Friesen and Wyman (1980) constructed a simulation of the reciprocal inhibition hypothesis using the same analog neurons—Lewis neuromimes (Lewis, 1968)—that Wilson and Waldron had used much earlier. Friesen and Wyman constructed a relatively precise model of the reciprocal inhibition hypothesis. They assigned relative synaptic strengths to each synapse in the network, using values calculated by Harcombe and Wyman (1977) from parameters of the motor patterns, and asked if this analog network displayed properties similar to the neurons in the fly. Neuromimes can run as long as the power is on, and can be adjusted to fire impulses at selected frequencies, so the simulation could run indefinitely. However, unlike the fly, the free-running analog circuit was a strictly determined device, and would lock into one output pattern unless perturbed by some extraneous event. Friesen and Wyman used two kinds of perturbations in different experiments—random, low frequency stimulation of one neuromime through an "excitatory synapse" and low-frequency antidromic stimulation of individual neuromimes. They then asked how similar were the probabilities of particular firing sequences in the fly and the model, and how similar were the responses of the fly and the model to antidromic stimulation? For proponents of the reciprocal inhibition hypothesis, the results were gratifyingly similar. The authors also asked how sensitive these results were to variations in parameters like synaptic strength and inherent firing frequency. They found that the stability of the output was relatively insensitive to these parameters, and they were able to predict from their results that the effects of the putative IPSPs should last at least 15% of the normal interspike interval in each unit. This is, in principle, a testable prediction.

However, this paper has not resolved the outstanding question about the relative merits of the two contradictory hypotheses. Because the synaptic parameters assigned were not determined by independent measurements in the fly, but, rather, were inferred from the motor pattern itself, and because the simulations were relatively insensitive to these parameters, the significance of the paper is limited to, at most, a test of the plausibility of the reciprocal inhibition hypothesis. The paper also did not attempt to model the electrical coupling hypothesis, or to see if the reciprocal inhibition model could generate results like those of Koenig and Ikeda (1980). Therefore, the reader has no new information with which to choose between these conflicting ideas.

4.1.4 Transients in the Receptor Network of Vertebrate Retinas

To choose to review a model of a receptor network in a book concerned with motor control may seem odd, but one of the best quantitative analyses of the contributions of active membrane properties to network dynamics was done on such a network, and the approach to experimental measurement and theoretical synthesis taken in that analysis could be applied successfully to some problems of motor-pattern generation. The rods and cones in vertebrate eyes are spaced in a regular mosaic, and are coupled together by weak electrical synapses. A small spot of light flashed onto the retina causes a voltage change not only in the illuminated receptors but also in receptors some distance away. Surprisingly, the time required following the onset of a flash to reach the peak of the voltage, was shorter in rods further away from a bar of light that in rods close to it (Detwiler, Hodgkin, and McNaughton, 1978).

Attwell and Wilson (1980) combined measurements of the currents in individual rods and of the coupling between pairs of rods to test the hypothesis that the surprising performance of the rod network was the result of the interaction of currents spreading through the electrical synapses and a membrane current, unfortunately called by them I_A. This is *not* the same I_A known in molluscan and vertebrate neurons. This study began with a careful physiological demonstration that individual rods are isopotential. This means that rods can properly be considered to be patches of membrane without important spatial structure, a simplification these authors exploited in their simulations. Attwell and Wilson measured the size and kinetics of the membrane current, I_A, and the attenuation of voltage responses in increasingly distant rods to current injected into one rod. They then used these various measurements to build a model to test their initial hypothesis.

The form of their model was a set of coupled differential equations that described the membrane potential of each rod in the network as a function of current and time. The equations included the kinetics of the membrane currents, and terms to account for current spread through gap junctions to neighboring rods. Several simplifications appeared in the model; the rods were considered to be uniform patches of membrane with I_A, and to

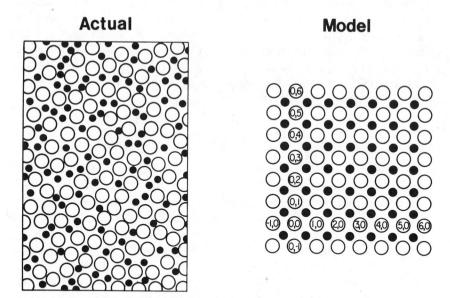

FIGURE 5. Comparison of actual and idealized arrangement of receptors in the retina. Actual arrangement is taken from a photomicrograph of an isolated flat-mounted retina focused at the level of the outer segments. The 120 rod outer segments in the field are shown as large open circles. The 107 cone outer segments are shown as small filled circles. Model: idealized arrangement of receptors assumed for computing the network behavior. Cones (filled circles) occupy the interstices of the square rod lattice (open circles). $\text{Rod}_{0,0}$ is the rod into which current is injected. Next neighbor rods are assumed to be coupled, so that $\text{rod}_{0,0}$ is coupled to $\text{rod}_{1,0}$, $\text{rod}_{0,-1}$, $\text{rod}_{-1,0}$ and $\text{rod}_{0,-1}$. Diagonal neighbors (e.g., $\text{rod}_{0,1}$ and $\text{rod}_{1,1}$) are assumed not to be directly coupled.

occur in a square lattice coupled by constant, uniform electrical synapses (Fig. 5). Electrical coupling to cones was ignored.

They then asked if their model could simulate their measured attenuation of response to injected current. Once they had tuned the parameter that described the resistance of the electrical coupling between rods, they found they could match the response of the retina satisfactorily, although this measured response had some significant nonlinearities (Fig. 6). At this point, they were ready to test their original hypothesis. To do so, they used an analytical function that described the photocurrent in an individual rod to simulate a bar of light shining on a row of rods, and calculated the time to peak voltage in rods increasingly distant from the bar. The time to peak was shorter the farther the rod was from the bar, as occurs in the retina and as predicted by their hypothesis (Fig. 7). This paradoxical behavior could be explained by an interaction between I_A in each rod and the rise-time of the spreading photocurrent, whose time-course is comparable to the time constant of I_A.

This is an excellent example of a model constructed both to test the plausibility of a hypothesis and to explore quantitatively its consequences. The rod I_A is an odd current whose amplitude when all channels are open is independent of membrane potential (see Attwell and Wilson, 1980), and it is not obvious that it would cause a resistively coupled network to behave as Detwiler et al. (1978) had reported. This quantitative simulation establishes that it does so.

Attwell, Wilson, and Wu (1984) extended this model by returning to the original assumption that rod-cone interactions were not significant factors in the performance of the rod network. Once they and their associates had described the membrane currents in isolated single- and double-cones, they incorporated this new information into an electrically coupled network of rods and cones, and calibrated the rod-cone coupling resistance by matching voltage-attenuation in their model to that measured with paired recordings from intact retina (Fig. 8). Then, they used the new model to test the hypothesis that the observed sensitivity to wavelength of rod and cone responses in the intact retina were caused by the synaptic network, and not by the intrinsic properties of either rods or cones. Their calculations of the rod and cone responses in the network, both for dim and bright lights, neatly predict the observed responses, and so support their hypothesis. The match between the observed and calculated responses also increases our confidence that this model is an accurate and reliable description of the receptor network. Attwell et al. then used it to calculate the spatial resolution of the rod network, and its responses to edges of light of different intensities moving at different speeds. Both of these calculations revealed that the model predicted the experimentally measured performance of the retina, and provided an explanation of this performance in terms of the circuit's organization and the membrane currents of individual receptors.

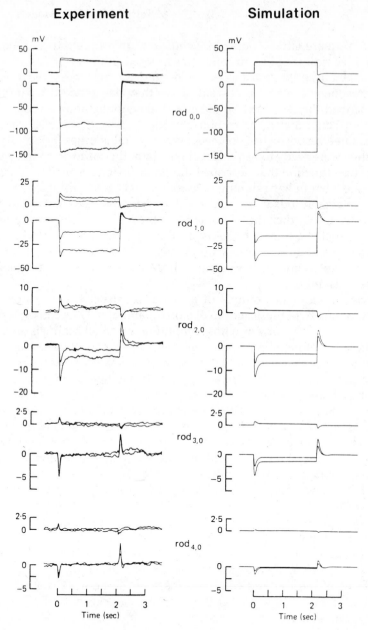

FIGURE 6 Measured and computed voltage responses of the rod network to injection of ±1 and ±2 nA current pulses into $rod_{0,0}$. Potentials measured with respect to resting potential. Pulse length was 2.14 s. Experiment: responses of rods at different distances from $rod_{0,0}$ (see Fig. 5 for nomenclature). At greater distances the responses become smaller and more transient, with a longer time-to-peak (e.g., for the 1 nA hyperpolarizing pulse the time to peak was 44 ms at $rd_{0,0}$ and 70 ms at $rod_{4,0}$. Depolarizing currents gave smaller responses than hyperpolarizing currents of the same magnitude. On terminating the 2 nA hyperpolarizing current pulse, the potential in $rod_{4,0}$ initially showed a positive overshoot which was followed by a small, but consistently observed, negative undershoot. From Attwell and Wilson (1980).

4.1.5   Escape Swimming in Tritonia

When the nudibranch *Tritonia diomedia* is confronted by a predator, it attempts to escape through a stereotyped sequence of swimming movements. The neural basis of this escape behavior has been studied by many workers (cf. Getting, 1983c, and this volume, for reviews) and a series of hypotheses based on experimental data have been proposed to explain it. Therefore, it is important to test quantitatively the ability of the more recent hypotheses to account for and explain the various parameters of swimming behavior. Getting (1983b) summarized the properties of the interneurons in the swim-circuit that he and his colleagues had described (Fig. 9A), and proposed that three factors—the network of monosynaptic connections, the dynamics of individual synaptic currents, and the accommodation characteristic of spike trains in certain neurons (Hume and Getting, 1982)—could together account quantitatively for the observed motor patterns. The plausibility of such a hypothesis can be tested by a simulation that includes accurate specifications of these factors. Getting constructed and tested a continuous mathematical model of the circuit (Fig. 9A) that condensed each group of neurons to an isopotential patch of membrane with complex synaptic conductances. He incorporated two currents into these membrane patches and included their temporal properties (Fig. 9B). He measured the input resistance, membrane time-constant, and resting potential of each kind of neuron, and incorporated these properties into the descriptions of each patch of membrane. Accommodation in each neuron was calibrated by fitting functions to experimental data and then simulated by an increase in potassium conductance. This is an example of

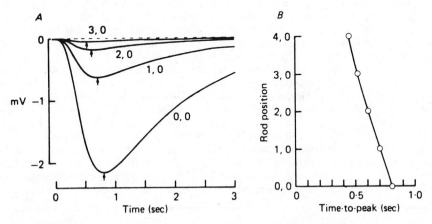

FIGURE 7. (A) Simulated photoresponses in the row of rods through $rod_{0,0}$ and $rod_{6,0}$, when a light bar falls on the row perpendicular to this through $rod_{0,0}$. Voltage response in $rod_{0,0}$ was taken from figure legend 6 of Detwiler et al. (1978). (B) Times-to-peak are shorter in the more distant rods, giving a negative conduction velocity as observed experimentally by Detwiler et al. (1978). This is produced by I_A. From Attwell and Wilson (1980).

EXPERIMENT   SIMULATION

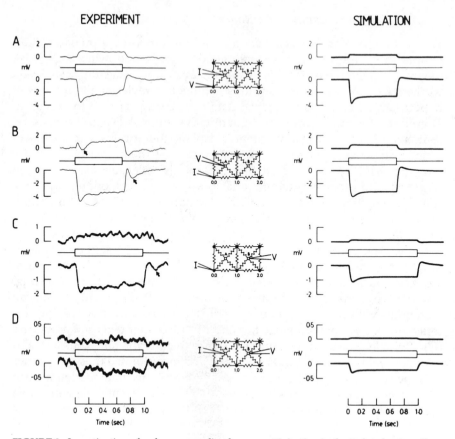

FIGURE 8. Investigation of rod-cone coupling by current injection in the isolated retina. Center insets: relative positions of the cells studied. Network geometry assumed is as described in the text. ●, denote rods, which are coupled to the four rods and the four cones around them. ○, denote cones, which are coupled only to the four rods around them. Resistors denote electrical synapses. Electrodes labelled I and V were sites of current injection and voltage recording respectively. Left-hand side: experimental results. (A) Response of a rod (resting potential −42 mV, denoted zero on the voltage scale) to injection of +1 nA (top trace) and −1 nA (bottom trace) into a next neighbor single cone (resting potential −41 mV). Current timing shown by center traces. (B) Response of a single cone to injection of ± 1 nA into a next neighbor rod. Same cells as in A. Arrows denote feed-back component of response. Two records averaged in A and B. (C) Response of a double cone to injection of ±1 nA into a rod 25 μm away. A transient feed-back hyperpolarization (arrow) was seen in this cone at the end of the −1 nA step, but not at the onset of the +1 nA step. (D) Response of a double cone to injection of ±1 nA into a single cone 15 μm away. Right-hand side: simulations of the data on the left from the properties of isolated rods and cones. From Attwell, et al. (1984).

436

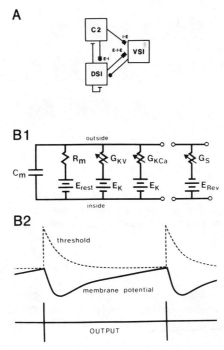

FIGURE 9. (A) Summary circuit diagram of the known monosynaptic connections between three populations of identified premotor interneurons that drive swimming in *Tritonia*. Excitatory connections are shown as T-bars, inhibitory connections as filled dots. Several of the monosynaptic connections are multicomponent and are indicated by mixed symbols. The temporal sequence for the multicomponent PSPs is indicated by the letter sequence: E, excitatory; I, inhibitory. (B) Conceptual basis for the reconstruction of neuron properties (B1) Equivalent circuit for a single neuron showing a single compartment that consists of the membrane resistance (R_m) in series with the resting potential (E_{rest}) paralleled by the input capacitance (C_m). The variable conductances (G_{KV} and G_{KCa}) and their associated potassium equilibrium potentials (E_K) represent the two time-dependent conductances added to mimic the time course of the spike afterpotential. Synaptic inputs to the compartment were added as a time-dependent conductance (G_s) associated with a reversal potential (E_{rev}). (B2) Representative time course of the threshold and membrane-potential variables during repetitive firing. When membrane potential equals the threshold value, the neuron is considered to have fired a spike, and the threshold variable is instantaneously elevated. Threshold then decays exponentially toward an asymptotic level (dotted line). At the same time, the two potassium conductances are activated to produce a membrane-potential trajectory similar to the spike afterpotential. Bottom trace shows the pulse output marking the time of threshold crossings. From Getting (1983).

the abstraction of lower-level phenomena necessary for successful modeling of higher-level hypotheses (Table 1).

The dynamics of each synapse were important to the hypothesis, so Getting then matched the PSPs in his model of each neuron to those recorded in real neurons in response to single presynaptic impulses by adjusting the amplitudes and time courses of the synaptic conductance. He

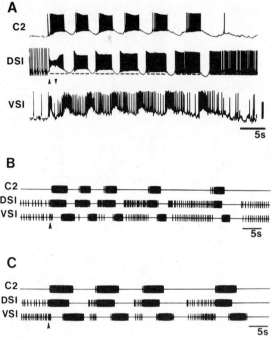

FIGURE 10. (A) Simultaneous intracellular recordings from three interneurons, a C2, DSI, and VSI, during a swim episode initiated by electrical stimulation of cerebral nerve 2 at 10 Hz for 1 s at arrows below the DSI trace. The dotted line under the DSI trace is a reference line at −45 mV to illustrate the ramp depolarization underlying the burst pattern. Voltage calibrations: 40 mV for C2 and DSI, 20 mV for VSI. (B) Simulated swim pattern. An extrinsic synaptic input to the DSI was stimulated at 10 Hz for 1 s at the arrow to produce a prolonged ramp depolarization of the DSI. Each vertical bar represents the time of firing for each of the three interneuron types. (C) Simulated swim with spike-frequency adaptation reduced by a factor of 100. This simulated swim was initiated with the same extrinsic stimulus as used in Figure 10B, and used the same synaptic strengths and time courses. Despite reduction of spike-frequency adaptation, the network was capable of producing repetitive cycles with the correct order of activation (DSI-C2-VSI); however, cycle period was substantially lengthened because of the increased burst durations of C2 and VSI. From Getting (1983).

assumed that the performance of each synapse during a train of presynaptic impulses would be adequately mimicked by summing individual postsynaptic currents.

   The results of this reconstruction of the swim network are instructive. The simulated network reproduces several characteristics of a real bout of swimming (Figs. 10A,B). The two patterns are not spike-for-spike identical, but this is not a serious criticism because *Tritonia*'s motor patterns are also highly variable at this level of detail. The model does satisfactorily reproduce burst durations and phases, and also the increase in period characteristic of the real pattern. The quantitative match of these parameters means that the three factors in the original hypothesis can collectively account for these features of the slug's behavior.

Getting then tested the necessity of accommodation by repeating the simulation with this feature of each neuron reduced one hundred-fold (Fig. 10C). This change alters both burst duration and period; the resulting pattern is less like that in the real animal. This result confirms that accommodation is a critical feature of these neurons, and that the cellular mechanisms that cause it are relevant to a full understanding of *Tritonia's* behavior. The result also supports Perkel and Mulloney's (1974) contention that slow active properties will determine the period of pattern-generating networks.

Getting's model, then, is a good example of a test of a quantitative hypothesis based on experimental data. This model is both more detailed and more specific than the ones constructed by Perkel and Mulloney (1974) but less complete than that of Attwell and Wilson (1980), in that it omits the voltage-dependent properties of these currents. Disparities between the performance of the model and the real circuit led to the prediction of another group of interneurons, a prediction that has been confirmed (Getting, 1983b). The simulation with reduced accommodation is also an example of the use of a well-founded model to simulate changes in the circuit that do not occur in nature, simulations that increase our understanding.

4.1.6 Recurrent Inhibition and Swimming in Leeches

Our final example considers normal swimming by the leech, a form of locomotion that requires coordinated movements by more than twenty segments of the animal's body. This is a centrally generated metachronal motor pattern that is produced by the chain of more than 20 ganglia in the ventral nerve cord (reviewed in Friesen and Stent, 1978; Kristan and Weeks, 1983). A sustained effort by Stent, Kristan, and their colleagues to discover how this motor pattern is generated has produced an important series of hypotheses about the organization of the leech's nervous system. They described, from experimental demonstrations of synaptic connections, a circuit of synapses among five pairs of neurons in each pair of adjacent ganglia. These circuits formed a concatenated chain that, they hypothesized, linked the individual segmental pattern generators together into a coordinated system, and produced both the basic motor pattern characteristic of each ganglion and the metachronal phase-shift between ganglia.

Friesen and Stent (1977) considered this circuit from the perspective of Szekely's recurrent inhibition results (1965). They began by constructing a discrete model of the five membered ring, each member of which had three possible states: firing, inhibited, and recovering from inhibition. The timing of transitions between states was determined by the time needed for each neuron to recover from the inhibited state to the firing state. They analyzed this circuit and its transitions graphically, and demonstrated that the hypothesis was inherently plausible. This graphical analysis of the dynamics of this complex system made their hypothesis and the evidence for it accessible to many readers.

To test their hypothesis further, they predicted that the intersegmental conduction delays that they had measured, 20 ms, would be the major determinant of the intersegmental phase lag that characterized the normal metachronal motor pattern. This then became a quantitative hypothesis, and to test its plausibility they constructed an analog form of the circuit, using Lewis neuromimes, that had about the correct period and the measured intersegmental delay. Any such concatenated chain will have edge-effects, the anomalous behavior of links at the end of the chain, and Friesen and Stent properly took these into account. They demonstrated graphically and with the analog chain that ganglia in the midst of such a concatenated chain will have metachronal phase-shifts of the correct sign and magnitude, and that the intersegmental delay in part determines this phase-shift. This paper, therefore, is a good example of the use of discrete models and analog models to test the plausibility of a hypothesis. It presents clearly Szekely's ideas (1965) on recurrent inhibition in the context of a physiologically identified circuit, and its graphical presentations of the model's predictions are very effective.

Subsequent experimental work on the leech nerve cord has demonstrated a property not predicted by the concatenated ring model; individual isolated ganglia can produce the fundamentals of the swimming motor program after the intersegmental connections have been cut (Weeks, 1981). This result means that each ganglion contains a system of neurons competent to generate the basic segmental swimming rhythm, even when the concatenated rings have been broken. The synapses made by neurons in the rings might reinforce the pattern-generating properties of this system; this has not yet been analyzed. However, the neurons that project between ganglia to form each concatenated ring have the properties required to coordinate the pattern-generating activity in these ganglia into their characteristic metachronal phase, and the concatenated ring model remains the most well-founded model of how a nervous system generates a metachronal motor pattern.

4.2   Models That Incorporate the Shapes of Neurons

The integrative properties of a neuron cannot be decided by study of its anatomy alone. The neuron's anatomical structure is important, but its specific membrane resistance, R_m, is equally so (Rall, 1977), and this parameter must be measured physiologically. The cases we have reviewed so far have not considered spatial or size-related features of neurons, but some hypotheses require us to include these features. In this section, we will review four examples of synthetic models that incorporate different degrees of structural detail to test hypotheses that involve the shapes of neurons. The examples are increasingly complex.

4.2.1   The Size Principle in Spinal Motor Neurons

Experimentalists have regularly observed that, within a pool of motor neurons, smaller neurons have lower thresholds to synaptic excitation, and that the order of recruitment of units within a pool proceeds from small to large. This observation is the size principle. Its significance and interpretation has been repeatedly discussed, but one central question that follows from the observation is whether it can be explained simply as the result of scaling a neuron's size according to some simple rule.

Zucker (1973) applied the principles of geometry and Ohm's law to the case of a spherical neuron with one dendrite on which the neuron receives synaptic input. He defined voltage-threshold and current-threshold properly, and asked under what conditions would a size principle be expected if the diameter of the soma and dendrite were varied. He constructed several alternative models that described different assumptions about the number of synaptic contacts on the dendrite, and the density of these contacts. This paper is an example of the use of simple mathematical models that have analytical solutions to explore alternative hypotheses. These alternative models could be manipulated algebraically, and analyzed without the need to solve them or to explore the ranges of parameters systematically. Zucker concluded that a size principle is possible only if particular physiological and anatomical conditions are true: either small neurons have lower voltage-thresholds, or small neurons have a higher density of excitatory synaptic contacts, or small neurons have a higher ratio of soma-to-dendrite input resistances than do large ones. These are specific predictions that are today experimentally testable. He demonstrated that no simple scaling rule will lead to a size principle. The paper is convincing because the solutions of the equations Zucker used are readily comprehensible.

4.2.2   Integration of Synaptic Currents

In thinking about synaptic integration in neural circuits, it is important to keep clear two related but distinct concepts that interact. Local circuits are synaptic circuits of neurons restricted to one region of the nervous system, like the retina. Both projection neurons and local neurons can be part of a local circuit (Shepherd, 1979). Subunits are isopotential regions within one neuron that are rather isolated electrically from other regions in that neuron (Koch et al., 1982). If subunits exist in neurons in local circuits, the subunits, and not the component neurons of which they are parts, are the appropriate level at which to analyse the physiological organization of the circuit. Yet, such an analysis is intrinsically more difficult than one where neurons are the fundamental units because subunits cannot be defined using only anatomical methods and because both the interactions of subunits and of neurons in the circuit must be grasped before the circuit can be understood. It is important, therefore, to see if meaningful subunits can be identified in interneurons, and if they are discovered, to see how they alter our concept of the local circuits in which they occur.

4.2.3 "Subunits" in Retinal Ganglion Cells

Ganglion cells integrate information from local interneurons in the inner plexiform layer of the retina. Koch, Poggio, and Torre (1982) suggested that the differences in linearity of responses to light observed in different kinds of retinal ganglion cells might arise from nonlinearities of synaptic integration in the dendrites of some of these cells. In particular, they suggested that some kinds of ganglion cells might have integrative subunits in their dendrites that performed local synaptic integration in relative isolation from other dendrites or the soma. To test this idea, they made detailed measurements of the dendrites of different anatomical classes of ganglion cells, using one Golgi-stained retina, and guessed that $R_m = 2.5$ kohm·cm². Using their anatomical data, they assigned values for the membrane resistances and coupling resistances of the different dendrites in each neuron, and then calculated steady-state voltage attenuations between each neuron's various parts to see if any subunits existed.*

Koch et al. (1982) used a sensible, quantitative definition of a "subunit" within a neuron, that should be widely adopted. They defined the input resistance of a region i to be

$$r_{ii} = \frac{V_i}{I_i} \tag{3}$$

where V_i is the voltage change at region i when current I_i is injected there. They defined the transfer resistance from region i to region j to be

$$r_{ij} = \frac{V_j}{I_i} \tag{4}$$

where V_j is the voltage change in region j that results from the current injected into region i. Notice the counterintuitive properties of these transfer resistances; the greater the transfer resistance, the smaller the voltage attenuation between regions, but considered from a structural perspective,

---

*This paper describes an interesting mathematical strategy that makes use of Green's functions to study the dynamics of integration in complicated dendrites (see also Koch and Poggio, 1985). However, the results they report consider only the steady-state voltage-transfers within the dendrites, and make no use of the elegant mathematics.

a greater resistance between two regions means they are farther apart or are connected by a finer process.

They then said that a subunit consists of all the regions of a neuron where

$$\frac{r_{ii}}{r_{ij}} \leq a, \text{ for } a > 1 \tag{5}$$

and

$$\frac{r_{ij}}{r_{is}} > c, \text{ for } c > 1 \tag{6}$$

Here, r_{ii} is the input resistance of region i, r_{ij} is the transfer resistance from region i to region j, r_{is} is the transfer resistance from region i to region s, the recording site, and a and c are criteria decided by the investigator. All this means that a subunit is a part of a neuron within which voltage attenuation is not larger than a, while attenuation between any part of the subunit and the recording site, s, is greater than c. Koch et al. set $c = 4$.

Their results showed that different anatomical classes of ganglion cells showed characteristically different numbers and patterns of subunit organization, and the authors continued on to a discussion of the sources of non-linearity in the retina. However, they did a critical test of their results; they recalculated each neuron with $R_m = 8$ kohm·cm² and discovered that most subunits disappeared. This is disturbing; their conclusions depend strongly on the value of this parameter, and there is no independent measurement or other rationale for selecting any value in a much broader range than that they explored. The measurement of R_m for different classes of ganglion cell in the cat is therefore an important experimental goal, one that must be accomplished before we can judge the biological significance of Koch et al.'s ideas about the origins of the observed nonlinearity.

4.2.4 Synaptic Integration in Flexor Motor Neurons

The fast flexor muscles of crayfish are innervated by segmental pools of motor neurons that include one peripheral inhibitor (Kennedy and Takeda, 1965). The responses of the flexor excitor (FE) and flexor inhibitor (FI) motor neurons to an impulse in their normal command interneurons differ in their magnitude and time-course (Roberts et al., 1982). The neurons also differ in their responses to certain unilateral synaptic input. Edwards and Mulloney (1987) suggested that both of these differences might be caused by differences in passive membrane properties and the integrative structures of these neurons. This is an inherently quantitative hypothesis that can be tested only by a quantitative comparison of the passive, or linear, integrative properties of these neurons.

Edwards and Mulloney tested this hypothesis by first measuring the voltage responses of these neurons to steps of current. From the log transform of these voltages, they obtained a series of exponentials and used this series to construct a three-compartment model of each neuron (Edwards and Mulloney, 1984). From the longest time constant, they calculated that R_m for FE was 12.9 $\pm$ 0.1 kohm·cm² but for FI was 37 $\pm$ 14 kohm·cm². It is important to note that the starting points for their subsequent structural models were these physiologically derived compartmental models that could reproduce the original physiological responses exactly.

To construct the necessary structural model of each neuron, they filled it with dye and measured accurately the length and diameter of each branch. They combined this quantitative anatomy and two assumptions: first, that the membrane's properties were uniform, and second, that the internal resistivity of the cytoplasm was 60 ohm/cm, to expand the initial three-compartment models into more elaborate multicompartmental models that described the branching structure of each neuron and yet faithfully reproduced the original voltage steps. The anatomical structures of each neuron and the corresponding multicompartmental model are shown in Figure 11.

With these two models as tools, they compared the responses of the FE and FI neurons to simulated synaptic currents from giant fiber input. These models are mathematical in form; they consist of a set of linear differential equations that can be solved using linear algebra to calculate the input resistance of any compartment and the voltage attenuation between any set of compartments (Perkel and Mulloney, 1978), and to calculate the time-courses of voltage changes in response to currents injected into any compartment (Perkel et al., 1981).

The model of the FE neuron readily predicted the time-course of the actual response of the FE neuron observed in physiological experiments when the synaptic currents were injected in regions 5, 7, 11, and 13. These compartments correspond to parts of branches that contact the giant axons that are the natural sources of synaptic excitation. The model of the FI neuron did not readily simulate the response of the FI neuron, but this was expected because the normal FI response is a complex of nearly synchronous PSPs from the giant fiber, from collateral-discharge interneurons and from FE motor neurons (Wine and Mistick, 1977). These asynchronous PSPs arise in unknown regions. The FI model did accurately predict the response to single giant spikes under conditions where the other parallel inputs had been experimentally eliminated.

The interesting conclusions of this work come from comparisons of the PSPs recorded in the soma, integrating segments and initial axon segments (IAS) of these two different neurons. In the FE model, the PSPs in the IAS and the soma are similar in size. In the FI model, however, the PSPs in the soma were about twice as large as those in the IAS because the larger diameter of the FI axon makes it a more effective current sink. Ex-

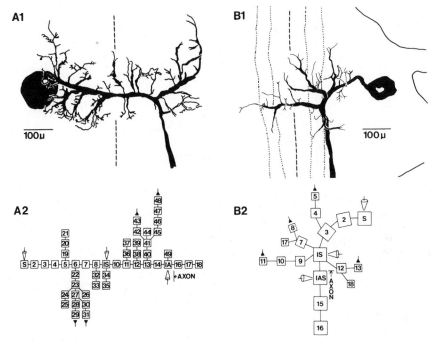

FIGURE 11. (A) Multicompartment models of FI and FE neurons. (A1) Camera lucida drawing of an FI neuron. (A2) Diagram of multicompartment model of the FI neuron. Each numbered or labelled box represents one region of the cell that is connected to ground by a parallel resistance and capacitance and to the other compartments by coupling resistances. The ▲ symbols identify dendritic compartments receiving "synaptic" current. S: soma; IS: integrating segment; IAS: initial axon segment. (B1) Camera lucida drawing of the stained FE neuron. The dots outline the axons of the two MG axons that contact the cell. (B2) Multicompartment model of the FE cell.

ploration of the responses of these models to synaptic input applied to individual dendrites revealed that the FE neuron's soma and IAS saw PSPs of similar size and time-course. The soma and IAS of the FI, on the other hand, showed major differences whose relative size depended on which branch was stimulated. PSPs arising on branches contralateral to the soma were smaller in the soma than in the IAS. PSPs arising ipsilateral to the soma were larger there than in the IAS (Fig. 12). Edwards tested these predictions in two experiments that recorded PSPs arising unilaterally from known sources, the stretch-receptor afferents. As predicted, PSPs arising contralateral to the soma were smaller, when recorded in the FI soma, than those arising ipsilateral to it. FE neurons respond equally well to EPSPs from stretch receptor afferents from either side of the body; FI neurons respond more readily to input from afferents contralateral to the FI soma.

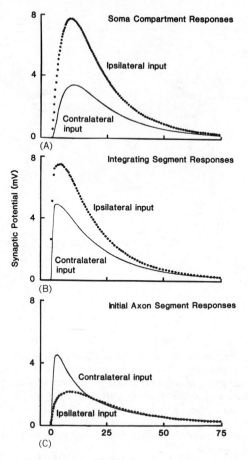

FIGURE 12. Synaptic integration in FI. (A) Responses of soma compartment (S) to 10 nA current pulses presented to ipsilateral dendritic compartments 27 and 29 (dots) and to contralateral dendritic compartments 41 and 46 (continuous). (B) Responses of integrating segment compartment (IS) to the same stimuli. (C) Responses of initial axon segment compartment (IAS) to the same stimuli.

These results confirm that the FE and FI neurons differ significantly in their integrative properties. The pattern of these differences is surprising; FI has a membrane time-constant three times that of FE, so FI's space constant should be longer than FE's (Jack et al., 1975), but other factors override this one. The large current sink formed by the FI axon dominates this neuron's integrative properties.

These results also illustrate several points related to the problem of modeling neuronal structure. Edwards and Mulloney chose to ignore these neurons' active response and the probable heterogeneity of their membranes. This choice was appropriate, given the hypothesis, and also prudent given the structural detail the models needed. Now that we have some foundation for confidence in these models, they are good starting points for models that have voltage-dependent conductances in the axon and IAS.

4.2.5 Synaptic Currents in Pyramidal Neurons

The fundamental integrative structures of pyramidal neurons in the guinea pig's hippocampus are now well described (e.g., Brown, Fricke, and Perkel, 1981). These interneurons would, therefore, be interesting subjects for the analysis of synaptic currents, if it were possible to voltage-clamp the sites at which the synapses occur. Johnston and Brown (1983) used both continuous mathematical models and analog models of these neurons to assess the errors that would occur in measurements of currents from mossy fiber synapses if the measurements were made from the neuron's soma (Figs. 13, 14). They used published values of the input resistance (R_N), time-constant (τ_m), electrotonic length (L) and ratio of dendritic conductance to somatic conductance (ρ)—all parameters defined in the context of an equivalent-cylinder model—to calibrate a compartmental model (Fig. 13) that had the same passive properties as a CA3 neuron. They then constructed two forms of this compartmental model. One was a continuous mathematical model suitable for computation of PSPs arising at different sites on the neuron. They used this to calculate the shape indices (Rall, 1977) of PSPs with a range of underlying conductance changes. Comparisons of these computed PSPs with those recorded in real neurons suggests that the mossy fiber synapses were located at sites equivalent to regions 1 and 2 of the model.

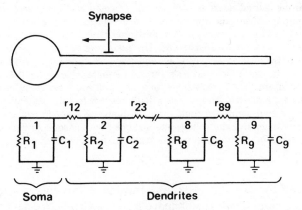

FIGURE 13. Compartmental representation of a hippocampal neuron. The average electrotonic structure of CA3 pyramidal neurons is represented by this nine-compartment model. Parameters of the model, L = 0.9, ρ = 1.5, τ_m = 24 ms, R_N = 35 Mohm, are very close to the average values for these parameters determined from 33 neurons in two independent investigations. Region 1 represents the soma and regions 2–9 represent the dendritic processes. From Johnston and Brown (1983).

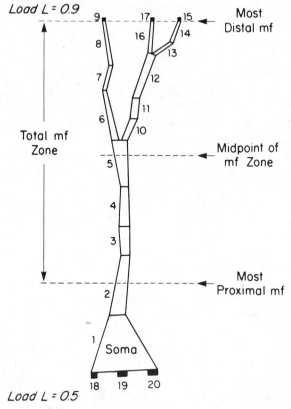

FIGURE 14. Branched compartmental digital model. The manner in which Johnston and Brown compartmentalized neurons is illustrated schematically. Parameters of each cmpartment were determined using measurements of the neuron's shape made from a camera lucida drawing, and values for R_m estimated from measured τ_m. For most compartments, R_i and C_i were calculated from its surface area and R_m. The linking resistances, r_{ij}, were calculated from measurements of the distance between the centers of each connected region. Compartments 9, 17, and 15 are the equivalent load resistances for a finite cable of $L = 0.9$, while compartments 18,19 and 20 are the load resistances for a cable of $L = 0.5$. Locations of the mossy fiber synaptic inputs are indicated. Those basilar dendrites that had the same diameter were collapsed into single equivalent-load compartments. Branched compartmental models such as this were used to determine the voltage attenuations from the soma to the different regions of the mossy fiber zone, and the electrotonic distances between these points. From Johnston and Brown (1983).

To measure the error in voltage-clamp measurements in such a neuron that occurs because of the distance from the electrode to each of its regions, Johnston and Brown constructed an accurate analog of their CA3 model (Fig. 13) and inserted it into their normal recording system, in series with the virtual-ground circuit. They used their standard recording electrode in their slice-chamber to try to clamp simulated synaptic currents introduced into different compartments of the analog model, and analysed the effectiveness of the clamp in different compartments as a function of the frequency of change in synaptic conductance. Therefore, they could say precisely how accurately they could measure synaptic currents of different durations at different points on the neuron's dendrites. The resulting plots of the relative error of their clamp in different regions of the model showed that the clamp failed dramatically as frequency and electrotonic distance increased, but that the regions on which mossy fiber synapses occurred could be clamped with reasonable accuracy, given their estimates of the spectral densities of currents at mossy fiber synapses. Furthermore, they could now define the magnitude of the errors in their measurements of these synaptic currents in the real neuron.

This elegant paper simplified a CA3 neuron by ignoring its active responses and the parts of its structure beyond the borders of mossy fiber synapses, but made careful use of both physiological and anatomical measurements to specify the parameters needed to test the ability of a voltage-clamp to measure the synaptic currents of mossy-fiber synapses. By comparing the performance of this well-calibrated model with PSPs from real CA3 neurons, Brown and Johnston were able to estimate parameters of synaptic currents before they attempted to measure them directly, and to define the limits within which their measurements would be accurate. The use of the analog form to measure the performance of their voltage-clamp apparatus greatly strengthened the reader's confidence in the accuracy and meaning of their subsequent experimental results (Brown and Johnston, 1983).

5   CONCLUSIONS

The purpose of computing is insight, not numbers (Hamming, 1973)

We have emphasized through this review the necessity of careful thinking at every stage in the construction and use of a synthetic model. Hamming's aphorism is true, and the insight comes from the careful construction and critical exploration of hypotheses. It is foolish to think that the computer will tell you the meaning of your data. Plant (1982) pointed out that ". . . the digital computer may be too much of a good thing. The ease with which the differential equations may be solved numerically may serve as a disincentive to the close inspection of the equations themselves."

To construct a useful synthetic model takes thought and time, but it is a necessary step in the analysis of any complex system. Synthetic models are not superfluous frills on an otherwise serious experimental science, nor are they the last choice of a neurobiologist frustrated by technical problems at the experimental bench. Good models clarify our descriptions, and force us to consider the consequences of ideas. They may also extend our understanding of how nervous systems work.

ACKNOWLEDGMENTS

We thank our colleagues Donald H. Edwards, Peter Getting, Esther Leise, and Martin Wilson for criticizing a draft of this paper, and the editors for their insightful suggestions.

Original research from our own laboratories was supported by USPHS NIH Grants NS12295 and NSF Grant BNS78 10516 to BM and by USPHS NIH Grant NS21376 and System Development Foundation Grant G283 to DHP.

REFERENCES

Adams, D. J., S. J. Smith, and S. H. Thompson (1980). Ionic currents in molluscan soma. *Ann. Rev. Neurosci.*, **3**:141–168.

Attwell, D. and M. Wilson (1980). Behavior of the rod network in the tiger salamander retina mediated by membrane properties of individual rods. *J. Physiol.*, **309**:287–315.

Attwell, D., M. Wilson, and S. M. Wu (1984). A quantitative analysis of interactions between photoreceptors in the salamander (*Ambystoma*) retina. *J. Physiol.*, **352**:703–737.

Bennett, M. V. L. (1971). Electroreception. In *Fish Physiology,* W. S. Hoad and D. J. Randall, eds. Academic Press, New York, pp. 493–574.

Brown, T. G. (1911). The intrinsic factors in the act of progression in the mammal. *Proc. Roy. Soc. Lond. B.*, **84**:308–319.

Brown, T. H., R. A. Fricke, and D. H. Perkel (1981). Passive electrical constants in three classes of hippocampal neurons. *J. Neurophysiol.*, **46**:812–827.

Brown, T. H. and D. Johnston (1983). Voltage-clamp analysis of mossy fiber synaptic input to hippocampal neurons. *J. Neurophysiol.*, **50**:487–507.

Byrne, G. C. (1981). Software for differential systems and applications involving macroscopic kinetics. *Comput. Chem.*, **5**:151–158.

Chay, T. R. and J. Rinzel (1985). Bursting, beating, and chaos in an excitable membrane model. *Biophys. J.*, **47**:357.

Churchhouse, R. F., ed. (1981). *Handbook of Applicable Mathematics,* vol. III, *Numerical Methods.* Wiley, Chichester.

DeStefano, J. J. III and E. M. Landaw (1984). Multiexponential, multicompartmental and noncompartmental modeling. I. Methodological limitations and physiological interpretations. *Am. J. Physiol.*, **246**:R651–R664.

Detwiler, P. B., A. L. Hodgkin, and P. A. McNaughton (1978). A surprising property of electrical spread in the network of rods in the toad retina. *J. Physiol.*, **274**:562–565.

Dodge, F. A. and J. W. Cooley (1973). Action potential of the motor neuron. I. *B. M. J. Res. Dev.*, **17**:219–229.

Edelson, D. (1981). Computer simulation in chemical kinetics. *Science*, **214**:981–986.

Edwards, D. H. and B. Mulloney (1984). Compartmental models of electrotonic structure and synaptic integration in an identified neuron. *J. Physiol.*, **348**: 89–113.

Edwards, D. H. and B. Mulloney (1987). Synaptic integration in excitatory and inhibitory crayfish motoneurons. *J. Neurophysiol.*, **57**:1425–1445.

Forsythe, G. E., M. A. Malcolm, and C. B. Moler (1977). *Computer Methods for Mathematical Computation*. Prentice-Hall, Englewood Cliffs, New Jersey.

Friesen, W. O. and G. S. Stent (1977). Generation of a locomotory rhythm by a neural network with recurrent cyclic inhibition. *Biol. Cybern.*, **28**:27–40.

Friesen, W. O. and G. S. Stent (1978). Neural circuits for generating rhythmic movements. *Ann. Rev. Biophys. Bioeng.*, **7**:37–61.

Friesen, W. O. and R. J. Wyman (1980). Analysis of *Drosophila* motor neuron activity patterns with neural analogs. *Biol. Cybern.*, **38**:41–50.

Getting, P. A. (1983a). Mechanisms of pattern generation underlying swimming in *Tritonia*. II. Network reconstruction. *J. Neurophysiol.*, **49**:1017–1035.

Getting, P. A. (1983b). Mechanisms of pattern generation underlying swimming in *Tritonia*. III. Intrinsic and synaptic mechanisms for delayed excitation. *J. Neurophysiol.*, **49**:1036–1050.

Getting, P. A. (1983c). Neural control of swimming in *Tritonia*. *Symp. Soc. Exp. Biol.*, **37**:89–128.

Glantz, R. M. and T. Viancour (1983). Integrative properties of crayfish medial giant neuron: steady-state model. *J. Neurophysiol.*, **50**:1122–1144.

Gorman, A. L. F. and M. Mirolli (1972). The passive electrical properties of the membrane of a molluscan neurone. *J. Physiol.*, **227**:35–49.

Hamming, R. W. (1973). *Numerical Methods for Scientists and Engineers*. McGraw-Hill, New York.

Harcombe, E. S. and R. J. Wyman (1977). Output pattern generation by *Drosophila* flight motoneurons. *J. Neurophysiol.*, **40**:1066–1077.

Hume, R. I., P. A. Getting, and M. A. Del Beccaro (1982). Motor organization of *Tritonia* swimming. I. Quantitative analysis of swim behavior and flexion neuron firing patterns. *J. Neurophysiol.*, **47**:60–74.

Hume, R. I. and P. A. Getting (1982). Motor organization of *Tritonia* swimming. III. Contribution of intrinsic membrane properties to flexion neuron burst formation. *J. Neurophysiol.*, **47**:91–102.

Jack, J. J. B., D. Noble, and R. Tsien (1975). *Electrical Current Flow in Excitable Cells*. Oxford University Press, Oxford.

Johnston, D. and T. H. Brown (1983). Interpretation of voltage-clamp measurements in hippocampal neurons. *J. Neurophysiol.*, **50**:464–486.

Kennedy, D. and K. Takeda (1965). Reflex control of abdominal flexor muscles in the crayfish. I. The twitch system. *J. Exp. Biol.*, **43**:211–227.

Keynes, R. D. and H. Martins-Ferreira (1953). Membrane potentials in the electroplates of the electric eel. *J. Physiol.*, **119**:315–351.

Kling, U. and G. Szekely (1968). Simulation of rhythmic nervous activities. I. Function of networks with cyclic inhibitions. *Kybernetic*, 5:89–103.

Koch, C., T. Poggio, and V. Torre (1982). Retinal ganglion cells: a functional interpretation of dendritic morphology. *Phil. Trans. Roy. Soc. Lond. B.*, 298:227–264.

Koch, C. and T. Poggio (1985). A simple algorithm for solving the cable equation in dendritic trees of arbitrary geometry. *J. Neurosci. Meth.*, 12:303–315.

Koenig, J. H. and K. Ikeda (1980). Neural interactions controlling timing of flight muscle activity in *Drosophila*. *J. Exp. Biol.*, 87:121–136.

Kristan, W. B. and J. C. Weeks (1983). Neurons controlling the initiation, generation and modulation of leech swimming. *Symp. Soc. Exp. Biol.*, 37:243–260.

Landaw, E. M. and J. J. DeStefano, III (1984). Multiexponential, multicompartmental, and noncompartmental modeling. II. Data analysis and statistical considerations. *Am. J. Physiol.*, 246:R665–R677.

Lewis, E. R. (1968). An electronic model of neuroelectric point processes. *Kybernetic*, 5:30–46.

Levine, J. D. (1973). Properties of the nervous system controlling flight in *Drosophila melanogaster*. *J. Comp. Physiol.*, 84:129–166.

McCulloch, W. S. and W. Pitts (1943). A logical calculus of the ideas immanent in nervous activity. *Bull. Math. Biophysics*, 5:115–133.

Mulloney, B. (1970). Organization of flight motor-neurons of *Diptera*. *J. Neurophysiol.*, 33:86–95.

Mulloney, B., D. H. Perkel and R. W. Budelli (1981). Motor pattern production: interaction of electrical and chemical synapses. *Brain Res.*, 229:25–33.

Partridge, L. D., S. H. Thompson, S. J. Smith, and J. A. Connor (1979). Current-voltage relationships of repetitively firing neurons. *Brain Res.*, 164:69–79.

Perkel, D. H. (1976). A computer program for simulating a network of interacting neurons. I. Organization and physiological assumptions. *Computers and Biomed. Res.*, 9:31–43.

Perkel, D. H. and B. Mulloney (1974). Motor pattern production in reciprocally inhibitory neurons exhibiting postinhibitory rebound. *Science*, 185:181–183.

Perkel, D. H. and B. Mulloney (1978a). Electrotonic properties of neurons: steady-state compartmental model. *J. Neurophysiol.*, 41:621–639.

Perkel, D. H. and B. Mulloney (1978b). Calibrating compartmental models of various neurons. *Am. J. Physiol.*, 235:R93–R98.

Perkel, D. H., B. Mulloney, and R. W. Budelli (1981). Quantitative methods for predicting neuronal behavior. *Neuroscience*, 6:823–838.

Plant, R. E. (1978). The effects of Ca^{++} on bursting neurons: a modelling study. *Biophys. J.*, 21:217–237.

Plant, R. E. (1979). The efficient numerical solution of biological simulation problems. *Computer Prog. In Biomed.*, 10:1–15.

Plant, R. E. (1981). Bifurcation and resonance in a model for bursting nerve cells. *J. Math. Biol.*, 11:15–32.

Plant, R. E. (1982). The analysis of models for excitable membranes: an introduction. *Lect. Math. Life Sci.*, 15:27–34.

Rall, W. S. (1969). Time constants and electrotonic length of membrane cylinders and neurons. *Biophys. J.*, **9**:1483–1508.

Rall, W. (1977). Core conductor theory and cable properties. In *Handbook of Physiology*, Sec. 1, E. R. Kandel, ed. pp. 39–98. Am. Physiol. Soc., Bethesda.

Rall, W. (1981). Functional aspects of neuronal geometry. In *Neurones without Impulses*, A. Roberts and B. M. H. Bush, eds., pp. 223–254. Cambridge U. P., Cambridge.

Roberts, A., F. B. Krasne, G. Hagiwara, J. J. Wine, and A. P. Kramer (1982). Segmental giant: evidence for a driver neuron interposed between command and motor neurons in the crayfish escape system. *J. Neurophysiol.*, **47**:761–781.

Schoener, T. W. (1972). Mathematical ecology and its place among the sciences. *Science*, **178**:389–391.

Shepherd, G. M. (1979). Functional analysis of local circuits in the olefactory bulb. In *The Neurosciences Fourth Study Program*, F. O. Schmitt and F. G. Worden, eds. MIT Press, Cambridge, pp. 129–144.

Smith, S. J. (1978). The Mechanism of Bursting Pacemaker Activity in Neurons of the Mollusc *Tritonia diomedia*, Ph.D. Thesis, University of Washington, Seattle.

Szekely, G. (1965). Logical network for controlling limb movements in urodela. *Acta. Sci. Hung.*, **27**:285–289.

Thompson, R. S. and W. G. Gibson (1981a). Neural model with probabilistic firing behavior. I. General considerations. *Math. Biosci.*, **56**:239–253.

Thompson, R. S. and W. G. Gibson (1981b). Neural model with probabilistic firing behavior. II. One- and two-neuron networks. *Math. Biosci.*, **56**:255–285.

Thompson, S. H. (1976). Membrane currents underlying bursting in molluscan pacemaker neurons. Ph.D. Thesis, University of Washington, Seattle.

Uspensky, J. V. (1948). *Theory of Equations*. McGraw-Hill, New York.

Weeks, J. C. (1981). Neuronal basis of leech swimming: Separation of swim initiation, pattern generation and intersegmental coordination by selective lesions. *J. Neurophysiol.*, **45**:698–723.

Wilson, D. M. (1966). Central nervous mechanisms for the generation of rhythmic behavior in arthropods. *Symp. Soc. Exp. Biol.*, **20**:100–228.

Wilson, D. M. and I. Waldron (1968). Models for the generation of the motor output pattern in flying locust. *Proc. IEEE*, **56**:1058–1064.

Wine, J. J. and D. C. Mistick (1977). Temporal organization of crayfish escape behavior: delayed recruitment of peripheral inhibition. *J. Neurophysiol.*, **40**:904–925.

Wyman, R. J. (1966). Multistable firing patterns among several neurons. *J. Neurophysiol.*, **29**:807–833.

Zucker, R. S. (1973). Theoretical implications of the size principle of motoneurone recruitment. *J. Theoret. Biol.*, **38**:587–596.

Chapter Twelve

ANALYTIC APPROACHES TO THE STUDY OF OUTPUTS FROM CENTRAL PATTERN GENERATORS

AFTAB E. PATLA

Department of Kinesiology
University of Waterloo
Waterloo, Ontario, Canada

1 INTRODUCTION

Tools and concepts from a wide variety of scientific fields are useful in trying to explain behavior in terms of the neuronal structures involved. This chapter examines the usefulness and limitations of a few analytical approaches from engineering and computer science as they apply to the understanding of one aspect of motor control: the neural control of rhythmic movements. In this approach, the functioning of the nervous system is often represented in terms of system block diagrams with several inputs and outputs, which converge and diverge (cf. Fentress, 1976; Houk and Rymer, 1981).

Rhythmic movements provide simpler interaction between the input and output. When activity is induced in isolated nervous systems, these networks receive relatively simple unpatterned input and produce a complex relatively detailed patterned output. Because these movements are easily elicited, readily related to normal behavior, and provide for repetitions to be observed and analysed, they have been studied more extensively than episodic behavior.

Numerous isolation, deafferentation, and fictive movement experiments have demonstrated that a number of rhythmic behaviors such as locomotion, breathing, feeding, and scratching are generated, in response to a simple tonic signal, by system units called "central pattern generators" (cf. Delcomyn, 1980; Grillner, 1985; Shik and Orlovsky, 1976; Stein, 1978; and other chapters: Getting, Grillner). One approach to understanding rhythmic movements is to use "simpler" neural systems which can be isolated and studied using known experimental techniques (cf. Selverston, 1980). The implicit belief is that once these simpler systems are understood completely, it will be possible to identify the principles of operation of the networks responsible for more complex rhythmic behaviors.

In complex mammalian systems this cell by cell analysis has not yet proved feasible, and the cells which form the pattern generator have not been identified to date. Nonetheless, functional subsystems and their interactions can be studied experimentally. In parallel with the experimental approach to understanding the structure and operation of rhythmic systems, analytical approaches, and computer simulations play an important complementary role. Analytical models, whether they are physical or mathematical in nature, focus experimental evidence into a coherent and hopefully parsimonious view. Simulations of models allow for predictions of outputs for a wide variety of inputs and discovery of inputs for a particular set of outputs. Our experiments are often most productive when guided by models.

In this chapter the power and limitations of some analytical techniques used to understand the principles of neuronal organization in central pattern generators are examined. This review largely draws upon data from mammalian locomotion including human locomotion. It is believed that vertebrate locomotion, a complicated and malleable behavior, may offer better hope for manipulation at the systems level (Loeb and Marks, 1980).

2   SYSTEM MODEL: A SCHEMATIC REPRESENTATION

The functional subsystems that constitute the control system for rhythmic movements are described in this section. This provides a framework for subsequent sections.

2.1   Inputs to the System

A necessary precursor to any system identification is a thorough knowledge about the inputs and the outputs of the system. The four major classes of input to the control system are: the tonic input to initiate and maintain rhythmic movements, patterned sensory input from the periphery, patterned input from the central nervous system, and coordinating signals between pattern generators for different appendages. Of these four classes of inputs, only the properties of tonic input are known best. The tonic input is a command signal that is needed to initiate and maintain activity such as locomotion. In crayfish, by activating appropriate command neurons, a rhythmic movement from a repertoire can be selected (Bentley and Konishi, 1978). Research in vertebrates has shown that, by changing the strength of the command signal, different speeds of locomotion can be elicited (Shik et al., 1966). The signal parameter that is responsible for initiation and maintenance of locomotion is the current level of the stimulus, with the stimulation frequency having very little effect (Shik et al., 1966). Therefore, this command signal can be characterized by a direct current input.

Some effects of patterned input from the peripheral and central nervous system on the output have been identified (cf. Andersson and Grillner, 1981; Dietz et al., 1979; Drew and Rossignol, 1984; Pearson, 1981; other chapters). Although not necessary for the production of rhythmic motor output, experiments have shown that these inputs are utilized on a cycle by cycle basis to provide normal patterned output. But the actual measurement and characterizations of these signals has been elusive. Only recently we have been able to monitor the activities of sensory receptors during movements such as locomotion (cf. Loeb et al., 1985). These inputs have been shown to be phasically active during particular phases of the movement cycle. Thus they cannot be represented as a d.c. signal.

During normal locomotion, the appendages of the animal maintain stable phase differences (Grillner, 1985; Shik and Orlovsky, 1976; Stein, 1976; von Holst, 1973). The stable phase difference between appendages is seen not only during normal locomotion, but also during forced coordination modes such as 2:1. This phase regulation suggests the presence of some coordinating signal between pattern generators (cf. Kulagin and Shik, 1970; Stein, 1977). In the swimmeret system of the crayfish, the existence of neural signals that regulate the phase difference has been observed (Stein, 1971). When this signal is abolished, the phase regulation is lost (Stein, 1971). It is interesting to note that modeling techniques, specifically the theory of coupled oscillators have been used to predict stable interoscillator phase differences (cf. Pavlidis and Pinsker, 1977; Stein, 1977; and other chapters). Since coordination between limbs exists in spinal and fictive preparations, the presence of a similar signal in mammals can be inferred. Moreover, the mechanism of phase transitions between two modes of locomotion is still not clearly understood (cf. Kelso, 1984; Haken et al., 1985).

To summarize, at present only the tonic input to the pattern generator is modeled. It is not productive at this stage to model other patterned inputs to the system, because not enough is known about their characteristics and effects on the output patterns.

2.2   The Outputs of the System

The outputs of the CPG are the rhythmic firing of the output neurons. These signals pass through various intervening processes and produce the rhythmic movements which can be described by the displacement (linear and angular) time curves of the various body segments (Fig. 1). In this section some of the intervening processes are identified and described, and their possible effects and contribution to the final output pattern are discussed. The discussion proceeds from the outside in.

Although the joint displacements are the final output of the system, we have to be careful in using them as a measure of motor output. Researchers have shown that identical joint kinematics can be produced by very different muscle activity and joint torque patterns. For example, even though the joint kinematics for forward and backward walking in humans are identical, the motor patterns as characterized by muscle activity profiles are different (Thorstensson, 1986). Even for the same movement such as normal locomotion, Winter (1984) has shown that the variability in the joint torque patterns is greater than the joint kinematic profiles.

The joint kinematics are caused by the net moments acting at each joint. It is relatively easy to determine using Newtonian mechanics, the net joint moments from the measured kinematics and any external force acting on the system (Bresler and Frankel, 1950). These joint moments for given kinematic trajectories are a function of the masses, moments of inertia of the musculoskeletal system, and the effects of gravity. Mochon and McMahon (1980) have shown that given the initial conditions at the onset of the swing phase of biped locomotion (established by the activity of the muscles in the stance phase), the leg then moves through the swing phase entirely under the action of gravity. Although their conclusion is not supported by other experimental data (cf. Winter and Robertson, 1978), their model forces us to examine how passive mechanical properties of the musculo-skeletal system can affect the generation of rhythmic movements.

Proceeding from the net joint moment to individual muscle force or moment contribution, one faces the problem of indeterminacy. Because of the number of muscles crossing a joint, there is no unique solution without imposing some criteria such as minimization of force or energy (cf. Chow and Jacobson, 1971; Crowninshield and Brand, 1981; Pedotti et al., 1978). The problem of identifying the correct criteria has been elusive (cf. Nelson, 1983). Others (cf. Pierrynowski and Morrison, 1985) have chosen a physiologically based model to determine muscular forces. One major problem has been lack of actual muscle force data during locomotion to compare with the obtained results, and determine the validity of the proposed models. For a given speed of locomotion, any partioning scheme would have to take into account the following: force/length/velocity relationship for a given neural input (Gordon et al., 1966; Hill, 1938); fibre type of the muscles; moment arm and the mechanical properties of the tendons and ligaments.

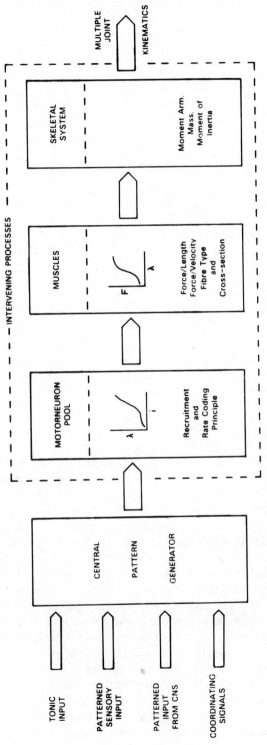

FIGURE 1. A schematic diagram showing various processes between the "CPG" output and the joint kinematics. Some of the nonlinearities, transformations and factors involved in these processes are included in each block. Starting with the central pattern generator, the various outputs are: (*a*) firing rate/time curves of the output neurons which may be the excitation current/time curves to the motoneuron pool; (*b*) motoneuron firing rate/time curves; and (*c*) muscle force/time curves, with many muscles affecting the displacement of any one joint.

459

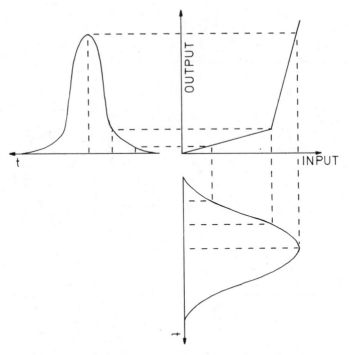

FIGURE 2. The effect of non-linearity on a simple sinusoidal input. The output in this case is no longer characterized by a single frequency; the power spectrum contains many frequency components.

For a given speed of locomotion, each muscle output can be represented by its force/time profile. The relation between the force generated and the firing rate of motoneurons is non-linear (Cooper and Eccles, 1930). Because of this nonlinearity, a pure sinusoidal input of the firing rate will produce a force/time waveform that is complex and contains more than the input frequency (Fig. 2). Thus, this nonlinearity can give rise to complexity in the shape of the waveform which is not present in the input.

Proceeding further inwards one is faced with the problem of determining the excitation to the entire motoneuron pool from the firing rate of the motoneurons. Kernell (1965) has shown a nonlinear relationship between the stimulating current and the firing rate (steady state and first impulse interval) for the hindlimb motoneurons of the cat. Once again, the nonlinearity will introduce frequencies that may not be present in the excitation current (Fig. 2). The recruitment and rate coding rules (cf. Henneman and Olson, 1965; Milner-Brown et al., 1973a,b) are built into the transformation from the excitation to the motoneuron pool to the firing of the motor units. Zheng et al. (1984) have proposed a physical model that simulates the recruitment principle. The model consists of a general input to the motoneuron pool and a number of devices in parallel to the input source. Each of the devices represents a motor unit and is composed of diodes in series with a threshold voltage and resistor. The current through each resistor represents the excitation current to that motor unit. By choosing appropriate values for the threshold, the motor units can be recruited according to the size principle. The nonlinear resistor in each device can modify the current and hence the firing rate of each motor unit. This model demonstrates how physical properties of components, and geometry of the circuit can produce the detailed output from a simple input.

It is clear that the neural control system for rhythmic movements can be studied at various levels. Each subsystem contributes to the final output, and to understand that we need to know more about input/output relationship for each system component.

3 SOME PROBLEMS IN SEARCH OF ANALYTICAL TECHNIQUES

The system block diagram (Fig. 1) clearly shows that there are convergent inputs and divergent outputs from the various subsystems. Depending on the level of analysis, we can measure firing rates of single neurons, muscle activity patterns, torque/time profiles, or displacement/time profiles. All these measures can be represented as a set of analog signals. In experiments we would like to make inferences about the organizational principles and structure of the control system from these sets of signals.

Some common experimental paradigms involved comparison of the muscle activity patterns before and after spinalization (cf. Belanger et al., 1986), deafferentation (cf. Grillner and Zangger, 1984), speed changes (cf. Halbertsma, 1983); and comparison of muscle activity patterns with the firing patterns of CNS neurons (cf. Drew et al., 1986). The types of questions that these experiments pose are: What are the patterns that the CPG generates in the absence of patterned input from the CNS or the periphery? How is the CPG for locomotion adapted for other rhythmic movements such as locomoting at different speeds? What is the relationship between firing patterns of the neurons in certain CNS pathways, and the muscle activity patterns? We are going to discuss specific examples which address these questions. These examples are representative of the work reported in the literature. As these examples illustrate, sophistication in measurements of multiple variables is usually coupled with simple and limited analyses of the data.

Drew et al. (1986) measured discharge patterns of reticulospinal and other reticular neurons in the CNS along with the muscle activity patterns during treadmill locomotion in cats. To correlate neuronal and muscular activity, rank-ordered raster displays were generated. These displays were triggered from the onset of each recorded muscle. Of the 97 reticulospinal neurons that were antidromically identified from the spinal cord, only 31%

were strictly related to the recorded EMGs. The discharge patterns of 34% of the neurons although modulated at the periodicity of the locomotor rhythm, were uncorrelated with any recorded EMGs. This type of analysis is unable to identify any complex relationship among the measured patterns. It is possible that the firing pattern of the locomotor related CNS neurons may be related to signals that are embedded in the muscle activity patterns, but in this case a simple correlation statistic will not uncover it.

Belanger et al. (1986) recorded muscle activity profiles before and after spinalization on the same cat. Qualitative analysis of the recorded data showed changes in the activity patterns of the sartorius, and the semitendinosus. It is clear that with this technique only gross changes in activity patterns of muscles can be noted. Where quantitative analyses have been done on similar types of problems, they have been conducted on a muscle by muscle basis. This is discussed in the next example.

Halbertsma (1983) studying speed related changes in muscle activity patterns measured the burst duration, peak level, average level, and total activity (area under the curve) for each muscle. Although adequate when quantifying activity of a single muscle, it is absolutely useless in identifying relationships among various muscle activity patterns. If we attempt to extrapolate the analysis to multiple activities by taking, for example, the durations between onset of one muscle activity and another, the number of measures become very large. Besides, even this does not allow us to determine if there is any common variance between different muscle activities. Standard statistical procedures are inadequate because we are dealing with a time series where the points on the muscle activity profile are not independent.

The implicit assumption in the analyses used in these examples is that the muscle activity profiles are independent activity patterns produced by a CPG. The number of synergists, both agonists and antagonists, involved in rhythmic movements such as locomotion, clearly suggests that these profiles are not independent. The major question that needs to be addressed is; how do we uncover the common or underlying feature signals among these activity patterns? It is possible, for example, that the locomotor related neurons in the CNS may correlate with these feature signals; or that changes after spinalization may be restricted to one of the feature signals, which, in turn, manifests itself in changes in a few muscle activity patterns; or that speed related changes may involve additional features generated by the nervous system. Pattern recognition techniques can help us address these hypotheses. A particular technique is described in the subsequent sections, along with some examples taken from human locomotion. These types of analyses can help us identify organizational principles and control strategies of the nervous system.

After we have identified these common or underlying feature signals, we have to determine structures or models that can generate these patterns. The major problem with the models in the literature has been that they have not been able to generate the detailed output patterns that are measured. In the last section, we discuss some requirements for these models, and explore a particular mathematical model that may be useful in this application.

4 PATTERN RECOGNITION: A TECHNIQUE FOR IDENTIFYING COMMON FEATURE SIGNALS AMONG A SET OF PATTERNS

Present techniques for analyzing a set of analog signals are clearly inadequate. Pattern recognition techniques offer a viable solution. To explain the concept, let us use a toy analog. We are all familiar with Lego sets that children (adults) can use to build a variety of structures such as house models. Suppose we were shown "n" different house models, and were asked to compare their structure. Based on our a priori knowledge about Lego sets, we can identify the parts or building blocks that are common to all houses, and parts that are particular to a model. This operation has allowed us to reduce these complex structures (houses) into a combination of fundamental parts. Thus building of these house models requires knowledge about the parts and the way they are combined.

When we want to analyse a set of analog time dependent signals, we are faced with the same problem. These signals are the "houses" of our analogy. What we need is to find the common features (signals) in these patterns. These features will be some time dependent signals. Along with identifying these features, we need to determine "combination rules" that have to be used to build our measured signals.

The major problem in identifying the common features is that we have no a priori knowledge about them. In the toy analogy, we have pieces such as a window or a door that we can use as a template to analyze the house structure. This information is not available to us when we analyze the set of analog signals representing the output of the control system. We have to perform some mathematical operations, similar to dismantling the house, to uncover these signals that can be used as building blocks, and also identify the combination rules.

Before we search for suitable techniques let us state our requirements. They are:

1. The technique should be able to identify the common feature signals among a set of measured analog signals and the rules for combining them to generate the measured signal.

2. The feature signals should be different from each other, i.e., they must be independent. If there is any covariance between them, clearly they can be further broken down into fundamental patterns. Because we have no a priori knowledge, we cannot specify the shapes of these feature signals.

3. The number of feature signals should be less than or equal to the number of measured signals. The rationale for this criterion is as follows. If the number of feature signals identified is greater than the number of measured signals, then we have lost economy in operation of the system. Instead of the system (CPG) having to generate the measured signals, it would be required to produce these larger set of feature signals. This criterion of economy imposed on the technique is similar to the classic minimization of degrees of freedom problem (Bernstein, 1967).

Having laid out these criteria, now we have to select a suitable pattern recognition algorithm. The most suitable is the Karhunen-Loeve expansion technique (cf. Patla, 1985). We will explain the implementation of this technique using an example from the study of human locomotion. The measurement procedure and step by step analysis of the data is explained. The mathematical procedure is described in Appendix 1. Further details can be obtained from standard pattern recognition text books (cf. Young and Calvert, 1974).

Myoelectric signals from seven muscles of the lower limb of human subjects were analyzed during walking at various speeds on a treadmill. The muscles studied were: tibialis anterior, soleus, medial gastrocnemius, vastus lateralis, rectus femoris, biceps femoris (long head) and erector spinae. The muscle activities were monitored using 4 mm surface electrodes in bipolar configuration (IVM, USA). The EMG amplifier included miniature preamplifiers taped near the electrode, and differential amplifiers (8 Hz–8 kHz, CMRR > 100 db). The full wave rectified and low pass filtered (4th order Butterworth filter, 10 ms, time constant) myoelectric signals were analog to digital converted (250 Hz, sampling frequency, record length = 16 s) along with the foot switch signal providing temporal information about heel contact and toe-off. Figure 3 shows a sample record when the subject was walking at his normal self paced speed.

These data, consistent with other studies, show very repeatable patterns suggesting the presence of a locomotor program (cf. Herman et al., 1976; Patla, 1985; Winter, 1983). The afferent connections between muscles of the lower limb in man are functionally significant (cf. Pierrot-Deseillgny, 1983) and in normal locomotion, peripheral input has been shown to play a role in shaping the normal locomotor output (cf. Dietz et al., 1979). The locomotor program may be considered to be similar to the CPG for locomotion in other animals.

The record shown in Figure 3 represents various muscle activities over approximately fifteen strides. Theoretical models for myoelectric signal generation (cf. DeLuca, 1979) have shown that appropriately processed EMG signals (full wave rectified and low pass filtered) reflect the neural input to the muscles. So these signals can be thought to represent neural activity profiles. On a stride by stride basis, there is variability which can

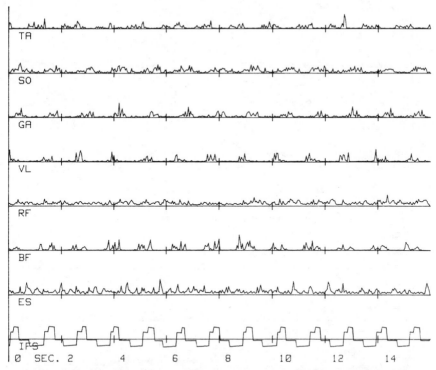

FIGURE 3. Filtered EMG signals recorded from seven muscles of the ipsilateral lower limb during treadmill locomotion at normal self paced speed. The muscles are: TA, tibialis anterior; SO, soleus; GA, medial gastrocnemius; VL, vastus lateralis; RF, rectus femoris; BF, biceps femoris (longhead); and ES, erector spinae. The last channel contains signal from the ipsilateral foot switch. The record duration is 16 seconds.

be assumed to be random. To determine the true muscle activity profile, we have to ensemble average the signals over a number of strides. Since the duration of individual strides may vary, before averaging we have to normalize each stride to 100%. This rubberbanding of individual strides may shorten some while lengthening the others. Each stride is represented by "N" points. In our example N was 100. The stride data in human locomotion study is usually normalized from heel strike to heel strike. After the normalization procedure, we can average each point along the stride and plot the mean and standard deviation (SD) points. This operation will give us an average activity profile for each muscle along with a ± 1 SD band around the curve. The data from Figure 3 was processed as discussed, and the results are shown in Figure 4. In the computer the average activity profiles are stored in a matrix of dimension "m" × "N", where "m" is the number of muscles and "N" is the number of points in each profile. Let us call this matrix I, representing input data. In this case m is

Input data

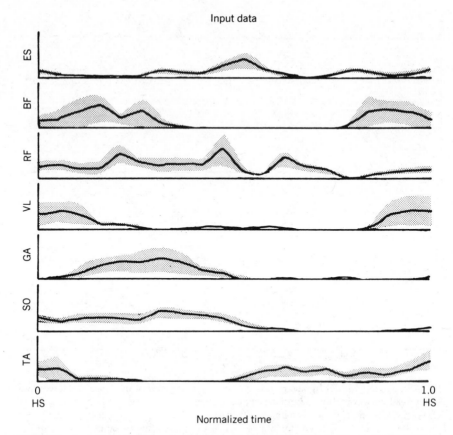

FIGURE 4. A plot of ensemble average of the seven muscle activity patterns shown in Figure 3. The muscle abbreviations are explained in Figure 3 caption. The average profile is shown as the solid line, while the shaded area represent ±1 SD band. The ±1 SD band is a measure of stride to stride variability. Each stride is normalized to 100%, from heel strike (HS) to heel strike. (Adapted from A. E. Patla, *J. Motor Behaviour,* **17**:443–461, 1985.)

7 and N is 100. The standard deviation of the activity profiles are stored in a matrix of similar dimension.

To identify the feature signals among this set of data, the following operations had to be done. First, the data for each muscle activity were normalized to their own peak value, and the d.c. bias (average value over the stride) was subtracted. Then, an autocorrelation matrix had to be calculated. This is done by multiplying the transpose of the matrix I with the matrix I. The transpose of matrix "I" called I^T, is a matrix of dimension "N" × "m". The product $[I]^T \cdot [I]$ is a matrix of dimension $[N \times N]$. After calculating this matrix, we calculate the eigenvalues and eigenvectors of this matrix using a standard algorithm. Definitions of eigenvalues and eigenvectors of a matrix can be found in any standard algebra textbook. Intuitively the largest eigenvector and associated eigenvalue will dominate the behaviour of subsequent operations associated with the data. Each eigenvector is a vector of dimension $[1 \times N]$ and has associated with it a eigenvalue. For this $[N \times N]$ matrix, the maximum number of "non zero" eigenvalues will be "m." Thus we will have maximum "m" eigenvectors.

The association between the eigenvectors/eigenvalues and the feature signals we are looking for is as follows. The eigenvectors are the "feature signals" among the set of input patterns. They are the bulding blocks or parts of the house in our toy analogy. Each eigenvector is a signal vector. These feature signals can be used to rebuild our set of input or measured patterns. The eigenvalue associated with each eigenvector is a measure of the fraction of total variance accounted for by each feature signal. Therefore, a large eigenvalue indicates that the feature is important or dominant. Since by definition, the eigenvectors are orthogonal, the feature signals are independent. The muscle activity profiles shown in Figure 4 were analyzed, and the feature signals were identified. The results are shown in Figure 5. For this set of signals, seven feature signals were identified. Beside each signal is the eigenvalue term expressed as a percentage. The first feature signal contributes 41.9% of the total variance while the seventh one contributes 1.8%. The feature signals are plotted in order of importance from the bottom up.

Let us now determine the rules by which these feature signals are combined to rebuild our set of measured patterns. Unlike building our Lego house where the rules for combining the parts can be complex, the measured patterns can be reconstructed by taking algebraic sum of appropriately weighted feature signals. The method of determining the weighting coefficients is explained in Appendix 1. Thus to reconstruct each measured pattern, a set of coefficients will be required. In our example, to reconstruct each muscle activity profile accurately, seven coefficients will be required. The reconstruction process is shown in the schematic diagram of Figure 6.

When we reconstruct the measured signals using all the identified feature signals, the results are identical to what we started out with. This is seen in Figure 6, where we used all seven feature signals to reconstruct the measured muscle activity patterns. As we have described, the feature signals identified are not necessarily equal in importance. The importance of the feature signal to the reconstruction process is measured by the associated eigenvalue. If we select less than the maximum number of feature signals identified to reconstruct the measured signals, there will be some error introduced. In our example, if we use only the first six feature signals the overall error will be 1.8%, while the first five feature signals will introduce an error of 4.8%. The overall error term is determined by summing the percent eigenvalues of the feature signals not used in the reconstruction of the measured signal. This error term does not indicate in which muscle activity pattern or where in time the error occurs. To better guide

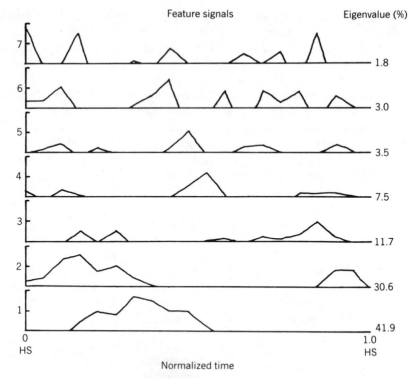

FIGURE 5. The plot of seven feature signals determined from the activity profiles shown in Figure 4. To determine these signals, a pattern recognition algorithm was used. Besides each feature signal, the eigenvalue expressed as a % value is listed. This value is a measure of the fraction of the total variance accounted by each feature signal. The signals are labelled from 1–7, 1 representing the most important feature signal, while 7 representing the least important signal. The x-axis is normalized time similar to Figure 4. The y-axis is normalized units. (Adapted from A. E. Patla, *J. Motor Behaviour*, **17**:443–461, 1985.)

our selection process, we approximate our measured patterns and plot it along with the one S.D. band of the measured signal. If the approximated patterns fall within the normal variability (± 1 SD), the number of features selected are deemed adequate.

In our example, the four most important feature signals were enough to approximate the measured signals (Patla, 1985), (Fig. 7). This suggests that the CPG has to generate only these four feature signals. The muscles that were monitored represent major flexors and extensors for each of the three joints of the lower limb, and, therefore, are a good representative sample. Thus the requirement that the CPG has to generate only four feature signals represents an economy in the operation of the control system.

The pattern recognition analyses, as discussed before, can be used to determine organizational principles within the locomotor program. The number and the specific shapes of the feature signals can suggest for ex-

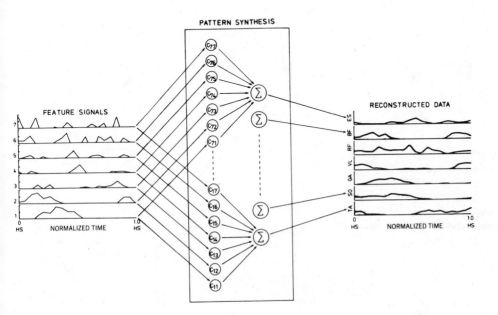

FIGURE 6. A schematic diagram showing how the feature signals are used in synthesis of the measured patterns. To generate each muscle activity profile, the feature signals are weighted (multiplied by a set of coefficients as shown) and summed together. In this case we use all the identified feature signals in the reconstruction process. The output is exactly similar to the input or measured data. The ± 1 SD band of the original data shown, is used as a guide for selecting the appropriate number of feature signals necessary for approximating the input data.

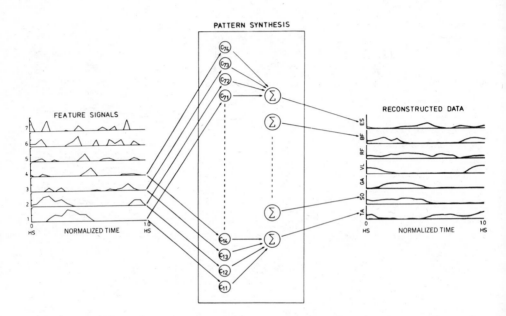

FIGURE 7. A schematic diagram showing the reconstruction process using only the first four feature signals (#1–#4). For each muscle activity, only first four coefficients are required. Since not all identified features signals are used in reconstruction, the output patterns are not exactly similar to the measured patterns. This is clear when you compare the average reconstructed profiles (solid line) in Figure 7 with the average reconstructed profiles in Figure 6. Because the reconstructed profiles fall within the ±1 SD band of the input data, the number of features selected are deemed adequate.

ample whether the CPG generates a general pattern for extensor and flexor activity. If the analyses had suggested that only two feature signals were required, they could represent general flexor and extensor activity patterns. If three feature signals were required, they could represent a general activation pattern for each of the three joints. Since the analyses revealed that four features were necessary, it suggests that the limb rather than the joint is controlled as a unit. A similar conclusion was arrived at when muscle activity patterns during locomotion over different slopes were analyzed (Patla, 1986).

Our analyses can be expanded to include the activity patterns for the different speeds of locomotion. We can then examine how the feature signals vary (Patla, 1985). In that study, individual muscle activity patterns over different speeds of locomotion were analyzed. Subjects were instructed to locomote on a treadmill at speeds ranging from $0.5 \times$ normal self-paced speed to twice the normal speed. This range thus included a very slow walk up to a slow jog. This allowed us to determine how the basic locomotor synergy is adapted for walking at various speeds. The analyses revealed that at least two feature signals per muscle were required to produce muscle activity profiles for different speeds of locomotion. This clearly rules out a simple gain control to change speed of locomotion. The phasic component of muscle activity patterns has to be modulated to accommodate different speeds of locomotion. Thus, more than one feature signal among the muscle activity patterns for different conditions, represents a different controlling strategy. We can examine the error (ME) introduced in reconstruction when only two features are used for the different muscles. This is a measure of modulation of the activity profiles over different locomotor speeds, and can provide interesting insights into the control of the different muscle activity patterns. The following trends were observed:

1. ME values for the extensor muscles were higher than for the flexor muscles.
2. ME values for the double jointed muscles in a synergistic group were higher than the single jointed muscles (gastrocnemius versus soleus; rectus femoris versus vastus lateralis).
3. ME values for the trunk muscle (erector spinae) was the highest.

These observations can be explained from a biomechanical perspective. The extensor muscles are mainly involved during the stance phase of locomotion which changes much more than the swing phase as the speed increases (cf. Grieve, 1968). The higher variability in the double jointed muscle can be attributed to its dual function during a stride. For example, the biceps femoris during stance phase extends the knee joint by backward rotation of the thigh (Winter, 1983), while flexing the knee during swing phase. The high variability in the trunk muscles can be explained as follows. The erector spinae muscle controls the large trunk mass, and any changes in this mass will be reflected in the activity of the trunk muscles.

Although the discussion concentrated on analyzing EMG signals, similar analysis could be carried out on any set of analog signals representing firing patterns of various cells, or the displacement signals of various joints, or the joint torque patterns. Now that we can identify the feature signals, we need to find structures that can generate these patterns in response to a tonic input.

5   CENTRAL PATTERN GENERATOR MODELS

The foregoing analysis suggests that the CPG generates a complex output. It does not simply alternate between flexors and extensors. Let us now turn our attention to qualities that model systems require, to generate such complex patterns. Since the central pattern generators produce rhythmic output patterns in response to a constant input signal, our efforts are directed towards understanding a system that functions as a neuronal oscillator. Neuronal oscillators used to model CPGs have to produce an output pattern that is rhythmic and complex in terms of the shape. Thus they have two functions: one as a time keeper, and the second as an information storage device (Pavlidis and Pinsker, 1977). The time keeping functions include maintaining the steady state periodicity of the behavior over a wide range, generating the transient response such as initiation or stopping, and coupling behavior between oscillators. The information aspect refers to the features of the output patterns. Since the output patterns are not simple sinusoid of one frequency, they have to be specified by their power spectrum. The neuronal oscillators have to encode this information. The models proposed fall into two main categories; analog, digital, and mathematical simulations of various neuronal networks (network models) and mathematical models in which the oscillators do not have their genesis in any particular neuronal network. In the following section the two classes of models that have been proposed are discussed, with particular emphasis on how they fulfill the two functions of the CPG.

5.1   Network Models

Researchers have classified the neuronal oscillator circuits into two main categories. The first class of neuronal oscillators relies on the endogenous oscillatory property of individual neurons to produce rhythmic output. There are neurons, for example, in the molluscan nervous system, which are capable of producing rhythmic bursts of impulses in the absence of any rhythmic synaptic input (cf. Friesen and Stent, 1978; Kristan, 1980). These rhythmic bursts have an ionic basis and involve changes in membrane conduction that are slow compared to the time course of a single action potential. The details of the operation of such neurons are discussed by Friesen and Stent (1978) and Kristan (1980). These endogenous bursters are thought to generate chronic rather than episodic rhythms (cf. Getting chapter).

The second class of neuronal oscillators that has been the subject of much research, consists of a network of interconnected, endogenously stable neurons. The rhythmic output of such an oscillator does not depend upon any endogenous oscillator neuron in its network, but rather on the pattern of interconnections (cf. Friesen and Stent, 1978; Kling and Szekely, 1968; Kristan, 1980; and other chapters). The oscillatory nature of such a circuit is therefore considered to be an emergent property of a network of neurons. Armed with this basic principle, researchers have tried to identify the combinations of network properties that would produce oscillatory output. The network properties that have been considered are: (a) the number of neurons, two or more than two; (b) the type of synaptic connections, i.e., excitatory, inhibitory, or excitatory and inhibitory; (c) synaptic property such as fatigue; and (d) the nature of the firing rate in a neuron in response to tonic excitation i.e., constant firing rate or frequency increasing linearly with time. Since there is no obvious basis for ranking these properties in terms of their desirability, it is not possible to select one network over the other based solely on these criteria, provided of course there is no similarities between the proposed network and biological reality. Thus, one has to examine the output patterns they can generate and based on this analysis classify the networks. Kristan (1980) has catalogued four properties of the output patterns that can be used to evaluate these networks. They are: (a) number of burst phases, one or more than one; (b) symmetrical or nonsymmetrical cycle; (c) range of periods, twofold or more than twofold; and (d) coordination modes. These properties have been used to determine the suitability of certain networks proposed as models for CPGs. Although an important first step, the properties listed are not detailed enough to properly classify the output patterns of the proposed networks. This can be explained by examining the first property.

The number of burst phases as defined by Kristan (1980) represents the number of impulse patterns that are not synchronous. This classification does not specify possible phase differences (the time difference between onsets of the two impulse bursts patterns expressed as a fraction of the cycle period) possible, nor does it specify the possibility and ranges of interpulse interval modulation within a burst. He dismisses the importance of specific impulse patterns within bursts in generating the movement (Kristan, 1980). To validate this assertion, one must demonstrate, for example, that when the motoneurons of the locust wing muscles are stimulated with bursts of various impulse patterns, the corresponding movements are identical. To be unable to account for the various impulse patterns observed during rhythmic movements seriously limits the usefulness of any model. It may be that these modulations of the inter-spike patterns within bursts are generated by the interneuronal circuits between the CPG and the motoneurons. But for systems such as the lobster stomatogastric rhythm generator where the motoneurons are part of the pattern generator (Selverston et al., 1976), the CPG must be able to produce the necessary impulse patterns within a burst of neuronal activity.

To date, the network simulation approach has explained the time keeper function to some degree in the steady state condition, but how information, such as the complex inter-pulse intervals or the phase differences between burst patterns, is encoded, has been ignored. Any proposed network models should require a minimum number of network properties, while the output of the network should be similar to the recorded output, thus maximizing the number of output properties.

5.2   Mathematical Models

Our efforts to identify neuronal networks for CPGs, specifically mammalian CPGs, have been hampered by lack of experimental techniques, and complexities of the nervous system. Mathematical models of oscillators that are not based on specific neuronal networks, offer a unique alternative to study organizational principles of CPGs. In this section we discuss various oscillator models, and explore their suitability as CPG analogs. To be a candidate for a model of a CPG, the oscillators must satisfy both time keeping and information storage functions. The major emphasis here is on whether the oscillator model is able to produce the complex output patterns that a CPG generates.

The use of mathematical models to study biological oscillators in general, and neural oscillators in particular, has been limited. Unlike sciences such as engineering where a complete description of an oscillator may require some obtainable parameter values, in neurobiology one usually starts with no knowledge about the state variables involved (Pavlidis, 1973). State variables are terms used in mathematics to describe the physical variables involved in an oscillator, and are affected by the oscillator themselves (Pavlidis and Pinsker, 1977). Because of our lack of knowledge about the state variables, it is difficult to write the equations describing the oscillator. Researchers studying biological rhythms have, therefore, tended to use a well known oscillator, such as the Van der Pol, to model these activities (cf. Sarna et al., 1971).

Instead of taking the indirect route to gain insights into the structure of the oscillator, it is possible to define the state variables of a neuronal oscillator and proceed forward. This approach has been used by Pinsker and Bell (1981) to study endogenous neuronal oscillators in Aplysia and by Patla et al (1985) to study the mammalian CPG. Both groups started with the assumption that the oscillator has one degree of freedom and can be described by two state variables. Pinsker and Bell (1981) used the membrane potential (u1) and its rate of change (u2) as the two state variables. Patla et al. (1985) used the instantaneous firing rate of the motoneuron pool (u1), and its rate of change (u2). The state of the system at any instant is described by a point in a plane whose coordinates are (u1,u2). As the state of the system changes, the point defines a trajectory. The family of all possible trajectories constitutes the system's phase plane. Thus, if a system behaves as an oscillator, the state of the system in that mode will traverse a closed trajectory, called a limit cycle. The nature of this limit cycle is defined by the oscillator equations.

Pinsker and Bell (1981) measured the membrane potential from a burst neuron and plotted it against its first derivative to give a phase plane portrait during oscillatory output. These trajectories were plotted for the free running oscillator before and after a change of system parameter, and also for phase resetting experiments produced by direct synaptic inhibition of an identified interneuron. As they point out, their analyses show the complex nature of the trajectories and although they speculate on the order of the system under study, no further information is gained over time domain plots.

The constraints on the oscillator equations that can be used to model biological oscillators with one degree of freedom are examined next. A system with one degree of freedom can be represented by the following generic pair of differential equations:

$$u1 = f1 \ (u1, \ u2) \tag{1}$$

$$u2 = f2 \ (u1, \ u2) \tag{2}$$

where $f1$ and $f2$ are functions of the two state variables $u1$ and $u2$.

For a linear undamped mechanical oscillator represented by a spring mass system, the motion of the system (output) can be completely described by knowing its displacement and velocity at any instant. The phase plane trajectory for the oscillatory behavior will be a circle (Figure 8A), with the origin being another stable point called a center (Pavlidis, 1973). The time domain output of the system is a sinusoidal displacement plot, the frequency determined by the values of the spring stiffness and the mass. Most biological oscillators have outputs that are not characterized by a sinusoid of one frequency. Thus, linear oscillators are an inadequate representation of the system. The nonlinear output of the oscillator necessitates the examination of the two classes of nonlinear differential equations: those arising from nonlinear conservative system and from nonlinear nonconservative systems. These two classes of nonlinear differential equations are discussed next.

A nonlinear conservative oscillator can be defined by the following equation:

$$\ddot{u} + p \ (u) = 0 \tag{3}$$

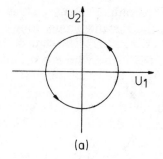

(a)

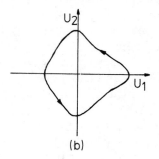

(b)

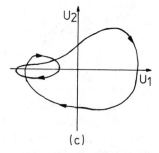

(c)

FIGURE 8. Phase plane plots for three types of oscillators: *(a)* linear undamped oscillator (for a mechanical analog U_1-displacement and U_2-velocity); *(b)* nonlinear conservative system; and *(c)* a biological oscillator.

where u is the output of the oscillator, and p is a nonlinear monotonic function. A mechanical analog of such a system would be a spring/mass system with the spring being nonlinear.

Integrating equation 3 we have:

$$\frac{1}{2}\dot{u}^2 + P(u) = T \tag{4}$$

where T is the integration constant and $P(u) = \int p(u)\,du$.

It is known that the period of the output is a function of the value of T. Thus, T can represent the level of tonic input to the oscillator. Although the output is nonlinear, the phase portrait during oscillation is symmetric about the u axis (Fig. 8B). The phase portraits for biological oscillators obtained by researchers show no such symmetry (Fig. 8C; Bardakjian et al., 1980; Patla et al., 1985; Pinsker and Bell, 1981). Thus these classes of oscillators are also inappropriate to model biological oscillators.

It is known that for endogenous (within the system) oscillations to occur, the nonlinear nonconservative system must have a stable limit cycle. These oscillators can be relaxation oscillators. Many biological rhythms such as the mammalian heart and the gastrointestinal signal, have been modeled using variants of the well known Van der Pol equation (Van der Pol and Van der Mark, 1928; Sarna et al., 1971). The two problems with relaxation oscillators such as the one represented by the Van der Pol equation are: (a) once the system is in the limit cycle no input is required to sustain the oscillations; and (b) although the output signal shape can be modified, there is no "direct" control over the details of the form, that is the frequency content, of the output pattern of the oscillator. The frequency content does not refer to the fundamental periodicity of the output, but rather to the frequencies that characterize the form of the output. Thus, they cannot be used to model the specific shape of the output signal (Patla et al., 1985; Pinsker & Bell, 1981) of CPGs for activities that also require constant tonic excitation such as locomotion in mammals (cf. Grillner, 1985). Some of the models discussed may be able to fulfill partly the time keeping role, but fall short of generating the features observed in the output patterns. A model that meets our criteria is discussed next.

Chua and Green (1974), and subsequently Bass (1975) and Bardakjian et al. (1983), have suggested a technique to synthesize system differential equations whose solution is a truncated Fourier series. Thus, the parameters of the oscillator will be the coefficients of a truncated Fourier series representation of the oscillator output. Bardakjian et al. (1983) have transformed this synthesized relaxation oscillator (SRO) to make it labile such that the system oscillates only in the presence of a stimulus (tonic input). The SRO thus meets our criteria for use as a model for CPG. It oscillates only in the presence of a stimulus, and it can generate any specified form of the output. The mathematical details of the labile SRO are explained in Appendix II.

The transformation techniques used in generating the differential equation, put in simple terms, allow a complex periodic waveform to be generated from its fundamental frequency signal and two nonlinear time independent shaping functions. The shaping functions are defined in Appendix 2. They are a function of the Fourier coefficients of the periodic signal that the CPG generates. The ability of the SRO to generate a complex (containing multiple frequency) time varying pattern from a simple (one frequency) time varying signal and two complex, but time indepen-

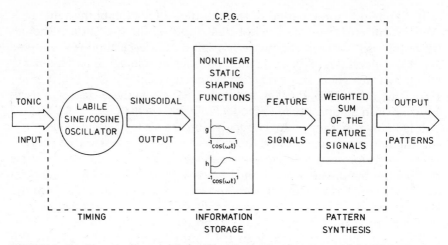

FIGURE 9. A schematic diagram of possible organizational structure of the CPG. The first two blocks, the labile sine/cosine relaxation oscillator (timing function) and the non-linear shaping functions (information storage) are a schematic representation of a labile synthesized relaxation oscillator. The oscillator generates the different feature signals. There are two static nonlinear shaping functions for each feature signal. These functions are dependent on the amplitude of the cosine waveform. The third block represents pattern synthesis. This component uses the feature signals to generate the output patterns of the CPG. The details of this reconstruction are shown in Figure 6 and 7.

dent static functions makes it very attractive to model CPGs (Patla et al, 1985).

The two stage process of generating the output provides a possibility of representing the CPG as two functional subsystems: (a) the fundamental frequency oscillator; and (b) the static nonlinear shaping functions (Patla et al., 1985). The fundamental frequency oscillator can be thought of as the time keeper, and the shaping functions as information storage devices (Fig. 9). We can use the labile sinusoidal relaxation oscillator model to study transient behavior of the CPGs, as well as examine the functioning of coupled CPGs. The shaping functions which mold the simple time varying signal into complex pattern thus provide the necessary encoding of activity patterns. As discussed by Patla et al. (1985), these subsystems can be realized using simple neuronal networks. For instance, the oscillator can be constructed from four neurons with inhibitory interconnections and the shaping functions can be realized with a set of parallel neurons with different thresholds, gain, and saturation values. Although by no means unique, these network analogs suggest an advantage of the SROs to model CPGs.

Besides the ability to find suitable network analogs to the system equations, another test of any model that represents the CPG could be to examine how it accommodates behaviors that are close to the natural rhythm. Thus, one could study how the model parameters change when the animal changes its speed of walking. Are the changes gradual? Can gradual change in system parameters for behaviors that are close to the natural rhythm be assumed as a criterion that a model should satisfy? Intuitively, one can argue that relatively small changes in speed (say, within the walking mode for an animal) should not require any abrupt changes in the system parameters. Patla et al. (1985) examined the oscillator parameters for three speeds of locomotion in cats and found the shaping functions to be relatively similar.

The synthesized relaxation oscillator outputs may represent the feature signals which are combined to produce the various output patterns of the central pattern generator. This allows the SRO to generate few feature signals that can be used to produce a larger set of activity patterns. Thus a CPG can be represented as three functional subsystems in cascade. The first two represent the SRO, while the third system represents the pattern synthesis that was discussed before (Fig. 6). The labile sine/cosine oscillator represents the time keeping function, and generates the fundamental periodicity of the output. The set of shaping functions for each feature signal are generated from the Fourier coefficients of the signal. These functions produce the detailed form of the feature signal from the sinusoidal output of the oscillator. The feature signals can be identified from the output patterns using the pattern recognition algorithm. The weighting coefficients identified with the pattern recognition algorithm are used in the synthesis of output patterns from the feature signals. This organizational scheme for a CPG is summarized in Figure 9.

6 SUMMARY

For proper system identification there is a need to characterize the inputs and outputs carefully. Efforts should be directed towards building a good database that can be used to build better models. Research in the area of understanding CPGs is at a stage where qualitative description of output patterns for instance, is not adequate. Pattern recognition techniques should be explored as a way to analyse a set of analog signals. The effects of various processes between the "CPG output" and the final behavior, which manifests itself in the kinematics of the various body segments, should be realized. Nonlinearities can introduce complexity that may not be present in the CPG input.

We began this chapter by arguing that analytical techniques borrowed from other disciplines, such as engineering and computer science, can help us better understand the control of rhythmic movements. The techniques discussed have allowed us to represent a CPG as three subsystems in cascade (Fig. 9). It is one model of organization within the CPG that can explain how complex output patterns are encoded within the nervous system. Further experimental work will be needed to validate this model. What this chapter has emphasized is that we have to develop models that go beyond just producing rhythmic output; they must be able to predict the output patterns we observe. Synergistic efforts that couple experimental work with analytical models are bound to yield better understanding of the nervous system.

ACKNOWLEDGMENTS

The author is grateful to Dr. R. B. Stein for giving him the opportunity to write this chapter. His constant encouragement is greatly appreciated. The author would also like to acknowledge the constructive comments and suggestions made by his colleagues Drs. F. Allard, J. Frank, C. MacKenzie, R. Norman, and D. Winter. The experimental work on human locomotion discussed in this chapter was supported by a grant from the Natural Sciences and Engineering Research Council of Canada.

APPENDIX 1: DETERMINATION OF FEATURES USING KARHUNEN–LOEVE EXPANSION

Let $o_i(t)$ $(i = 1,2, \ldots ,m)$ be a set of time dependent functions represented by N discreet sampling points. Then these functions can be represented as column vectors:

$$o_i = \begin{bmatrix} o_i(t_1) \\ o_i(t_2) \\ \cdot \\ \cdot \\ o_i(t_N) \end{bmatrix} \qquad (i = 1,2, \ldots ,m) \qquad (1)$$

These functions can be expanded as a linear combination of basis functions (features), $u_j(t)$ $(j = 1,2, \ldots ,m)$, as follows:

$$o_i = \sum_j c_{ij} \cdot u_j \qquad (2)$$

where u_j is a vector representation of the jth basis function as shown below:

$$u_j = \begin{bmatrix} u_j(t_1) \\ u_j(t_2) \\ \cdot \\ \cdot \\ u_j(t_N) \end{bmatrix} \qquad (j = 1,2, \ldots ,m) \qquad (3)$$

The coefficients c_{ij} in equation 2 are given by the following equation:

$$c_{ij} = u_j^T \cdot o_i \qquad (4)$$

where the vector u_j^T represents the transpose of vector u_j.

The basis functions $u_j(t)$ ($j = 1, 2, \ldots, m$) are the eigenvectors of the autocorrelation matrix, s, and are calculated as follows:

$$s = E_i [o_i \cdot o_i^T] \qquad (5)$$

where o_i^T is the transposed vector of o_i, and E represents the operation in which the expected value (average) of the sum in the square bracket is taken.

Since the basis functions are eigenvectors they are mutually orthonormal. Thus,

$$u_j^T \cdot u_j = \begin{cases} 1 & \text{for } i = j \\ 0 & \text{for } i \neq j \end{cases} \qquad (6)$$

The basis functions u_j can be calculated using a standard subroutine for evaluating the eigenvectors. From equations 4 and 6, the expansion of the time functions o_i given by equation 2 follows. Further details about the Karhunen–Loeve expansion technique can be found in the book by Young and Calvert (1974).

APPENDIX 2: EQUATIONS FOR A LABILE SYNTHESIZED RELAXATION OSCILLATOR

It is well known that any periodic stable waveform can be represented by a finite Fourier series. Thus, the output of the oscillator, $u(t)$, can be represented by the following series

$$u(t) = a_0 + \sum_{k=1}^{m} (a_k \cdot \cos(k\omega t) + b_k \cdot \sin(k\omega t)) \qquad (1)$$

where a_0 represents the d.c. value of the waveform, a_k is the cosine coefficient, b_k is the sine coefficient, and ω is the fundamental frequency.

The series in equation 1 is a linear sum of the harmonics. Using the Chebyshev polynomials of the first and the second kind, T_k and U_k, any harmonic can be represented as a function of the fundamental frequency as shown below:

$$\cos(k\omega t) = T_k (\cos(\omega t)) \qquad (2)$$

and

$$\sin(k\omega t) = \sin(\omega t) \cdot U_{k-1}(\cos(\omega t)) \qquad (3)$$

Substituting equations 2 and 3 in 1 we have

$$u(t) = a_0 + \sum_{k=1}^{m} \left[a_k \cdot T_k(\cos(\omega t)) + b_k \cdot \sin(\omega t) \cdot U_{k-1}(\cos(\omega t)) \right] \qquad (4)$$

The series defined by equation 4 is a sum of nonlinear functions of sinusoids at the fundamental frequency. Let us define two functions $g(.)$ and $h(.)$ as follows:

$$g(x_2) = a_0 + \sum_{k=1}^{m} a_k \cdot T_k(x_2) \qquad (5)$$

$$h(x_2) = \sum_{k=1}^{m} b_k \cdot U_{k-1}(x_2) \qquad (6)$$

where $x_2 = \cos(\omega t)$
    Equation 4 can then be rewritten as

$$u(t) = g(x_2) + x_1 \cdot h(x_2) \qquad (7)$$

where $x_1 = \sin(\omega t)$
    Equation 7 suggests a way of generating any periodic waveform using a sine/cosine fundamental frequency generator and the two nonlinear functions $g(.)$ and $h(.)$.
    A relaxation oscillator that can produce sine and cosine functions has been modified by Bardakjian et al. (1983) to make it stimulus dependent. This oscillator is defined by the following set of equations.

$$\dot{x}_1 = \omega \cdot [x_2 + x_1 (St - x_1^2 - x_2^2)] \qquad (8)$$

$$\dot{x}_2 = \omega \cdot [-x_1 + x_2 (St - x_1^2 - x_2^2)] \qquad (9)$$

where $St = (Ti - Th)$, Ti = tonic input (stimulus), Th = excitation threshold, $\dot{x}_1$ = first derivative of x_1 with respect to time, and $\dot{x}_2$ = first derivative of x_2 with respect to time. The system defined by equations 8 and 9 oscillates only in the presence of an input stimulus. The phase plane portrait of this oscillator is a circle. Chua and Green (1974) and Bass (1975) have shown how a simple transformation can be used to embed the nonlinearities $g(.)$ and $h(.)$ in the system defined by equations 8 and 9. Once these nonlinearities are embedded, the relaxation oscillator defines a complex limit cycle (see, for example, Fig. 8C).

REFERENCES

Andersson, O. and S. Grillner (1981). Peripheral control of the cat's step cycle 1. Phase dependent effects of ramp-movements of the hip during "fictive locomotion." *Acta Physiol. Scand.*, **113**:89–101.

Bardakjian, B. L. and S. K. Sarna (1980). A computer model of human colonic electrical control activity (ECA). *IEEE Trans. Biomed. Engn.*, **27**:193–202.

Bardakjian, B. L., T. Y. El-Sharkawy, and N. E. Diamant (1983). On a population of labile synthesized relaxation oscillators. *IEEE Trans. Biomed. Engn.*, **30**:696–701.

Bass, S. C. (1975). The mathematical and laboratory generation of prescribed periodic waveforms. *IEEE Trans. Circuits Systems.*, **22**:603–610.

Belanger, M., T. Drew, J. Provenchar, and S. Rossignol (1986). The study of locomotion and cutaneous reflexes in the same cat before and after spinalization. *Soc. Neurosci. Abstr.*, **241**:13.

Bentley, D. and M. Konishi (1978). Neural control of behaviour. *Ann. Rev. Neurosci.*, **1**:35–39.

Bernstein, N. (1967). *The Coordination and Regulation of Movements*, Pergamon, Oxford, U.K.

Bresler, B. and J. P. Frankel (1950). The forces and moments in the leg during level walking. *Trans. Am. Soc. Mech. Engineers.*, **72**:27–36.

Chow, C. K. and D. H. Jacobson (1971). Studies of human locomotion via optimal programming. *Math. Biosci.*, **10**:239–306.

Chua, L. O. and D. N. Green (1974). Synthesis of nonlinear periodic systems. *IEEE Trans. Circuits Systems*, **21**:286–294.

Cooper, S. and J. C. Eccles (1930). The isometric responses of mammalian muscles. *J. Physiol.*, **69**: 377–385.

Crowninshield, R. D. and R. A. Brand (1981). A physiologically based criterion of muscle force prediction in locomotion. *J. Biomech.*, **14**:793–802.

Delcomyn, F. (1980). Neural basis of rhythmic behaviour in animals. *Science.*, **210**:492–498.

DeLuca, C. J. (1979). Physiology and mathematics of myoelectric signals. *IEEE Trans. Biomed. Eng.*, **26**:313–325.

Dietz, V., D. Schmidtbleicher, and J. Noth (1979). Neuronal mechanisms of human locomotion. *J. Neurophysiol.*, **42**:1212–1222.

Drew, T. and S. Rossignol (1984). Phase-dependent responses evoked in limb muscles by stimulation of medullary reticular formation during locomotion in thalamic cats. *J. Neurophysiol.*, **52**:653–675.

Drew, T., R. Dubuc, and S. Rossignol (1986). Discharge patterns of reticulospinal and other reticular neurons in chronic, unrestrained cats walking on a treadmill. *J. Neurophysiol.*, **55**:375–401.

Fentress, J. C. (1976). *Simpler Networks and Behaviour*. Sinauer Associates, Sunderland, Mass.

Friesen, W. O. and G. S. Stent (1978). Neural circuits for generating rhythmic movements. *Annu. Rev. Biophys. Bioeng.*, **7**:37–61.

Gordon, A. M., A. F. Huxley, and F. J. Julian (1966). The variation in isometric tension with sarcomere length in vetebrate muscle fibres. *J. Physiol.*, **184**:170–192.

Grieve, D. W. (1968). Gait patterns and the speed of walking. *Biomed. Eng.*, **3**:119–122.

Grillner, S. (1985). Neurobiological bases of rhythmic motor acts in vertebrates. *Science.*, **228**:143–149.

Grillner, S. and P. Zangger (1984). The effect of dorsal root transection on the efferent motor pattern in the cat's hindlimb during locomotion. *Acta Physiol. Scand.*, **120**:393–405.

Haken, H., J. A. S. Kelso, and H. Bunz (1985). A theoretical model of phase transitions in human hand movements. *Biol. Cybern.*, **51**:347–356.

Halbertsma, J. (1983). The stride cycle of the cat: The modelling of locomotion by computerized analysis of automatic recordings. *Acta Physiol. Scand. (Suppl.)*, **521**:1–75.

Henneman, E. and C. B. Olson (1965). Relations between structure and function in the design of skeletal muscle. *J. Neurophysiol.*, **28**:581–598.

Herman, R., R. Wirta, S. Bampton, and F. R. Finley (1976). Human solutions for locomotion: Single limb analysis. In *Neural Control of Locomotion*, R. M. Herman, S. Grillner, P. S. G. Stein, and D. G. Stuart, eds. Plenum Press, New York, pp. 13–15.

Hill, A. V. (1938). The heat of shortening and the dynamic constants of muscle. *Proc. Roy. Soc. London*, **126**:136–195.

Houk, J. C. and W. Z. Rymer (1981). Neural control of muscle length and tension. In *Motor Control*, V. B. Brooks, ed. American Physiological Society Handbook of Physiology, Bethesda, Md.

Kelso, J. A. S. (1984). Phase transitions and critical behaviour in human bimanual coordination. *Am. J. Physiol.: Reg. Integ. Comp. Physiol.*, **15**:R1000–R1004.

Kernell, D. (1965). The adaptation and the relation between discharge frequency and current strength of cat lumbosacral motoneurons stimulated by long-lasting injected currents. *Acta Physiol. Scand.*, **65**:65–73.

Kling, V. and G. Szekely (1968). Simulation of rhythmic nervous activities. I. Function of networks with cyclic inhibitions. *Kybernetik*, 5:89–103.

Kristan, W. B. (1980). Generation of rhythmic motor patterns. In *Information Processing in the Nervous System*, H. M. Pinsker and W. D. Willis, Jr., eds. Raven Press, New York, pp. 241–261.

Kulagin, A. S. and M. L. Shik (1970). Interaction of symmetrical limbs during controlled locomotion. *Biophysics*, **15**:171–178.

Loeb, G. E. and W. B. Marks (1980). Epistemology and heuristics in neural network research. *Behavioral and Brain Sciences*, 3:556–557.

Loeb, G. E., J. A. Hoffer, and C. A. Pratt (1985). Activity of spindle afferents from cat anterior thigh muscles. I. Identification and patterns during normal locomotion. *J. Neurophysiol.*, **54**:549–564.

Milner-Brown, H. S., R. B. Stein, and R. R. Yemm (1973). The orderly recruitment of human motor units during voluntary isometric contractions. *J. Physiol.*, **230**:350–370.

Milner-Brown, H. S., R. B. Stein, and R. R. Yemm (1973). Changes in firing rate of human motor units during linearly changing voluntary contractions. *J. Physiol.*, **230**: 371–390.

Patla, A. E. (1985). Some characteristics of EMG patterns during locomotion: Implications for the locomotor control process. *J. Motor Behav.*, **17**:443–461.

Patla, A. E., T. W. Calvert, and R. B. Stein (1985). Model of a pattern generator for locomotion in mammals. *Am. J. Physiol.: Reg. Integ. Comp. Physiol.*, **248**:R484–R494.

Patla, A. E. (1986). Effects of walking on various inclines on EMG patterns of lower limb muscles in humans. *Human Movement Science.*, **5**:345–357.

Pavlidis, T. (1973). *Biological Oscillators: Their Mathematical Analysis.* Academic Press, New York.

Pavlidis, T. and H. M. Pinsker (1977). Oscillator theory and neurophysiology. *Fed. Proc.*, **36**:2033–2035.

Pearson, K. G. (1981). Function of sensory input in insect motor systems. *Can. J. Physiol. Pharmacol.*, **59**:660–666.

Pedotti, A., V. V. Krishnan, and L. Stark (1978). Optimization of muscle-force sequencing in human locomotion. *Math. Biosci.*, **38**:57–76.

Pierrot-Deseilligny, E., C. Bergego, and L. Mazieres (1983). Reflex control of bipedal gait in man. In *Motor Control Mechanisms in Health and Disease*, J. E. Desmedt, ed. Raven Press, New York, pp. 699–716.

Pierrynowski, M. R. and J. B. Morrison (1985). A physiological model for the evaluation of muscular forces in human locomotion: Theoretical aspects. *Math. Biosci.*, **75**:69–101.

Pinsker, H. M. and J. Bell (1981). Phase plane description of endogenous neural oscillators in Aplysia. *Biol. Cybern.*, **39**:211–221.

Sarna, S. K., E. E. Daniel, and Y. J. Kingma (1971). Simulation of slow wave electrical activity of small intenstine. *Am. J. Physiol.* **220**:166–175.

Selverston, A. J., D. F. Russell, J. P. Miller, and D. G. Kling (1976). The stomatogastric nervous system: Structure and function of a small neural network. *Progress in Neurobiology,* **6**:1–75.

Selverston, A. (1980). Are central pattern generators understandable? *Behavioral Brain Sciences,* **3**:535–571.

Shik, M. L., and N. G. Orlovskii (1976). Neurophysiology of locomotor automatism. *Physiol. Rev.*, **56**:465–501.

Shik, M. L., F. V. Severin, and G. N. Orlovskii (1966). Control of walking and running by means of electrical stimulation of the mid-brain. *Biophysics USSR.*, **11**:756–765.

Stein, P.S.G. (1971). Intersegmental coordination of swimmeret motoneuron activity in crayfish. *J. Neurophysiol.*, **34**:310–318.

Stein, P. S. G. (1976). Mechanisms of interlimb phase control. In *Neural Control of Locomotion*, R. M. Herman, S. Grillner, P. S. G. Stein, and D. G. Stuart, eds. Plenum, New York, pp. 465–469.

Stein, P. S. G. (1977). Application of the mathematics of coupled oscillator systems to the analysis of neural control of locomotion. *Federation Proceedings,* **36**:2056–2059.

Stein, P. S. G. (1978). Motor systems, with special reference to the control of locomotion. *Am. Rev. Neurosci.*, **1**:61–81.

Thorstensson, A. (1986). How is the normal locomotor program modified to produce backward walking? *Exp. Brain Res.*, **61**:664–668.

Van der Pol, B. and J. Van der Mark (1928). The heart beat considered as a relaxation oscillator and an electrical model of the heart. *Phil. Mag. (Suppl.)*, **6**:763–775.

Van Holst, E. (1973). *The Behavioral Physiology of Animals and Man*. Methuen & Co. Ltd., London, U.K.

Winter, D. A. (1983). Biomechanical motor patterns in normal walking. *J. Motor Behav.*, **15**:302–330.

Winter, D. A. (1984). Kinematic and kinetic patterns in human gait: Variability and compensatory effects. *Human Movement Science.*, **3**:51–76.

Winter, D. A. and D. G. E. Robertson (1978). Joint torque and energy patterns in normal gait. *Biol. Cybern.*, **29**:137–142.

Young, T. Y. and T. W. Calvert (1974). *Classification, Estimation and Pattern Recognition*. Elsevier, New York.

Zheng, Y. F., H. Hemami, and B. T. Stokes (1984). Muscle dynamics, size principle and stability. *IEEE Trans. Biomed. Engn.*, **31**:489–497.

INDEX

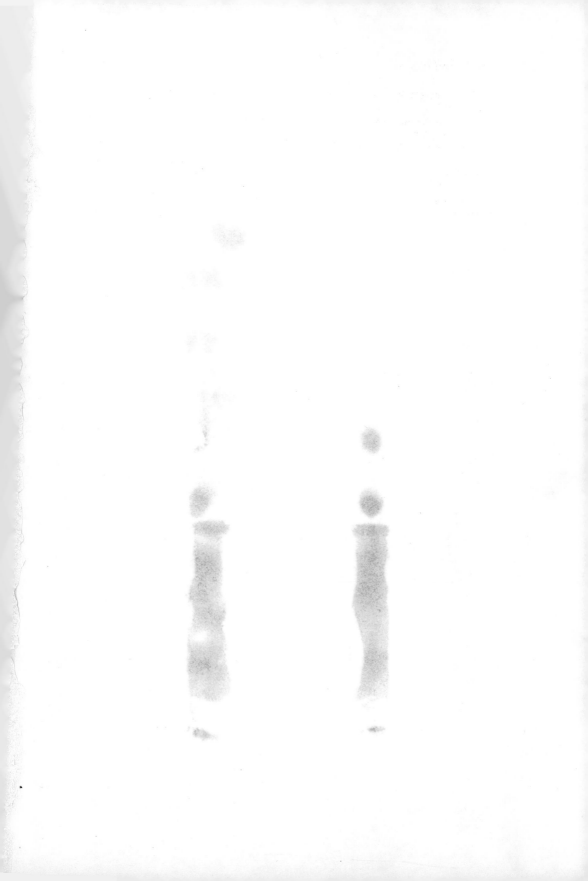